Contents

I. Critical Care Principles

II. Medical Considerations

III. Surgical Considerations

IV. Appendices

Contributing Authors

Shihab U. Ahmed, M.D., M.P.H., *Instructor of Anesthesia, Harvard Medical School; Assistant in Anesthesia, Department of Anesthesia and Critical Care, Massachusetts General Hospital, Boston, Massachusetts 02114*

Rae M. Allain, M.D., *Instructor in Anesthesia, Harvard Medical School; Assistant in Anesthesia, Department of Anesthesia and Critical Care, Massachusetts General Hospital, Boston, Massachusetts 02114*

Keith Baker, M.D., Ph.D., *Assistant Professor of Anesthesia, Harvard Medical School; Assistant in Anesthesia, Department of Anesthesia and Critical Care, Massachusetts General Hospital, Boston, Massachusetts 02114*

Luca M. Bigatello, M.D., *Assistant Professor of Anesthesia, Harvard Medical School; Assistant in Anesthesia, Department of Anesthesia and Critical Care, Massachusetts General Hospital, Boston, Massachusetts 02114*

James G. Cain, M.D., *Assistant Professor, Department of Anesthesiology and Critical Care, West Virginia School of Medicine, Morgantown, West Virginia 26506-9134*

John L. Chow, M.D., M.S., *Instructor of Anesthesia, Harvard Medical School; Assistant in Anesthesia, Department of Anesthesia and Critical Care, Massachusetts General Hospital, Boston, Massachusetts 02114*

Fritz Daudel, M.D., *Assistant in Anesthesia, Department of Anesthesia and Critical Care, Massachusetts General Hospital, Boston, Massachusetts 02114*

Kevin C. Dennehy, M.B, B.Ch., F.F.A.R.C.S.I., *Clinical Instructor of Anesthesia, Harvard Medical School; Assistant in Anesthesia, Department of Anesthesia and Critical Care, Massachusetts General Hospital, Boston, Massachusetts 02114*

Randall O. Dull, M.D., Ph.D., *Assistant Professor, Department of Anesthesia and Critical Care Medicine, Johns Hopkins University School of Medicine, Baltimore, Maryland 21287*

Peter F. Dunn, M.D., *Instructor of Anesthesia, Harvard Medical School; Assistant in Anesthesia, Department of Anesthesia and Critical Care, Massachusetts General Hospital, Boston, Massachusetts 02114*

Mustapha Ezzeddine, M.D., *Formerly, Clinical Fellow in Neurology, Harvard Medical School; Formerly, Stroke Service, Massachusetts General Hospital, Boston, Massachusetts 02114*

Robert L. Goulet, M.S., R.R.T.,   *Senior Therapist,*
Department of Respiratory Care, Massachusetts General
Hospital, Boston, Massachusetts 02114

David Greer, M.D., M.A.,   *Clinical Fellow in Neurology,*
Harvard Medical School; Assistant in Critical Care and
Stroke Neurology, Massachusetts General Hospital, Boston,
Massachusetts 02114

Kenneth L. Haspel, M.D.,   *Instructor of Anesthesia, Harvard*
Medical School; Medical Director, Post Anesthesia Care Unit,
Assistant in Anesthesia, Massachusetts General Hospital,
Boston, Massachusetts 02114

Judith Hellman, M.D.,   *Instructor of Anesthesia, Harvard*
Medical School; Assistant in Anesthesia, Department of
Anesthesia and Critical Care, Massachusetts General
Hospital, Charlestown, Massachusetts 02129

Dean Hess, Ph.D., R.R.T.,   *Assistant Professor of Anesthesia,*
Harvard Medical School; Assistant Director of Respiratory
Care, Massachusetts General Hospital, Boston,
Massachusetts 02114

Horacio Hojman, M.D.,   *Instructor in Clinical Surgery,*
UMass Medical Center, Worcester, Massachusetts 01655

William E. Hurford, M.D.,   *Associate Professor of Anesthesia,*
Harvard Medical School; Director, Critical Care, Department
of Anesthesia and Critical Care, Massachusetts General
Hospital, Boston, Massachusetts 02114

Robert M. Insoft, M.D.,   *Department of Pediatrics,*
Massachusetts General Hospital, Boston, Massachusetts 02114

Jean Kwo, M.D.,   *Instructor in Anesthesia, Harvard Medical*
School; Assistant in Anesthesia, Department of Anesthesia
and Critical Care, Massachusetts General Hospital, Boston,
Massachusetts 02114

Stephanie L. Lee, M.D., Ph.D.,   *Assistant Professor of*
Medicine, Tufts School of Medicine; Director, Thyroid
Disease Center, New England Medical Center, Boston,
Massachusetts 02111

Bonnie T. Mackool, M.D., M.S.P.H.,   *Instructor, Harvard*
Medical School; Director, Consultation and Inpatient Service,
Department of Dermatology, Massachusetts General Hospital,
Boston, Massachusetts 02114

Ricardo Martinez-Ruiz, M.D.,   *Instructor in Anesthesia,*
Harvard Medical School; Assistant in Anesthesia, Department
of Anesthesia and Critical Care, Massachusetts General
Hospital, Boston, Massachusetts 02114

Colin T. McDonald, M.D.,   *Instructor in Neurology, Harvard Medical School; Attending Physician in Neurology, Department of Neurology, Massachusetts General Hospital, Boston, Massachusetts 02114*

Luat T. Nguyen, M.D.,   *Staff Anesthesiologist, Sacred Heart Medical Center, Eugene, Oregon 97401*

Laura E. Niklason, M.D., Ph.D.,   *Assistant Professor, Department of Biomedical Engineering, Duke University; Assistant Professor, Department of Anesthesiology, Duke University Medical Center, Durham, North Carolina 27710*

Jeffrey A. Norton, M.D.,   *Instructor of Anesthesia, Harvard Medical School; Assistant in Anesthesia, Department of Anesthesia and Critical Care, Massachusetts General Hospital, Boston, Massachusetts 02114*

Robert A. Peterfreund, M.D., Ph.D.,   *Assistant Professor of Anesthesia, Harvard Medical School; Associate Anesthetist, Department of Anesthesia and Critical Care, Massachusetts General Hospital, Boston, Massachusetts 02114*

Richard M. Pino, M.D., Ph.D.,   *Assistant Professor of Anesthesia, Harvard Medical School; Assistant in Anesthesia, Department of Anesthesia and Critical Care, Massachusetts General Hospital, Boston, Massachusetts 02114*

Brian J. Poore, M.D.,   *Cardiac Anesthesiologist, St. Thomas Hospital, Nashville, Tennessee 37205*

John A. Powelson, M.D.,   *Instructor in Surgery, Harvard Medical School; Clinical Director, Renal Transplant Surgery, Brigham and Women's Hospital, Boston, Massachusetts 02115*

Jesse D. Roberts, Jr., M.D., M.S.,   *Assistant Professor of Anaesthesia, Harvard Medical School; Assistant Anesthetist and Pediatrician, Departments of Anesthesia and Pediatrics, Massachusetts General Hospital, Boston, Massachusetts 02114*

Jonathan Rosand, M.D.,   *Clinical Fellow of Neurology, Harvard Medical School; Assistant in Neurology, Department of Neurology, Massachusetts General Hospital, Boston, Massachusetts 02114*

Adam Sapirstein, M.D.,   *Instructor in Anesthesia, Harvard Medical School; Assistant in Anesthesia, Department of Anesthesia and Critical Care, Massachusetts General Hospital, Boston, Massachusetts 02114*

David Schinderle, M.D.,   *Resident, Department of Anesthesiology, Duke University Medical Center, Durham, North Carolina 27710*

Lee H. Schwamm, M.D., *Associate Program Director, Massachusetts Institute of Technology–Clinical Research Center; Assistant Professor of Neurology and Associate Director, Acute Stroke Service, Massachusetts General Hospital, Boston, Massachusetts 02114*

Alan Z. Segal, M.D., *Assistant Professor of Neurology, Department of Neurology, Cornell University Medical College; Assistant Attending Neurologist, New York Presbyterian Hospital, New York, New York 10021*

Kenneth E. Shepherd, M.D., *Assistant Professor of Clinical Anesthesia, Harvard Medical School; Assistant in Anesthesiology, Department of Anesthesia and Critical Care, Massachusetts General Hospital, Boston, Massachusetts 02114*

Robert L. Sheridan, M.D., *Associate Professor of Surgery, Harvard Medical School; Burn and Trauma Services, Massachusetts General Hospital; Assistant Chief of Staff, Shriners Burns Hospital, Boston, Massachusetts 02114*

Thomas Suarez, M.D., *Department of Anesthesia, Sinai Hospital of Baltimore, Baltimore, Maryland 21215*

B. Taylor Thompson, M.D., *Associate Professor of Medicine, Pulmonary and Critical Care Unit, Harvard Medical School; Director, Medical Intensive Care Unit, Pulmonary and Critical Care Unit, Massachusetts General Hospital, Boston, Massachusetts 02114*

To-Nhu Vu, M.D., *Instructor of Anesthesia, Harvard Medical School; Clinical Assistant, Department of Anesthesia and Critical Care, Massachusetts General Hospital, Boston, Massachusetts 02114*

John L. Walsh, M.D., *Instructor of Anesthesia, Harvard Medical School; Assistant Anesthetist, Department of Anesthesia and Critical Care, Massachusetts General Hospital, Boston, Massachusetts 02114*

Ralph L. Warren, M.D., *Assistant Professor of Surgery, Harvard Medical School; Associate Visiting Surgeon, Director of Trauma and Surgical Critical Care, Massachusetts General Hospital, Boston, Massachusetts 02114*

Maria M. Zestos, M.D., *Interim Chief, Department of Anesthesia, Children's Hospital of Michigan, 3901 Beaubien Street, Detroit, Michigan 48201*

Preface

Critical care medicine is an interdisciplinary art. The *Critical Care Handbook of the Massachusetts General Hospital, Third Edition,* was written as a multidisciplinary guide to the care of critically ill patients. It is designed to be an initial source of information for practitioners, residents, and medical students in anesthesia, medicine, and surgery; for nurses, respiratory therapists, and other health care professionals involved in the care of the critically ill; and for primary care physicians who might need an introduction to current critical care practice. It emphasizes the physiologic principles and fundamental approaches to the care of the critically ill patient. We realize, however, that no pocket-sized volume can completely cover all the topics of critical care medicine. Topics such as nursing care, design and administration of critical care units, health policy and resource management, and so on, have not been included. Instead, we have chosen to cover the most common problems encountered by house-staff in the everyday care of critically ill patients. This is a book to be used at the bedside, rather than kept on the bookshelf.

The authors are internists, pulmonologists, neurologists, surgeons, anesthesiologists, pediatricians, and respiratory therapists who are involved in the day-to-day care of critically ill patients. We have provided specific suggestions for approaches to common problems ranging from respiratory failure to rashes. These suggestions primarily reflect current clinical practices at our hospital; other methods undoubtedly are equally effective and we have endeavored to include them. As with our other manuals, the *Critical Care Handbook* is meant to stimulate reading in more complete textbooks and current journals and continual study of medical physiology and pharmacology as it applies to critically ill patients. It is a beginning, not an end.

Such a handbook is always a work-in-progress. Critical care medicine is a rapidly changing field. This edition of the handbook has been completely rewritten, expanded, and reorganized. We have enlisted over three dozen authors who were given the daunting task of covering complex topics in great detail while using the fewest possible number of words. Each of their contributions has been reviewed and edited to the best of our abilities. In addition, some source material from prior editions and from our companion handbook, *Clinical Anesthesia Procedures of the Massachusetts General Hospital, Fifth Edition,* has been included verbatim when appropriate. The integral contributions of the editors and authors of these handbooks are gratefully acknowledged.

We acknowledge the continuing guidance and support of Warren M. Zapol, M.D., and are most grateful for the excellent secretarial and editorial assistance of Ms. Rita Prevoznik. We especially thank R. Craig Percy and his colleagues at Lippincott Williams & Wilkins for their support and encouragement of this project.

Critical Care Principles

Hemodynamic Monitoring

John Walsh and Randall Dull

I. **The cardiovascular system** perfuses organs to maintain function and viability. The goal of cardiovascular hemodynamic monitoring is to maintain adequate organ perfusion and system stability.

    A. Signs and symptoms of individual organ dysfunction can result from inadequate end-organ flow:

        1. **Central Nervous System (CNS).** Decreased mental status.

        2. **Cardiac.** Chest pain, ischemia on electrocardiography (ECG), and wall motion abnormalities on echocardiography.

        3. **Renal.** Decreased urine output, increased blood urea nitrogen (BUN) to creatinine ratio, and decreased fractional excretion of sodium.

        4. **Gastrointestinal.** Abdominal pain, decreased bowel sounds, and hematochezia.

        5. **Periphery.** Cool limbs, poor capillary refill, and weak pulses.

    B. **End-organ blood flow** is determined by that organ's perfusion pressure divided by its resistance to flow. In most cases, the perfusion pressure is the difference between the arterial pressure and venous pressure; in cases of increased intracranial pressure (ICP), the cerebral perfusion pressure is the difference between the arterial pressure and the ICP. Because the arterial pressure is time varying, **mean arterial pressure** (MAP) is generally chosen as a static substitute for defining an average perfusion pressure.

II. **Monitoring arterial blood pressure.** In the normal state, most organs can maintain relatively constant blood flow over a wide range of perfusion pressures (i.e., **autoregulation**). Blood pressure is monitored to ensure that an adequate perfusion pressure exists. In some pathologic states, however, a low perfusion pressure can be sufficient to provide adequate flow; conversely, a high perfusion pressure can be inadequate if an organ's resistance to flow is great.

    A. **Noninvasive blood pressure (NIBP)** measurement involves occluding an artery by a pressurized cuff and then measuring the oscillations in cuff pressure, or the pressure at which flow resumes through the artery as the cuff is deflated. Multiple techniques exist for determining blood pressure by this method:

        1. **Automated techniques** are the most common methods for NIBP measurement in the intensive care unit (ICU). Typically, the cuff is inflated approximately 40 mm Hg above the previous systolic pressure (or approximately 170 mm Hg initially) and then incrementally deflated while sensing

pressure oscillations in the cuff. The mean arterial blood pressure (MAP) correlates well with the lowest pressure at which maximal oscillations occur. The systolic and diastolic pressures are determined by an algorithm, but they generally correlate with the initial rise and final fall of oscillations about the maximum oscillations.

a. Limitations

    (1) Cuff size. The cuff should cover approximately two thirds of the upper arm or thigh; that is, the width of the cuff should be 20% greater than the diameter of the limb. A cuff that is too narrow can produce falsely high measurements; a cuff that is too wide can produce falsely low values.

    (2) Dysrhythmias, such as atrial fibrillation, can make a measured value difficult to interpret.

    (3) Movement. Motion artifact is rejected by some instruments, but it still increases the cycle time.

    (4) Rapid pressure changes. Venous congestion can occur if the instrument is set to cycle too frequently; cycle times less than 2 minutes apart should be avoided for routine monitoring. Some instruments have a "STAT" mode, which cycles rapidly to give a fairly continuous measure of systolic pressure.

    (5) Very low or high blood pressures may not correlate with intraarterial measurements.

2. Auscultation of Korotkoff's sounds. An occlusive cuff is inflated above the systolic blood pressure. As the cuff is slowly (3–5 mm Hg/s) deflated, a pressure will be reached at which blood begins to flow turbulently through the artery. The pressure at which the sound of this turbulent flow is heard through a stethoscope is the systolic blood pressure. As the pressure in the cuff decreases below the diastolic blood pressure, the sounds muffle or disappear.

a. Limitations

    (1) Requires a human operator.

    (2) Vasoconstriction can decrease flow, making the sounds difficult to hear.

    (3) Prone to observer error.

    (4) Rapid deflation can produce an erroneously low pressure reading.

3. Palpation or Doppler detection of flow. As the cuff is deflated, the distal pulse is palpated or detected by Doppler ultrasound. The pressure in the cuff at which the pulse is first detected correlates with the systolic blood pressure. This technique only measures systolic blood pressure.

4. **Tonometry** is a variant of the oscillometric method, in which the artery is only partially occluded and oscillations in arterial pulsation are measured. Most commonly, the radial artery is chosen. This method offers the advantage of continuous pressure measurement. The measurements are affected by motion and uncertain at extremes of pressure.

B. **Invasive blood pressure monitoring** most commonly measures pressure directly by means of an indwelling arterial catheter coupled through fluid-filled tubing to an external pressure transducer. The transducer converts the pressure into an electrical signal that is subsequently filtered and displayed on a screen.

1. **The clinical indications** for invasive arterial monitoring include:
   a. Necessity for rigorous **control of blood pressure** (e.g., arterial aneurysms).
   b. Hemodynamically unstable patient.
   c. Necessity for frequent arterial blood sampling.
2. **A disposable transducer** is connected to a pressurized bag of saline or heparinized saline. The line is continuously flushed at 3 ml/h to prevent clot formation at the tip of the cannula.
3. **Tubing** should be rigid and as short as possible for proper transmission of the pressure wave. Air bubbles should be meticulously purged from the system.
4. **The signal** from the well-prepared transducer set-up should have a relatively flat frequency response below 20 Hz and, consequently, provide an accurate representation of the pressure for all physiologic heart rates.
5. The system should be electronically **zeroed** when the transducer is open to air. This can be done with the transducer at any height. When measuring pressures, the transducer should remain at a stable height with respect to the patient. This is generally chosen as the height of the coronary sinus. In practice, the 4th intercostal space, midaxillary line is a reasonable approximation.

C. **Interpretation of the blood pressure** depends on the clinical question being asked.
1. The systolic blood pressure can be of interest when monitoring patients with aneurysms in whom a sudden high pressure might induce a rupture.
2. The mean arterial pressure is the pressure most accurately measured, and it can be the most useful measurement for assessing perfusion pressure of vital organs.

III. **Monitoring central pressures and cardiac output**
A. **Central venous pressure (CVP)**
1. **CVP is measured** by coupling the intravascular space through a fluid-filled tube to an external pressure transducer. The intravascular space is

typically monitored at the junction of the superior vena cava and the right atrium. The transducer is set up in the same way as the arterial line; special care is taken to ensure that the transducer is maintained at the same level with respect to the patient during sequential measurements (e.g., at the level of the coronary sinus).

2. **Waveform.** A CVP trace contains three positive deflections, waves **a, c,** and **v** (Fig. 1-1). These correspond approximately with atrial contraction, change in shape of the heart in systole, including tricuspid bulging, and right atrial filling.

3. **Value.** The CVP is often read after the a-wave and before the c-wave to reflect presystolic right ventricular pressure. To reflect transmural filling pressure, the CVP, as with all central vascular pressures, is read at end-expiration. **The CVP is normally on the order of 2 to 6 mm Hg.**

   a. If the waveform does not contain pathologic waves a or v, the difference between the **mean value** (at end-expiration) and the value between waves a and c is usually small and clinically unimportant.

4. **Physiologic interpretation** (Fig. 1-2). By itself, the CVP does not indicate the volume status of the

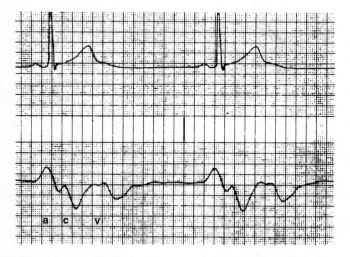

Fig. 1-1. A normal central venous pressure tracing is shown in the bottom half of the figure with its corresponding electrocardiogram in the top half. Waves a, c, and v on the venous pressure tracing are labeled. The x descent occurs between waves c and v; the y descent occurs after the v-wave. (From Kaplan JA. *Cardiac anesthesia*, 2nd ed. Philadelphia: WB Saunders, 1987:186.)

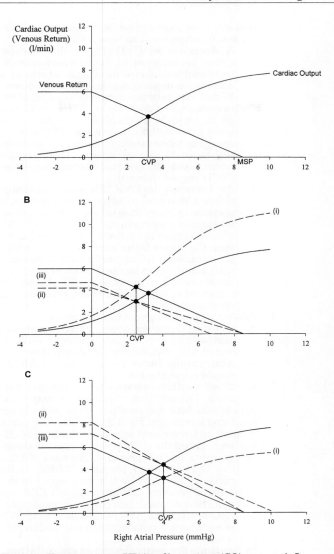

Fig. 1-2.   Venous return (VR)/cardiac output (CO) curves. A. In steady-state, VR = CO. Thus, the measured central venous pressure (CVP) will occur at that point on the independent axis where the VR and CO curves cross. B. A fall in CVP could be caused by an increase in cardiac performance (i), an increased impedance to venous return (ii), a decrease in the mean systemic pressure (MSP) (iii), or a combination of these. C. An increase in CVP could be caused by a decrease in cardiac performance (i), a decreased impedance to VR (ii), an increase in MSP (iii), or a combination of these.

patient; some assumption, or assessment, of the cardiac function needs to be included.

    a. A decrease in CVP (Fig. 1-2B) indicates either an increase in cardiac performance, increased impedance to venous return, or a decrease in mean systemic pressure (volume). With a concomitant increase in blood pressure, the reason for a decrease in CVP is most likely an increase in cardiac performance; if the blood pressure falls, the drop in CVP is likely caused by a decrease in volume or by increased resistance to venous return. This analysis assumes that the systemic vascular resistance (SVR) has not changed.

    b. An increase in CVP (Fig. 1-2C) indicates either a decrease in cardiac performance, a decrease in impedance to venous return, or an increase in mean systemic pressure (volume). With a concomitant decrease in blood pressure, the reason for an increase in CVP is likely decreased cardiac performance, whereas with a concurrent increase in blood pressure, the reason for an increase in CVP is probably increased volume or decreased resistance to venous return.

5. Effects of pathology on interpretation

    a. Cannon a-waves occur when the atrium contracts against a closed tricuspid valve. It occurs with atrioventricular dissociation.

    b. Abnormally large v-waves occur with tricuspid regurgitation.

6. Effect of positive airway pressure on interpretation. The addition of positive airway pressure affects both the cardiac output and venous return relationships (Fig. 1-3). The Starling curve is based on transmural pressure, which is the difference between the atrial pressure and the transmitted extra-cardiac pressure. Because of this, positive end-expiratory pressure (PEEP) shifts the curve to the right by a degree equal to the transmitted pressure. At high levels of PEEP, the curve can be depressed, reflecting increased right-ventricular afterload. The net result is that CVP increases, whereas venous return and cardiac output decreases.

7. Indications for central venous cannulation

    a. Measurement of right ventricular filling pressures as a guide to intravascular volume, impedance to venous return, and right ventricular function.

    b. Injection of dye for **cardiac output determination (see below).

    c. Provide access for administration of drugs or parenteral nutrition into the central circulation.

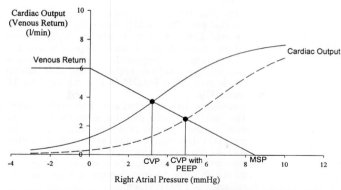

Fig. 1-3. Effect of positive end-expiratory pressure (PEEP) on the venous return/cardiac output curves. PEEP has the effect of shifting the Starling curve to the right by a degree equal to the transmitted extra-cardiac pressure. At high levels of PEEP (>15 cm H_2O), the curve can be depressed secondary to increased right ventricular afterload. The central venous pressure measured is consequently higher. MSP, mean systemic pressure.

       d. **Provide intravenous (IV) access** for patients with poor peripheral veins.

B. **Pulmonary artery catheter (PAC).** The PAC is a catheter that passes sequentially through the vena cava, right atrium, right ventricle, and into the pulmonary artery. The PAC provides useful information, including the CVP, pulmonary artery pressure (PAP), pulmonary artery occlusion pressure (PAOP), mixed-venous blood chemistries, and cardiac output (CO).

    1. **Measuring PAP and PAOP.** As with the CVP, the PAP and PAOP are determined by coupling the intravascular space through a fluid-filled tube to an external pressure transducer. For an accurate measure of PAOP, the tip of the catheter should reside in a lung zone where pulmonary venous pressure is greater than alveolar pressure (West zone III), which, because the design of the catheter, is the usual case.

        a. **Waveform.** The morphology of the PAP waveform is similar to that of the systemic arterial waveform, but is smaller and precedes it slightly. When the balloon at the tip of the catheter is inflated, the catheter occludes flow in the artery and the morphology of the waveform changes to more closely approximate that of the CVP. Waves a and v, as well as x- and y-descents, are present; the c-wave, however, often is not apparent.

        b. **Value. The PAP is normally 15 to 25 mm Hg systolic and 5 to 12 mm Hg diastolic.**

The **PAOP** provides an estimate of the left-atrial pressure (LAP). Because of the interposed lung, this estimate is delayed and dampened. Waves a and c typically are not very large. Consequently, the mean pressure at end-expiration reflects the left atrial pressure. **The PAOP is normally 5 to 12 mm Hg.**

2. **Physiologic interpretation.** The performance of the left ventricle can be described by two curves: the end-systolic pressure-volume relationship and the diastolic pressure-volume relationship (Fig. 1-4). To the extent that the PAOP reflects left-ventricular end-diastolic pressure, an assessment of left-sided heart function may be made by the change in PAOP value.

   a. **An increase in PAOP** may reflect a decrease in diastolic compliance, an increase in end-diastolic volume, or both (Fig. 1-4).

   b. **A decrease in PAOP** may reflect an increase in diastolic compliance, a decrease in end-diastolic volume, or both (Fig. 1-4).

3. **Effects of pathology** on interpretation

   a. **A poorly compliant ventricle can be responsible for a large a-wave.** The best measure of left-ventricular end-diastolic pressure (LVEDP) in this case is the peak of the a-wave. Atrioventricular dissociation can also produce large a-waves, but the LVEDP in this case should be measured before the a-wave.

   b. **Mitral regurgitation can result in abnormally large v-waves.**

   c. **Ventricular interdependence.** When the right ventricle (RV) dilates (e.g., in response to acute pulmonary hypertension or pulmonary embolus), the interventricular septum stiffens and shifts toward the left ventricular (LV) cavity. The altered septal behavior decreases LV diastolic compliance. Left-ventricular end-diastolic pressure for a given end-diastolic volume increases as a result.

4. **Indications.** Pulmonary artery catheters should be used only if the potential benefit in terms of diagnosis or guidance of treatment outweighs the risk of insertion and complications associated with their use (see below). Possible indications include acute myocardial infarction (MI) with shock, unexplained hypotension, multiorgan dysfunction, and PA hypertension.

5. **Additional types of PACs include:**

   a. **Venous infusion port** (VIP, VIP+) catheters that provide additional ports.

   b. **Paceports** that provide specially positioned ports to pass temporary pacing wires or infuse drugs.

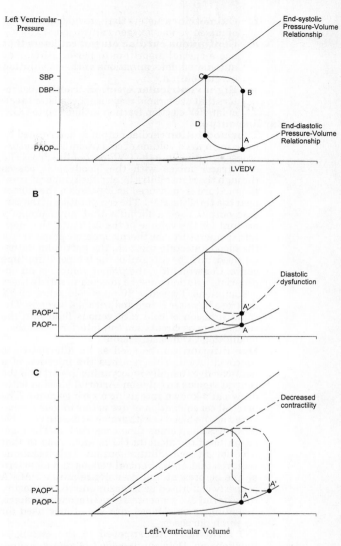

Fig. 1-4.   Left ventricular pressure–volume relationships. The cardiac cycle (A-B-C-D-A) is limited by the end-systolic pressure-volume relationship (describing the contractility) and the end-diastolic pressure-volume relationship. The pulmonary artery occlusion pressure (PAOP) approximates the left-ventricular end-diastolic pressure. An increase in PAOP may be ascribed to decreased diastolic compliance (*panel B*), an increase in left ventricular end-diastolic volume (LVEDV) (*panel C*), or a combination of both. An increase in LVEDV often results from decreased contractility in the setting of a properly performing right ventricle (*panel C*). SBP, systolic blood pressure; DBP, diastolic blood pressure.

c. **Oximetric** catheters that provide monitoring of mixed venous oxygen saturation.

d. **Continuous cardiac output** catheters that use a special algorithm to perform frequent automated determinations of thermodilution cardiac output.

e. **Right ventricular ejection fraction** catheters that use a rapid response thermistor to calculate RV ejection fraction in addition to CO.

C. **Cardiac output**

1. **Thermodilution** cardiac output is determined by injecting a fixed volume of cold (room temperature or less) solution into the CVP port of the PAC. The cold tracer mixes with the blood as it passes through the right ventricle, and the temperature of the mixture is measured as it passes a thermistor near the tip of the PAC. The computation of the cardiac output uses a formula that must properly account for the volume of the injectate, the injectate temperature, the thermodynamic properties of the blood, injectate solution, the particular catheter used, and the integral of the temperature-time curve. Consequently, the proper volume of an appropriate solution must be injected to satisfy these assumptions. Typically, 10 ml of cold saline or 5% dextrose in water is injected within 4 seconds. The rapid infusion of cold intravenous fluid into the central venous circulation can interfere with thermodilution CO measurements.

2. **Dye dilution** can be used as an alternative to thermodilution. This requires the injection of a nontoxic dye (usually indocyanine green) into the central venous circulation. Arterial blood is withdrawn at a known rate using a syringe pump. The arterial concentration of dye is continuously measured as the blood is withdrawn and a curve of dye concentration versus time constructed. The algorithm used to calculate CO is analogous to that used for a thermodilution output. This technique requires that both a central venous and an arterial line be present, but does not require a PAC. A properly calibrated sensor is required to measure the arterial dye concentration. Alternative tracers, including radioisotopes, are sometimes used for research purposes.

3. **CO is usually interpreted** in the setting of hypotension. Determining the CO allows diagnosis of a low tone state [low systemic vascular resistance (SVR)], a low CO, or both. If the CO is low, a concurrent measurement of heart rate (HR) will help determine whether the reason is related to the heart rate or to ventricular performance (i.e., **stroke volume = CO/HR**).

4. **Physiologic interpretation**

a. **Respiration.** During spontaneous breathing, negative intrathoracic pressure enhances venous return and increases LV afterload. During positive pressure breathing, inspiration reduces venous return and LV afterload. Cardiac output can vary over the respiratory cycle, depending on the mode of ventilation and baseline levels of venous return and cardiac performance. Accordingly, the timing of injection affects the interpretation of a thermodilution CO measurement. If a consistent trend is desired, **it is probably best to inject at a constant point in the respiratory cycle, usually at end-expiration.** If an average over the respiratory cycle is desired, it is usual to take the mean of three measurements obtained at random times throughout the respiratory cycle.

   b. **Tricuspid regurgitation** can produce both erroneously high and low readings. Rarely do they vary more than 20% from the actual value.

   c. **Intracardiac shunts** also produce erroneous measurements.

IV. Cardiac echocardiography

   A. **Mechanism.** Echocardiography (Echo) uses high frequency (2.5–10 MHz) ultrasonic waves to generate images of the heart and surrounding structures. The two common approaches used in the ICU are transthoracic and transesophageal.

   B. Echo can provide many of the parameters that a PAC can provide (e.g., estimates of cardiac ejection and blood flow), but it is far more expensive and labor intensive to use as a continuous monitor in the ICU.

   C. Echo can also provide information that a PAC cannot, such as valvular function, assessment of ventricular contractility, diastolic relaxation, and assessment of the pericardium. Intracardiac structures such as vegetations, tumor, or thrombus can be visualized. Consequently, echo can be invaluable for intermittent assessment of cardiac function and diagnosis of cardiac and pericardial pathology.

   D. **Indications** include assessment of:
      1. Low CO accompanied by unexplained high filling pressures.
      2. Valvular lesions and intracardiac shunts.
      3. Pericardial disease.
      4. Intracardiac thrombus.
      5. Suspected vegetations.

V. Electrocardiogram (ECG). The ECG is used to determine heart rate and to detect and diagnosis dysrhythmias, pacemaker function, and myocardial ischemia. The presence of an ECG signal does not guarantee cardiac contraction or output. The ECG findings can also suggest electrolyte abnormalities.

   A. **Mechanism of measurement**
      1. **Electrode application.** Because the ECG is a small electrical signal (about 1 mV), its measure-

ment is susceptible to electrical interference from improper application of electrodes. Electrodes should have adequate gel and be applied to a clean, dry skin area.

2. **Electrode location.** For the ECG to be interpreted properly, the electrodes must be placed in consistent locations. The limb leads must be located on or near their appropriate limbs, and the precordial lead typically over V5 (5th intercostal space, anterior axillary line).

3. **Calibration** of the ECG signal should be checked with the internal calibration button. A 1-mV signal should produce a 1-cm deflection.

4. **Mode.** Most monitors have a diagnostic and monitor mode. The monitor mode filters out more noise because of a narrower frequency bandpass (0.5–40 Hz); it consequently creates a more stable tracing for simple rhythm monitoring. The diagnostic mode, with a wider bandpass (0.05–100 Hz), should be used whenever evaluating ST-segment changes for ischemia. Newer monitors permit continuous analysis and trending of ST-segment changes.

B. **Rhythm detection.** Lead II is most commonly monitored because the P wave is easily seen, allowing detection of dysrhythmias. Inferior ischemia can also be detected.

C. **Ischemia detection.** Typically, a five-lead system is used (with simultaneous monitoring of leads II and V5) in patients with significant cardiac disease. This combination provides 80% to 96% sensitivity to detect ischemic events (V5 alone, 75% to 80%; II alone, 18% to 33%). Lead V5 is monitored to detect myocardial ischemia, because most of the left ventricular myocardium lies beneath it. If only a three-lead electrode system is available, a modified V5 lead is obtained by placing the right arm lead under the right clavicle, the left arm lead in the V5 position, and the left leg lead as usual while monitoring lead I.

VI. **Procedures**

A. **Arterial cannulation**

1. **Location.** The radial artery is most commonly used. Other sites include the ulnar, brachial, axillary, femoral, and dorsalis pedis arteries. With increasing distance from the heart, systolic blood pressure increases, MAP generally decreases, and the pressure waveform displayed on the monitor narrows.

2. **Radial artery catheter insertion technique**

a. Immobilize the forearm and hand with the wrist slightly hyperextended over a padded arm board (Fig. 1-5). The thumb can be extended to place the volar surface of the wrist exactly parallel to the floor. Palpate the radial artery medial to the head of the radius.

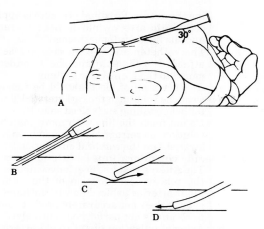

Fig. 1-5. Percutaneous radial artery cannulation. A. Direct threading method. B–D. Transfixing method. The positioning of the hand and forearm is the same for both methods.

   b. After preparing the skin, a 25-gauge needle is used to raise a skin wheal with 1% lidocaine. A 15-gauge needle skin puncture facilitates catheter passage.

   c. Select the appropriate-sized catheter (22- to 24-gauge for infants, 20- to 22-gauge for larger children, and 18- or 20-gauge for adults).

   d. **Transfixion method.** The catheter is advanced slowly and completely through the artery. Although blood often shows in the hub of the needle, it may not with the 22- or 24-gauge needle. The needle is removed from the cannula (keeping it sterile for possible reuse), and the catheter is firmly connected to a T-connector stopcock and flush syringe. The system should allow blood to flow back into the syringe. The catheter is lowered almost parallel to the skin of the wrist and slowly withdrawn until blood pulsates freely in the system. The catheter is then advanced into the vessel. The catheter should be flushed free of blood and the stopcock turned off until it is connected to the transducer. A sterile arterial guidewire can be used if catheter insertion is difficult.

   e. **Direct threading technique.** The needle is advanced slowly until the artery is entered and free flow of blood is observed. The catheter is advanced over the needle while rigidly fixing the needle. Proximal pressure is applied to occlude the artery while the needle is removed and the flush system attached.

f. The catheter and T-connector are securely attached to the skin and the T-connector is joined to the transducer system.

g. At least 2 ml of blood should be removed to clear the volume in the catheter and T-connector before taking each blood sample.

h. Do not flush the line with more than 3 ml of solution, as retrograde flow has been demonstrated into the cerebral circulation.

3. Specific considerations for arterial cannulation

a. The **Allen's test** has been advocated to assess the relative contribution of the radial and ulnar arteries to blood flow to the hand. However, it does not accurately predict complications and is not performed routinely.

b. Arterial pulsation distal to old arterial cannulation sites can represent collateral flow. Proximal pulsation should be assessed before insertion to confirm that thrombosis has not occurred.

c. Whenever a left- versus right-sided disparity occurs in measured blood pressure, in general, pressure should be measured on the side with the higher pressure.

d. For femoral and axillary arterial pressure measurement, a 6-inch 18-gauge catheter is inserted by Seldinger technique after cannulation by a 2-inch, 18- or 20-gauge catheter.

e. **Damped waveforms** can be caused by proximal pressure on the artery, transducer malfunction, and mechanical problems such as air and clot. The catheter should aspirate and flush easily. It may require repositioning, rewiring, or replacing with a larger gauge or longer cannula. Blood pressure should be measured by another technique in the interim.

4. Complications are rare, but they include thrombosis, distal ischemia, infection, and fistula or aneurysm formation. If the hand or digit appears ischemic, the cannula should be removed as soon as possible. In this case, if the radial artery was cannulated, do not choose the ipsilateral ulnar artery as the alternative site.

B. Insertion of central venous catheters

1. Sites. The internal jugular vein, subclavian vein, external jugular vein, cephalic vein, axillary vein, and femoral vein all provide access to the central circulation. **Portable two-dimensional ultrasound imaging** (e.g., Siterite, Dymax Corporation, Pittsburgh, PA) can be used to define the anatomy of central vessels and determine their patency. Subsequently, cannulation can be performed under ultrasonic guidance or visualization.

2. **Cannulation of the right internal jugular vein** (Seldinger technique) (Fig. 1-6).

   a. An oxygen mask is applied, and the patient's head is turned toward the left and slightly extended. The neck is cleaned with an antiseptic solution.

   b. A person wearing a sterile gown and gloves drapes the area with sterile towels to expose the suprasternal notch, clavicle, lateral border of the sternocleidomastoid (SCM) muscle, and the lower border of the mandible.

   c. The midpoint between the mastoid process and the sternal attachment of the SCM is located.

   d. The internal jugular vein can be entered medial to the SCM at this point (anterior approach) or, more laterally, at the apex of the two heads of the SCM (central approach). The external jugular vein should be identified to avoid puncture.

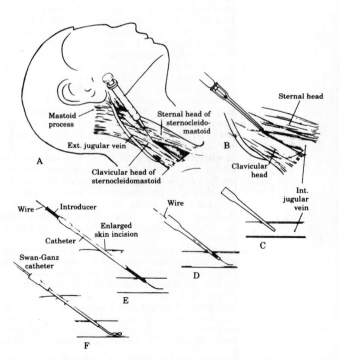

Fig. 1-6. Cannulation of the right internal jugular vein. (Seldinger technique). See text for details.

    e. The patient is placed in the Trendelenburg position, unless contraindicated by conditions such as intracranial hypertension and congestive heart failure.

    f. The carotid artery is gently palpated, and the skin and deep tissues are infiltrated with 1% lidocaine just lateral to the carotid artery. A finder needle (22- or 25-gauge) is advanced laterally to the artery at a 30-degree angle to the skin, pointing approximately toward the ipsilateral axilla (anterior approach) or nipple (central approach) until venous blood is aspirated.

    g. A Valsalva maneuver can increase vein size during difficult cannulations.

    h. This needle is removed, and an 18-gauge thin wall needle (or IV catheter) is inserted at the same angle and depth. Blood should be easily aspirated when the vein is entered.

    i. The syringe is removed and a guidewire is advanced through the needle or catheter while the ECG is observed. The wire should pass easily. The thin wall needle (or catheter) is removed over the guidewire. The insertion site can be superficially enlarged with a No. 11 scalpel blade inserted parallel to the skin and pointed laterally (to avoid the carotid artery). With countertraction on the skin, a dilator is advanced over the wire; gentle twisting of the dilator can aid insertion. While maintaining proximal control of the guidewire at all times, the dilator is withdrawn, a catheter passed, and, the wire removed. Infusion ports are flushed after residual air is aspirated. The catheter is secured to the skin, and an occlusive dressing is applied.

    j. A **chest radiograph** should be obtained to check the position of the radiopaque catheter and to exclude a pneumothorax. Correct tip position is at the junction of the SVC and the right atrium. Make sure that the tip of a catheter placed via the left jugular vein does not abut against the wall of the SVC at a steep angle.

3. **The external jugular vein** runs superficially from the edge of the mid-SCM toward the clavicle laterally. An external jugular catheter can be inserted in a manner similar to that described above in section VI.B.2. Occlusion of the vein at the clavicle will make it larger and less mobile. The external jugular vein bends to join the subclavian vein. Consequently, threading the catheter centrally can be more difficult. A "J"-shaped guidewire should be used.

4. **The subclavian vein** crosses under the clavicle just medial to the midclavicular line. The needle

is inserted inferior to the outer third of the clavicle. The periosteum of the clavicle is identified
with the needle and the tip "walked" posteriorly
under the clavicle and directed toward the sternal
notch. It should remain close to the posterior edge
of the clavicle to avoid a pneumothorax. The catheter is inserted into the vein as described in section
VI.B.2.

5. **The basilic vein** can be used as well. Long
catheters threaded through an introducer needle
are made for this purpose. Alternatively, a 20-inch
16-gauge catheter can be introduced sterilely
through a 2-inch 14-gauge catheter placed in the
vein. If the catheter is difficult to thread, the arm
can be abducted and the head turned toward the
side of the insertion to decrease the incidence
of catheter passage up into the jugular vein. A
140-cm guidewire can also be used.

6. **Percutaneously inserted central catheters
(PICC)** also can be inserted via peripheral arm
veins. Single and double lumen catheters are available. These provide long-term IV access for infusion of drugs and total parenteral nutrition and
have low rates of complications and infections.

7. **Cannulation of the femoral vein** can be accomplished by entering the vein just medial to the
femoral artery (inferior to the inguinal ligament)
and proceeding as described in section VI.B.2. The
leg should be slightly abducted before insertion.

8. **Complications of CVP catheter insertion** and
use include:
    a. Dysrhythmias, both atrial and ventricular,
    which generally are short-lived and corrected
    by withdrawing the catheter.
    b. Carotid or subclavian artery puncture. If un-
    noticed, a large IV catheter can be threaded
    into the artery and cause damage requir-
    ing surgical repair. Attention must be paid
    throughout the cannulation to the color and
    pulsations of the blood. The color or oxygen
    saturation of a venous sample drawn through
    the finder or thin-wall needle can be compared
    with a simultaneously drawn arterial sample.
    With the patient breathing an enriched oxy-
    gen concentration, a difference in saturation is
    usually apparent. Additionally, the pressure
    in the finder needle or cannula can be mea-
    sured by connecting it to a pressure transduc-
    er or to a free-flowing IV fluid bag. Whenever
    an arterial cannulation suggestion remains, a
    fresh puncture site should be sought. In anti-
    coagulated patients, subclavian vein cannula-
    tion has a higher risk of hemorrhage than that
    done in the jugular veins, because of the diffi-
    culty in compressing the subclavian artery in

case of puncture. Hence subclavian vein cannulation may be contraindicated in patients on anticoagulation medication.

   c. Pneumothorax, pericardial tamponade, hemothorax, hydrothorax, chylothorax, infection, and air embolism.

C. Pulmonary artery catheter (PAC) insertion (Fig. 1-7). The right internal jugular vein is used most commonly because of easy access from the head of the patient and the lower incidence of pneumothorax, but all the aforementioned access sites can be used. Once inserted, most catheters terminate in the right PA.

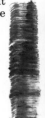

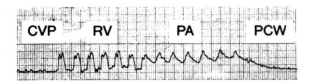

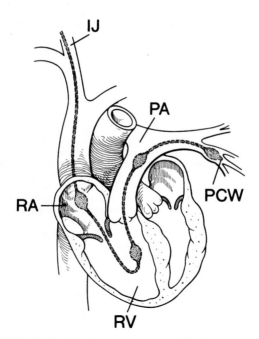

Fig. 1-7.   **Characteristic pressure waves seen during insertion of a pulmonary artery catheter. CVP, central venous pressure; IJ, internal jugular; RA, right atrium; RV, right ventricle; PA, pulmonary artery; PCW, pulmonary capillary wedge**

1. Oxygen is supplied by face mask, and the ECG is monitored. The Seldinger technique is used as described in section VI.B.2. The dilator–introducer assembly is placed over the wire, with care not to burr the end of the introducer as it is manipulated through skin and soft tissue.

2. The wire and dilator are removed from the introducer, and the side port of the introducer is aspirated for blood and then flushed. The patient can now be taken out of the Trendelenburg position.

3. A **protective sheath** is placed over the PAC so that the distal 70 cm will remain sterile. The PAC is then checked for symmetric balloon inflation with 1.5 ml of air. The PA and CVP lumens are flushed with saline and attached to calibrated pressure transducers through three-way stopcocks. Raising and lowering the PAC distal end while observing the resulting change in the pressure tracing can serve as a quick test of the calibration and sensitivity of the system before insertion.

4. The PAC can be held over the patient to observe its natural curve, which is designed to facilitate flotation through the heart. **The PAC is inserted to a depth of 20 cm;** the monitor should confirm **a CVP waveform.** The balloon is inflated with 1.0 to 1.5 ml of air, and the PAC is advanced until **a right ventricular pressure waveform** is seen. This should occur **at a depth of approximately 30 to 35 cm.**

5. The PAC is then advanced until **a PA tracing is obtained (at about 40–45 cm).** Premature ventricular contractions often are encountered.

6. The PAC is inserted until **a PAOP tracing is obtained (at a depth of about 50–55 cm).** The PA tracing should reappear with deflation of the balloon. If it does not, withdraw the catheter slightly until the PA tracing reappears.

7. The sterile sheath is connected to the introducer, and an occlusive tape is applied at the sheath's proximal end, allowing the position of the PAC to be adjusted approximately 10 cm. The introducer is secured to the skin, a sterile occlusive dressing applied, and the PAC secured to the patient.

8. During PAC insertion, it may be difficult to pass the catheter into the right ventricle and PA because of balloon malfunction, valvular lesions, a low-flow state, or a dilated right ventricle. The monitoring equipment should be rechecked for calibration and scale. Inflating the balloon with a full 1.5 ml of air, slow PAC advancement, and large inspirations by the patient to augment blood flow may be helpful. The PAC may have to be withdrawn to a depth of 20 to 30 cm, rotated slightly, and readvanced.

9. The PAC is placed with **fluoroscopic visualiza-tion** when a permanent pacemaker has been placed within the past 6 weeks, when selective PA placement is necessary (e.g., a patient undergoing a right pneumonectomy), or if a PAC is required in the presence of significant structural abnor-malities (e.g., Eisenmenger complex).

10. **Complications** include:

a. **A transient right bundle branch block.** In the patient with first-degree block and left bundle branch block, insertion of the PAC can result in complete heart block. Appropriate medications (e.g., isoproterenol) and pacing capability (e.g., external transcutaneous, transvenous pacer, or Paceport PAC) should be available.

b. **Pulmonary artery rupture or infarction.** Balloon inflation should be slow, stopped im-mediately when a PAOP tracing is obtained, and never kept inflated for an extended period because of the possibility of PA rupture or infarction. PA pressures always should be monitored when a PAC is in place. A persis-tent "wedge" waveform occurrence indicates that the catheter should be pulled back immediately.

c. **PACs may rarely knot.** Fluoroscopic guid-ance may be needed to untangle and remove the catheter.

d. **Balloon rupture.** At no time should the bal-loon be filled with more than 1.5 ml of air.

e. Other complications as previously described for CVP catheters (see section VI.B.8.).

SELECTED REFERENCES

Jacobsohn E, Chorn R, O'Connor M. The role of the vasculature in regulating venous return and cardiac output: historical and graph-ical approach. *Can J Anaesth* 1997;44:849–867.

Lake CL. *Clinical monitoring for anesthesia and critical care,* 2nd ed. Philadelphia: WB Saunders, 1994.

Mark JB. *Atlas of cardiovascular monitoring.* New York: Churchill Livingstone, 1998.

Pagel PS, Grossman W, Haering JM, et al. Left ventricular diastolic function in the normal and diseased heart (Part 1). *Anesthesiology* 1993;79:836–854.

Pagel PS, Grossman W, Haering JM, et al. Left ventricular diastolic function in the normal and diseased heart (Part 2). *Anesthesiology* 1993;79:1104–1120.

Perret C, Tagan D, Feihl F, et al. *The pulmonary artery catheter in critical care.* Oxford: Blackwell Science, 1996.

Sagawa K, Maughan L, Suga H, et al. *Cardiac contraction and the pres-sure-volume relationship.* Oxford: Oxford University Press, 1988.

Respiratory Monitoring

Dean Hess

I. **Monitoring** is a continuous, or nearly continuous, evaluation of the physiologic function of a patient in real time to guide management decisions—including when to make therapeutic interventions and assessment of those interventions. The decision to monitor, as with any other clinical decision, should be based on clinical indications.

   A. **Safety.** Monitoring is often performed to assure patient safety. For example, pulse oximetry is used to detect hypoxemia and airway pressure is monitored to detect a mechanical ventilator disconnection. Although monitoring has improved safety during anesthesia, its impact on patient outcome in the intensive care unit (ICU) is less clear.

   B. **Assess interventions.** Invasive and noninvasive monitoring is commonly used in the ICU to assess patient response to clinical interventions. Titration of the fraction of inspired oxygen (FIO_2) is commonly guided by pulse oximetry; the level of pressure support is guided by respiratory rate; and the inspiratory to expiratory (I:E) ratio is guided by measurement of intrinsic-positive end-expiratory pressure (auto-PEEP).

II. **Gas exchange**

   A. **Arterial blood gases and pH.** Although arterial blood gas analysis may be used excessively, it is the gold standard for assessment of pulmonary gas exchange.

      1. **PaO_2.** The normal arterial PO_2 (PaO_2) is 90 to 100 mm Hg breathing room air at sea level.

         a. **Decreased PaO_2 (hypoxemia)** occurs with pulmonary diseases resulting in shunt ($\dot{Q}_S/\dot{Q}_T$), ventilation/perfusion ($\dot{V}/\dot{Q}$) mismatch, hypoventilation, and diffusion defect. A low mixed venous PO_2 (e.g., decreased cardiac output) will magnify the effect of shunt on PaO_2. The PaO_2 is also decreased with decreased inspired oxygen (e.g., at high altitude).

         b. **Increased PaO_2 (hyperoxemia)** can occur when breathing supplemental oxygen. The PaO_2 also increases with hyperventilation.

         c. **Effect of FIO_2.** The PaO_2 should always be interpreted in relation to the level of supplemental oxygen. For example, a PaO_2 of 95 mm Hg breathing 100% oxygen is different than a PaO_2 of 95 mm Hg breathing room air (21% oxygen).

      2. **PCO_2.** The arterial PCO_2 ($PaCO_2$) reflects the balance between carbon dioxide production ($\dot{V}CO_2$) and alveolar ventilation ($\dot{V}_A$): $PaCO_2 = (\dot{V}CO_2/\dot{V}_A)(0.863)$. $PaCO_2$ varies directly with carbon dioxide production

and inversely with alveolar ventilation. Note that Pa_{CO_2} is determined by alveolar ventilation and not minute ventilation *per se*. Minute ventilation affects Pa_{CO_2} only to the extent that it affects the alveolar ventilation.

3. **Arterial pH** is determined by bicarbonate (HCO_3^-) concentration and Pa_{CO_2}, as predicted by the **Henderson-Hasselbalch equation:**

$$pH = 6.1 + \log\left(\frac{HCO_3^-}{[0.03 \times Pa_{CO_2}]}\right)$$

See Table 2-1 for a classification of acid-base disturbances, Table 2-2 for common clinical causes of acid-base disturbances, and Table 2-3 for the expected degree of compensation for acid-base disorders.

B. **CO-oximetry.** Spectrophotometric analysis of arterial blood is used to measure levels of oxyhemoglobin (oxygen saturation of hemoglobin), carboxyhemoglobin (carbon monoxide saturation of hemoglobin), and methemoglobin (amount of hemoglobin in the oxidized ferric form rather than the reduced ferrous form).

1. **Oxyhemoglobin** (HbO_2) measured by CO-oximetry is the gold standard for determination of oxygen saturation and is superior to other means of determining oxygen saturation, such as that calculated empirically by a blood gas analyzer or that measured by pulse oximetry. The normal HbO_2 is about 97%.

Table 2-1. Classification of acid-base disorders

Disorder	pH	Pa_{CO_2}	HCO_3^-
Respiratory acidosis			
Uncompensated	↓↓	↑↑	N
Partially compensated	↓	↑↑	↓
Fully compensated	N	↑↑	↑↑
Respiratory alkalosis			
Uncompensated	↑↑	↓↓	N
Partially compensated	↑	↓↓	↓
Fully compensated	N	↓↓	↓↓
Metabolic acidosis			
Uncompensated	↓↓	N	↓↓
Partially compensated	↓	↓	↓↓
Fully compensated	N	↓↓	↓↓
Metabolic alkalosis			
Uncompensated	↑↑	N	↑↑
Partially compensated	↑	↑	↑↑
Fully compensated	N	↑↑	↑↑

N, normal.

Table 2-2. Common causes of acid-base disturbances

Respiratory acidosis
Respiratory center depression
Disruption of neural pathways affecting respiratory muscles
Neuromuscular blockade
Respiratory muscle weakness
Pulmonary disease

Respiratory alkalosis
Respiratory center stimulation (anxiety, hypoxia, disease)
Iatrogenic (mechanical ventilation)

Metabolic acidosis
Normal anion gap
  Diarrhea
  Acetazolamide (Diamox)
  Renal tubular acidosis
Increased anion gap
  Lactic acidosis
  Ketoacidosis
  Renal failure
  Poisoning: methanol, ethylene glycol, aspirin

Metabolic alkalosis
Hypokalemia
Nasogastric suctioning or vomiting
Contraction alkalosis
Bicarbonate administration
Steroid therapy
Citrate, acetate, lactate administration

Table 2-3. Expected compensation for acid-base disturbances[a]

Respiratory acidosis
$\Delta HCO_3^- = 0.10 \times \Delta PaCO_2$ (acute)
$\Delta HCO_3^- = 0.35 \times \Delta PaCO_2$ (chronic)

Respiratory alkalosis
$\Delta HCO_3^- = 0.2 \times \Delta PaCO_2$ (acute)
$\Delta HCO_3^- = 0.5 \times \Delta PaCO_2$ (chronic)

Metabolic acidosis
$\Delta PaCO_2 = 1.2 \times \Delta HCO_3^-$

Metabolic alkalosis
$\Delta PaCO_2 = 0.9 \times \Delta HCO_3^-$

[a] If the acid-base status exceeds the expected level of compensation, a mixed acid-base disturbance is present.

2. **Carboxyhemoglobin** (HbCO) levels should be measured whenever carbon monoxide inhalation is suspected. Endogenous carboxyhemoglobin levels are 1% to 2% and can be elevated in cigarette smokers and those living in polluted environments. Because carboxyhemoglobin does not transport oxygen, the HbO$_2$ is effectively reduced by the HbCO level.

3. **Methemoglobin.** The iron in the hemoglobin molecule can be oxidized to the ferric form in the presence of a number of oxidizing agents, the most notable being nitrates. Because methemoglobin (metHb) does not transport oxygen, the HbO$_2$ is effectively reduced by the metHb level.

C. **Continuous blood gas monitoring**

1. **Principles of operation.** Intraarterial blood gas systems use optical biosensors called "fluorescent optodes." The optode consists of a miniaturized probe containing a fluorescent dye. Fluorescence is augmented with an increase in hydrogen ion concentration or PCO_2 and quenched with an increase in PO_2. Photosensors are used to quantify the signal to measure pH, PCO_2, and PO_2. Systems for continuous blood gas monitoring use a probe that passes through an arterial catheter and resides in the arterial lumen. In an alternative approach, blood is withdrawn into the optode chamber from an arterial catheter whenever blood gas analysis is desired.

2. **Limitations.** A major limitation of these systems is their cost, which is very high. Whether the benefits of continuous (or on-demand) blood gas analysis outweigh the costs and technical constraints has not yet been determined.

D. **Point-of-care blood gas monitoring** is performed near the site of patient care. Point-of-care analyzers are available to measure blood gas tensions and pH. These analyzers can also measure electrolytes, glucose, lactate, urea nitrogen, and hematocrit.

1. **Advantages.** Point-of-care analyzers are small and portable (some are hand-held), they require small blood volumes (several drops), and report results quickly (a few minutes). They are relatively easy to use (e.g., self-calibrating) and, typically, use a disposable cartridge that contains the appropriate biosensors.

2. **Disadvantages.** The cost-to-benefit ratio of these devices is unclear. For example, the disposable cartridges are expensive. Further, appropriate documentation for compliance with CLIA-88 or JCAHO requirements is necessary, which involves two levels of quality-control checks at least twice daily. Instrument maintenance and quality control can be labor-intensive and confusing for those who are unfamiliar with these procedures.

E. **Pulse oximetry**
1. **Principles of operation.** The pulse oximeter passes two wavelengths of light (e.g., 660 nm and 940 nm) from light-emitting diodes through a pulsating vascular bed to a photodetector. A variety of probes are available in disposable or reusable designs; they include digital probes (finger or toe), ear probes, and nasal probes.
2. **Accuracy.** Pulse oximeters use empiric calibration curves developed from studies of healthy volunteers. The accuracy of pulse oximetry is ±4% to 5% at saturations >80% (and less at lower saturations). The implications of this accuracy relate to the oxyhemoglobin dissociation curve (Fig. 2-1). If the pulse oximeter displays an oxygen saturation (SpO_2) of 95%, the true saturation could be as low as 90% or as high as 100%. This range of SpO_2 translates to a PO_2 range from as low as approximately 60 mm Hg to >150 mm Hg.
3. **Limitations** of pulse oximetry should be recognized and understood by everyone who uses pulse oximetry data.
   a. **Saturation versus PO_2.** Because of the shape of the oxyhemoglobin dissociation curve, pulse oximetry is a poor indicator of hyperoxemia. It is also an insensitive indicator of hypoventilation. If the patient is breathing supplemental oxygen, significant hypoventilation can occur without desaturation.

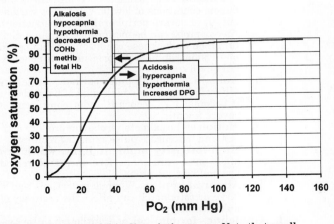

Fig. 2-1. **Oxyhemoglobin dissociation curve.** Note that small changes in oxygen saturation relate to large changes in PO_2 when the saturation is >90%. Also note that the saturation can change without a change in PO_2 if a shift occurs in the oxyhemoglobin dissociation curve.

b.   **Differences between devices and probes.**
Calibration curves vary from manufacturer to
manufacturer. The output of the light-emitting
diodes of pulse oximeters varies from probe to
probe. For these reasons, the same pulse oximeter and probe should be used for each SpO_2
determination for a patient.

c.   **The penumbra effect** occurs when the pulse
oximeter probe does not fit correctly and light is
shunted from the light-emitting diodes directly
to the photodetector.

d.   **Dyshemoglobinemia.** Pulse oximeters only
use two wavelengths of light and, therefore,
evaluate only two forms of hemoglobin—
oxyhemoglobin and deoxyhemoglobin. Carboxyhemoglobinemia and methemoglobinemia
result in significant inaccuracy of pulse oximetry. Carboxyhemoglobinemia produces a SpO_2
greater than the true oxygen saturation and
methemoglobinemia causes the SpO_2 to move
toward 85%. Fetal hemoglobin does not affect
the accuracy of pulse oximetry.

e.   **Endogenous and exogenous dyes and
pigments** such as intravascular dyes (particularly methylene blue) and nail polish can
affect the accuracy of pulse oximetry. Hyperbilirubinemia does not affect the accuracy of
pulse oximetry.

f.   **Skin pigmentation.** The accuracy and performance of pulse oximetry is affected by deeply
pigmented skin.

g.   **Perfusion.** Pulse oximetry becomes unreliable
during conditions of low flow (e.g., low cardiac
output or severe peripheral vasoconstriction).
An ear probe can be more reliable than a digital probe under these conditions. A dampened
plethysmographic waveform suggests poor signal quality.

h.   **Anemia.** Although pulse oximetry is generally reliable over a wide range of hematocrit,
it becomes less accurate under conditions of
severe anemia.

i.   **Motion** of the oximeter probe can produce artifact and inaccurate pulse oximetry readings.

j.   **High-intensity ambient light,** which can
affect pulse oximeter performance, is corrected
by shielding the probe.

k.   **Abnormal pulses.** Venous pulsations and a
large dicrotic notch can affect the accuracy of
pulse oximetry.

4.   **Guidelines for clinical use.** Although pulse oximetry improves the detection of desaturation, little
evidence indicates that its use improves outcome.
Despite this, pulse oximetry has become a standard
of care in the ICU (particularly for mechanically

ventilated patients). Pulse oximetry is useful to titrate supplemental oxygen in mechanically ventilated patients. A $SpO_2 \geq 92\%$ reliably predicts a $PaO_2 \geq 60$ mm Hg in white patients ($SpO_2 \geq 95\%$ in black patients). SpO_2 should be periodically confirmed by blood gas analysis.

F. Capnometry

1. **Capnometry** is the measurement of CO_2 at the airway. **Capnography** is the display of a CO_2 waveform called the **capnogram** (Fig. 2-2). The PCO_2 measured at end-exhalation is called the **end-tidal PCO_2** ($PetCO_2$).

2. **Principles of operation.** Quantitative capnometers measure CO_2 using the principles of infrared spectroscopy, Raman spectroscopy, or mass spectroscopy. Nonquantitative capnometers indicate CO_2 by a color change of an indicator material. Mainstream capnometers place the measurement chamber directly on the airway, whereas sidestream capnometers aspirate gas through tubing to a measurement chamber in the capnometer.

3. The **end-tidal PCO_2** represents alveolar PCO_2; it is determined by the rate at which CO_2 is added to the alveolus and the rate at which CO_2 is cleared from the alveolus. Thus, the $PetCO_2$ is a function of the $\dot{V}/\dot{Q}$. With a normal $\dot{V}/\dot{Q}$, the $PetCO_2$ approximates the $PaCO_2$. With a high $\dot{V}/\dot{Q}$ (dead space), the $PetCO_2$ is lower than the $PaCO_2$. With a low $\dot{V}/\dot{Q}$, $PetCO_2$ approximates the mixed-venous PCO_2. The $PetCO_2$ can be as low as the inspired PCO_2 (zero) or as high as the mixed venous PCO_2. Changes in $PetCO_2$ can be caused by changes in CO_2 produc-

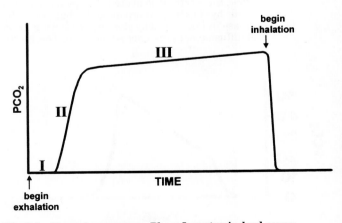

Fig. 2-2.   Normal capnogram. Phase I: anatomic dead space; phase II: transition from dead space to alveolar gas; phase III: alveolar plateau.

tion, changes in CO_2 delivery to the lungs, or changes in alveolar ventilation. The gradient between $PaCO_2$ and $PetCO_2$ is normally small (< 5 mm Hg). However, the $P(a\text{-}et)CO_2$ is increased with diseases that increase dead space and it can occasionally be negative.

4. **Abnormal capnogram.** The shape of the capnogram can be abnormal in some conditions (Fig. 2-3).

5. **Limitations.** Clinical interest has been expressed in using $PetCO_2$ as a noninvasive indicator of $PaCO_2$. Unfortunately, however, considerable intra- and interpatient variability exists in the relationship between $PaCO_2$ and $PetCO_2$. The $P(a\text{-}et)CO_2$ is often too variable in critically ill patients to allow precise prediction of $PaCO_2$ from $PetCO_2$.

6. **Guidelines for clinical use.** The utility of $PetCO_2$ to predict $PaCO_2$ is limited in the ICU. Capnometry is useful to detect esophageal intubation. End-tidal CO_2 monitoring to confirm tracheal intubation is generally regarded as a standard of care. Commercially available low-cost disposable devices produce a color change in the presence of exhaled CO_2. Capnometry has been used to evaluate pulmonary blood flow during resuscitation, but this application has not received widespread clinical use.

G. **Transcutaneous blood gas monitoring.** Transcutaneous PO_2 ($PtcO_2$) and transcutaneous PCO_2 ($PtcCO_2$) have been commonly monitored in the neonatal ICU, but has had limited acceptance in the care of adults.

1. **Principles of operation.** The $PtcO_2$ electrode uses a polarographic principle and the $PtcCO_2$ uses a Severinghaus electrode. To produce a $PtcO_2$ similar to PaO_2, the electrode is heated. The increase in PO_2 caused by heating approximately balances the decrease in PO_2 caused by skin oxygen consumption and diffusion of oxygen across the skin. The $PtcCO_2$

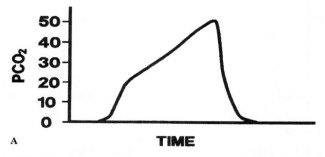

A

Fig. 2-3.   **Abnormal capnograms. A. Increased phase III that occurs with obstructive lung disease.**

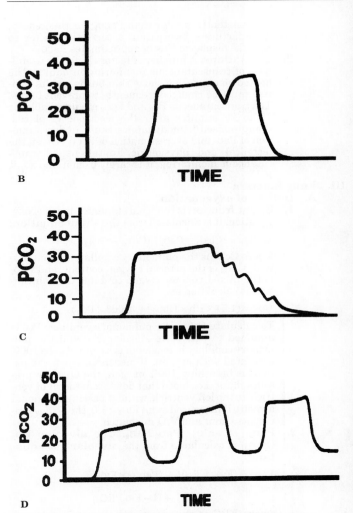

Fig. 2-3. *Continued.* B. "Curare cleft" that occurs with partial recovery from neuromuscular blockade. C. Cardiac oscillations. D. Rebreathing with a shift of the capnogram from baseline.

is consistently greater than $PaCO_2$; for this reason, manufacturers incorporate a correction factor so that the displayed $PtcCO_2$ approximates $PaCO_2$.

2. **Limitations.** A number of factors limit the usefulness of transcutaneous monitoring in adults. The heated electrode can cause skin burns and its position must be changed frequently to prevent burns. The transcutaneous PO_2 and PCO_2 are unreliable for 15 to 20 minutes after the electrode is placed. Compromised hemodynamics cause underestimation of PaO_2 and overestimation of $PaCO_2$. Given the technical and physiologic limitations of transcutaneous monitoring, it is rarely used in the adult ICU.

III. **Lung function**
   A. **Indices of oxygenation**
      1. **Shunt fraction** is the "gold standard" index of oxygenation. It is calculated from **the shunt equation:**

$$\dot{Q}_S/\dot{Q}_T = (Cc'O_2 - CaO_2)/(Cc'O_2 - C\bar{v}O_2)$$

where $Cc'O_2$ is the pulmonary capillary oxygen content, CaO_2 is the arterial oxygen content, and $C\bar{v}O_2$ is the mixed venous oxygen content. Oxygen content is calculated as:

$$CO_2 = (1.34 \times Hb \times HbO_2) + (0.003 \times PO_2)$$

To calculate $Cc'O_2$, the pulmonary capillary PO_2 is assumed to equal the alveolar PO_2 and the pulmonary capillary hemoglobin is assumed to be 100% saturated with oxygen. If measured when the patient is breathing 100% oxygen, the $\dot{Q}_S/\dot{Q}_T$ represents shunt (i.e., blood that flows from the right ventricle to the left ventricle without passing functional alveoli). If measured at an $FIO_2 < 1.0$, the $\dot{Q}_S/\dot{Q}_T$ represents shunt and $\dot{V}/\dot{Q}$ mismatch.

      2. **PAO_2, $P(A-a)O_2$, PaO_2/PAO_2.** The **alveolar PO_2 (PAO_2)** is calculated from the **alveolar gas equation:**

$$PAO_2 = (FIO_2 \times EBP) - (PaCO_2 \times FIO_2$$

$$+ [1 - FIO_2/RQ])$$

where EBP is the effective barometric pressure (barometric pressure minus water vapor pressure) and RQ is the respiratory quotient. For calculation of PAO_2, an RQ of 0.8 is commonly used. For $FIO_2 \geq 0.6$, the effect of RQ on the alveolar gas equation becomes:

$$PAO_2 = (FIO_2 \times EBP) - PaCO_2$$

For $FIO_2 < 0.6$, the alveolar gas equation becomes:

$$PAO_2 = (FIO_2 \times EBP) - (1.2 \times PaCO_2)$$

An increased difference between PAO_2 and PaO_2, the **$P(A-a)O_2$ gradient,** can be caused by shunt,

$\dot{V}/\dot{Q}$ mismatch, or diffusion defect. The $P(A-a)O_2$ is normally ≤ 10 mm Hg breathing room air and ≤ 50 mm Hg breathing 100% oxygen. The **PaO_2/PAO_2** can also be calculated and is normally >0.75 at any FIO_2.

   3. **PaO_2/FIO_2** is the easiest of the indices of oxygenation to calculate. The acute respiratory distress syndrome is associated with a $PaO_2/FIO_2 < 200$ and acute lung injury is associated with a $PaO_2/FIO_2 < 300$.

B. **Indices of ventilation**
   1. **Dead space** (V_D/V_T) is calculated from the **Bohr equation,** which measures the ratio of dead space to total ventilation:

$$V_D/V_T = (PaCO_2 - P\bar{E}CO_2)/PaCO_2$$

where $P\bar{E}CO_2$ is the mixed exhaled PCO_2. To determine $P\bar{E}CO_2$, exhaled gas is collected in a bag from the expiratory port of the ventilator and its CO_2 concentration is measured with a blood gas analyzer or capnometer. The normal V_D/V_T is 0.3 to 0.4.

IV. **Lung mechanics**
A. **Plateau pressure** (Pplat) is the mean peak alveolar pressure during mechanical ventilation.
   1. **Measurement.** Pplat is measured by applying an end-inspiratory breath-hold for 0.5 to 2 seconds. During the breath-hold, pressure equilibrates throughout the system so that the pressure measured at the proximal airway approximates the peak alveolar pressure (Fig. 2-4). For valid measurement of Pplat, the patient must be relaxed and breathing in synchrony with the ventilator.
   2. **An increased Pplat** indicates a greater risk of alveolar over-distension during mechanical ventilation. Many authorities recommend that Pplat be maintained ≤ 35 cm H_2O. This assumes that chest wall compliance is normal. Higher plateau pressures may be necessary if chest wall compliance is decreased (e.g., abdominal distension).
B. **Auto-PEEP**
   1. **Measurement.** Auto-PEEP is measured by applying an end-expiratory pause for 0.5 to 2 seconds. The pressure measured at the end of this maneuver that is in excess of the PEEP set on the ventilator represents the amount of auto-PEEP. For this measurement to be valid, the patient must be relaxed and breathing in synchrony with the ventilator— active breathing will invalidate the measurement. Measurement of auto-PEEP during active breathing requires the use of an esophageal balloon.
   2. **Clinical implications.** Auto-PEEP is determined by the ventilator settings (tidal volume and expiratory time) and lung function (airways resistance and lung compliance). The level of auto-PEEP can be decreased by reducing the minute ventilation with either a decrease in tidal volume or respira-

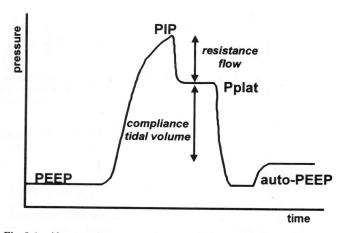

Fig. 2-4. Airway pressure waveform. Peak alveolar pressure (Pplat) is determined by applying an end-inspiratory breath-hold and auto-PEEP is determined by applying an end-expiratory breath-hold. The difference between peak inspiratory pressure (PIP) and Pplat is determined by resistance and end-inspiratory flow and the Pplat-PEEP difference is determined by compliance and tidal volume. PEEP, positive end-expiratory pressure; PIP, peak inspiratory pressure.

tory rate (permissive hypercapnia). Increasing the expiratory time will decrease the level of auto-PEEP, which can be achieved by changing the I:E ratio (i.e., shortening the inspiratory time) or decreasing the respiratory rate. The level of auto-PEEP can also be reduced by decreasing airways resistance (i.e., secretion clearance or bronchodilator administration).

C. **Esophageal pressure**
   1. **Measurement.** Esophageal pressure is measured from a balloon containing a small volume of air (<1 ml) placed into the lower esophagus. The measurement and display of esophageal pressure is facilitated by commercially available systems.
   2. **Clinical implications.** Esophageal pressure changes reflect changes in pleural pressure, but the absolute esophageal pressure does not reflect absolute pleural pressure. Changes in esophageal pressure can be used to assess (a) respiratory effort and work-of-breathing during spontaneous breathing and assisted modes of ventilation, (b) chest wall compliance during full ventilatory support, and (c) auto-PEEP during spontaneous breathing and assisted modes of ventilation. If exhalation is passive, the change in esophageal (i.e., pleural) pressure required to reverse flow at the proximal airway (i.e., trigger the ventilator) reflects the

amount of auto-PEEP. Negative esophageal pressure changes that produce no flow at the airway indicate failed trigger efforts, that is, the patient's inspiratory efforts are insufficient to overcome the level of auto-PEEP and trigger the ventilator (Fig. 2-5). Clinically, this is recognized as a patient respiratory rate (observed by inspecting chest wall movement) that is greater than the trigger rate on the ventilator.

D. Compliance (the inverse of elastance) is the change in volume (usually tidal volume) divided by the change in pressure required to produce that volume.

    1. Respiratory system, chest wall, and lung compliance.

        a. Respiratory system compliance is most commonly calculated in the ICU:

$$Crs = \Delta V / \Delta P = \text{tidal volume} / (\text{Pplat} - \text{PEEP})$$

        Respiratory system compliance is normally 100 ml/cm H_2O and reduced to 50 to 100 ml/cm H_2O in mechanically ventilated patients. Respiratory system compliance is determined by the compliance of the chest wall and the lungs.

        b. Chest wall compliance is calculated from changes in esophageal pressure (pleural pres-

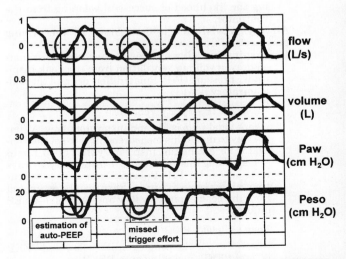

Fig. 2-5. Use of esophageal pressure to determine auto-PEEP. The change in esophageal pressure required to trigger the ventilator is the level of auto-PEEP. Also note the presence of missed trigger efforts in which the inspiratory effort of the patient is not sufficient to overcome the amount of auto-PEEP.

sure) during passive inflation. Chest wall compliance is normally 200 ml/cm H_2O, which can be decreased by abdominal distension, chest wall edema, chest wall burns, and thoracic deformities (e.g., kyphoscoliosis). Chest wall compliance is also decreased with an increase in muscle tone (e.g., a patient who is bucking the ventilator). Chest wall compliance is increased with flail chest and paralysis.

   c. **Lung compliance** is calculated from changes in transpulmonary pressure. **Transpulmonary pressure** is the difference between alveolar pressure (Pplat) and pleural pressure (esophageal). Normal lung compliance is 200 ml/cm H_2. Lung compliance is decreased with pulmonary edema (cardiogenic or noncardiogenic), pneumothorax, consolidation, atelectasis, pulmonary fibrosis, pneumonectomy, and mainstem intubation. Lung compliance is increased with emphysema.

  2. When compliance is decreased, greater transpulmonary pressure is required to deliver a given tidal volume into the lungs. Thus, a decreased compliance will result in higher Pplat and PIP. To avoid dangerous levels of airway pressure, lower tidal volumes are used to ventilate the lungs of patients with decreased compliance. Deceased lung compliance also increases the work-of-breathing, decreasing the likelihood of successful weaning from the ventilator.

E. **Airways resistance** is determined by the driving pressure and the flow:

  1. **Inspiratory airways resistance** can be estimated during volume ventilation from the peak inspiratory pressure (PIP–Pplat) difference and the end-inspiratory flow:

$$Rinsp = (PIP - Pplat)/\dot{V}end\text{-}insp$$

where $\dot{V}end$-insp is the end-inspiratory flow. A simple way to make this measurement is to set the ventilator for a constant inspiratory flow of 60 L/min (1 L/s). Using this approach, the inspiratory airways resistance is the PIP–Pplat difference. The **expiratory airways resistance** (Rexp) can be estimated from the peak expiratory flow and the Pplat–PEEP difference:

$$Rexp = (Pplat - PEEP)/\dot{V}exp$$

where $\dot{V}exp$ is the peak expiratory flow and PEEP is total PEEP (including auto-PEEP).

  2. **Common causes** of increased airways resistance are bronchospasm and secretions. Resistance is also increased with a small inner diameter endotracheal tube. For intubated and mechanically ventilated patients, airways resistance should be < 10 cm H_2O/L/s at a flow of 1 L/s. Expiratory airways resistance is typically greater than inspiratory airways resistance.

F. **Work of breathing**
1. **The Campbell diagram** (Fig. 2-6) is used to determine the work-of-breathing. The Campbell diagram includes the effects of chest wall compliance, lung compliance, and airway resistance on the work-of-breathing. Work-of-breathing is increased with decreased chest wall compliance, decreased lung compliance, or increased airways resistance.
2. **Clinical implications.** Work-of-breathing requires special equipment and an esophageal balloon to quantify, and for that reason it is not frequently measured. Moreover, it is not clear that measuring work-of-breathing improves patient outcome. It may be useful to quantify patient effort during mechanical ventilation, but this can often be achieved by simply observing the respira-

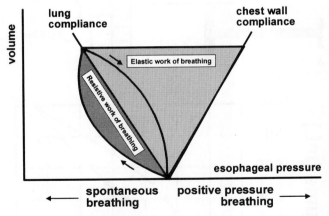

Fig. 2-6. Campbell diagram. The chest wall compliance curve is determined by plotting volume as a function of esophageal pressure during positive pressure breathing with the chest wall relaxed. The lung compliance curve is determined from the point of zero flow at end-exhalation to the point of zero flow at end-inhalation during spontaneous breathing. Because of airways resistance, the esophageal pressure is more negative than predicted from the lung compliance curve. The areas indicated on the curve represent elastic work-of-breathing and resistive work-of-breathing. Note that a decreased chest wall compliance will shift that compliance curve to the right, thus increasing the elastic work-of-breathing. A decrease in lung compliance shifts that curve to the left, also increasing the work-of-breathing. An increased airways resistance causes a more negative esophageal pressure during spontaneous breathing, increasing the resistive work-of-breathing.

tory variation on a central venous pressure tracing. Large inspiratory efforts produce great negative deflections of the central venous pressure
trace during inspiratory efforts. Increasing the
level of ventilatory assistance should reduce these
negative deflections.

G. The **static pressure–volume curve** measures the
pressure–volume relationship of the respiratory system.

1. **Measurement.** A calibrated syringe and pressure
manometer are used to determine the pressure volume curve (Fig. 2-7A). The patient is preoxygenat-
ed with 100% oxygen and the syringe is filled with
oxygen. The patient is disconnected from the ventilator and allowed to exhale to resting end-expiratory lung volume (functional residual capacity).

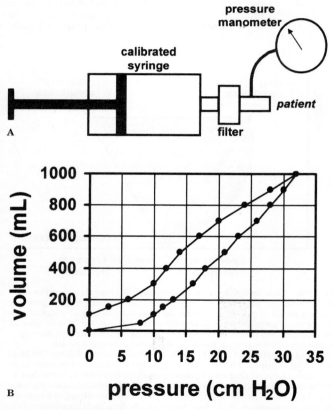

Fig. 2-7.   A. Super-syringe set-up to measure static compliance.
B. Static pressure-volume loop showing inflation and deflation
curves.

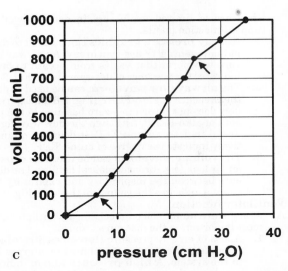

Fig. 2-7. *Continued* C. Inspiratory pressure-volume curve showing a lower inflection point at 8 cm H_2O and an upper inflection point at 25 cm H_2O.

The syringe is attached to the airway and the pressure is measured at 50- to 100-ml step changes in volume from the syringe. Both the inflation and deflation pressure– volume curve can be measured (Fig. 2-7B).

2. **Lower and upper inflection points** can be determined from the pressure–volume curve (Fig. 2-7C). It has been suggested that the level of PEEP should be set above the lower inflection point to avoid alveolar collapse and Pplat should be set below the upper inflection point to avoid alveolar over-distension. Important limitations are seen to the clinical use of pressure–volume curves: accurate measurements require heavy sedation (and often paralysis); it is unclear whether the inflation or deflation curve should be assessed; it can be difficult to determine precisely the inflection points; the respiratory system pressure–volume curve can be affected by both the lungs and the chest wall; and the pressure–volume curve models the lungs as a single compartment.

H. **Ventilator graphics,** typically scalar graphs of pressure, flow, and volume, can be displayed by many microprocessor-based ventilators. Flow–volume and pressure–volume graphics can also be displayed, but these are less useful. Dynamic pressure–volume loops typically reflect how the ventilator delivers flow, and

they are of limited usefulness to detect lower and
upper inflection points.

1. **Airway pressure graphics** can be used to detect
    patient–ventilator dys-synchrony. An airway pres-
    sure waveform that varies from breath to breath
    indicates the presence of dys-synchrony (Fig. 2-8A).
2. The **airway flow waveform** can be used to detect
    the presence of auto-PEEP (Fig. 2-8B). Expiratory
    flow does not return to a zero baseline in the pres-
    ence of auto-PEEP. Although the flow waveform is
    useful to detect auto-PEEP, it does not quantita-
    tively indicate the degree of auto-PEEP.
3. The **volume waveform** can be useful in detecting
    an air leak (e.g., bronchopleural fistula). The differ-
    ence between the inspiratory and expiratory tidal
    volume indicates the volume of the leak (Fig. 2-8C).

V. **Ventilator function**
    A. **Alarms** are numerous on mechanical ventilators. The
        most important is the disconnect alarm.
        1. A loss of airway pressure **(low-pressure alarm)**
            indicates a ventilator disconnect or a gross leak
            in the system. A **high pressure alarm** indicates
            an elevated airway pressure. The high-pressure
            alarm also serves to cycle the ventilator to the
            expiratory phase to avoid injury caused by over-
            pressurization of the lungs. Appropriate setting of
            the high-pressure alarm is particularly important
            during volume ventilation. Common causes of a
            high-pressure alarm are obstruction of the venti-
            lator circuit or the patient's airways (e.g., kinked
            ventilator circuit, kinked endotracheal tube, sec-
            retions, bronchospasm), a sudden decrease in lung
            compliance (pneumothorax, mainstem intubation,
            congestive heart failure), or patient–ventilator dys-
            synchrony ("bucking the ventilator").
        2. **Expired tidal volume** should be monitored during
            volume ventilation to detect a leak. During pressure
            ventilation, the tidal volume should be monitored to
            detect changes in respiratory system compliance,
            resistance, auto-PEEP, or patient breathing efforts.
        3. FIO_2. Although the blenders in mechanical ventila-
            tors are reliable, it is prudent to monitor FIO_2 in
            mechanically ventilated patients.
    B. **Inspired gas conditioning.** Because the upper airway
        is bypassed, the inspired gas is warmed and humidified
        during mechanical ventilation. Traditionally, this has
        been accomplished using an active heated humidifier.
        Recently, passive humidifiers (artificial noses) have
        been increasingly used during mechanical ventilation.
        1. **Airway temperature** is typically monitored dur-
            ing mechanical ventilation when active humidifiers
            are used. High temperatures should be monitored
            to avoid airway burns and low temperatures should
            be monitored to avoid delivery of inadequately
            humidified gas.

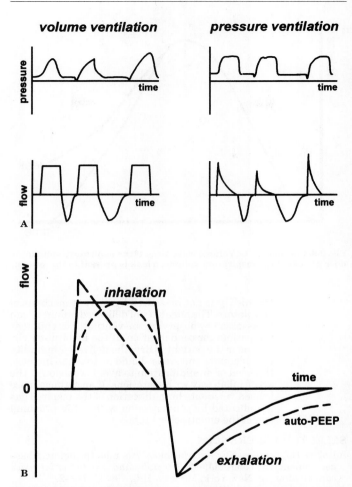

Fig. 2-8. A. Patient-ventilator dys-synchrony. During volume ventilation, the pressure waveform varies from breath-to-breath. During pressure ventilation, the flow waveform varies from breath-to-breath. B. Flow waveform. The inspiratory flow is determined by the flow setting on the ventilator. Expiratory flow should return to zero. If the expiratory flow does not return to zero, auto-PEEP is present.

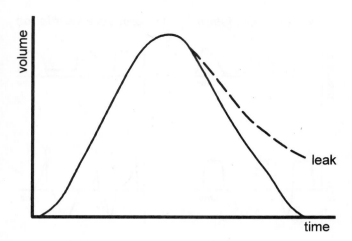

Fig. 2-8. *Continued*   **C. Volume waveform. If the expiratory volume does not equal the inspiratory volume, a leak is present in the system.**

2. **Humidity** is not measured by current mechanical ventilators. The adequacy of delivered humidity can be assessed by observing the ventilator circuit near the patient for condensation. If the inspiratory circuit near the patient is dry, the delivered humidity is inadequate and steps should be taken to increase the level of humidification to avoid occlusion of the artificial airway with secretions. If an artificial nose is used, adequate humidification of the inspired gas is indicated by condensation within the proximal end of the endotracheal tube.

SELECTED REFERENCES

Adrogue HJ, Madias NE. Arterial blood gas monitoring: acid-base assessment. In: Tobin MJ, ed. *Principles and practice of intensive care monitoring.* New York: McGraw-Hill, 1998:217–242.

Ahrens T. Utilization of intensive care unit technology. *New Horiz* 1998;6:41–51.

Banner MJ, Jaeger MJ, Kirby RR. Components of the work of breathing and implications for monitoring ventilator-dependent patients. *Crit Care Med* 1994;22:515–523.

Bhavani-Shankar K, Kumar AY, Moseley HS, et al. Terminology and the current limitations of time capnography: a brief review. *J Clin Monit* 1995;11:175–182.

Burton SL, Hubmayr RD. Determinants of patient-ventilator interactions: bedside waveform analysis. In: Tobin MJ, ed. *Principles and practice of intensive care monitoring.* New York: McGraw-Hill, 1998:655–666.

Cardoso MM, Banner MJ, Melker RJ, et al. Portable devices used to detect endotracheal intubation during emergency situations: a review. *Crit Care Med* 1998;26:957–964.

Franklin ML. Transcutaneous measurement of partial pressure of oxygen and carbon dioxide. *Respir Care Clin N Am* 1995;1:119–131.

Hanly PJ. Transcutaneous monitoring of carbon dioxide. In: Tobin MJ, ed. *Principles and practice of intensive care monitoring.* New York: McGraw-Hill, 1998:401–414.

Hanning CD, Alexander-Williams JM. Pulse oximetry: a practical review. *BMJ* 1995;311:367–370.

Hess D, Kacmarek RM, Stoller JK. Perspectives on monitoring in respiratory care. In: Kacmarek RM, Hess D, Stoller JK, eds. *Monitoring in respiratory care.* St. Louis: Mosby—Year Book, 1993:1–12.

Hess D, Kacmarek RM. Techniques and devices for monitoring oxygenation. *Respir Care* 1993;38:646–671.

Hess D. Capnography: technical aspects and clinical applications. In: Kacmarek RM, Hess D, Stoller JK, eds. *Monitoring in respiratory care.* St. Louis: Mosby—Year Book, 1993:375–406.

Hess DR, Branson RD. Noninvasive respiratory monitoring equipment. In: Branson RD, Hess DR, Chatburn RL, eds. *Respiratory care equipment.* Philadelphia: JB Lippincott Company, 1995:247–282.

Hess DR. Capnometry. In: Tobin MJ, ed. *Principles and practice of intensive care monitoring.* New York: McGraw-Hill, 1998:377–400.

Hess DR. Respiratory care monitoring. In: Burton GG, Hodgkin JE, Ward JJ, Hess DR, Pilbeam SP, Tietsort JA, eds. *Respiratory care. A guide to clinical practice,* 4th ed. Philadelphia: JB Lippincott, 1997:309–332.

Hess DR. Selection of monitoring equipment. In: Tobin MJ, ed. *Principles and practice of intensive care monitoring.* New York: McGraw-Hill, 1998:1469–1480.

Hutchison DCS, Gray BJ. Transcutaneous and transconjunctival oxygen monitoring. In: Tobin MJ, ed. *Principles and practice of intensive care monitoring.* New York: McGraw-Hill, 1998:289–302.

Jubran A, Tobin MJ. Monitoring during mechanical ventilation. *Clin Chest Med* 1996;17:453–473.

Jubran A. Pulse oximetry. In: Tobin MJ, ed. *Principles and practice of intensive care monitoring.* New York: McGraw-Hill, 1998:261–288.

Kacmarek RM, Hess DR. Airway pressure, flow and volume waveforms, and lung mechanics during mechanical ventilation. In: Kacmarek RM, Hess D, Stoller JK, eds. *Monitoring in respiratory care.* St. Louis: Mosby—Year Book, 1993:497–544.

Koff PB, Hess D. Transcutaneous oxygen and carbon dioxide measurements. In: Kacmarek RM, Hess D, Stoller JK, eds. *Monitoring in respiratory care.* St. Louis: Mosby—Year Book, 1993:349–376.

Kufel TJ, Grant BJB. Arterial blood gas monitoring: respiratory assessment. In: Tobin MJ, ed. *Principles and practice of intensive care monitoring.* New York: McGraw-Hill, 1998:197–216.

Mahutte CK. Continuous intravascular and on-demand extravascular arterial blood gas monitoring. In: Tobin MJ, ed. *Principles and practice of intensive care monitoring.* New York: McGraw-Hill, 1998:243–260.

Mathews PJ Jr. CO-oximetry. *Respir Care Clin N Am* 1995;1:47–68.

Pierson DJ. Goals and indications for monitoring. In: Tobin MJ, ed. *Principles and practice of intensive care monitoring.* New York: McGraw-Hill, 1998:33–44.

Ranieri VM, Dambrosio M, Brienza N. Intrinsic PEEP and cardiopulmonary interaction in patients with COPD and acute ventilatory failure. *Eur Respir J* 1996;9:1283–1292.

Ranieri VM, Grasso S, Fiore T, et al. Auto-positive end-expiratory pressure and dynamic hyperinflation. *Clin Chest Med* 1996;17: 379–394.

Rossi A, Polese G, Brandi G, et al. Intrinsic positive end-expiratory pressure (PEEPi). *Intensive Care Med* 1995;21:522–536.

Rossi A, Polese G, Milic-Emili J. Monitoring respiratory mechanics in ventilator-dependent patients. In: Tobin MJ, ed. *Principles and practice of intensive care monitoring.* New York: McGraw-Hill, 1998:553–596.

Schmitz BD, Shapiro BA. Capnography. *Respir Care Clin N Am* 1995; 1:107–117.

Stock MC. Capnography for adults. *Crit Care Clin* 1995;11:219–232.

Truwit JD, Rochester DF. Monitoring the respiratory system of the mechanically ventilated patient. *New Horiz* 1994;2:94–106.

Wahr JA, Tremper KK, Diab M. Pulse oximetry. *Respir Care Clin N Am* 1995; 1:77–105.

Zijlstra WG, Maas AH, Moran RF. Definition, significance and measurement of quantities pertaining to the oxygen carrying properties of human blood. *Scand J Clin Lab Invest Suppl* 1996;224: 27–45.

Zin WA, Milic-Emili J. Esophageal pressure measurement. In: Tobin MJ, ed. *Principles and practice of intensive care monitoring.* New York, McGraw-Hill, 1998:545–552.

Airway Management

Peter F. Dunn, Robert L. Goulet,
Kenneth L. Haspel, and William E. Hurford

Endotracheal intubation is required to provide a patent airway when patients are at risk for aspiration, when airway maintenance by mask is difficult, and when prolonged mechanical ventilation is required. This chapter discusses the evaluation of the airway, techniques for endotracheal intubation, and management of the chronically instrumented airway.

I. **Indications for endotracheal intubation**
   A. **Normal respiratory function** requires a patent airway, adequate respiratory drive, neuromuscular competence, intact thoracic anatomy, normal lung parenchyma, and the ability to cough, sigh, and defend against aspiration. Impairments in these parameters, singularly or in combination, can result in the need for endotracheal intubation and ventilatory support.
   B. **Endotracheal intubation**
      1. Provides relative protection against pulmonary aspiration.
      2. Maintains a patent conduit for respiratory gas exchange.
      3. Provides a means for coupling the lungs to mechanical ventilators.
      4. Establishes a route for clearance of secretions.

II. **Airway evaluation.** A systematic evaluation of the need for tracheal intubation is essential. The need for intubation can be immediate (e.g., cardiopulmonary arrest); emergent (e.g., impending respiratory failure); or urgent (e.g., decreased level of consciousness with inadequate airway control).
   A. **If cardiopulmonary resuscitation is underway,** bag-mask ventilation with 100% oxygen, followed by intubation, is required (see Chapter 15). Otherwise, perform a rapid evaluation to determine the need for intubation.
   B. **Apply oxygen by face mask.** The potential improvement in systemic oxygenation can allow more time to evaluate the patient and consider options.
   C. **Assess level of consciousness.** Obtundation, stupor, or coma can result from respiratory difficulties (e.g., hypoxemia or hypercapnia), or from metabolic, pharmacologic, and neurologic problems. Depressed consciousness can lead to airway obstruction, pulmonary aspiration, atelectasis, and pneumonia.
   D. **Integument. Cyanosis** is present when at least 5 g/dl of deoxyhemoglobin is present. Thus, in anemia, cyanosis can be absent despite a low oxygen saturation.

With polycythemia, small decreases in oxygen saturation can manifest as cyanosis. Cold, diaphoretic skin suggests intense autonomic stress or circulatory failure.

E.   **Respiration**

1.   Respiratory efforts should be noted, with particular attention paid to the rate and depth of thoracic movements. **Slow, deep respirations** (< 10/min) suggest opioid effect or central nervous system (CNS) disorder. **Tachypnea** (> 35/min) is a nonspecific finding that can be present with disorders that cause decreased respiratory system compliance [e.g., pulmonary edema, consolidation, acute respiratory distress syndrome (ARDS)] or increased respiratory load (e.g., increased dead space, fever). It is a common finding in pulmonary embolism and with respiratory muscle fatigue.

2.   **An absent gag reflex** or the inability to maintain an adequate airway in all head positions, or both, indicates the need for intubation.

3.   **Evaluation for upper airway obstruction** includes visual (laryngeal tug, chest wall retraction, chest or abdomen discoordination), tactile (air flow felt by placing a hand in front of the patient's mouth and nose, position of trachea in the neck), and auscultory (stridor, absent breath sounds), which are indicators of either complete or partial obstruction. In the absence of coexisting processes (e.g., cervical spine injury) and depending on the cause of the obstruction (e.g., depressed mental status), obstruction can be relieved by extending the head at the atlanto-occiptal joint, performing a chin lift, jaw thrust, and inserting an oral or nasal airway prior to intubation (see below).

4.   **Examine respiratory excursions** for symmetry, timing, and coordination. A pneumothorax, splinting, or large bronchial obstruction can cause side-to-side asymmetry. A long inspiratory time suggests upper airway or other extrathoracic obstruction; a prolonged expiratory time suggests intrathoracic obstruction, bronchospasm, or both. Discordant breathing efforts or the use of accessory muscles suggest respiratory muscle weakness or fatigue. Long inspiratory or expiratory pauses (e.g., Cheyne-Stokes asthma or apneustic breathing) are caused by brainstem or metabolic abnormalities and depressant drugs.

5.   **Auscultate** the chest for symmetric breath sounds, bronchospasm, rhonchi, or rales, which are suggestive of secretions or pulmonary edema.

6.   **Pulse oximetry** aids in assessing the adequacy of oxygenation.

F. **The cause of respiratory failure** usually is apparent. Readily reversible causes of respiratory failure can be addressed prior to intubation. Timely reversal can circumvent the need for intubation in cases of opioid or benzodiazepine-induced respiratory depression, residual pharmacologic neuromuscular blockade, pneumothorax, acute pulmonary edema, or mucous plugging of the airway.

G. **Arterial blood gas** (ABG) tensions and pH may be helpful in measuring disease severity, documenting changes in condition over time, or assessing the efficacy of interventions. The use of ABGs, however, should not substitute for clinical evaluation of the patient or delay needed interventions.

III. **Preparation for endotracheal intubation**

A. **A focused history and physical examination,** which can be obtained quickly while preparing the equipment needed for intubation (see below), includes:

1. **Assessment of airway anatomy.** A receding mandible (**micrognathia**); small oropharynx; protruding, prominent upper incisors; and a short, muscular "bull" neck are associated with potentially difficult laryngoscopy and intubation. Temporomandibular joint or cervical spine immobility can make visualization of the glottis difficult. If these are recognized, alternative or additional intubation techniques can be used (**see section V.A.**).

2. **Medication allergies**

3. **Assessment of aspiration risk,** including the time since last gastric intake; trauma, recent vomiting, upper gastrointestinal (GI) bleeding, hemoptysis, bowel obstruction, esophageal reflux history, morbid obesity, diabetes mellitus, and depressed mental status.

4. **Cardiovascular status:** angina-ischemia, infarction, dysrhythmias, congestive heart failure, aneurysms, and hypertension.

5. **Neurologic status:** increased intracranial pressure (ICP), ischemic symptoms, intracranial aneurysm and hemorrhage.

6. **Musculoskeletal status:** neck and mandibular immobility or instability, neuromuscular disorders (especially recent cord denervation injuries, recent crush injuries, and burns).

7. **Coagulation status:** platelet count, anticoagulation therapy, or coagulopathy (especially if a nasal intubation is anticipated).

8. **Past intubation problems,** including a history of periglottic or subglottic stenosis. This history is not entirely reliable because many other factors (e.g, airway edema, trauma, hemoptysis) may have intervened.

B. **Intubation method.** In an emergency, options are limited by the requirements for experience, expedience, and availability of specialized equipment. The most useful techniques are the following:

1. **Orotracheal intubation** is performed with direct laryngoscopy.
   a. **Advantages** include ease and minimal equipment needs. It is the most familiar technique, allowing endotracheal tube (ETT) placement under direct vision.
   b. **Disadvantages.** Adequate mandible and neck mobility are necessary to allow direct visualization. Topical, regional (block), or general anesthesia is often required.
2. **Nasotracheal intubation** can be performed as a blind procedure, guided by breath sounds, or under direct vision with laryngoscope or fiberoptic bronchoscope.
   a. **Advantages.** Blind placement can be performed in a neutral head and neck position without general anesthesia or muscle paralysis. Nasotracheal intubation can be performed when the oral route is difficult or impossible (i.e., in a patient with limited mouth opening). A nasal tube also does not interfere with surgical repair of the mandible or oropharynx.
   b. **Disadvantages.** It is more difficult to place the tube quickly. Spontaneous respiration must be present to guide the tube for blind placement. Placement by direct vision with the laryngoscope, with or without the Magill forceps, has the same disadvantages as the orotracheal intubation method. Tube diameter is limited by choanal size. Severe nasal hemorrhage, which can be life threatening, can occur. Transient bacteremia commonly occurs during the intubation. Once placed, a nasally placed tube tends to soften and kink in the nasopharynx, which can increase airway resistance, making passage of a suction catheter more difficult. Nasal intubation is relatively contraindicated if initial examination suggests nasopharyngeal injury, nasal polyps, basilar skull fracture, epistaxis, coagulopathy, planned systemic anticoagulation or thrombolysis (i.e., the patient with an acute myocardial infarction), or immunocompromise. Sinusitis and otitis occur frequently with nasal intubation.
3. **Fiberoptic laryngoscopes** consist of glass fibers that are bound together to make a flexible unit (the insertion tube) used to transmit light and images. Flexible fiberoptic laryngoscopy can be performed orally or nasally.
   a. **Advantages.** It is very useful with distorted anatomy or in patients requiring

maximal head and neck stability (i.e., unstable neck fractures).

b. **Disadvantages.** More skill is required than with other techniques. Fiberoptic intubation is not the technique of choice for emergency intubation of apneic patients. In patients with upper airway bleeding or vomiting, visualizing hypopharyngeal anatomy is difficult because of the limited capacity to clear secretions with the suction channel of the fiberscope.

4. **The laryngeal mask airway (LMA)** can be an important adjunct for establishing an emergency airway, especially in patients in whom mask ventilation is difficult or impossible and traditional endotracheal intubation has been unsuccessful.

a. **Advantages.** The LMA is a fast and reliable method of establishing an airway when other methods have failed. Endotracheal intubation subsequently can be done by placing an ETT through the lumen of the LMA, with or without the assistance of a fiberoptic bronchoscope.

b. **Disadvantages.** The LMA does not protect the airway against aspiration of gastric contents. The LMA may not be tolerated by an awake or agitated patient.

5. **Airway support devices** such as oral or nasopharyngeal airways do not prevent aspiration or guarantee continued airway patency. At best, they are temporary measures.

IV. **Techniques for airway management**

A. **Make thorough preparations for intubation** prior to the initial attempt. Time spent in establishing the best possible intubating conditions usually is well spent. Equipment required for intubation is listed in Table 3-1.

1. **Minimal equipment** includes a Yankauer tipped suction catheter, laryngoscope with an appropriate blade (usually Macintosh 3 or Miller 2 for adults and Miller 1 for small children), and an appropriately sized ETT with a stylet inserted and the cuff checked by briefly inflating it with approximately 10 ml of air.

2. **Check that suction is available and functioning** in the form of a Yankauer or "tonsil tip" suction device.

3. **An appropriate size** for the endotracheal tube depends on the patient's age, body habitus, and indication for intubation. A 7-mm endotracheal tube is a reasonable choice for most women and an 8-mm endotracheal tube for most men. Suggested pediatric tube sizes are listed in Table 3-2.

**Table 3-1.   Suggested contents
of an emergency intubation kit**

Equipment	Drugs
Intravenous catheters (14–22 g)	Atropine
Laryngoscope blades:	*cis*-atracurium
Macintosh 2,3,4	Ephedrine
Miller 0,1,2,3	Epinephrine
Endotracheal tubes	Esmolol
(3–8 mm inner diameter)	Ethyl aminobenzoate
Syringes (12 ml)	(Hurricaine) spray
Magill forceps	Etomidate
Colorimetric end-tidal CO_2	Glycopyrrolate
detectors	Labetalol
Nasal airways	Lidocaine (1% and 4%)
Oral airways	Lidocaine ointment
Tape	Midazolam
Yankauer suction catheters	Naloxone (Narcan)
Tube changers	Oxymetazoline (Afrin) spray
Guidewires	Pancuronium
Q-tip swabs	Phenylephrine
Nasogastric tubes	Phenylephrine/lidocaine spray
Jet ventilator	Propofol
	Propranolol
	Saline
	Succinylcholine
	Surgi-lube
	Viscous lidocaine

Table 3-2.   Pediatric endotracheal tube sizes[a]

Age	Size (mm)
Premature infant	2.5
Term infant	3.0
1–4 mo	3.5
4 mo to 1 y	4.0
1.5–2.0 y	4.5
2.5–3.5 y	5.0
4–6 y	5.5
7–9 y	6–7.0

[a] Tube size should be adjusted to provide airway leak pressures of less than
25 cm H_2O; all tubes uncuffed.

The absence of air leaking past the ETT during positive-pressure ventilation with the cuff down indicates too tight a fit at the laryngeal or tracheal level. For an emergent intubation, a tube 0.5 mm smaller than usual will facilitate intubation.

4. **Position the patient**
   a. In the supine position, the pharyngeal and laryngeal axes of the patients are offset, which makes it extremely difficult to have a good view of the glottis during direct laryngoscopy (Fig. 3-1). Positioning the patient in the so-called "sniffing" position, with the occiput elevated by folded blankets and the head in extension, aligns the oral, pharyngeal, and laryngeal axes so that the pathway from the lips to the glottis is nearly a straight line.
   b. Move the **bed** away from the wall and remove the headboard to allow access to the patient's head. If the headboard is fixed, or if the patient is in an unusual location or traction, move the patient diagonally in the bed to afford access to the patient and airway. Adjust the height of the bed so that the patient's head is at your midchest level.
   c. **The trauma patient** presents special challenges. All patients with multiple trauma, head, or facial injury must be presumed to have a cervical spine injury until such is excluded by a full evaluation. In such patients, excessive motion of the spine can produce or exacerbate a spinal cord injury. During airway manipulations, an assistant should stabilize the head and neck in a neutral position by maintaining in-line cervical traction. Note that the greatest cervical displacement appears to occur during bag and mask ventilation, and that orotracheal intubation causes no more cervical displacement or neurologic sequelae than nasotracheal intubation.

B. **Ventilation** should be assisted (or maintained) and 100% oxygen administered by mask and self-inflating bag (e.g., Ambu or Laerdahl) as soon as the airway is clear. In the obtunded patient, the airway can be opened with a gentle chin lift and the mask applied tightly over the patient's nose and mouth.
   1. **An oropharyngeal airway (OPA)** can facilitate the establishment of a patent airway in the obtunded patient when proper head positioning and chin lift and jaw thrust alone are ineffective. The adult OPA sizes are 80 mm, 90 mm, and 100 mm, (Guedel sizes 3, 4, and 5, respectively), which reflect the length from the flange

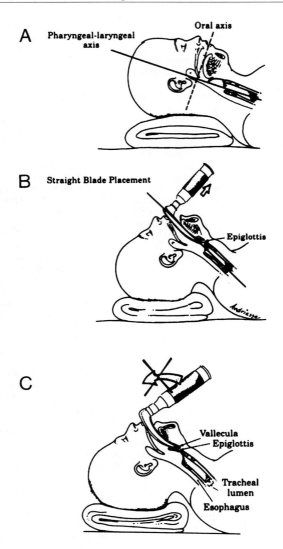

A   Pharyngeal-laryngeal
    axis

Oral axis

B   Straight Blade Placement

Epiglottis

C

Vallecula
Epiglottis

Tracheal
lumen

Esophagus

Curved Blade Placement

Fig. 3-1.   A. The "sniffing position" aligns the oral, pharyngeal, and
laryngeal axes for visualization of the glottis during laryngoscopy.
B. The handle of the laryngoscope should be lifted in the direction
of its long axis to view the glottis. C. The laryngoscope should not
be used as a lever to prevent damage to teeth or the alveolar ridge.

to the distal tip. The size can be estimated by measuring the OPA from the ear lobe to the corner of the patient's lips. The device is normally inserted backward along the hard palate and rotated into position as it approaches the posterior wall of the pharynx. Improperly placed, the OPA may obstruct the airway by pushing the tongue posteriorly or by pressing the epiglottis against the glottic opening. The OPA can induce vomiting or laryngospasm in an awake or semiconscious patient.

2. **A nasopharyngeal airway** should be considered as an adjunct to mask ventilation in patients with intact oropharyngeal reflexes or in whom mouth opening is impossible. The adult sizes range from 6.0 mm to 9.0 mm, which indicate the internal diameter of the tube. The tube should be well lubricated and gently inserted through the naris, along the floor of the nasal cavity (parallel to the hard palate), until the flange rests against the outer naris. **Coagulopathy** is a relative contraindication to its use, as is a basilar skull fracture (especially involving the ethmoid bone). Although the risk is less than with an OPA, vomiting and laryngospasm can still occur in some patients.

C. **An intravenous** (IV) line should be freely running and its adequacy demonstrated prior to laryngoscopy. In cases of cardiac arrest, in which the administration of sedatives and paralytic agents are unnecessary, intubation may precede the establishment of adequate IV; the endotracheal tube can be used as an alternative drug administration route (see Chapter 15).

D. **Monitoring during intubation** should include continuous electrocardiography (ECG), pulse oximetry, and frequent blood pressure measurements.

E. **Orotracheal intubation**
1. **The laryngoscope** is composed of a handle, which usually contains batteries for the light source, and a laryngoscope blade, which usually contains a light bulb in the distal third of the blade. The **Macintosh** and **Miller** blades are most commonly used.
   a. **The Macintosh blade** is curved, and its tip is inserted into the vallecula (the space between the base of the tongue and the pharyngeal surface of the epiglottis) (Fig. 3-2). Pressure against the hyoepiglottic ligament elevates the epiglottis to expose the larynx. The Macintosh blade provides a good view of the oro- and hypopharynx, thus allowing more room for ETT passage with diminished epiglottic trauma. Size ranges vary from 1 to 4, with most adults requiring a Macintosh No. 3 blade.

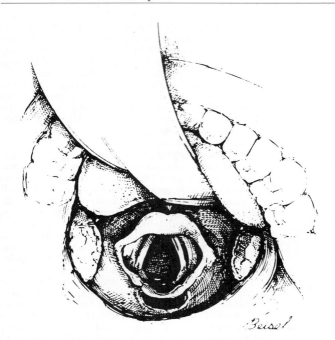

Fig. 3-2. View of the glottis by direct laryngoscopy with a Macintosh blade. Notice that the tip of the blade has been placed in the vallecula (the tip of the Miller blade is placed under the epiglottis, lifting it to view the glottis).

       b. **The Miller blade** is straight, and it is passed so that the tip lies beneath the laryngeal surface of the epiglottis. The epiglottis is then lifted to expose the vocal cords. The Miller blade allows better exposure of the glottic opening but provides a smaller passageway through the oro- and hypopharynx. Size ranges vary from 0 to 3, with most adults requiring a Miller No. 2 or No. 3 blade.

  2. **A malleable stylet** inserted through the ETT (without extending past the tip) can be used to provide a 40- to 80-degree anterior bend 2 to 3 inches from the tip of the ETT ("hockey stick" configuration), which allows passage of the tube along the posterior aspect of the epiglottis and facilitates intubation under difficult circumstances.

  3. **Laryngoscopy.** Hold the laryngoscope in your left hand close to the junction of the blade and the handle. Open the patient's mouth with your right hand by applying a scissoring motion with your thumb and index finger on the patient's upper and lower premolars or gums. Insert the laryngoscope into the right side of the patient's mouth, taking care to avoid the teeth and pinching the lips between the blade and teeth. If using a Macintosh blade, insert it without resistance along the curve of the anterior pharynx. Once the blade is inserted, sweep the blade to the midline, using the large flange of the blade to push the tongue out of the way. The epiglottis and vallecula will be visualized. Advance the blade into the vallecula and lift the handle in a direction parallel to its long axis to expose the vocal cords and laryngeal structures. If using a Miller blade, the tip of the blade is placed past the vallecula and is used to compress and elevate the epiglottis on lifting the handle. The laryngoscope blade should never be used as a lever, with the upper teeth or maxilla as the fulcrum, because damage to the maxillary incisors or gingiva can result.

4. **If the cords cannot be visualized**
   a. Secondary to vomitus or foreign material, suctioning or manual extraction is required.
   b. Because of the anterior position of the larynx, apply pressure to the thyroid or cricoid cartilages or change to a straight blade.
   c. Increase head flexion.
   d. Remove the laryngoscope and ventilate the patient with bag and mask. **Do not permit hypoxemia during a prolonged laryngoscopy in a patient who is easily ventilated by mask.**

5. **To insert the endotracheal tube,** hold it in your right hand as you would hold a pencil and advance it through the oral cavity from the right corner of the mouth, and then through the vocal cords. Place the proximal end of the endotracheal tube cuff just below the vocal cords, remove the stylet (if used), and note the markings on the tube in relation to the patient's incisors or lips. In the average adult, the proper depth of insertion, measured at the upper incisors, is approximately 21 cm for women and 23 cm for men. Inflate the cuff just to the point of obtaining a seal in the presence of 20 to 30 cm H_2O positive airway pressure.

6. **Esophageal intubation remains one of the most common mistakes in airway management associated with a fatal outcome.** No single technique for verifying endotracheal placement is foolproof.
   a. **Verification of proper endotracheal tube position** usually includes the persistent detection of carbon dioxide (CO_2) in

end-tidal samples of exhaled gas and auscultation over the stomach and both lung fields.

   b. **The measurement of the CO_2 concentration** in exhaled gas has become a standard for verifying tracheal placement of an endotracheal tube. In the absence of a capnometer, disposable colorimetric CO_2 detectors can be used to confirm the presence of CO_2. This technique is not foolproof; CO_2 will not be present if pulmonary circulation is absent (i.e., in a dead patient or in the absence of adequate chest compressions during cardiopulmonary circulation).

   c. **Small concentrations of CO_2** can be detected after an esophageal intubation, especially if bag and mask ventilation has insufflated previously exhaled air into the stomach. With an esophageal intubation, the amount of CO_2 detected in exhaled gas should decrease with repetitive breaths. With an endotracheal intubation, the end-tidal CO_2 concentration should be stable during repetitive exhalations. If it is not, additional confirmation is necessary.

7. **Physical signs and symptoms** of an endotracheal intubation include observation of the tube passing through the vocal cords and of chest and abdominal movement with ventilation; auscultation of breath sounds over both the right and left chest as well as the abdomen; palpation of the abdomen and of the trachea as the tube is passed. The exhaled tidal volume also can be measured; it is reduced with an esophageal intubation. Water vapor may be observed to fill the endotracheal tube on expiration and disappear on inspiration after proper placement. Other techniques for confirming endotracheal tube placement include fiberoptic endoscopy; the use of a self-inflating bulb (the esophageal detector) or an airflow whistle on the proximal end of the endotracheal tube; and chest radiography. Although any or all of these tests can be performed, any single test lacks adequate predictive value to reliably exclude an esophageal intubation.

8. **In the absence of direct visualization** of the endotracheal tube passing between the vocal cords, maintain a very high index of suspicion of incorrect tube placement for the first several minutes following intubation. Only after adequate oxygenation and ventilation appear certain (i.e., after several minutes), it is safe to leave the patient under the care of others.

9. **If the tube position is uncertain** despite these manuevers or the patient's condition is deteriorating without a readily explained cause (e.g., pneumothorax), **remove the tube** and reinsti-

tute bag and mask ventilation prior to another intubation attempt. If the patient regurgitates through an ETT placed in the esophagus, some advocate leaving the esophageal tube in place to act as a conduit for vomitus. This is acceptable only if the tube does not interfere with repeat visualization of the cords.

10. **If the tube has been advanced too far,** the right mainstem bronchus may be selectively intubated, resulting in absence of breath sounds over the left lung field and the right apex. Listening for breath sounds high in each axilla can decrease the chances of being misled by transmitted breath sounds from the opposite lung. Pull the tube back, with the cuff deflated, while ventilating and auscultating the left lung field until left-sided breath sounds are heard.

11. **When the ETT is in good position,** securely fasten it with tape, preferably to taut skin overlying bony structures. Note the depth of the tube at the incisors or gums in the patient's chart along with a description of the procedure.

12. **Obtain a chest radiograph** following intubation to confirm tube position and bilateral lung expansion. The distal end of the tube should rest within the midtrachea, which is approximately 5 cm above the carina in the adult.

F. **Nasotracheal intubation**
   1. **Nasal mucosal vasoconstriction and anesthesia** are achieved with a solution of 0.25% phenylephrine, 3% lidocaine, or 2% lidocaine with 1:200,000 epinephrine using cotton-tipped swabs. Even during general anesthesia, vasoconstriction with a topical solution such as oxymetazoline oxymetolazone (Afrin, Schering-Plough Healthcare Products, Inc., Memphis, TN) is advisable.

   2. **Common endotracheal tube sizes** are 6.0 to 6.5 mm for women and 7.0 to 7.5 mm for men. Insertion to a depth of 26 cm, measured at the naris (in women) and 28 cm (in men) usually results in proper positioning.

   3. **General preparations** are as described for orotracheal intubation.

   4. **Nasal passage** of the tube. Generously lubricate the nares and tube. Initially probe the nasopharynx with a well-lubricated nasal airway to establish which naris has greater patency. If both nares are patent, the right naris is preferred because the bevel of most ETTs, when introduced through the right naris, faces the flat nasal septum, reducing damage to the turbinates. Advance the tube in a direction that is perpendicular to the face and parallel to the hard palate. Inexperienced operators often tend to direct the tube cephalad, which tends to damage the

turbinates. As the tube is passed into the naso-pharynx, it may impact against the posterior nasopharyngeal wall. Retract the tube slightly, extend the patient's neck, and re-advance the tube. Forcible advancement of the tube at this point risks tearing the mucosa and creating a false passage. After passage through the naris into the pharynx, advance the tube through the glottic opening.

5. **Tracheal insertion** can be accomplished by several methods.

   a. **A Magill forceps** can be used to guide the tube into the trachea while direct laryngoscopy is performed. The laryngoscopic technique is the same as that used for oral intubation. The forceps direct the tip of the endotracheal tube anteriorly and through the glottis. Grasp the tube with the forceps proximal to the endotracheal tube cuff. This reduces the chance of damaging the endotracheal tube cuff during insertion and permits the distal end of the tube to be inserted through the glottic opening. An assistant should advance the tube under the direction of the laryngoscopist.

   b. **Blind techniques** require a spontaneously breathing patient. Listen for breath sounds at the proximal end of the tube while advancing the ETT during inspiration. A cough followed by a deep inhalation, condensate forming in the tube during exhalation, and loss of voice suggest tracheal entry. Sudden loss of breath sounds suggests passage into the esophagus, vallecula, or piriform recess.

     (1) **Extending the neck or providing cricoid pressure** can help direct the tube away from the esophagus.

     (2) **Anterior flexion** directs the tube away from the vallecula.

     (3) **Tilting (not rotating) the head** toward the side of the tube insertion and rotating the tube toward the midline directs the tube away from the piriform recess.

     (4) **Inflating the cuff** of the ETT helps lift it off the posterior wall of the pharynx and directs the tube through the cords in a patient with an anterior larynx. In this instance, the cuff is deflated as the tube passes between the cords.

   c. **The Endotrol** tracheal tube (Mallinckrodt, Inc., Glens Falls, NY) has a cord running up the concave side from the proximal end to the tip of the tube. Pulling on a ring attached to the proximal end of the cord flexes the tube anteriorly, which may direct the tip toward the glottis. It is sometimes useful for blind nasal intubation, especially when the neck cannot be manipulated.

   d. **A fiberoptic bronchoscope** can be used to direct the ETT into the trachea (see below).

G. Fiberoptic intubation can be used for both nasal and oral endotracheal intubation. It should be considered as a first option rather than as a last resort when a difficult airway is anticipated. Fiberoptic intubation should be considered for patients with known or suspected cervical spine pathology, head and neck tumors, morbid obesity, or a history of difficult ventilation or intubation. Before attempting emergency fiberoptic intubation, acquire facility with its use on mannequins and elective intubations.

   1. **Standard equipment** for oral or nasal fiberoptic intubation includes a sterile fiberoptic scope with light source, an oral bite block or Ovassapian airway, topical anesthetics and vasoconstrictors, and suction.

   2. **Technique.** To perform a fiberoptic intubation, place an endotracheal tube over a lubricated fiberoptic scope, attach suction tubing to the suction port; grasp the control lever with one hand and use the other hand to advance and maneuver the insertion tube. An oral Ovassapian airway is helpful and well tolerated for oral laryngoscopy. Administration of an anticholinergic solution can help dry secretions that may obscure the view. After the administration of topical or general anesthesia, flex the tip of the insertion tube scope anteriorly and position it within the hypopharynx. Advance the scope toward the epiglottis. To avoid entering the piriform fossa, keep the insertion tube of the fiberoptic scope in the midline as it is advanced. If the view becomes impaired, retract the scope until the view clears, or remove it and clean the lens, and then reinsert it in the midline. As the tip of the scope slides beneath the epiglottis, the vocal cords will be seen. Advance the scope with the tip in a neutral position until tracheal rings are noted. Then, stabilize the scope and advance the endotracheal tube over the insertion tube and into the trachea. Sometimes the tip of the endotracheal tube becomes caught against the arytenoids during advancement. If resistance occurs, turning the endotracheal tube 90 degrees counterclockwise will allow passage through the vocal cords.

   3. **Nasal intubation** can be performed similarly. Anesthetize and vasoconstrict the nasal mucosa, as discussed. With the ETT loaded on the scope, pass the scope under direct vision through the nasopharynx and into the trachea. Tongue retraction is usually not needed, but occasionally may be helpful. Maintain the scope's position in the trachea while an assistant passes the ETT over the scope and through the nose.

4. **An alternate technique** involves passage of the nasotracheal tube into the oropharynx as in blind nasal intubation. Lubricate the scope, pass it through the ETT, and guide the tube's passage through the cords and position within the trachea under direct vision.

H. **The laryngeal mask airway** has assumed an important role in airway management in the operating room and as an emergency airway adjunct in other locations.

1. LMAs come in both pediatric and adult sizes (Table 3-3). The most common adult sizes are 3 and 4.

2. With minimal experience, the LMA can be easily placed (Fig. 3-3) and an airway established in most patients. The most common causes of failure include the folding of the LMA cuff back on itself in the oropharynx and the folding of the epiglottis down over the larynx by the tip of the LMA. These can be overcome by keeping the cuff pressed against the hard palate during insertion and using the correct size LMA. The LMA should not be placed in patients with intact upper airway reflexes.

3. The LMA does not protect against the possibility of gastric aspiration and is not suitable for long-term mechanical ventilation. An ETT can be placed through the lumen of the LMA, either blindly or with the aid of a fiberscope. The **Fast-trach LMA** (The Laryngeal Mask Company, LTD., San Diego, CA) is specially designed to permit subsequent endotracheal intubation through the LMA. The LMA also can be used as a temporary airway until a tracheostomy can be performed.

Table 3-3.   Laryngeal mask airway sizes

Patient age, size	LMA size	Cuff volume	ETT size (ID)
Neonates/infants, to 5 kg	1.0	Up to 4 ml	3.5 mm
Infants, 5–10 kg	1.5	Up to 7 ml	4.0 mm
Infants/children, 10–20 kg	2.0	Up to 10 ml	4.5 mm
Children, 20–30 kg	2.5	Up to 14 ml	5.0 mm
Children, 30 kg to small adults	3.0	Up to 20 ml	6.0 cuffed
Average adults	4.0	Up to 30 ml	6.0 cuffed
Large adults	5.0	Up to 40 ml	7.0 cuffed

LMA, laryngeal mask airway; ETT, endotracheal tube; ID, inner diameter.

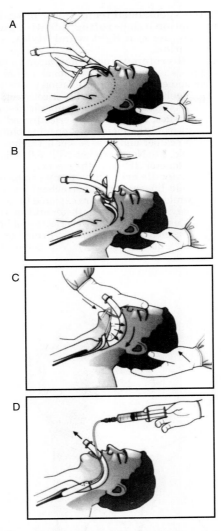

Fig. 3-3.   A. With the head extended and the neck flexed, carefully flatten the laryngeal mask airway (LMA) tip against the hard palate. B. With the index finger, push the LMA in a cranial direction following the contours of hard and soft palate. C. Maintaining pressure with the finger on the tube in the cranial direction, advance the mask until definite resistance is felt at the base of the hypopharynx. D. Inflation without holding the tube allows the mask to seat itself optimally. (From A.I.J. Brain, LMA instruction manual. 1996; with permission).

I. **Other specialized techniques for endotracheal intubation** include **retrograde wire-guided intubation,** use of a **light wand stylet,** and **tactile intubation.**

J. **Cricothyrotomy** is performed as an emergency procedure when ventilation via mask or LMA is impossible and endotracheal intubation is unsuccessful.

　1. **Technique.** Localize the cricothyroid notch (Fig. 3-4). Incise the skin and superficial subcutaneous tissues, and pierce the cricothyroid membrane. Expand the membrane opening bluntly or with a scalpel and pass a small tracheostomy tube (No. 4 to No. 6) or a cut ETT [6.0 or 6.5 mm inner diameter (ID)] into the trachea.

　2. **A needle cricothyrotomy** can be used to provide life-saving transtracheal jet oxygenation while other means are explored to secure the airway. A 14-gauge IV catheter attached to a syringe is used to puncture the cricothyroid membrane. Tracheal placement is confirmed by aspirating air from the catheter. The needle is removed

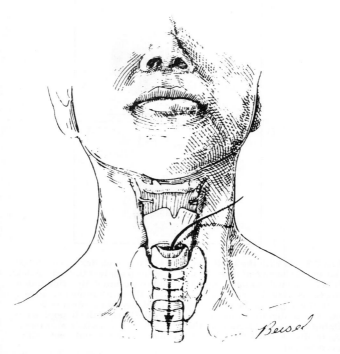

Fig. 3-4. The cricothyroid membrane is the entry point of an artificial airway during cricothyrotomy.

and air again aspirated from the catheter. With the catheter firmly maintained in position, then attach it by tubing to a jet ventilator or, if unavailable, to a wall oxygen flowmeter opened to its maximal setting. By cyclically interrupting the flow of oxygen, gas flow is delivered at a 1:2 ratio of inspiration to expiration (1 second on; 2 seconds off). The chest should be seen to rise and fall with each jet.

3. **Complications.** The flow from the wall at 50 psi can exceed 500 ml/s. Inadequate time for expiration can result in high airway pressures and barotrauma, leading to poor venous return and pneumothorax. Other complications of this technique are subcutaneous and mediastinal emphysema, tracheal mucosal trauma, bleeding, and misplacement of the catheter.

K. **Emergency tracheostomy** entails significant time and risk of bleeding that usually precludes its use as an emergency airway technique.

V. **Pharmacologic aids to intubation** include neuromuscular blocking drugs (NMBDs), sedatives, narcotics, and general and local anesthetics (see Chapters 5, 6, and 7).

A. **Neuromuscular blocking drugs** induce compete respiratory arrest and abolish protective airway reflexes. Because laryngoscopy and intubation can be extremely painful and distressing, **patients who are chemically paralyzed must be obtunded or pharmacologically sedated. When pharmacologic paralysis is required to secure the airway, patient survival depends on rapid and skillful laryngoscopy and intubation.** NMBDs are slow in onset; for that reason, they are dangerous for the patient who cannot tolerate even a few seconds of depressed ventilation.

1. **Succinylcholine** (1.0–1.5 mg/kg IV), with its rapid onset and brief duration of action, is the NMBD of choice for emergent endotracheal intubation in many patients. See Chapter 7 for important contraindications.

2. **Nondepolarizing muscle relaxants** typically have relatively slow onsets and long durations of action. Some newer NMBDs have relatively rapid onsets (e.g., rocuronium) and brief durations of action (e.g., mivacurium). These agents can also be useful for intubation in selected patients. See Chapter 7 for additional details concerning the use of these agents.

3. **When rapid airway control is needed and succinylcholine is contraindicated,** large doses of **vecuronium** (0.25 mg/kg IV), or *cis*-**atracurium** (> 0.2 mg/kg IV) can be used to decrease the onset of neuromuscular blockade to 1 to 1.5 minutes. Both drugs have relatively prolonged durations of action. High-dose **ro-**

curonium (1.2 mg/kg IV) provides intubating conditions after 60 to 90 seconds (comparable to succinylcholine) without significant cardiac effects, but it also has a prolonged duration of action.

4. **All patients requiring emergent airway management are probably at risk for aspiration of gastric contents.** Thus, when paralysis is chosen, the intubation should follow a "**rapid sequence.**" Administer the neuromuscular blocking agent immediately after rendering the patient rapidly unconscious with a drug such as propofol, etomidate, or ketamine. Apply cricoid pressure (**the Sellick maneuver**) with the onset of unconsciousness. To minimize gastric insufflation and the risk of regurgitation, under ideal circumstances, avoid positive-pressure ventilation until the airway is secured by an endotracheal tube. If the intubation is not immediately successful, positive-pressure ventilation can be administered via bag and mask while maintaining cricoid pressure or via a laryngeal mask airway.

B. **Sedative-hypnotics, analgesics, and amnestics** are used during airway manipulation primarily to blunt autonomic responses and to obtund consciousness, pain, and recall (see Chapter 5).

C. **Benzodiazepines,** especially midazolam or diazepam, are frequently used for IV sedation and amnesia during endotracheal intubation. Onset is rapid (60–90 seconds) and duration is brief (20–60 minutes) following single-dose administration (**see Chapter 5**). Cardiovascular side effects are minimal. For sedation, incremental doses of midazolam (0.5 to 1.0 mg IV) or diazepam (2 mg IV) can be repeated until the desired effect is achieved. The dose for induction of anesthesia is 0.1 to 0.2 mg/kg IV for midazolam or 0.3 to 0.5 mg/kg for diazepam.

D. **Opioids.** Fentanyl and morphine are commonly used for analgesia, sedation, and cough suppression during endotracheal intubation. Intravenous fentanyl has a rapid onset (1 minute) and in usual doses (50–500 μg) has a brief duration of action. Intravenous morphine (2–10 mg) has a longer peak onset time (5–10 minutes) and a longer duration of action (1–3 hours) (see Chapter 5 for additional details). Newer opioids—**alfentanil, sufentanil,** and **remifentanil**—offer more rapid onset times (30–60 seconds) and shorter durations with conventional doses than fentanyl, but they are rarely indicated for endotracheal intubation.

E. **Beta-adrenergic blocking drugs** such as **esmolol** (10–20 mg IV in the adult) can blunt the cardiovascular response to laryngoscopy and intubation. Doses should be titrated to effect.

F. **Lidocaine** (1.0–1.5 mg/kg IV) can augment anesthesia and blunt the hemodynamic response to intubation. Lidocaine must be administered several minutes prior to laryngoscopy to be maximally effective.

G. **Oropharyngeal topical anesthesia** can be provided with viscous lidocaine, aerosol anesthetic sprays, or inhalation of aerosolized lidocaine. Topical anesthesia with unmetered aerosol sprays poses a risk of overdose and toxicity.

H. **Glossopharyngeal nerve blocks, superior laryngeal nerve blocks, and translaryngeal ("transtracheal") blocks** are occasionally useful in selected patients. In general, these blocks diminish the ability to guard against aspiration. Nerve blocks are relatively contraindicated in patients with coagulopathy.

VI. **Special intubation situations**

A. **A difficult intubation** is defined as the inability to place an ETT after three attempts by an experienced laryngoscopist. Unfortunately, no single clinical examination can predict accurately those patients in whom laryngoscopies will be difficult.

1. **The American Society of Anesthesiologists (ASA) Difficult Airway Algorithm** (Fig. 3-5) outlines protocols to be used when a difficult airway is encountered. Although the algorithm was designed initially to aid the decision-making process when a difficult airway is encountered in the operating room, it is also useful for emergent airway situations in other locations such as the intensive care unit (ICU).

   a. For a patient with a recognized difficult airway and spontaneous respirations, the choices for establishing a secure airway include awake direct laryngoscopy, fiberoptic laryngoscopy, blind nasal intubation, or an elective surgical airway.

   b. When intubation attempts have failed and spontaneous or assisted ventilation is absent, quick action is required to establish oxygenation and ventilation by other means. The ASA Difficult Airway Algorithm mentions three temporary means for delivering oxygen and eliminating carbon dioxide: the laryngeal mask airway, the Combitube, and transtracheal jet ventilation via cricothyrotomy.

2. **Back-up personnel** should be called if a difficult intubation is anticipated (e.g., patients with severe facial injuries, airway burns, or unstable cervical spin injuries).

3. **Use of the LMA should be considered** when mask ventilation is inadequate and endotracheal intubation has failed.

4. **A surgical airway** should be considered if intubation has failed and the airway cannot be maintained with bag and mask or LMA. A surgical cricothyrotomy should be performed by person-

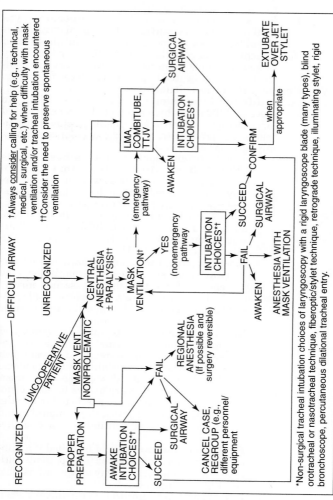

nel with previous training in the technique. In the absence of a physician specifically trained in cricothyrotomy, a **needle or catheter percutaneous cricothyrotomy** should be considered when bag and mask or LMA ventilation and attempts at intubation have been unsuccessful. When performed under emergency conditions, serious complications, including bleeding and subcutaneous emphysema, are common with this technique and can make a subsequent surgical cricothyrotomy impossible.

B. **A full stomach, vomiting, and airway bleeding** increase the hazards of pulmonary aspiration during intubation. If intubation is anticipated, oral and gastric feedings should be discontinued for 8 hours prior to intubation; however, this is seldom practical. If present, the nasogastric tube should be placed on suction. The elective placement of a nasogastric tube to drain the stomach prior to intubation can be effective for liquid gastric contents, but its presence is not a guarantee of an empty stomach.

   1. **With obtundation or neuromuscular incompetence,** the presence of oral foreign matter requires immediate oral intubation with laryngoscopic visualization. Suction with a Yankauer tip should be available. During intubation, estimate severity of aspiration and determine the pH of the suctioned material.

   2. **In the conscious patient,** awake intubation is generally preferred unless contraindicated by cardiovascular or neurologic problems. Topical local anesthesia makes the procedure more comfortable, although its use decreases protective airway reflexes, increasing the risk of aspiration.

   3. **A "rapid sequence" intubation** (see above) is performed if general anesthesia is required. The technique is similar to a rapid-sequence induction.

   4. **Increased intracranial pressure (ICP)** (see Chapter 11). Pain or tracheal stimulation can increase ICP, even in comatose individuals. Intubation should be accomplished with minimal stimulation in any patient at risk for increased ICP. Adjuncts to consider to facilitate intubation include local anesthetic blocks, general anesthesia, including barbiturates, etomidate, or opioids; intravenous lidocaine; and the use of neuromuscular blockade.

C. **Myocardial ischemia or recent infarction** demands that heart rate and blood pressure be maintained within a narrow range. Hypertension (or hypotension) and tachycardia can exacerbate myocardial ischemia. Pharmacologic adjuncts to consider during endotracheal intubation include deep opioid anesthesia, local anesthetic blockade of airway reflexes, and the use of adequate β-adrenergic blockade. A pharmacologic method of treating hypotension (e.g., phenylephrine) and hypertension (e.g., nitroglycerin) should be immediately available.

D. **Neck injury** with potentially unstable cervical vertebrae presents the risk of precipitating or aggravating spinal cord damage during intubation. The head, neck, and thorax should be maintained in a neutral "in-line" position. Oral intubation is preferred during emergent situations. During intubation, a second individual should provide light in-line traction to maintain the head and neck in a neutral position. Flexion and anterior head motion pose the greatest risks for cord injury. Extension is less of a hazard; however, it should be minimized. If the intubation is difficult or the pharyngeal and vocal cord anatomy is not easily visualized, it is prudent to use an awake fiberoptic intubation (oral or nasal), intubate through an LMA (with or without fiberoptic assistance), or to proceed to a cricothyrotomy in more emergent situations.

E. **Oropharyngeal and facial trauma.** The nasal route is relatively contraindicated if a possibility of cranial vault disruption exists, because of the potential for tubes and catheters to penetrate the brain. Once the airway is secured, a fiberoptic nasal intubation can be performed electively, if needed, to facilitate operative repair. In the case of a massively disrupted face, a cricothyrotomy or tracheostomy may be preferable.

F. **Emergency neonatal and pediatric intubations** (see Chapter 39). Children generally are less cooperative than adults, making certain techniques (e.g., awake fiberoptic intubation) difficult. Hypoxemia occurs more rapidly during apnea in children than in adults. In addition, the tracheal cartilage in prepubertal individuals is not fully developed, predisposing them to tracheal malacia and stenosis. Cuffed ETTs are usually avoided because the cuff material requires a smaller tube size in already narrow airways, and because of the risk of tracheal damage from mucosal ischemia from compression by the inflated cuff. Tubes placed in pediatric patients should have a leak of air regurgitating back around the tube into the pharynx with positive-pressure ventilation. A leak at less than 25 cm H_2O of positive airway pressure is optimal. A greater leak makes ventilation more difficult; a lesser leak is likely to cause tracheal edema on extubation and to increase the risk of tracheal damage.

G. **Immunocompromised patients** require intubation with a technique that minimizes tracheal contamination. Aspiration is disastrous in this population, and nasal intubation should be avoided because of the risks of sinusitis and bacteremia. Perform intubation under direct vision, with care taken to keep the ETT as sterile as possible prior to passage through the cords.

VII. Endotracheal and tracheostomy tubes

   A. Tube materials

     1. Polyvinyl chloride (PVC) tubes are disposable, flexible, and transparent; they are the current standard.

     2. Silicone tubes are softer than PVC, but they are more likely to kink.

     3. Armored or anode tubes have metal coil-reinforced bodies with a rubber, silicone, or PVC coating. They are less likely to kink than PVC, but they are more flexible, usually requiring a stylet for placement.

   B. Cuff designs

     1. High-pressure, low-compliance cuffs have a small surface area of contact with the trachea and can produce tracheal damage more easily than low-pressure cuffs. High-pressure cuffs can be found on certain specialty tubes. Some low-pressure cuffs (e.g., those found on double-lumen endobronchial tubes) can generate high pressures if overinflated.

     2. Low-pressure, high-compliance cuffs are found on standard disposable ETTs. They present a high surface area for tracheal contact at relatively low cuff pressures, preserving tracheal mucosal blood flow.

     3. Foam filled cuffs, as seen on some **Bivona** tubes (Bivona, Inc., Gary, IN), are sometimes used in patients with tracheal dilatation or in patients who require high cuff pressures to attain a seal (Fig. 3-6). The cuff is deflated for insertion, then left open to atmosphere and allowed to inflate passively within the trachea. A minimal cuff volume is required to ensure acceptable lateral wall pressures. Air and moisture are periodically aspirated from the cuff. If the cuff requires additional air to create a seal, the tube takes on the characteristics of the standard high-compliance tube.

     4. Lanz cuffs have a balloon within a shield pilot valve system to buffer the cuff pressure. The pilot system has a thick plastic guard surrounding a highly compliant inner balloon that distends at pressures above 28 cm H_2O, relieving high tracheal cuff pressure. The tracheal cuff is similar to the standard low-pressure, high-compliance cuffs found on other disposable tubes. Creating a seal at high airway pressures can be difficult with these cuffs.

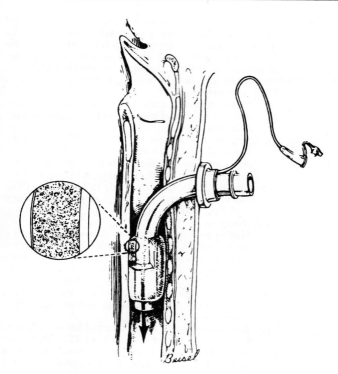

Fig. 3-6.   Bivona FomeCuff (Bivona, Inc., Gary, IN).

C. **Tracheostomy tube designs.** Many tracheostomy
    tubes are available (see Fig. 3-7). Representative tubes
    include:
    1. **Portex disposable inner cannula (DIC).** The
        body of the DIC tube has a uniform radius of
        curvature, designed to accept a thin-walled, non-
        pliable inner cannula. With the inner cannula in-
        serted, the inner diameter of the tube is reduced
        by 1 ml. This tube is available in fenestrated and
        nonfenestrated, cuffed and uncuffed, versions.
    2. **Portex Blue Line.** The body of this tube ex-
        tends straight toward the anterior tracheal sur-
        face prior to initiating its curvature.
    3. **Portex Extra Long.** This tube is designed for
        the patient with a large neck. The distance be-
        tween tracheostomy tube flange and initiation
        of curvature is longer than the standard tra-
        cheostomy tube.
    4. **Shiley single cannula tube (SCT).** This tube
        is longer in vertical dimension (see Table 3-4)

Portex D.I.C.

Portex Blue Line

Portex Extra Long

4 cuffless Shiley

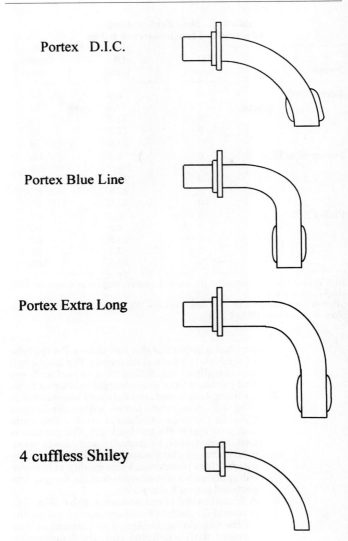

Fig. 3-7. Tracheostomy tube designs.

**Table 3-4.   Size designations
of standard tracheostomy tubes**

Name	ID (mm)	OD (mm)	Length (mm)
Portex DIC[a]	6	8.5	64
	7	9.9	70
	8	11.3	73
	9	12.6	79
	10	14.0	79
Portex Blue Line	6	8.3	55
	7	9.7	75
	8	11.0	82
	9	12.4	87
	10	13.8	98
Shiley SCT	6	8.3	67
	7	9.6	80
	8	10.9	89
	9	12.1	99
	10	13.3	105

DIC, disposable inner cannula; ID, inner diameter; OD, outer diameter; SCT, single cannula tube.
[a] Portex fenestrated tubes are made from the DIC body. An inner cannula in place decreases the ID by 1 mm.

and has a larger volume cuff than a Portex tube of equivalent internal diameter. The larger cuff usually allows the Shiley tube to seal at lower cuff pressure than a similarly sized Portex tube.

5. **Talking tracheostomy tube** or Communitrach (Fig. 3-8). A separate lumen within the body of the tube provides a dedicated air flow that exits just proximal to the tracheal cuff. The gas flow is patient-controlled by fingertip and passes retrograde through the glottis and pharynx, allowing intermittent phonation. Voice quality varies considerably and secretions can occlude the gas flow port and prevent phonation.

6. **A fenestrated tracheostomy tube** (Fig. 3-9) is useful for patients who can spend some time off the ventilator. Designed to function in conjunction with a deflated cuff, the fenestration allows additional gas flow through the lumen of the tube to the pharynx. In conjunction with a one-way speaking valve (e.g., the Passy-Muir valve), excellent phonation is possible. A removable inner cannula blocks this fenestration, and it is used when the patient is receiving mechanical ventilation. An uncuffed fenestrated tube can be used for selected patients who do not require the tracheostomy to facilitate mechanical ventilation or protect the airway. Occlusion

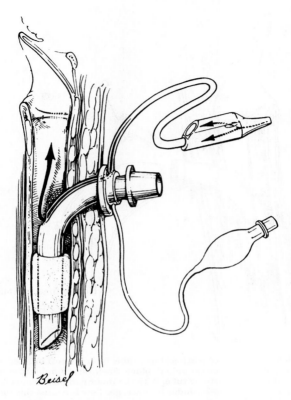

Fig. 3-8.   Talking tracheostomy tube.

of the fenestration with secretions or by tissue of the tracheal wall because of tube malposition is a common problem.

7. **Sizes** of tracheostomy tubes vary, depending on the manufacturer and style of tube (Table 3-4).

VIII. **Maintenance of endotracheal and tracheostomy tubes**

A. **General care**

1. **Suctioning.** The pharynx and trachea of intubated patients may require suctioning to clear secretions.

2. **Cuff pressures** should be kept less than 30 cm H_2O and monitored routinely. Increased occlusion pressures may suggest the need for a larger tube or a similarly sized tube with a larger cuff.

3. **Securing the tube.** Tape or a tube holder should be reapplied as needed. For an oral tube,

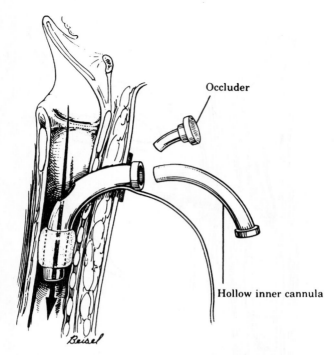

Fig. 3-9. Fenestrated tracheostomy tube. With the cuff inflated and the long, hollow inner cannula in place, function is similar to standard cuffed tracheostomy tube. With the inner cannula removed, the cuff deflated, and the occluder in place, gas flow is routed through the glottis and pharynx.

avoid excessive pressure on the lips. Patients with **nasotracheal tubes** should be periodically assessed for sinusitis, otitis media, and necrosis of the nares.

B. **Common endotracheal and tracheostomy tube problems**

1. **Cuff leaks** are usually evident as audible pharyngeal gas flow diverted anteriorly around the cuff during positive-pressure ventilation. A large leak may prompt urgent reintubation with a new tube. Usually, however, addition of a small volume of air to the cuff recreates a seal. Causes of persistent cuff leaks include:

a. **Supraglottic cuff position.** A cuff that holds air but does not seal the airway may be within or above the vocal cords. Cuff position can be evaluated by chest radiograph or

laryngoscopic examination. Deflate the cuff;
advance the tube and reconfirm intratracheal placement.

   b. Damaged cuff system. A cuff unable to
hold any air is likely to require immediate
replacement. Slow cuff leaks allow time for
further evaluation. Small leaks can occur
from the pilot valve or balloon, the cuff, or
cuff–tube interface.

   c. Tracheal dilation as a cause of persistent
cuff leaks often can be diagnosed with the
aid of a chest radiograph. The tissue–air
interface at an inflated cuff is visible radiographically as a widened trachea. A larger
tube, or one with a larger cuff volume, may
be required. Alternatively, a foam cuff tube
(e.g., Kamman-Wilkinson or Bivona) can be
tried.

  2. Airway obstruction is an emergency fore-
warned by the high pressure limit alarm during
volume ventilation, or by low volume alarms
during pressure ventilation. Quickly evaluate
the airway. A kinked tube may allow manual
ventilation, but not allow a suction catheter to
pass. Manipulation of the head and neck can
temporarily increase flow through a kinked tube.
Inability to manually ventilate requires immediate tube replacement.

C. Endotracheal tube changes are indicated for
mechanical tube failure, changing tube size, or position (e.g., nasal to oral). Common techniques for tube
changes include:

  1. Direct laryngoscopy

  2. Bronchoscopic change. With a new ETT
loaded onto the fiberscope, the fiberscope is
advanced to the cords. After the pharynx and
supraglottic areas are suctioned, an assistant
deflates the cuff on the indwelling ETT and the
fiberscope is advanced through the cords and
into the trachea. While the endoscopist maintains intratracheal visualization of the fiberscope position, the assistant slowly withdraws
the old ETT and the new ETT is advanced over
the fiberscope into the trachea. This technique
is particularly useful in patients in whom direct
laryngoscopy is contraindicated or technically
difficult.

  **3. Specially designed long malleable stylets
(tube changers)** can be used to perform tube
changes blindly or under direct vision. Pass
the stylet through the existing ETT and remove the tube, being careful not to dislodge
the stylet. Then slip a new ETT into the trachea over the stylet. Many tube changers have

a lumen for oxygen administration or, if necessary, jet ventilation.

   4. **When changing nasal tubes,** change to an oral tube as an intermediate step rather than attempt placement of bilateral nasal tubes.

IX. **Tracheostomy** is usually performed as an open surgical procedure. Percutaneously placed tracheostomy, however, is increasingly common at many institutions.

   A. **Advantages** of tracheostomy over translaryngeal intubation include:
      1. Improved patient comfort.
      2. Decreased risk of laryngeal dysfunction and damage.
      3. Improved oral hygiene.
      4. Improved ability to communicate, including the ability to phonate when the cuff can be deflated.

   B. **Disadvantages** of tracheostomy include:
      1. Possibility of tracheal stenosis at the stoma site.
      2. Stomal infection, which can secondarily infect nearby open skin areas and vascular catheters.
      3. Erosion of neighboring vascular tissue can lead to hemorrhage.
      4. Operative complications.
      5. Scarring and granulation tissue at the stoma site.

   C. **Deciding the appropriate time** for conversion from ETT to tracheostomy is a controversial issue. It is generally accepted—but not proved—that incidence and severity of glottic damage are related to duration of intubation. In clinical practice, elective tracheostomy is considered after 3 weeks of translaryngeal intubation.

   D. **Replacement of tracheostomy tubes**
      1. **Changing an "immature" tracheostomy tube.** The tract for the tracheostomy tube can be extremely difficult to cannulate in the initial postoperative period. If a tracheostomy change is required before the stoma is 7 to 10 days old, the tube should be changed over a malleable stylet and provisions made available for immediate orotracheal intubation in case the tract is lost. It is preferable for the surgeon who performed the tracheostomy to be present because exploration of the tract may be necessary.
      2. **Tracheostomy tube changes.** Proper cleanliness, function and mobility of the appliance should be assessed regularly and the appliance changed as needed.
         a. Be prepared to perform an orotracheal intubation, if necessary.
         b. Administer 100% oxygen.
         c. Clean the tracheostomy site and suction the patient.
         d. Check the new tube and test for cuff integrity. Insert the obturator through the lumen of the new tube to provide a smooth surface at the tip of the tracheostomy tube.

    e. Deflate the cuff and remove the existing tube. Expect some resistance to decannulation as the deflated cuff is pulled past the anterior tracheal wall.

    f. Visualize the stoma tract and insert the new tube. Inflate the cuff and be prepared to ventilate manually with 100% oxygen.

    g. Evaluate for proper intratracheal placement, as for any endotracheal tube (see section IV. E.).

E. **Airway bleeding.** Suctioning of blood from the airway requires prompt evaluation.

    1. Commonly, this bleeding represents **mucosal erosion** from the repeated trauma of suctioning. Fiberoptic bronchoscopy is the most direct means of assessment. If the source is not obvious, pull the tube back with the bronchoscope in place to view the trachea underlying the cuff. If, after examination, the cause of the persistent bleeding is in doubt, obtain a repeat examination by an otorhinolaryngoloist. If bleeding is not significant, a period of healing without irritation is warranted. Alternatively, a tracheostomy tube or ETT can be placed distal to the area of erosion until healing occurs.

    2. With tracheostomy, the risk of erosion into the mediastinal blood vessels exists. If this occurs, the patient can **exsanguinate.** If bleeding continues and is of sufficient quantity, a risk is seen of clotting within the ETT and airway obstruction. Emergent orotracheal intubation and surgical exploration may be necessary.

F. **Decannulation** is considered once indications for airway support are no longer present. The patient should be adequately oxygenated and ventilated, and be able to clear secretions and protect the lungs from aspiration.

    1. **Vocal cord dysfunction** and aspiration can occur from prolonged intubation. Such dysfunction can spontaneously resolve within several weeks following extubation.

        a. **Continued presence of a tracheostomy tube** can increase the chance of aspiration by mechanical interference with coordinated swallowing. Decreasing this potential problem may involve inserting a smaller uncuffed tracheostomy tube (such as a No. 4 Shiley) to decrease the mechanical stresses caused by movement of the tracheostomy tube during swallowing. The smaller tube will maintain stomal patency and allow suctioning of the airway.

        b. **A nasogastric tube** can contribute to decreased coordination during swallowing.

   c. **Protecting such patients from aspiration** can involve:
    (1) Tracheostomy. A cuffed tracheostomy tube can be used to prevent gross aspiration until cord function improves.
    (2) Extubation, prohibiting oral intake, with enteral or parenteral feeding, until the patient is no longer at risk. An enteral feeding tube should be located in the duodenum to decrease the chance of reflux and aspiration.
   d. **Consultation with a speech and swallowing therapist** is appropriate. Coordination of swallowing can be assessed by fiberoptic visualization or radiographically by a modified barium swallow. Patient education and training can reduce the risks of aspiration and improve swallowing.
  2. The following airway appliances may be considered as the patient progresses toward decannulation:
   a. **Fenestrated tracheostomy tubes** allow breathing either through the tracheostomy or through the natural airway. The patient can speak normally when the inner cannula is removed, the cuff is down, and the opening of the tube either occluded or fitted with a one-way speaking valve. A fenestrated tube provides no protection against aspiration when configured in this manner.
   b. **A small cuffless tracheostomy tube,** such as the 4 CFS Shiley (Fig. 3-7), is often the last airway appliance used prior to decannulation. Most often, it serves as a safety device and as a conduit for suction. Resistance to airflow around such tubes, even when the tube is capped, is seldom clinically significant.

SELECTED REFERENCES

Benumof JL, Dagg R, Benumof R. Critical hemoglobin desaturation will occur before return to an unparalyzed state following 1 mg/kg intravenous succinylcholine. *Anesthesiology* 1997;87:979–982.

Benumof JL. The LMA and the ASA difficult airway algorithm. *Anesthesiology* 1996;84:686–689.

Benumof JL, Scheller MS. The importance of transtracheal jet ventilation in the management of the difficult airway. *Anesthesiology* 1989;71:769–778.

Bishop MJ, Weymuller Jr. EA, Fink BR. Laryngeal effects of prolonged intubation. *Anesth Analg* 1984;63:335–342.

Brain AIJ, Denman WT, Goudsouzian NG. *Laryngeal mask airway instruction manual.* Berkshire, UK: Brain Medical Ltd., 1996:21–25.

Cousins MJ, Bridenbaugh PO. *Neural blockade in clinical anesthesia and management of pain,* 2nd ed. Philadelphia: Lippincott, 1988: 533–576.

Deutschman CS, Wilton P, Sinow J, et al. Paranasal sinusitis associated with nasotracheal intubation: a frequently unrecognized and treatable source of sepsis. *Crit Care Med* 1986;14:111–114.

Dorsch JA, Dorsch SE. Endotracheal tubes. *Understanding anesthesia equipment,* 3rd ed. Baltimore:Williams & Wilkins, 1994:439–541.

El-Gaqnzouri AR, McCarthy RJ, Tuman KJ, et al. Preoperative airway assessment: predictive value of a multivariate risk index. *Anesth Analg* 1996;82:1197–1204.

Eubanks DH, Bone RC. Airway management. *Comprehensive respiratory care: a learning system,* 2nd ed. St. Louis:CV Mosby, 1990.

Fluck Jr. RR, Hess DR, Branson RD. Airway and suction equipment. In: Branson RD, Hess DR, Chatburn RL, eds. *Respiratory care equipment.* Philadelphia: Lippincott, 1995:116–144.

Hauswald M, Sklar DP, Tandberg D, et al. Cervical spine movement during airway management: cinefluoroscopic appraisal in human cadavers. *Am J Emerg Med* 1991;9:535–538.

Hurford WE. Nasotracheal intubation. *Respir Care* 1999;44:643–649.

Hurford WE. Orotracheal intubation outside the operating room: anatomic considerations and techniques. *Respir Care* 1999;44: 615–629.

McKourt KC, Salomela L, Miraklew RK, et al. Comparison of rocuronium and suxamethonium for use during rapid induction of anaesthesia. *Anaesthesia* 1998;53:867–871.

Mehta S, Mickiewicz M. Pressure in large volume, low pressure cuffs: its significance, measurement, and regulation. *Intensive Care Med* 1985;11:267–272.

Ovassapian A, Randel GI. The role of the fiberscope in the critically ill patient. *Crit Care Clin* 1995;11:29–51.

Roberts JT. *Clinical management of the airway.* Philadelphia: WB Saunders, 1994.

Weis FR, Hatton MN. Intubation by use of the light wand: experience in 253 patients. *J Oral Maxillofac Surg* 1989;47:577–580.

Whited RE. A prospective study of laryngotracheal sequelae in long term intubation. *Laryngoscope* 1984;94:367–377.

Wilson, DJ. Airway appliances and management. In: Kacmarek RM, Stoller JK, eds. *Current respiratory care.* Philadelphia: BC Decker, 1988:80–89.

Wilson RS. Tracheostomy and tracheal reconstruction. In: Kaplan JA, ed. *Thoracic anesthesia.* New York: Churchill Livingstone, 1991: 441–461.

Mechanical Ventilation

Ricardo Martinez-Ruiz, Luca M. Bigatello, and Dean Hess

I. **Mechanical ventilation** provides artificial support of gas exchange.
   A. **Indications**
      1. **Hypoventilation**
         a. **Arterial pH** rather than $Paco_2$ should be evaluated to treat hypoventilation. Chronic compensated hypercapnia usually is a stable condition that does not require mechanical ventilatory support.
         b. **Hypoventilation resulting in an arterial pH of less than 7.30** often is considered an indication for mechanical ventilation, but other considerations such as patient's fatigue and associated morbidity may prompt initiation of mechanical ventilation at a higher or lower pH.
      2. **Hypoxemia**
         a. **Supplemental oxygen** should be administered to all hypoxemic patients.
         b. Patients with **hypoxemic respiratory failure** caused by atelectasis, pulmonary edema, or both can benefit from **continuous positive airway pressure (CPAP)** administered by face mask.
         c. **Endotracheal intubation and mechanical ventilation** should be considered for severe hypoxemia ($Spo_2 < 90\%$) unresponsive to more conservative measures.
      3. **Respiratory fatigue**
         a. **Excessive work of breathing** (e.g., tachypnea, dyspnea, use of accessory muscles, nasal flaring, diaphoresis, tachycardia) may be an indication for mechanical ventilation before abnormalities of gas exchange occur.
      4. **Airway protection**
         a. Mechanical ventilation can be initiated in patients who require endotracheal intubation for airway protection, even in the absence of respiratory abnormalities (e.g., decreased mental status or increased aspiration risk).
         b. **The presence of an artificial airway** is not an absolute indication for mechanical ventilation. For example, many long-term tracheostomy patients do not necessarily require mechanical ventilation.

B. **Goals of mechanical ventilation**
   1. Provide adequate alveolar ventilation (P_ACO_2).
   2. Provide adequate oxygenation.
   3. Promote patient-ventilator synchrony.
   4. Apply positive end-expiratory pressure (PEEP) to maintain alveolar recruitment.
   5. Use the lowest possible FIO_2.
   6. Avoid alveolar overdistension.
   7. Avoid auto-PEEP.

II. **The ventilator system** (Fig. 4-1).
   A. **The ventilator** is powered by gas pressure and electricity. Gas pressure provides the energy required to inflate the lungs. Gas flow is controlled by electronics (microprocessor).
   B. **An inspiratory valve** controls flow and pressure during the inspiratory phase. The expiratory valve is closed during the inspiratory phase.
   C. **The expiratory valve** controls PEEP. The inspiratory valve is closed during the expiratory phase.
   D. **The ventilator circuit** delivers flow between the ventilator and the patient.
      1. Because of gas compression and the elasticity of the circuit, the patient does not receive part of the gas volume delivered from the ventilator. This **compression volume** is typically about 3 to 4 ml/cm H_2O. Some ventilators compensate for this, whereas others do not.
      2. The volume of the circuit through which the patient rebreathes is **mechanical dead space.** Mechanical dead space should be less than 50 ml.
   E. **Gas conditioning**
      1. **Bacterial filters** are placed in the inspiratory and expiratory limbs of the circuit.
      2. **The inspired gas** is actively or passively humidified.
         a. **Active humidifiers** pass the inspired gas over a heated water chamber for humidifica-

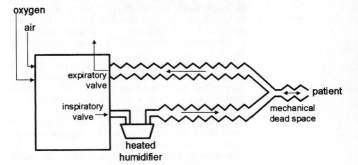

Fig. 4-1. **Simplified block diagram of mechanical ventilator system.**

tion. Some active humidifiers are used with a **heated circuit** to decrease condensate within the circuit.

   b. Passive humidifiers (artificial noses) are inserted between the ventilator circuit and the patient. They trap heat and humidity in the expired gas, which is returned on the subsequent inspiration. Passive humidification is satisfactory for many patients, but it is less effective than active humidification; it increases the resistance to inspiration and expiration, and increases mechanical dead space.

   c. Water droplets present in the inspiratory circuit near the patient (or in the proximal endotracheal tube when a passive humidifier is used) suggest that the inspired gas is adequately humidified.

III. Classification of mechanical ventilation

   A. Negative-versus positive-pressure ventilation

      1. The **iron lung** and **chest cuirass** create negative pressure around the thorax during the inspiratory phase. Although useful for some patients with neuromuscular disease requiring long-term ventilation, these devices are almost never used in the intensive care unit (ICU).

      2. Positive-pressure ventilation applies positive pressure to the airway during the inspiratory phase. Positive-pressure mechanical ventilation is used almost exclusively in the ICU.

      3. Exhalation occurs passively with both positive-pressure ventilation and negative-pressure ventilation.

   B. Invasive versus noninvasive ventilation

      1. Invasive ventilation is delivered through an endotracheal tube or a tracheostomy tube.

      2. Although mechanical ventilation through an artificial airway remains the standard in the most acutely ill patients, **noninvasive positive-pressure ventilation (NPPV)** can be used successfully in some patients with rapidly reversible conditions, such as an exacerbation of chronic obstructive pulmonary disease (COPD) or acute congestive heart failure. Many patients, however, are seen for whom NPPV is not appropriate (Table 4-1).

         a. Noninvasive ventilation can be applied with a nasal or an oronasal mask. Oronasal masks are often preferred in acutely ill dyspneic patients, in whom mouth leak is often problematic.

         b. Although portable pressure ventilators are available for NPPV, any ventilator can be used to provide this therapy.

         c. Pressure support ventilation is most commonly used for NPPV.

Table 4-1. Patient selection for noninvasive positive pressure ventilation

Indications
Respiratory distress with dyspnea, use of accessory muscles, abdominal paradox
pH <7.35 with Pa_{CO_2} >45 mm Hg
Respiratory rate >25/min

Relative contraindications
Respiratory arrest
Unstable cardiovascular status
Uncooperative patient
Facial, esophageal, or gastric surgery
Craniofacial trauma or burns
High aspiration risk
Unable to protect airway
Anatomic lesion of upper airway
Extreme anxiety
Massive obesity
Copious secretions

C. **Full versus partial ventilation**
   1. **Full ventilatory support** provides the entire minute ventilation with no interaction between the patient and the ventilator. This usually requires sedation (see Chapter 5) and sometimes neuromuscular blockade (see Chapter 7). Full ventilatory support is indicated for patients with severe respiratory failure, patients who are hemodynamically unstable, patients with complex acute injuries while they are being stabilized, and all patients receiving paralysis.
   2. **Partial ventilatory support** provides a variable portion of the minute ventilation, with the remainder provided by the patient's inspiratory effort. The patient–ventilator interaction is important during partial ventilatory support.
      a. Partial ventilatory support is indicated for patients with moderately acute respiratory failure or patients who are recovering from respiratory failure (e.g., during ventilator weaning).
      b. **Advantages** of partial ventilatory support include avoidance of muscle atrophy during long periods of mechanical ventilation, preservation of the ventilatory drive and breathing pattern, decreased requirement for sedation and neuromuscular blockade, and a better hemodynamic response to positive-pressure ventilation.

IV. Phase variables
  A. The **trigger variable** starts inspiration.
    1. The trigger variable is time when the ventilator initiates the breath.
    2. When the patient initiates the breath, the ventilator detects either a pressure change (**pressure-trigger**) or a flow change (flow-trigger or **flow-by**).
    3. The **trigger sensitivity** is set to prevent excessive patient effort but avoid auto-triggering. Pressure sensitivity is commonly set at 0.5 to 2 cm H_2O and flow triggering is set at 2 to 3 L/min.
    4. Both pressure-triggering and flow-triggering are often equally effective when sensitivity is optimized and closely monitored.
  B. The **control variable** remains constant throughout inspiration, regardless of impedance. Most common are volume control and pressure control (Table 4-2).
    1. **Volume-controlled ventilation.** The term "volume-control" is commonly used, although the ventilator actually controls flow (the time derivative of volume).
      a. With volume-controlled ventilation, **tidal volume delivery is constant** regardless of changes in airways resistance or respiratory system compliance.
      b. A decrease in respiratory system compliance or an increase in airways resistance results in an increased peak airway pressure during volume-controlled ventilation.
      c. With volume-controlled ventilation, the **inspiratory flow is fixed** regardless of patient effort. This can induce patient–ventilator dyssynchrony.
      d. Inspiratory flow patterns during volume-controlled ventilation include constant flow (square wave) (Fig. 4-2), decelerating flow (Fig. 4-3), and flow approximating a sine wave.

Table 4-2.   Volume-controlled versus pressure-controlled ventilation

	Pressure-controlled ventilation	Volume-controlled ventilation
Tidal volume	Variable	Set
Peak inspiratory pressure	Set	Variable
Plateau pressure	Set	Variable
Inspiratory flow	Decelerating and variable	Set
Inspiratory time	Set	Set
Respiratory rate	Minimum set (patient can assist)	Minimum set (patient can assist)

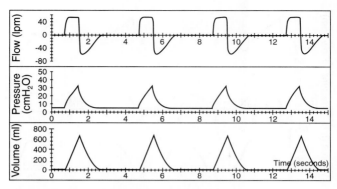

Fig. 4-2. Constant flow volume ventilation.

    e. **The inspiratory time** during volume-controlled ventilation is determined by the inspiratory flow, inspiratory flow pattern, and tidal volume.

    f. Volume-controlled ventilation is preferred when a constant minute ventilation is desirable (e.g., patients with intracranial hypertension).

  2. Pressure-controlled ventilation

    a. With pressure-controlled ventilation (Fig. 4-4), **the pressure applied to the airway is constant** regardless of the airways resistance or respiratory system compliance.

    b. **The inspiratory flow** during pressure-controlled ventilation is decelerating and determined by the pressure setting, airways

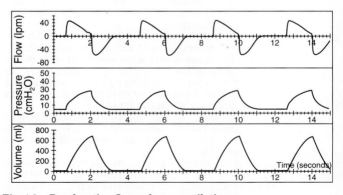

Fig. 4-3. Decelerating flow volume ventilation.

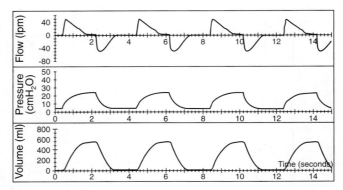

Fig. 4-4.   Pressure-controlled ventilation.

resistance, and respiratory system compliance. With low respiratory system compliance [e.g., acute respiratory distress syndrome (ARDS)], flow decelerates rapidly. With high airways resistance (e.g., COPD), flow decelerates slowly.

c. **Factors that affect tidal volume** during pressure-controlled ventilation are respiratory system compliance, airways resistance, and pressure setting. Increasing the inspiratory time will affect tidal volume during pressure-controlled ventilation only if the end-inspiratory flow is not zero.

d. Unlike volume-controlled ventilation, **inspiratory flow is variable** during pressure-controlled ventilation. Increased patient effort will increase the flow from the ventilator and the delivered tidal volume.

e. The variable flow with pressure-controlled ventilation can improve patient–ventilator synchrony.

f. With pressure-controlled ventilation, **the inspiratory time is set** on the ventilator.

g. **Pressure-controlled ventilation is desirable** to avoid alveolar overdistension in patients with acute lung injury because the peak alveolar pressure cannot be greater than the pressure set on the ventilator.

3. The choice of volume-controlled versus pressure-controlled ventilation usually is the result of clinician familiarity, institutional preferences, or personal bias.

C. **Limit** is the variable that cannot be exceeded during inspiration. This is often the same as the control variable, but it is not always the variable that terminates inspiration.

 D. **Cycle** is the variable that terminates inspiration, which is commonly volume, time, or flow.
V. **Modes of ventilation.** The combination of the various possible breath types and phase variables determines the mode of ventilation.
 A. **Controlled mechanical ventilation**
   1. All breaths are delivered by the ventilator and patient triggering is not possible.
   2. Setting the ventilator sensitivity so triggering is not possible generally is not done.
   3. Controlled mechanical ventilation usually requires sedation and sometimes neuromuscular blockade.
 B. **Assist-control ventilation (A/C)** (Fig. 4-5).
   1. **The patient can trigger** ventilation at a rate greater than that set on the ventilator, but always receives at least the set rate.
   2. All breaths, whether ventilator-triggered or patient-triggered, are delivered at the set volume (and flow) or the set pressure control (and inspiratory time). That means A/C allows the patient to vary the respiratory rate, but not the breath delivery after the ventilator is triggered.
   3. Triggering at a rapid rate can result in hyperventilation, hypotension, and dynamic hyperinflation.
 C. **Synchronized intermittent mandatory ventilation (SIMV)** (Fig. 4-6).
   1. With SIMV, the patient receives the mandatory set tidal volume (and flow) or the set pressure control (and inspiratory time) at the rate set on the ventilator.
   2. The mandatory breaths are synchronized with patient effort.
   3. Between the mandatory breaths, the patient can breath spontaneously.

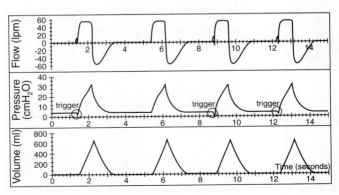

Fig. 4-5. Assist-control ventilation.

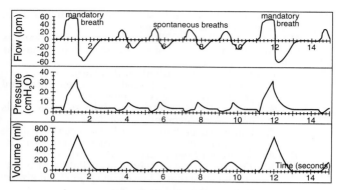

Fig. 4-6. Synchronized intermittent mandatory ventilation.

4. The spontaneous breaths can be pressure-supported breaths (Fig. 4-7).
5. The patient's inspiratory efforts can be as great during the mandatory breaths as the spontaneous breaths. Thus, it is a myth that SIMV rests the patient during the mandatory breaths and works the patient during the spontaneous breaths.
6. The different breath types during SIMV can induce patient–ventilator dyssynchrony.
7. Note that the A/C and SIMV become synonymous if the patient is not triggering the ventilator (e.g., with neuromuscular blockade).
D. **Pressure-support ventilation (PSV)** (Fig. 4-8)
1. **The patient's inspiratory effort** is assisted by the ventilator at a preset pressure with PSV.

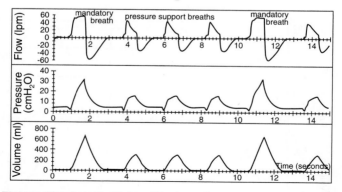

Fig. 4-7. Synchronized intermittent mandatory ventilation with pressure support.

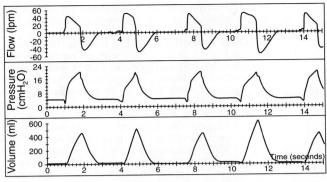

Fig. 4-8.   Pressure-support ventilation.

2.   The ventilator delivers breaths only in response to patient effort. Thus, appropriate apnea alarms must be set on the ventilator.

3.   The ventilator cycles to the expiratory phase when the flow decelerates to a ventilator-determined value (e.g., 5 L/min or 25% of the peak inspiratory flow).

4.   The tidal volume, inspiratory time, and respiratory rate can vary with PSV.

5.   **Tidal volume** is determined by the level of pressure support, lung mechanics, and inspiratory effort of the patient.

6.   Because PSV is flow cycled, the ventilator may not cycle correctly in the presence of a leak (e,g., bronchopleural fistula). A secondary time cycle will terminate inspiration at 3 to 5 seconds (depending on the ventilator).

7.   **If the patient actively exhales,** the ventilator will pressure cycle to the expiratory phase.

E.   **Continuous positive airway pressure (CPAP)**

1.   With CPAP, the ventilator provides no inspiratory assistance.

2.   Strictly speaking, CPAP applies a positive pressure to the airway. Current ventilators, however, allow the patient to breath spontaneously without applying positive pressure to the airway (CPAP = zero).

3.   The demand valves of modern ventilators offer little resistance to breathing; they should not increase the patient work of breathing and result in fatigue. This is particularly true with flow-triggering (flow-by).

F.   **Dual control modes.** Although the ventilator is capable of controlling only pressure or volume at any given time, recently developed modes allow the ventilator to switch between pressure control and volume control, either within a delivered breath or from breath to breath.

1. **Dual control within the breath.** These modes are known as **volume-assured pressure support (VAPS)** and **pressure augmentation.**

   a. Both of these techniques can operate during mandatory breaths or pressure-supported breaths.

   b. Once the breath is triggered, the ventilator targets the pressure support setting. This portion of the breath is pressure controlled and is associated with a rapid variable flow, which may reduce the work of breathing.

   c. As the pressure support level is reached, the ventilator's microprocessor determines the volume that has been delivered from the machine, compares this measurement to the desired tidal volume, and determines if the minimal desired tidal volume will be reached.

   d. If the delivered tidal volume and set tidal volume are equivalent, the breath is a pressure-support breath.

   e. If the patient's inspiratory effort is diminished, as the flow decelerates and reaches the set peak flow setting, the breath changes from a pressure-limited to a volume-limited breath. Flow remains constant, increasing the inspiratory time until the volume has been delivered. During this time, the pressure will rise above the pressure support setting. A similar condition can occur with an acute decrease in lung compliance or an increase in airways resistance.

2. **Dual control breath-to-breath**

   a. **Volume support (VS).** This mode alters the level of pressure support on a breath-to-breath basis to maintain a clinician-selected tidal volume. The maximal pressure change from breath to breath is less than 3 cm H_2O and can range from 0 cm H_2O above PEEP to 5 cm H_2O below the high pressure alarm setting.

   b. **Pressure-regulated volume control (PRVC).** This mode is a form of pressure-limited, time-cycled ventilation that uses tidal volume as a feedback control for continuously adjusting the pressure limit. The pressure limit will increase or decrease at less than 3 cm H_2O per breath in an attempt to deliver the desired tidal volume. The pressure limit will fluctuate between 0 cm H_2O above the PEEP level to 5 cm H_2O below the high-pressure alarm setting.

G. The choice of ventilation mode depends on the capability of the ventilator, the experience and preference of the clinician, and, most importantly, the needs of the patient. Rather than relying on a single "best" mode of ventilation, determine the mode that is most appropriate for each situation.

VI. Specific ventilator settings

A. **A tidal volume** target of 6 to 10 ml/kg ideal body weight is used.

1. Tidal volume targets have decreased in recent years because of concerns related to **ventilator-induced lung injury (VILI).**

2. Use a tidal volume of 6 ml/kg for patients with **ARDS.**

3. Use a tidal volume of 6 to 8 ml/kg with **obstructive lung disease.**

4. Use a tidal volume of 8 to 10 ml/kg with **neuromuscular disease** or **postoperative ventilatory support.**

5. **Monitor the plateau pressure** and consider tidal volume reduction (permissive hypercapnia) if the plateau pressure is more than 35 cm H_2O.

6. Because lung injury is a function of transalveolar pressure, a higher plateau pressure may be safe if chest wall compliance is decreased.

B. **Respiratory rate**

1. The respiratory rate and tidal volume determine **minute ventilation.**

2. Set the rate at 12 to 15/min to achieve a minute ventilation of 7 to 10 L/min.

   a. With low tidal volumes and a low pH, a higher respiratory rate may be necessary.

   b. A lower respiratory rate may be necessary to avoid auto-PEEP.

3. Adjust the rate to achieve the desired pH and $Paco_2$.

4. Avoid high respiratory rates that produce auto-PEEP.

5. **A high minute ventilation** (>10 L/min) results from increased carbon dioxide production or a high dead space.

C. **Inspiratory:expiratory (I:E) ratio**

1. **Inspiratory time** is determined by flow, tidal volume, and flow pattern during volume ventilation. Inspiratory time is set directly with pressure-control ventilation.

2. **Expiratory time** is determined by the inspiratory time and respiratory rate.

3. The expiratory time generally should be longer than the inspiratory time (e.g., I:E of 1:2).

4. **The expiratory time should be lengthened** (e.g., higher inspiratory flow, lower tidal volume, lower respiratory rate) if the blood pressure drops in response to positive-pressure ventilation or if auto-PEEP is present.

5. **Longer inspiratory times** increase mean airway pressure and can improve PaO_2 in some patients.
    a. Little role for an inverse I:E (I:E >1:1) is seen.
    b. When long inspiratory times are used, hemodynamics and auto-PEEP must be closely monitored.

D. Oxygen concentration (FIO_2)
1. Initiate mechanical ventilation with an FIO_2 of 1.0.
2. Titrate the FIO_2 using pulse oximetry.
3. Inability to reduce the FIO_2 to less than 0.60 indicates the presence of shunt (intrapulmonary or intracardiac).

E. Positive end-expiratory pressure
1. **The use of PEEP can increase oxygenation** in lung diseases characterized by alveolar collapse. Positive end-expiratory pressure maintains alveolar recruitment, increases the functional respiratory capacity, decreases intrapulmonary shunt, and can improve lung compliance. Because lung volumes are typically decreased with acute respiratory failure, it is reasonable to use a PEEP of at least 3 to 5 cm H_2O with the initiation of mechanical ventilation for most patients.
2. **Maintaining alveolar recruitment** in disease processes (e.g., ARDS) can decrease the likelihood of ventilator-associated lung injury.
3. A number of methods have been used to titrate the best level of PEEP.
    a. PEEP can be titrated to a desired level of oxygenation, such as the level of PEEP that allows the FIO_2 to be decreased to 0.6 without hemodynamic compromise.
    b. PEEP can be set 2 to 3 cm H_2O above the lower inflexion point of the pressure-volume curve.
    c. In patients with COPD, PEEP can be used to improve the patient's ability to trigger the ventilator.
    d. In patients with left ventricular failure, PEEP can improve cardiac performance by decreasing venous return and left ventricular afterload.
4. **Deleterious effects of PEEP**
    a. PEEP can **decrease cardiac output.** Hemodynamics should be monitored during PEEP titration.
    b. High levels of PEEP can result in **alveolar overdistension** during the inspiratory phase. It may be necessary to decrease the tidal volume with high PEEP.
    c. PEEP can **worsen oxygenation with unilateral lung disease** because it results in a redistribution of pulmonary blood flow to the unventilated lung units.

VII. Complications of mechanical ventilation
A. Ventilator-induced lung injury
1. **Overdistension injury** occurs if the lung parenchyma is subject to an abnormally high transpulmonary pressure.
   a. Overdistension injury produces inflammation and increased alveolar-capillary membrane permeability.
   b. Tidal volume is not a good indicator of the risk of overdistension lung injury because the distribution of the tidal volume in the lungs is not known (i.e., healthy alveoli may receive much of the tidal volume and become overdistended).
   c. Some authorities have recommended that the plateau pressure be maintained at 35 cm H_2O or less to prevent overdistension injury.
   d. Because the risk of overdistension lung injury is related to transpulmonary pressure, higher plateau pressures may be safe if chest wall compliance is reduced (e.g., abdominal distension, chest wall burns, chest wall edema, obesity).
2. **Derecruitment injury**
   a. PEEP levels that are not sufficiently high to maintain alveolar recruitment can result in alveolar opening and closing with each respiratory cycle. This can result in inflammation and increased alveolar-capillary membrane permeability.
   b. This injury can be avoided by using appropriate levels of PEEP with ARDS—often 10 to 15 cm H_2O, and occasionally 15 to 20 cm H_2O.
3. **Oxygen toxicity**
   a. High concentrations of oxygen for long periods can cause lung damage.
   b. Although it is prudent to reduce the FIO_2 provided that arterial oxygenation is adequate, the precise role of oxygen toxicity in patients with acute lung injury is unclear.
   c. Appropriate levels of inspired oxygen should never be withheld for fear of oxygen toxicity.
B. Patient-ventilator dyssynchrony
1. **Trigger dyssynchrony** refers to the inability of the patient to trigger the ventilator.
   a. Trigger dyssynchrony can be caused by an **insensitive trigger setting** on the ventilator. This is corrected by adjusting the trigger sensitivity.
   b. An alternative approach to triggering may be tried, such as flow instead of pressure triggering.
   c. A common cause of trigger dyssynchrony is the presence of **auto-PEEP.** If auto-PEEP is

present, the patient must generate sufficient inspiratory effort to overcome the auto-PEEP before triggering can occur. Techniques to decrease the level of auto-PEEP should be used (e.g., administer bronchodilators, increase expiratory time). In patients with expiratory flow limitation (e.g., COPD), increasing the set PEEP on the ventilator can counterbalance the auto-PEEP and improve trigger synchrony.

2. **Flow dyssynchrony**
   a. During volume ventilation, the ventilator flow is fixed and may not meet the patient's inspiratory flow demands. The inspiratory pressure waveform will demonstrate a characteristic scalloped pattern.
   b. Flow dyssynchrony can be improved during volume ventilation by increasing the inspiratory flow or changing the inspiratory flow pattern.
   c. Switching from volume control to a pressure-limited mode, in which flow rates are variable, can be helpful.

3. **Cycle dyssynchrony** occurs when the patient's expiratory effort begins before the end of the inspiratory phase set on the ventilator. Cycle dyssynchrony occurs during volume-controlled or pressure-controlled ventilation if the inspiratory time is too long. This is corrected by shortening the inspiratory time.
   a. With high airways resistance and high lung compliance (e.g., COPD), a prolonged time may be required for the inspiratory flow to decelerate to the flow cycle set on the ventilator during pressure support. If the inspiratory time is longer than neural inspiration, the patient will actively exhale to terminate the inspiratory phase. This can be avoided by using pressure control rather than pressure support. Set the inspiratory time so that the inspiratory phase terminates before flow reaches zero or before the patient actively exhales.
   b. Some recently manufactured ventilators allow the clinician to adjust the termination flow during pressure support to improve synchrony.

C. **Auto-PEEP**
   1. **Auto-PEEP** is the result of gas trapping (dynamic hyperinflation) caused by insufficient expiratory time, increased expiratory airflow resistance, or both. The pressure exerted by this trapped gas is called auto-PEEP.
   2. The increase in alveolar pressure caused by auto-PEEP can adversely affect hemodynamics.
   3. The presence of auto-PEEP can produce trigger dyssynchrony as discussed above.

4. **Detection of auto-PEEP**
   a. Some ventilators allow auto-PEEP to be measured directly.
   b. In spontaneously breathing patients, auto-PEEP can be measured using an **esophageal balloon.**
   c. The **patient's breathing pattern** can be observed. If exhalation is still occurring when the next breath is delivered, auto-PEEP is present.
   d. **Inspiratory efforts that do not trigger the ventilator** suggest the presence of auto-PEEP.
   e. If flow graphics are available on the ventilator, it can be observed that **expiratory flow** does not return to zero before the subsequent breath is delivered.

5. **Factors affecting auto-PEEP**
   a. **Physiologic factors.** A high airways resistance or high respiratory system compliance increases the likelihood of auto-PEEP.
   b. **Ventilator factors.** A high tidal volume, high respiratory rate, or prolonged inspiratory time will increase the likelihood of auto-PEEP. Reducing the minute ventilation decreases the likelihood of auto-PEEP.

D. **Barotrauma**
   1. **Alveolar rupture** during positive-pressure ventilation can lead to air extravasation through the bronchovascular sheath into the pulmonary interstitium, mediastinum, pericardium, peritoneum, pleural space, and subcutaneous tissue.
   2. Sudden hemodynamic instability in a mechanically ventilated patient should raise the suspicion of a **tension pneumothorax.**

E. **Hemodynamic perturbations**
   1. Positive-pressure ventilation increases intrathoracic pressure and **decreases venous return.** Right ventricular filling is limited by the reduced venous return.
   2. When alveolar pressure exceeds pulmonary venous pressure, pulmonary blood flow is affected by alveolar pressure rather than by left atrial pressure, producing an **increase in pulmonary vascular resistance.** Consequently, right ventricular afterload increases and right ventricular ejection fraction falls.
   3. **Left ventricular filling is limited** by reduced right ventricular output and decreased left ventricular diastolic compliance.
   4. Increased right ventricular size affects left ventricular performance by shifting the interventricular septum to the left.
   5. **Intravascular volume replacement** counteracts the negative hemodynamic effects of PEEP.

   6. Increased intrathoracic pressure can **improve left ventricular ejection fraction and stroke volume.** This beneficial effect can be significant in patients with poor ventricular function.

F. Nosocomial pneumonia (see Chapter 28)

   1. Mechanically ventilated patients are at risk for ventilator-associated pneumonia.

   2. Ventilator-associated pneumonia is most often related to aspiration of secretions around the cuff of the endotracheal tube. Thus, ventilator-associated pneumonia is more likely endotracheal tube-associated pneumonia.

   3. Because the source of ventilator-associated pneumonia is usually not the ventilator *per se,* the tubing and humidifier on the ventilator do not need to be changed at regular intervals.

VIII. Discontinuation of mechanical ventilation

   A. Assessment of weaning readiness is the most important aspect of the discontinuation of mechanical ventilation.

   1. Resolution of the cause of respiratory failure.

   2. Cessation of deep sedation and neuromuscular blockade.

   3. Absence of sepsis.

   4. Stable cardiovascular status.

   5. Correction of electrolyte and metabolic disorders.

   6. Adequate arterial oxygenation (e.g., $PaO_2 > 60$ mm Hg with $FIO_2 \leq 0.5$ and PEEP ≤ 5 cm H_2O).

   7. Adequate respiratory muscle function.

   B. Weaning parameters

   1. Traditional weaning parameters (e.g., vital capacity, maximal inspiratory force, minute ventilation) are poor predictors of weaning success.

   2. The rapid shallow breathing index (RSBI) has been shown to be predictive of weaning success.

   a. The patient's respiratory rate and minute ventilation are measured for 1 minute during spontaneous breathing.

   b. The respiratory rate is divided by the tidal volume (expressed in liters).

   c. A RSBI of 105 or less is reasonably predictive of weaning success.

   3. Spontaneous breathing trial

   a. A spontaneous breathing trial can be performed if the patient meets the criteria for weaning readiness and has an RSBI less than 105.

   b. Prospective, controlled studies have shown that approximately 75% of patients can be extubated if they successfully complete a spontaneous breathing trial.

   c. The spontaneous breathing trial can be conducted with the patient breathing spontaneously while attached to the ventilator

(CPAP mode),
H₂O), or discon~~Ventilation~~

attached to a T-
supplemental ox

(1) **A 30-minu**~~PSV (5–7 cm~~
ing trial is ~~dilator and~~
(e.g., 2 h). ~~idity and~~

(2) The spontaneou
be terminated if ~~ath-~~
of respiratory dis~~rial~~
greater than 35/mi.
heart rate faster tha,
ute or 20% change fro
blood pressure greate.
or less than 90 mm H₆
phoresis.

C. Weaning techniques

1. Ventilator weaning is conducted if the
   fails the spontaneous breathing trial.

2. Weaning can be provided with a **gradual reduction of rate with SIMV** (SIMV weaning), a
   gradual reduction of pressure with PSV (pressure support weaning), or with **periodic spontaneous breathing trials** (T-piece weaning).
   Prospective controlled trials have reported the
   poorest weaning outcomes with SIMV.

3. The choice of PSV or T-piece weaning is a matter
   of clinician preference.

4. If one approach to weaning is not successful, it is
   prudent to select a different approach. Nevertheless, a standardized approach using specific
   protocols appears to wean patients more quickly
   from mechanical ventilation.

D. Failure to wean

1. **Reasons for weaning failure** include:
   a. Insufficiently treated pulmonary disease.
   b. Auto-PEEP and hyperinflation.
   c. Concomitant cardiac disease.
   d. Nutrition and electrolyte imbalance.
   e. Inadequate rest following an exhausting
      spontaneous breathing trial.
   f. Severe muscle weakness following neuro-
      muscular disease or polyneuropathy of criti-
      cal illness (see Chapter 30).

2. **Long-term ventilatory requirements**
   a. Some patients require a prolonged time
      (weeks or months) to wean. These patients
      can benefit from care in a specialized long-
      term ventilator weaning facility.
   b. Because of the nature of their disease, some
      patients will not wean from mechanical ven-
      tilation. If desirable, mechanical ventilation
      can be continued in a long-term care facility
      or at home.

NCES

M. *Essentials of mechanical ventilation.* New
98   ., 1996.

J, eds. Recent advances in mechanical ventilation.
1996;17(3):355–619.

nciples and practice of mechanical ventilation. New
w-Hill, 1994.

rinciples and practice of intensive care monitoring. New
raw-Hill, 1998.

Sedation

William E. Hurford

Posttraumatic stress disorder is common in survivors of critical illness. Among patients with acute respiratory distress (ARDS), those recalling multiple distressing experiences during their intensive care unit (ICU) stay had the highest degree of impairment after recovery from their acute illness. Treatment of anxiety and delirium, provision of adequate analgesia, and, when necessary, amnesia is not only humane, but may reduce the incidence of posttraumatic stress disorders in survivors.

I. **Definitions**
   A. **Anxiety** specifically describes an unpleasant alteration of mood and emotions that is not accompanied by cognitive dysfunction. The patient continues to think and comprehend normally.
   B. **Delirium** describes a second common indication for sedation. Delirium, as with anxiety, is characterized by an unpleasant alteration of mood. Unlike anxiety, an acute confusional state with cognitive impairment accompanies delirium. The distinction of cognitive impairment is important in making the proper diagnosis and prescribing appropriate therapy.
   C. Both anxiety and delirium often, but not necessarily, are accompanied by **agitation,** which is simply excessive motor activity resulting from any type of internal discomfort. Agitation can accompany delirium, pain, fear of death, and so on. It is a nonspecific symptom, but one that attracts much attention in the critically ill patient.
   D. It may be necessary to provide **anesthesia.** An anesthetic state renders the patient unconscious, relieves pain, provides muscle relaxation, and blunts undesirable reflexes such as tachycardia and hypertension.
   E. **Sedation** is the induction of a relaxed, calm state that is free from anxiety. Sedation is a vague term that covers a variety of states of consciousness and responsiveness.
      1. **Light sedation** or **conscious sedation** denotes that the patient can respond to verbal stimuli and follow commands appropriately.
      2. **Deep sedation** implies unresponsiveness to verbal stimuli, but responsiveness to touch, pain, or other noxious stimuli. The goals for providing sedation to a patient are extremely variable. It may be desirable simply to induce a calm, relaxed state, or it may be necessary to provide deep sedation or general anesthesia.
      3. Several rating scales have been developed to communicate a patient's level of sedation more easily.

One of the most common scales, the **"Ramsay scale,"** (Table 5-1) simply rates the patient's level of arousal from anxiety or agitation (level 1) to deep sedation (levels 4 and 5) to anesthetized (level 6).

4. The desired duration of sedation may last from a few minutes to months. The desired depth and duration of sedation often dictate the choice of drug.

II. Drug choice

A. **Choosing a drug** is often complex. Ideally, the pharmacokinetics of the drug should be considered, including its plasma half-life, volume of distribution; the formation of active metabolites; the pharmacodynamics, or effect of the drug in the individual patient; side effects and cost. Drug costs can vary widely.

B. **Problems with relying on pharmacokinetic data to sedate critically ill patients include:**

1. Published pharmacokinetic data are usually derived from healthy volunteers.
2. Actual pharmacokinetic values vary widely among individual patients.
3. Drug volume of distribution, effect, and elimination are often affected by liver, renal disease, sepsis, and so forth.
4. The drug concentration at the active site may not be reflected by the serum concentration of the drug.
5. The initial effect of the drug is often terminated by redistribution in tissues rather than by metabolism or end-organ elimination.
6. Many metabolites are biologically active.

C. **Intravenous infusions (IV) of short-acting drugs** (e.g., propofol, alfentanil) are extremely titratable to effect; they are convenient and accumulate minimally. Such infusions are indicated for short-term use (< 48 hours) or in patients with severe liver and or renal disease. They are usually not appropriate for routine long-term use, because rapid reversal of the drug effect is usually unnecessary or undesirable in such situations. The pharmacokinetics and pharmacodynamics of such drugs vary widely among individ-

Table 5-1.   Ramsay sedation scale

Level	Response
1	Anxious, agitated, restless
2	Cooperative, oriented, tranquil
3	Responds to commands only
4	Asleep, brisk response to stimulus
5	Asleep, sluggish response to stimulus
6	Unarousable

From Ramsay MA, Savege TM, Simpson BR, Goodwin R. *Controlled sedation with alphaxalone-alphadolone.* BMJ 1974;2:656–659, with permission.

uals; prolonged effects can occur; and the drugs are usually expensive.

    D. **Pharmacologic sedation** can be achieved by selecting a small number of drugs from a few classes.

        1. **Benzodiazepines** (e.g., diazepam, midazolam, or ativan) are indicated to treat anxiety.

        2. **Haloperidol,** a butyrophenone, is commonly used to treat delirium.

        3. Deep sedation and anesthesia commonly are provided by a combination of a **hypnotic** (e.g., thiopental, propofol, and ketamine), a benzodiazepine, and an opioid (e.g., morphine, fentanyl).

III. Benzodiazepines

    A. **Types.** Benzodiazepines are often divided into short- and long-acting groups, based on pharmacokinetic values in normal individuals (see Table 5-2). Their duration of action in critically ill patients is unpredictable.

    B. **Side effects** of benzodiazepine administration can be desirable and include amnesia and respiratory depression. Some patients, especially those with delirium, can become disinhibited when benzodiazepine is administered. Intravenous preparations of diazepam are prepared in propylene glycol, which can produce pain on injection and thrombophlebitis. An emulsified preparation of diazepam, **Dizac,** is well tolerated and has a reduced incidence of such side effects.

    C. **The effects of benzodiazepines dissipate** mostly through redistribution from plasma to tissues. With repeated doses, organ elimination becomes more important. Benzodiazepines are conjugated in the liver to glucuronides and eliminated by the kidney. Organ elimination is slowed in the elderly and in critically ill patients (especially those with sepsis). Pharmacogenetic abnormalities, which account for slowed metabolism of midazolam, occur in 6% to 10% of patients.

    D. **Flumazenil** is a specific benzodiazepine receptor antagonist. Its duration of action is less than 1 hour, so a persistent effect may require a continuous infusion. It is expensive, and its acute administration has been associated with seizures and pulmonary edema. It should be used with caution (if at all) and titrated to effect.

IV. Delirium

    A. **Occurrence.** Delirium is an acute confusion state that occurs in approximately 10% to 15% of acute medical and surgical patients. Its incidence is increased in the elderly. Delirium is present in almost all patients with more than 40% burns.

    B. **Clinical features** of delirium include disorientation, altered perceptions, arousal and psychomotor abnormalities, decreased attention, impaired memory, disorganized thinking and speech, dysgraphia, and a disturbed sleep-wake cycle. The course is fluctuating and characterized by lucid intervals.

    C. **Risk factors.** Delirium is thought to result from vulnerability on the part of the patient (e.g., cognitive

Table 5-2.   Common benzodiazepines used in the intensive care unit

Drug	Adult dosage (range)	Half-life (h)	Active metabolites
Long acting			
Chlordiazepoxide (Librium)	15–100 mg/d	5–25	Desmethylchlordiazepoxide Demoxepam N-desmethyldiazepam
Diazepam (Valium, Dizac)	6–40 mg/d	20–50	N-desmethyldiazepam N-methyloxazepam (temaxepam) Oxazepam
Flurazepam (Dalmane)	15–60 mg/d	40–114	N-desalkylflurazepam
Alprazolam (Xanax)	0.75–4 mg/d	12–15	None
Short acting			
Lorazepam (Ativan)	2–6 mg/d	10–20	None
Midazolam (Versed)	2.5–30 mg/d	1–4	Alpha-hydroxymidazolam
Oxazepam (Serax)	30–120 mg/d	3–6	None

impairment, severe illness, visual impairment, and so on) and hospital-related insults (e.g., medications and procedures). The precise cause is entirely unclear. Inouye and Charpentier developed a predictive model for the occurrence of delirium in hospitalized general medical patients aged more than 70 years. Among the risk factors were the use of physical restraints, malnutrition, three or more medications added over the last 24 hours, the use of a bladder catheter, and any iatrogenic event. A greater number of factors was associated with an increased incidence of new-onset delirium (zero factors, 4%; one to two factors, 20%; three or more factors, 35%).

D. **Organic causes of delirium,** which must always be considered, include drug withdrawal, Wernicke's encephalopathy, hypertensive encephalopathy, hypoglycemia, hypoperfusion, hypoxemia, intracranial bleeding, meningitis or encephalitis, and side effects of medications.

E. **Intravenous haloperidol** is the drug of choice for the treatment of critically ill patients with delirium. Haloperidol is a butyrophenone with potent antipsychotic properties. Although it is an α-1 adrenergic antagonist, it has few hypotensive side effects. It has little apparent effect on ventilation. Extrapyramidal side effects are uncommon in the critically ill patient, perhaps because of concurrent use of benzodiazepines or beta-blockers. Prolongation of the QT interval and serious ventricular dysrhythmias, notably torsade-de-pointes, have been described in patients following haloperidol administration. Monitoring the QT interval of the electrocardiogram is advisable when high doses of haloperiodol are used. Haloperidol has been associated with neuroleptic malignant syndrome. It also decreases the threshold for seizures and should be used cautiously in patients with delirium tremens.

F. **Administration of haloperidol.** The starting dose for haloperidol is 0.5 to 1.0 mg, depending on level of agitation, age, and degree of illness. Although not approved by the Food and Drug Administration, the IV route appears preferable in the critically ill patient because absorption is assured. Side effects can be reduced with IV administration. Because the onset of action is approximately 11 minutes, allow 20 minutes between doses. For continued agitation, double the previous dose. No specific upper limit is seen. Supplemental anxiolytics, analgesics, or both may be necessary. After the patient is calm for 24 hours, reduce the dose by 50% every 24 hours, and taper over 3 to 5 days. Usually only two to three doses per day are necessary because the serum half-life is 14 hours.

V. **Anesthesia and deep sedation**

A. **Components of anesthesia** include unconsciousness, amnesia, analgesia, and the avoidance of unwanted reflexes.

B. **Sedatives and hypnotics** are used to induce amnesia, sleep, and unconsciousness.

   1. **Barbiturates** were classically used to induce amnesia and unconsciousness. They are not analgesic and have profound vasodilatory and myocardial depressant properties. In individuals who are hypovolemic or have preexisting myocardial dysfunction, barbiturates can cause lethal hypotension. Their effects are initially dissipated by redistribution, followed by slow hepatic clearance. Tolerance develops rapidly. Barbiturates decrease intracranial pressure (see Chapters 11 and 29). **Sodium thiopental** is the most commonly used IV barbiturate; it has a brief duration of action (3 to 4 minutes) because of redistribution. The induction dose of anesthesia in healthy patients is 4 mg/kg IV. This dosage must be decreased, depending on the cardiovascular status.

   2. **Propofol** (2,6-di-isopropylphenol) produces rapid induction and emergence of anesthesia; it accumulates minimally and has little "hangover" effect. As with sodium thiopental, it is not an analgesic. Propofol also reduces intracranial pressure. Its disadvantages include hypotension (decreased peripheral tone), pain on injection, respiratory depression, and expense. Importantly, because it is dissolved in a soya bean emulsion, which supports bacterial growth, contamination of propofol can occur if it is not handled with strictly aseptic technique. The dose for induction of anesthesia is 2 to 2.5 mg/kg IV in healthy patients. Infusions of 25 µg/kg/min to 75 µg/kg/min IV can be used for continuous deep sedation.

   3. **Ketamine** (1–3 mg/kg IV or 5–8 mg/kg intramuscularly) produces a dissociative state rather than anesthesia. Following ketamine administration, arousal can be slow and hallucinations problematic. Ketamine can increase cerebral metabolic rate and aggravate intracranial hypertension. Because ketamine has sympathomimetic and vagolytic actions, its side effects are useful in situations where an increased heart rate is desirable. Ketamine causes minimal respiratory depression, making it occasionally useful for brief periods of deep sedation in spontaneously breathing patients.

   4. **Etomidate** is an imidazole hypnotic agent used for induction of anesthesia (0.1–0.3 mg/kg IV). Etomidate has minimal cardiovascular depressant effects and decreases cerebral blood flow and metabolism in a dose-dependent manner. It is not an analgesic. Myoclonus, nausea and vomiting, venous irritation, and adrenal suppression are important side effects.

C. **Opioids** provide both analgesia and sedation, but do not provide reliable amnesia. Because they have potent antitussive and respiratory depressant effects, opioids are often used to improve a patient's tolerance for mechanical ventilation. These same sedative and respiratory depressant effects, however, can interfere with weaning if not carefully titrated. Chest wall rigidity, especially with high doses of fentanyl and other potent opioids, can occur. Gastrointestinal motility is decreased and the resulting constipation can be severe. Tolerance can develop with prolonged administration. Common opioids are listed in Table 5-3.

1. **Morphine** is first conjugated in the liver and then excreted unchanged in the urine. Elimination can be delayed in renal failure. The morphine-6-glucouronide metabolite is biologically active. During acidemia, the duration of action of morphine and its metabolites is prolonged in the brain.

2. **Fentanyl** has a relatively short duration of action after a single dose because of its high lipid solubility and redistribution into tissues. With repeated or continuous administration, hepatic metabolism becomes responsible for the termination of the drug's effect. Under these conditions, the elimination half-life of fentanyl is longer than that of morphine (2–16 hours vs. 1.5–6 hours).

3. **Meperidine** is also metabolized in the liver. The clearance of an active metabolite, normeperidine, is dependent on renal function. Normeperidine can accumulate with repetitive doses or in patients with decreased renal function. Use with caution (if at all) in patients with hepatic or renal failure or seizure disorders. Normeperidine, which is a central nervous system stimulant, can precipitate twitching, tremor, or seizures. Monoamine oxidase (MAO) inhibitors, fluoxetine, and other serotonin uptake inhibitors greatly potentiate the effects of meperidine.

D. **Anesthetic depth** can be difficult to judge in critically ill patients. Assurance of adequate anesthetic level and amnesia is extremely important, especially if the patient is also pharmacologically paralyzed. The use of processed electroencephalographic monitoring [Bispectral Index (BIS) monitoring] can be useful for maintaining a particular level of anesthesia, but it has not been fully evaluated in critically ill patients.

VI. **Brief summary of practice guidelines adopted by the Society of Critical Care Medicine**

A. **Morphine sulfate** is the preferred analgesic agent for critically ill patients.

B. **Fentanyl** is the preferred analgesic agent for critically ill patients with hemodynamic instability, and for patients manifesting symptoms of histamine release with morphine or morphine allergy.

C. **Hydromorphone** (Dilaudid) can serve as an acceptable alternative to morphine.

Table 5-3.   Common opioids used in the intensive care unit

Drug	Adult dose[a] (mg)	Pediatric dose[a] (mg/kg)	Duration of action (h)	Approximate conversion factor	Metabolism	Comments
Codeine			4		Hepatic to morphine	Avoid IV route due to large histamine release and cardiovascular effects
Parenteral	—	—		0.08		
Oral	15–60	0.5–1		0.05		
Fentanyl (Sublimaze)			0.5–2		Hepatic	Rapid IV injection can result in skeletal muscle and chest wall rigidity
Parenteral	0.050–0.10	0.001–0.002		80		
Transdermal patch	—	—		80		25, 50, 75, or 100 µg/h
Hydromorphone (Dilaudid)			4		Hepatic; eliminated in urine, principally as glucuronide conjugates	Pediatric use not well established
Parenteral	1–4	0.05–0.1		4		
Oral	1–4	0.05–0.1		1.33		

Meperidine (Demerol)

	Dose (mg)	Dose (mg/kg)	Half-life (h)	Metabolism	Comments
Parenteral	50–150	1–1.5	3–4	Hepatic; normeperidine (active metabolite) is dependent on renal function and can accumulate with high doses or in patients with decreased renal function	Use with caution in patients with hepatic or renal failure or seizure disorders or receiving high dosages; normeperidine (a metabolite and CNS stimulant) can accumulate and precipitate twitching, tremor, or seizures. MAO inhibitors, fluoxetine, and other serotonin uptake inhibitors greatly potentiate the effects of meperidine
Oral	50–150	1–1.5			Not recommended

0.1
0.03

(continued)

Table 5-3. *Continued*

Drug	Adult dose[a] (mg)	Pediatric dose[a] (mg/kg)	Duration of action (h)	Approximate conversion factor	Metabolism	Comments
Methadone (Dolophine)			4–12 h, increases to 22–48 h with repeated doses			Phenytoin, pentazocine, and rifampin can increase the metabolism of methadone and may precipitate withdrawal. Increased toxicity: CNS depressants, phenothiazines, tricyclic antidepressants, and MAO inhibitors can potentiate the adverse effects of methadone
Parenteral	2–10	—		1.0		
Oral	2–10	—		0.7		

Morphine					In the liver via glucuronide conjugation; excreted unchanged in urine	Histamine release. Can cause hypotension in patients with acute myocardial infarction
Parenteral	5–10	0.1–0.2	4–5	1.0		
Oral[b]	10–30	0.20–0.5		0.33		
Oxycodone (Percocet and others)						
Oral	5	0.05–0.15	4	0.33	Hepatic	

IV, intravenous; CNS, central nervous system; MAO, monoamine oxidase.

Published tables vary widely in suggested equi-analgesic doses. Titration to clinical responses is always necessary. Recommended doses do not apply to patients with hepatic or renal insufficiency or other conditions affecting drug metabolism and kinetics. Pediatric doses should not be applied to infants < 6 months of age.

[a] These doses (oral, intravenous) are recommended starting doses for acute pain. Optimal doses for each patient are determined by titration and the maximal dose is limited by adverse effects. Any oral or parenteral analgesic may be converted into its intramuscular morphine equivalent by multiplying the dose by the conversion factor.

[b] Controversy exists concerning actual conversion factor (3:1 ratio).

   D. Midazolam or propofol are preferred only for the
       short-term (< 24 hours) treatment of anxiety in the crit-
       ically ill adult.
   E. Lorazepam is the preferred agent for the prolonged
       treatment of anxiety in the critically ill adult.
   F. Haloperidol is the preferred agent for the treatment
       of delirium in the critically ill patient.

SELECTED REFERENCES

Ariano RE, Kassum DA, Aronson KJ. Comparison of sedative recov-
    ery time after midazolam versus diazepam administration. *Crit
    Care Med* 1994;22:1492–1496.

Bennett SN, McNeil MM, Bland, LA, et al. Postoperative infections
    traced to contamination of an intravenous anesthetic, propofol.
    N Engl J Med 1995;333:147–154.

Bion JF, Logan BK, Newman PM, et al. Sedation in intensive care:
    morphine and renal function. *Intensive Care Med* 1986;12:359–365.

Bodenham A, Park GR. Reversal of prolonged sedation using flumaze-
    nil in critically ill patients. *Anaesthesia* 1989;44:603–605

Carrasco G, Molina R, Costa J, et al. Propofol vs. midazolam in short-,
    medium-, and long-term sedation of critically ill patients. *Chest* 1993;
    103:557–564.

Cassem NH, Hackett TP. Psychiatric consultation in a coronary care
    unit. *Ann Intern Med* 1971;75:9–14.

Forsman A, Öhman R. Pharmacokinetic studies on haloperidol in
    man. *Current Therapeutic Research* 1976;20:319–336.

Glass P, Bloom M, Kearse L, et al. Bispectral analysis measures seda-
    tion and memory effects of propofol, midazolam, isoflurane, and
    alfentanil in healthy volunteers. *Anesthesiology* 1997;86:836–847.

Hansen-Flaschen JH, Brazinsky S, Basile C, et al. Use of sedating
    drugs and neuromuscular blocking agents in patients requiring
    mechanical ventilation for respiratory failure: a national survey.
    JAMA 1991;266:2870–2875.

Inouye SH, Bogardus ST, Charpentier PA, et al. A multicomponent
    intervention to prevent delirium in hospitalized older patients.
    N Engl J Med 1999;340:669–676.

Inouye SK, Charpentier PA. Precipitating factors for delirium in hos-
    pitalized elderly persons: predictive model and interrelationship
    with baseline vulnerability. *JAMA* 1996;275:852–857.

Kress JP, O'Connor MF, Pohlman AS, et al. Sedation of critically ill
    patients during mechanical ventilation: a comparison of propofol
    and midazolam. *Am J Respir Crit Care Med* 1996;153:1012–1018.

Menza MA, Murray GB, Holmes VF, et al. Decreased extrapyramidal
    symptoms with intravenous haloperidol. *J Clin Pyschiatry* 1987;
    48:278–280.

Park GR, Gray PA. Infusions of analgesics, sedatives and muscle
    relaxants in patients who require intensive care. *Anaesthesia* 1989;
    44:879–880.

Schelling G, Stoll C, Haller M, et al. Health-related quality of life and
    posttraumatic stress disorder in survivors of the acute respiratory
    distress syndrome. *Crit Care Med* 1998;26:651–659.

Shader RI, Greenblatt DJ. Use of benzodiazepines in anxiety dis-
    orders. *N Engl J Med* 1993;328:1398–1405.

Shapiro BA, Warren J, Egol AB, et al. Practice parameters for intra-venous analgesia and sedation for adult patients in the intensive care unit: an executive summary. *Crit Care Med* 1995;23:1596–1600.

Tesar GE, Murray GB, Cassem NH. Use of high-dose intravenous haloperidol in the treatment of agitated cardiac patients. *J Clin Psychopharmacol* 1985;5:344–347.

Analgesia

Shihab U. Ahmed, Jeffrey A. Norton,
and To-Nhu Vu

I. **Acute pain: physiology and anatomy**
   A. **Acute postincisional or posttraumatic pain** arises from activation of the peripheral nociceptors. These nociceptors are terminal branches of small sensory, unmyelinated C-fibers and thinly myelinated A-delta nerve fibers. Many of these nociceptors are polymodal, meaning that they can be stimulated by mechanical, cold, heat, or chemical modalities, and they are innervated by C-fibers.
   B. Two types of **A-fiber** mechano and heat nociceptors exist:
      1. **Type I fibers** have a very high threshold under normal conditions; thus, they are called high threshold mechanoreceptors.
      2. **Type II fibers** have a substantially lower threshold, and much shorter duration between stimulus onset and receptor activation. Type II fibers are thought to cause initial highly localized, sharp pain of short duration (first pain).
   C. **Sensitization** of nociceptors, which occurs with local tissue injury and inflammation, is characterized by a decrease in threshold and increased response to super threshold stimuli (**hyperalgesia**). With tissue injury, there is a collection of algogenic mediators, most notably prostanoids, kinins, serotonin, hydrogen and potassium ions, substance P, nitric oxide, and other cytokines. These chemical mediators play a major role in peripheral hyperalgesia by their action on the nociceptors. Peripheral hyperalgesia has been divided into primary and secondary hyperalgesia. Primary hyperalgesia occurs at the site of tissue injury and secondary hyperalgesia occurs in uninjured skin surrounding the injured site.
   D. **Visceral nociceptors,** like somatic nociceptors, are nerve endings of the primary sensory afferent fibers. Primary visceral afferent fibers frequently travel along the sympathetic efferent fibers. Most of these visceral nociceptors are polymodal and respond to smooth muscle spasm, ischemia, distention, or inflammation.
   E. **Acute postoperative and posttraumatic pain** is nociceptive in nature, secondary to the activation of both somatic and visceral nociceptors by tissue injury and inflammation. **Somatic** pain is characteristically well localized and sharp compared with visceral, which tends to be less well defined and diffuse. **Visceral pain** can cause referred pain to the cutaneous

dermatomes because of the convergence of visceral and somatic afferent fibers in the spinal cord.

II. **Chronic pain issues in the intensive care unit (ICU) setting.** Patients in the ICU have pain resulting from multifactorial causes. In addition to the acute postoperative nociceptive pain, patients in the ICU often have pre-existing chronic painful conditions.

A. **Neuropathic pain,** defined as pain resulting from lesions of the peripheral or central nervous systems, is an important type of chronic pain.

1. The sources of neuropathic pain are numerous, including cerebrovascular accident, myelopathy, radiculopathy, plexopathy, and neuropathy. Patients with certain previous surgical procedures (e.g., mastectomy, thoracotomy, and limb amputation) have a high incidence of chronic pain because of the high risk of neural tissue trauma associated with these procedures. In patients with malignancies, neuropathic pain can result from nerve injury secondary to chemotherapy, radiation, or tumor invasion or compression.

2. Neuropathic pain is often characterized as sharp, burning, lancinating, or shock-like. Allodynia, hyperalgesia, and radicular symptoms are other features of neuropathic pain.

B. **Perioperative nociceptive pain** can sensitize the peripheral and central nervous systems. Although the transition from acute to chronic pain is not well defined, subsequent paradoxical generation of abnormal nerve impulses results in painful sensations. Nociceptive input can also trigger abnormal sympathetic efferent activity, leading to sympathetically maintained pain.

1. Patients with chronic pain often have significant **myofascial pain** resulting from abnormal posturing, bracing, and positioning.

2. **Emotional and psychological factors** contribute to chronic pain. Because chronic pain is often a confluence of multiple factors, its treatment requires a multidisciplinary approach with inputs from the pain specialist, physical therapist, and psychiatrist.

3. **Preemptive analgesia** and adequate pain control after an operation can decrease the incidence of long-term pain.

III. **Pharmacological intervention**

A. **Opioid analgesics** are efficacious for controlling acute nociceptive pain but are less effective for neuropathic pain. They can be agonists, antagonists, or mixed agonist–antagonists. The agonists' analgesic effects are derived from their interactions at the mu opioid receptors. The most commonly used agonists in the ICU are morphine, fentanyl, hydromorphone, methadone, and meperidine (see Chapter 5, Table 5-3 for oral and intramuscular doses). They are often administered intravenously to achieve rapid onset, better availability, and easier titration.

1. Dosage titration is based on the severity of the patient's pain and on the patient's general physical condition and age. The goal is to provide adequate pain relief while minimizing side effects.

2. If one opioid fails to provide adequate analgesia, rotation of opioids is indicated. Because of incomplete cross-tolerance among opioids, substituting one opioid for another can improve analgesic effect and reduce toxicity.

3. **Morphine sulfate,** the oldest agent in use, is the standard against which other narcotics are compared. Morphine is given in doses ranging from 0.02 to 0.05 mg/kg intravenously (IV) every 2 to 4 hours. The peak onset time is 20 minutes, and the duration of action is up to 4 to 5 hours. Large doses of morphine can lead to histamine release, decreased peripheral vascular resistance, and reduce blood pressure in hypovolemic patients.

   a. **Morphine-6-glucoronide,** an active metabolite, can accumulate with repeat administration in patients with renal disease.

4. **Fentanyl,** a synthetic opioid, is approximately 75 to 80 times more potent than morphine. The dose for fentanyl is 0.5 to 2.0 µg/kg IV every 2 hours; onset is 30 seconds; and duration of action is 1 to 2 hours.

5. **Hydromorphone,** another commonly used opioid, is four times more potent than morphine. The dose for hydromorphone is 2 to 15 µg/kg IV every 4 to 6 hours. The central nervous system onset time is 15 minutes, and duration of action is 4 to 5 hours.

6. **Methadone** is equipotent to morphine. The dose is 0.05 to 0.1 mg/kg every 4 to 12 hours. Because of the long half-life (15 to 40 hours) and the potential for drug accumulation, methadone is not recommended as an initial therapy.

7. **Meperidine** is also not considered to be first-line therapy because of its active metabolite, **normeperidine.** Normeperidine has a half-life of 15 to 20 hours. In patients with renal disease, normeperidine can accumulate and cause seizures. Concurrent administration of meperidine with monoamine oxidase inhibitors can result in hyperpyrexia, seizures, delirium, respiratory depression, or excitation. Unlike other opioids, meperidine causes tachycardia and mydriasis. The usual dose is 0.5 to 1.0 mg/kg IV every 2 to 4 hours. The onset of action is 10 minutes; duration of action is 3 to 5 hours.

B. **Agonist–antagonists** are not commonly used in the ICU setting. They act as agonists at the kappa receptor to provide analgesia and antagonists at the mu receptors. They have low efficacy, can reverse analgesia, and can cause withdrawal symptoms in patients chronically treated with opioids.

C. Antagonists, such as **naloxone,** can be used in the setting of opioid overdose. The dose is titrated carefully to reverse respiratory depression without precipitating withdrawal.

D. In addition to the intravenous route, opioid analgesics can be administered intramuscularly (IM), orally, and transdermally. No advantage is seen to using the IM route over IV administration.

    1. The intramuscular route is unreliable because of the variability in onset, degree, and duration of analgesia.

    2. For patients who are able to take oral medications and have reliable intestinal absorption, consider the use of oral maintenance opioids (e.g., oxycontin, MS-Contin, and methadone).

    3. Transdermal preparations include the fentanyl patch. This patch is recommended for patients with chronic stable pain who cannot take oral medications. The starting dose is 25 to 50 µg/h, changed every 72 hours. The onset of analgesic action is 12 hours.

IV. Patient-controlled analgesia. When compared with conventional intermittent dosing of opioids, **patient controlled analgesia** (PCA) provides superior pain relief, better patient satisfaction, and less fluctuations in plasma opioid concentrations. The PCA infusion pump allows patients to have control over their pain. Metaanalyses of 15 randomized control trials showed that patients prefer PCA to intermittent dosing. The pump can be programmed to deliver a set dose at a specific interval (lock-out period), a continuous background infusion (basal rate), and a maximal hourly dosage. Commonly used drugs include morphine and hydromorphone.

A. For **morphine,** patients can be given loading doses of 2 mg IV every 5 minutes to a maximal dose of 10 mg. Then, the PCA pump is set for a bolus of 1 to 2 mg, lockout of 5 to 10 minutes, no basal infusion, and an hourly limit of 10 mg.

B. For **hydromorphone,** the settings are 0.25 to 0.5 mg bolus, lockout of 10 minutes, no basal infusion, and an hourly limit of 3 to 4 mg.

C. Patients must be educated to the proper use of PCA and must be cognitively and physically able to use the pump. As with any route of administration, special care should be exercised in patients with advanced liver, lung, and kidney diseases; patients with head injury; patients who are hypovolemic; and the elderly. Respiratory depression is greater than 1% during PCA with a continuous background infusion, and 0.2% with no basal rate. Continuous basal infusions are suggested only when patients have been on long-term opioids.

V. Nonopioid adjuvants

A. Adjuvant analgesics are used to optimize pain relief and to reduce opioid toxic effects. They include nonsteroidal antiinflammatory agents (NSAIDs), tricyclic antidepressant drugs, and membrane stabilizers.

B. **Ketorolac tromethamine (toradol)** is the most commonly used parenteral NSAID. In one study, ketorolac (10 to 30 mg) was equal in analgesic effect to 12 mg of morphine. The dose for ketorolac is 15 to 30 mg every 6 hours. To minimize adverse side effects, ketorolac should be given for 5 days or less. The side effects of NSAIDs, in general, include gastric ulceration and bleeding, and renal and hepatic dysfunction.

C. **Cyclooxygenase II (COX-2) inhibitors** are selective NSAIDs with minimal gastrointestinal side effects.

D. For patients with significant neuropathic pain, **membrane stabilizers** (gabapentin, mexiletine, lamotrigine, topiramate) and **tricyclic antidepressants** (amitriptyline, nortriptyline, desipramine) have been shown to be effective. These agents are selected based on their side effect profiles. They are titrated slowly to minimize sedation.

VI. **Neuraxial analgesia**

A. In the ICU setting, intrathecal or epidural administration of local anesthetics or opiates can provide excellent analgesia for postoperative patients as well as for those who have suffered traumatic injuries. These techniques are particularly desirable in patients who have undergone major vascular, thoracic, abdominal, or orthopedic procedures. Increasing data support reduced hospitalization times and fewer perioperative complications for patients undergoing thoracic and abdominal surgical procedures when epidural analgesia was included in the anesthetic plan.

B. **Intrathecal analgesia** can be an effective way to achieve analgesia, although not as widely used as the epidural route. Intrathecal agents are used increasingly in the treatment of chronic cancer pain. This application often requires the implantation of an indwelling pump to provide a continuous infusion of low-dose local anesthetic, opiate, or clonidine.

C. **Epidural analgesia** has been reported to improve postoperative cardiovascular, pulmonary, gastrointestinal, immunologic, and hemostatic function, particularly in high-risk patients. Postoperative pain triggers the body's stress response and activates the autonomic nervous system. In addition to pain relief, epidural analgesia has been shown to reduce these organ system responses to surgery. Epidural opioids can produce analgesia without motor or sympathetic blockade.

1. Three methods of epidural drug administration currently are commonly used: bolus, continuous infusion, and patient-controlled epidural analgesia (PCEA). These methods can be used to administer local anesthetic, opiate, or a combination of the two.

a. **Bolus injections** are most commonly used for the long-acting drugs, such as morphine. Although requiring no special equipment, bolus injection of medications can result in overmedication of patients which, in turn, results in potentially excessive levels of drug, particularly morphine. Because of poor lipid solubility, higher single doses of morphine are needed to penetrate the dura and spinal cord. **Respiratory depression** can occur for up to 12 hours after a single epidural bolus of morphine, and it can persist as long as 16 to 18 hours. This risk appears to be less likely with administration of fentanyl or hydromorphone.

b. **Continuous infusions** of epidural analgesics avoid the initial high peaks associated with bolus administration of drug. Although requiring an infusion pump, its inconvenience can be outweighed by reduced side effects and a more continuous level of analgesia. Spinal cord levels of opiate can accumulate with continuous epidural infusion, so it is essential to monitor a patient's mental status and respiratory rate. Lipid soluble agents (e.g., fentanyl, alfentanil, and sufentanil) are often infused continuously because of their short duration of action. High systemic levels of these drugs can occur because of rapid uptake by epidural vessels. Blood levels of fentanyl, for example, have been shown to increase over time.

c. **Patient-controlled epidural analgesia (PCEA)** combines a continuous infusion of epidural analgesia with a patient-controlled option for administering bolus doses of medication for increasing pain such as that associated with movement. As with traditional intravenous PCA, PCEA appears to reduce dose requirements for analgesics when compared with continuous infusion techniques.

2. **Local anesthetics** are commonly combined with epidural opiates to achieve synergetic effects. The addition of local anesthetics to epidural opiate infusions has been shown to result in earlier discharge times in patients having abdominal surgery.

a. **Bupivacaine,** in concentrations of 0.0625 to 0.1%, has been the most popular choice for local anesthetic. Often bupivacaine is combined with fentanyl in dosages ranging from 4 to 10 µg/ml, hydromorphone (0.025 to 0.05 mg/ml), or morphine (0.1 mg/ml).

b. **Ropivacaine,** with reportedly less motor blockade, is becoming more widely used for continuous epidural infusion; it is also used in combination with opioids.

c. **Common side effects** of epidural administration of local anesthetics include hypotension, numbness, and urinary retention. Motor block of the legs can be observed in lower thoracic or lumbar epidural blockade.

3. **Placement of epidural catheters.** Patients can be placed in the lateral decubitus or sitting position to locate the epidural space and place an epidural catheter. Helpful landmarks include the inferior border of the scapula—corresponding to T7—and the iliac crests—corresponding to L4. Utilize the spinous processes as midline landmarks and identify the appropriate interspace. Placing the catheter at the middle of the level where analgesia is required is optimal. Infiltrate the skin with 1% lidocaine, using first a 25-gauge needle, and then a slightly longer 22-gauge needle, to anesthetize the subcutaneous fat and tissue. Using a slightly longer needle helps define the anatomy of intraspinous ligaments and bony structures. Advance a 17-gauge epidural needle in the midline, using a more acute angle when approaching the thoracic epidural space than when approaching the lumbar epidural space. A paramedian approach to the epidural space can be used when a midline approach is technically difficult (e.g., in higher thoracic levels where intervertebral spaces are narrower). The epidural space is located using a loss or resistance to air technique. On locating the epidural space, the catheter is threaded 3 to 5 cm into the space. Both the distance from skin to epidural space and the depth of catheter insertion should be recorded so that subsequent movement of the catheter can be detected. Careful aspiration on the catheter, testing for cerebrospinal fluid or blood, must be performed prior to the administration of a test dose of anesthetic—typically 3 ml of 1% lidocaine with epinephrine. The catheter is secured with a transparent dressing, which permits inspection of the insertion site.

4. **Complications of epidural analgesia** can occur from placement of the catheter or from the injection of local anesthetics and opioids.

   a. **Inadvertent dural puncture** leading to postdural puncture headache is the most common complication of epidural catheter placement. The incidence of dural puncture has been reported to be between 0.16% to 1.3%. Development of headache occurs in 16% to 86%.

   b. **Paresthesias** (usually self-limiting) and neurologic injury are estimated to occur in 0.01% to 0.001% of cases.

   c. Although extremely rare, **paraplegia** can result from the development of epidural hematoma. **Epidural abscess** is an extremely rare cause of paraplegia associated with epidural analgesia.

    d. Puncture of epidural blood vessels during catheter placement is estimated to occur in 3% to 12% of cases, but formation of symptomatic epidural hematomas associated with epidurals is exceedingly rare. The risk of epidural hematoma formation appears to be increased in patients who are anticoagulated, including those receiving low molecular weight heparin.

    e. Local anesthetic complications include accidental intrathecal or intravascular injection of anesthetics, which can produce high spinal anesthesia, dysrhythmias, seizures, and cardiovascular collapse. Use of a test dose of anesthetic with epinephrine, as well as smaller incremental volumes of anesthetic, help minimize these risks. Motor and autonomic blockade can result from continuous infusion of even low concentrations of local anesthetics; this can lead to hypotension, urinary retention, and motor weakness and impair patient mobility. Use of thoracic epidural catheters has been shown to be associated with lower rates of complications (e.g., motor weakness or hypotension) than lumbar epidural catheters.

    f. Opioid-related complications include respiratory depression, pruritis, nausea, and urinary retention. Respiratory depression is sometimes delayed and appears to be dose dependent. Although all commonly used epidural opioids have been reported to cause respiratory depression, morphine carries the highest risk, with an incidence of delayed respiratory depression of less than 1%. Other complications of epidural opioid administration include pruritus (28% to 100%); nausea (30% to 100%); and urinary retention (15% to 90%). Morphine appears to have the highest incidence of these side effects, and fentanyl the lowest. Little evidence supports the idea that combinations of local anesthetic and opioids reduce the incidence of these complications, although the addition of local anesthetics can reduce epidural opioid usage by as much as 50%.

VII. Peripheral nerve blocks. Peripheral nerve blocks provide a unique way to control pain following surgery or trauma. They can be administered as a single injection or by continuous infusion. In cases where a neuraxial block or parenteral opioid is contraindicated or suboptimal, peripheral nerve blockade can be useful.

    A. Intercostal nerve blocks can provide excellent pain control for thoracic or abdominal incisions or rib fractures. Intercostal nerve blocks can provide unilateral analgesia and may reduce cardiovascular and respiratory risks for some critically ill patients. Placement of a catheter in the intercostal space avoids repeated injections and provides prolonged analgesia.

1. This block can be performed with the patient in the prone, supine, lateral, or sitting position. In the prone, lateral, or sitting position, the block is performed 7 to 8 cm from the posterior midline at the angle of the ribs. For the supine position, this block is performed at the posterior axillary line to include the lateral cutaneous branch. An abdominal incision may require blocking T5 to T12 bilaterally; for thoracotomy, select two ribs above and two below on the same side of the incision. After raising a skin wheal with lidocaine, a 22-gauge needle is advanced perpendicular to the skin over the lower edge of the rib. After contacting the rib, the needle is "walked" off the inferior margin of the rib until it just slips off the rib and into the subcostal groove. After a negative aspiration for blood, fluid, or air, 3 to 5 ml of 0.5% bupivacaine (usually with 1:200,000 epinephrine) is slowly injected. The procedure is repeated at each interspace to be blocked. If prolonged pain control is desired, a 20-gauge peripheral nerve block catheter or an epidural catheter can be threaded 3 to 5 cm into the intercostal space via an 18-gauge short bevel or Tuohy needle. An intermittent injection of 20 ml 0.5% bupivacaine (usually with 1:200,000 epinephrine) can be administered through the catheter every 7 to 8 hours.

2. **Limitations of intercostal blocks** include potential local anesthetic toxicity with multiple blocks, need for repeated blocks, and difficulty blocking upper thoracic segments because of interference from the scapula. The block may not provide analgesia to the posterior chest wall.

B. **The brachial plexus** or its peripheral branches can be blocked to provide pain control for upper extremity fractures or postoperative pain. An interscalene approach is recommended if shoulder or proximal arm analgesia is required; an axillary approach is sufficient for pain below the elbow.

1. For an **interscalene block,** the patient should be supine, the head resting on a flat surface and turned 45 degrees toward the opposite side. The interscalene groove is identified by palpating the posterior border of the clavicular head of the sternocleidomastoid muscle at the level of the cricoid cartilage and then rolling the operator's finger slightly laterally. Having the patient lift his or her head off the bed or take a deep inspiration can be helpful in identifying the interscalene groove. A skin wheal is raised with lidocaine at this level. A 2.5-cm, 22-gauge needle is advanced into the groove, perpendicular to the skin. Stimulation of

the plexus results in a paresthesia or muscle twitch below the shoulder. A paresthesia to the upper back requires that the needle be repositioned. A nerve stimulator set to deliver 0.5 to 0.7 mA may be helpful to elicit a motor response. After identifying the plexus, 30 to 40 ml of local anesthetic is injected in divided doses with frequent aspiration. Complications of this procedure include pneumothorax and intrathecal, epidural, or intraarterial injection. Because the ispilateral phrenic nerve is often also blocked, caution should be used in patients with lung disease.

2. An **axillary block** can be performed to relieve pain below the elbow. A transarterial approach can be performed if the patient is not coagulopathic. The patient is placed in a supine position with the arm abducted to 90 degrees. The axillary artery is palpated against the humeral head. A 23-gauge, 2.5-cm needle is advanced through anesthetized skin and toward the axillary artery. Aspirate continuously while advancing the needle slowly. When arterial blood is seen, advance the needle until blood is no longer aspirated. A total volume of 20 to 25 ml of local anesthetic is injected behind the artery, and another 10 to 15 ml is injected in front of the artery, carefully aspirating to avoid intraarterial injection. Injecting 5 ml of local anesthetic in a fan pattern just superior to the artery can block the musculocutaneous nerve. The intercostobrachial nerve can be blocked by a subcutaneous injection of 5 ml of local anesthetic placed directly interior to the axillary artery and extending to the interior border of the axilla. After the injections, the arm is adducted and gentle pressure is applied to reduce hematoma formation.

C. **Lower extremity peripheral nerve blocks** include a "three-in-one" femoral nerve block, sciatic nerve block at the popliteal fossa, and ankle blocks.

1. **A "three-in-one" femoral nerve block** can control pain involving the hip, femoral shaft, or knee. The femoral pulse is palpated with the patient in the supine position. A skin wheal is raised 1 to 2 cm lateral to the pulse, and 1 to 2 cm below the inguinal ligament. A 22-gauge insulated block needle connected to the peripheral nerve stimulator is advanced cephalad at a 30-degree angle to the skin. A loss of resistance sensation will be felt twice: first, as the needle advances through the fascia lata and then as it advances through the fascia iliaca. After a quadriceps femoris response in the form of cephalad knee cap movement is elicited by a nerve stimulator output of 0.5 mA, 20 to 30 ml of local anesthetic is injected. Firm pressure is applied just distal to the puncture site during injection to help cephalad spread of anesthetic. Contraindications

for this technique include previous femoral vascular graft or renal transplant. Complications, which are rare, include hematoma, intravascular injection, and nerve injury.

2. **A popliteal sciatic nerve block** is useful to provide foot and ankle analgesia. Along with the femoral nerve block, this block provides reliable analgesia below the knee joint. The traditional approach to popliteal fossa block is done with the patient lying prone and the knee flexed 30 degrees. This outlines the borders of the popliteal fossa, which is bordered by the popliteal skin crease inferiorly, the long head of the biceps femoris laterally, and the superimposed tendons of the semimembranosus and semitendinosus muscles medially. The needle insertion site is 6 to 7 cm above the popliteal skin crease and 1 cm lateral to midline. An insulated peripheral nerve block needle, connected to a nerve stimulator, is advanced at a 45-degree angle to the skin with the tip directed cephalad and anterior. Either dorsal or plantar flexion is elicited by a current output of 0.5 mA or less. After proper positioning of the needle, 30 to 40 ml of local anesthetic is injected. The popliteal fossa contains a large amount of fatty tissue, and close proximity of the needle tip to the nerve is important for a successful block. For patients who cannot lie in the prone position, a supine approach to the nerve has been described. The patient's affected lower extremity is flexed at both the hip and knee joints, and then supported by an assistant. The needle then is advanced as in the classic approach. It is important to remember that the saphenous nerve, which is a branch of the femoral nerve, also needs to be blocked to provide complete analgesia below the knee. This can be performed by injecting 10 ml of local anesthetic in the deep subcutaneous tissue between the medial surface of the tibial condyle and the superimposed tendons of the semimembranosus and semitendinosus muscles.

SELECTED REFERENCES

Ballantyne JC. Postoperative patient-controlled analgesia: meta-analyses of initial randomized control trials. *J Clin Anesth* 1993; 5:182–193.

De Leon-Casasola OA. Clinical outcome after epidural anesthesia and analgesia in high-risk surgical patients. *Reg Anesth* 1996;21(6S): 144–148.

De Leon-Casasola OA, Lema MJ. Postoperative epidural opioid analgesia: what are the choices? *Anesth Analg* 1996;83:867–875.

Haasio J, Rosenberg PH. Continuous supraclavicular brachial plexus anesthesia. *Techniques in Regional Anesthesia and Pain Management* 1997;1:157–162.

Jensen TS. Mechanisms of neuropathic pain. In: Wall PD, Melzack R, eds. *Textbook of pain,* 3rd ed. New York: Churchill Livingstone, 1994:77–86.

Levy MH. Pharmacologic treatment of cancer pain. *N Engl J Med* 1996;335:1124–1132.

Liu SS, Carpenter RL, Neal JM. Epidural anesthesia and analgesia. *Anesthesiology* 1995;82:1474–1506.

Mulroy MF. Epidural opioid delivery methods: bolus, continuous infusion, and patient-controlled epidural analgesia. *Reg Anesth* 1996; 21(6S):100–104.

Reisine T, Pasternak G. Opioid analgesics and antagonists. In: Goodman GA, Hardman JG, Limbird LE, eds. *The pharmacologic basis of therapeutics,* 9th ed. New York: McGraw-Hill, 1996; 674–715.

Sidebotham D, Dijkhiuzen MRJ, Schug SA. The safety and utilization of patient-controlled analgesia. *J Pain Symptom Manage* 1997;14: 202–209.

Singelyn FJ, Gouverneur JM. Continous "3-in-1" block as postoperative pain treatment after hip, femoral shaft, or knee surgery: a large scale study of efficacy and side effects. *Anesthesiology* 1994;81:1054–1067.

Singelyn FJ, Aye F, Gouverneur JM. Continuous popliteal sciatic nerve block: an original technique to provide postoperative analgesia after foot surgery. *Anesth Analg* 1997;84:383–386.

Volka JD, Hadzic A, Koorn R, et al. Supine approach to the sciatic nerve in popliteal fossa. *Can J Anaesth* 1996;43:964–967.

Williams JT. The painless synergism of aspirin and opium. *Nature* 1997;390:557–558.

Neuromuscular Blockade

William E. Hurford

I. **Possible indications for pharmacological paralysis**
   A. **Improve patient-ventilator synchrony.** Many patterns of mechanical ventilation such as the use of inverse inspiratory:expiratory ratios and permissive hypercapnia are difficult for patients to tolerate, despite deep sedation.
   B. **Patients with increased airway resistance** (e.g., asthmatics) or patients with decreased elastic recoil of their lungs (e.g., those with severe emphysema) may require prolonged expiratory times. These patients are particularly susceptible to generating intrinsic positive end-expiratory pressure (PEEP). Spontaneous respiratory efforts may not trigger the inspiratory valve of the ventilator; they can lead to poor coordination with the ventilator and can increase the level of intrinsic PEEP. Neuromuscular blockade (NMB) may be required to permit low respiratory rates and prolonged expiratory times.
   C. **Patients with severe head injuries** often require intubation and mechanical ventilation for airway protection and hyperventilation. When these patients have a concurrent lung injury, the requirement for hyperventilation can involve strategies to minimize ventilator-associated lung injury. Routine use of neuromuscular blocking drugs (NMBDs) can, however, be associated with additional complications.
   D. **Reduction of a patient's oxygen consumption** is a rare indication for the use of NMBDs in patients with severe respiratory failure. The increased oxygen consumption and carbon dioxide production of a hypermetabolic or febrile state can jeopardize oxygenation. Such patients may benefit from active cooling. Shivering during active cooling can produce great increases rather than decreases of oxygen consumption. Nondepolarizing NMBDs can eliminate shivering during active cooling and thus reduce oxygen consumption.
   E. **Muscular spasms associated with tetanus,** which can interfere with mechanical ventilation, rarely cannot be controlled without the use of NMBDs.
   F. **No clinical evidence** supports the use of NMBDs to decrease the incidence of barotrauma during mechanical ventilation. Administering NMBDs to patients who already have synchronous mechanical ventilation does not improve their pulmonary gas exchange.
II. **Difficulties with neuromuscular blockade**
   A. **Disconnection** from the ventilator can be fatal. The patient may not have sufficient neuromuscular reserve to breathe spontaneously if NMBDs are used.

B. **Gas distribution** within the lung is altered with positive-pressure ventilation compared with spontaneous ventilation. Worsening of gas exchange can occur in some patients.

C. **Neurologic and psychologic evaluation** of the patient is hindered by neuromuscular blockade. Normal muscular responses and reflexes are eliminated.

D. **Pain and anxiety** may go undetected if a patient is pharmacologically paralyzed. Additional sedative and analgesic medications (see Chapters 5 and 6) must be administered to assure that the patient is not awake or in pain while NMBDs are used.

E. **Coughing** and clearance of airway secretions by the patient are eliminated.

F. **Reversal** of neuromuscular blockade can be difficult and prolonged.

G. **Severe myopathies and neuropathies** have been associated with the use of NMBDs in critically ill patients.

III. **Choice of neuromuscular blocking drug**

A. In selecting a NMBD, consideration is given to the anticipated duration of neuromuscular block, the patient's state of health, as well as the cost, hemodynamic side effects, and metabolism (Tables 7-1 and 7-2). For example, rocuronium, an intermediate-acting, nondepolarizing relaxant with a fast onset time, may be suitable for rapid sequence induction when succinylcholine administration is contraindicated, but its expense prohibits its use for long-term infusions.

B. **Succinylcholine** is a depolarizing muscle relaxant with an onset time of 60 seconds and a clinical duration of 5 to 10 minutes. It is indicated for facilitation of emergent endotracheal intubation.

1. **Succinylcholine is contraindicated in many critically ill patients.** Muscles of patients who have been at bedrest, immobilized, burned, suffered crush injuries (although succinylcholine appears safe in the acute setting), or those with significant paralysis or paresis have an increased number of extra-junctional acetylcholine receptors. Administration of a depolarizing agent can result in an unexpectedly large increase in potassium release, with life-threatening or fatal hyperkalemia. The consequences of this potassium release are increased in patients with preexisting hyperkalemia or renal failure. Prolonged paralysis can occur in those patients with genetic or drug-induced (e.g., echothiophate, neostigmine) pseudocholinesterase deficiency. A history of malignant hyperthermia is an absolute contraindication to the use of succinylcholine.

2. **Succinylcholine transiently increases intraocular and intracranial pressure** and has been considered relatively contraindicated in these settings. Many reports indicate its safe use after open eye injuries or in the setting of intracranial hyper-

Table 7-1.   Common neuromuscular blocking drugs

Drug	Indication	Customary intubating dose (mg/kg IV)	Maintenance infusion	Cost
cis-Atracurium	Intubation and maintenance for ≤2 h, or with compromised renal or hepatic function, or when changes in BP or HR ≥20% are undesirable	0.15–0.2	2 µg/kg/min	++
Mivacurium	Intubation and maintenance for ≤1 h with normal renal and hepatic function	0.15–0.25	10 µg/kg/min	+++
Pancuronium	Intubation and/or maintenance for >2 h. Combination with *d*-tubocurarine produces negligible changes in HR or BP.	0.08–0.1	1 µg/kg/min	+
Rocuronium	Rapid sequence induction, when succinyl-choline is contraindicated	0.6–1.2	0.01–0.012 mg/kg/min	+++
Succinylcholine	Routine or rapid sequence intubation	1.0	NA	+
d-Tubocurarine	Maintenance for >2 h	0.5–0.6	0.08–0.12 mg/kg/h	+
Vecuronium	Intubation and maintenance for ≤2 h and when changes in BP or HR of ≥20% are undesirable	0.1–0.2	1 µg/kg/min	+++

IV, intravenous; BP, blood pressure; HR, heart rate.
Doses are customary and not necessarily equipotent. A large variability in response to NMBDs is found among patients. Response should be monitored and doses individually adjusted.

Table 7-2. Elimination and cardiovascular side effects of common neuromuscular blocking drugs

Drug	Elimination	Histamine release[a]	Ganglionic effects	Vagolytic activity	Sympathetic stimulation
cis-Atracurium	80% Hofmann elimination; remainder renal and hepatic elimination	0	0	0	0
Mivacurium	Hydrolysis by plasma cholinesterase	+	0	0	0
Pancuronium	70% to 80% renal; remainder hepatic metabolism and biliary excretion	0	0	+	+
Rocuronium	Hepatic	0	0	0	0
Succinylcholine	Hydrolysis by plasma cholinesterase	±	+	0	0
d-Tubocurarine	70% renal; remainder biliary excretion	++	—	0	0
Vecuronium	80% renal; remainder hepatic metabolism and biliary excretion	0	0	0	0

[a] Histamine release is dose- and rate-dependent and less pronounced when drugs are given slowly.

tension, especially if adequate anesthesia is administered prior to the succinylcholine.

C. **Nondepolarizing NMBDs** are quartenary ammonium compounds with either a steroidal (e.g., vecuronium, pancuronium, rocuronium, pipecuronium) or benzoisoquinoline structure (*d*-tubocurarine, atracurium, *cis*-atracurium, mivacurium, doxacurium). Although these drugs typically have relatively slow onsets and long durations of action, some newer agents are notable for relatively fast onset (e.g., rocuronium) or short durations of action (e.g., mivacurium). Relaxants associated with histamine release (e.g., *d*-tubocurarine, atracurium, mivacurium, see Table 7-2) may be associated with hypotension, especially with large bolus doses. Pancuronium is associated with tachycardia caused by its vagolytic effect. *cis*-Atracurium, vecuronium, and rocuronium have minimal cardiovascular side effects.

D. **Few studies** exist to guide therapy. Much of the decision-making process is a matter of extrapolation from studies of healthy patients undergoing surgery and the clinical experience of particular physicians (i.e., local custom). Most clinical experience with neuromuscular blocking drugs among intensive care units (ICU) has been with pancuronium and vecuronium. Current concerns are prolonged duration of action, the development of poorly understood myopathies and neuropathies, and cost.

E. **Metabolism and excretion.** *d*-Tubocurarine, doxacurium, pancuronium, and pipecuronium are renally excreted and should be avoided in anephric or renal failure patients (see Table 7-2). Vecuronium and rocuronium are excreted primarily in the bile and should be used with caution in patients with liver failure. The elimination of atracurium and *cis*-atracurium is organ independent, and mivacurium is metabolized by pseudocholinesterase.

F. **Vecuronium** is popular because of its benign hemodynamic profile and the fact that it is perceived to have an intermediate duration of action. Reports of prolonged paralysis in patients with renal failure were followed by confirmatory studies in patients with normal renal function receiving long-term neuromuscular blockade with **pancuronium** or vecuronium. This prolonged effect appeared to be related to the accumulation of the 3-desacetyl metabolite.

G. ***cis*-Atracurium** (Nimbex) is an intermediate-duration NMBD. This drug is a stereoisomer of **atracurium,** but is three times as potent on a milligram-per-milligram basis. As with atracurium, it degrades by Hofmann elimination. Because of this, its duration of action is largely independent of renal or hepatic function. Histamine release or cardiovascular side effects do not occur with *cis*-atracurium administration. The drug is currently less expensive than equivalent doses of atracurium or vecuronium, and has replaced atracurium in clinical

practice. A study comparing the recovery times of vecuronium with *cis*-atracurium in patients in the ICU reported that recovery of neuromuscular function was
more rapid with *cis*-atracurium.

H. ***d*-Tubocurarine** (*d*-TC) is the oldest of the NMBDs in
current clinical use. Although now rarely administered,
its low cost makes it an attractive option for producing
long-acting neuromuscular blockade. It is minimally
metabolized, instead depending on renal and hepatic
clearance and redistribution to terminate its effect.
Accumulation can occur in renal failure. *d*-Tubocurarine
can cause histamine release, which can produce skin
flushing, hypotension, and bronchoconstriction. Significant histamine release has been documented only with
intermittent intravenous (IV) dosing and appears to be
dependent on the dose and rate of infusion. Lower histamine levels can occur with continuous *d*-TC infusions
and their effects can be partially blunted by concurrent
administration of drugs with H_1 or H_2 receptor blocking
activity. Continuous infusions of *d*-TC at rates averaging
15 mg/h appear reasonably well tolerated. Patients
receiving a cumulative dose of ≥ 800 mg or an infusion for
≥ 60 h, however, have an eightfold increased likelihood of
prolonged neuromuscular failure. In addition, high doses
of *d*-TC can block autonomic ganglions, producing systemic hypotension and profound mydriasis, which can
confound neurologic examination of the patient.

I. **Pipecuronium** and **doxacurium** are long-acting
agents that have no cardiovascular side effects. Their
high cost limits their use in critically ill patients.

J. **Mivacurium** is an intermediate-acting agent that is
hydrolyzed by plasma cholinesterase. It is expensive
and in high doses can cause histamine release.

K. **Neuropathic and myopathic changes** have been
associated with the administration of NMBDs in critically ill patients. Pathologic changes include marked
atrophy of type I and type II muscle fibers, destructive
myopathy, and relatively intact nerves. The cause of
neuromuscular failure remains unclear. The use of
vecuronium, pancuronium, and high doses of steroids,
appears to be associated with its occurrence. Neuromuscular blocking drugs, corticosteroids, and the underlying disease process can act synergistically to produce
neuromuscular injury.

1. **Critical illness polyneuropathy,** a disorder of the
spinal cord and the peripheral nerve, has been associated with NMBD use, but it can occur in their
absence. Patients develop muscle weakness, wasting, impaired tendon reflexes, and difficulty weaning
from respiratory support.

2. Critically ill patients subjected to prolonged neuromuscular blockade agents are probably at risk for
neurologic complications regardless of the agent
used. Because of this, it appears prudent to minimize both the dose and duration of the NMBDs.

IV. Delivery

 A.   Intermittent versus continuous administration

1.   Intermittent dosing regimens can be problematic if the patient's muscular activity interferes with mechanical ventilation. Doses administered on a regular schedule may maintain neuromuscular blockade more effectively. Intermittent dosing can precipitate dose related side-effects and can produce peak plasma levels of the drug that are far in excess of those required. Intermittent dosing regimens, therefore, have the potential to overdose the patient and prolong the duration of the block.

2.   Continuous infusions of NMBDs have the theoretical advantage of providing a constant drug level and a more reliable degree of neuromuscular block. Issues concerning the pharmacokinetics and pharmacodynamics of NMBDs complicate the use of continuous infusions in critically ill patients.

 a.   Accumulation of NMBDs and their metabolites has been described for pancuronium, vecuronium, and atracurium. *cis*-Atracurium and *d*-TC have not been well studied, but they appear to accumulate in renal failure.

 b.   Tachyphylaxis occurs during long-term administration. *d*-Tubocurarine infusions can accentuate the upregulation of acetylcholine receptors at the muscle membrane in models of burn injury. Even subparalytic doses of NMBDs are probably sufficient to alter acetylcholine receptor number or function. Some advocate the use of scheduled periods of muscle relaxant abstinence to prevent prolonged block or neuromuscular failure. The strategy of these "drug holidays" is not supported by clinical or laboratory studies.

 c.   Drug interactions, major changes of acid-base status, temperature, and volumes of drug distribution can affect the degree of neuromuscular blockade. These interactions usually are of minor significance in the acute setting. Their importance in critically ill patients is uncertain and has not been well studied.

 d.   Synergistic effects occur when a steroidal NMBD (e.g., pancuronium and vecuronium) is administered along with a benzylisoquinoline NMBD (e.g., *d*-tubocurarine, atracurium, and *cis*-atracurium). Blocking drugs with similar chemical structure have additive effects.

 B.   Monitoring of neuromuscular function. The response to peripheral nerve stimulation can be quantified to judge the extent of neuromuscular blockade and determine the requirement for additional NMBD.

1.   The **adductor pollicis muscle** response to ulnar nerve stimulation at the wrist is used most often to

assess neuromuscular function. Cutaneous electrodes are placed over the ulnar nerve at the wrist and attached to a pulse generator, which delivers a graded impulse of electrical current at a specified frequency. Evoked muscle tension can be estimated by feeling for thumb adduction or measured by using a force transducer. Tension and twitch height decrease with the onset of neuromuscular blockade. If the ulnar nerve is unavailable, other sites can be used (e.g., facial nerve).

2. The response to **train-of-four** twitches (supramaximal stimuli at a frequency of 2 Hz repeated at intervals no less than 10 seconds apart) is most commonly assessed. Responses at this frequency show fade during partial curarization. During nondepolarizing neuromuscular blockade, elimination of the fourth response corresponds to 75% depression of the first response when compared with control. Disappearance of the third, second, and first responses corresponds to 80%, 90%, and 100% depression of the first twitch, respectively. The ratio of the height of the fourth to the first twitch correlates with the degree of clinical recovery. The train-of-four is the most useful method for clinical monitoring, because it does not require a control height, it is not as painful as tetanic stimuli, and it does not induce changes in subsequent recovery. It is not helpful in quantifying the degree of depolarizing blockade because no fade will be evident.

3. Because a safe and reliable dose cannot be predicted, a reliable technique is needed to determine the degree of neuromuscular block. A belief exists that careful monitoring with a peripheral nerve stimulator assures adequate blockade and reduces the complications of overdosage and myopathy. Monitoring the twitch response of a critically ill patient, however, can be problematic. The twitch response is affected by the patient's temperature, amount of local tissue edema, electrolyte abnormalities, and concurrent medications. Interobserver variability in the interpretation of the twitch response is also a problem. These problems are generally surmountable.

4. The correct level of neuromuscular blockade to use in the treatment of a critically ill patient is unknown. Some practitioners believe that some indications require superpharmacologic diaphragmatic paralysis. To achieve this level of chemical blockade, the twitch response to peripheral nerve stimulation must be abolished. This is necessary because the adductor pollicis is more sensitive to pharmacologic neuromuscular blockade than the diaphragm. Other practitioners believe that most patients can be appropriately managed with a level of blockade that produces one or two residual twitches with a train-of-four stimuli, which is our clinical practice. It

assures that overdosage (> 100% block) is not occurring and permits the patient to move slightly in response to noxious stimuli to indicate if the level of sedation, analgesia, or both is inadequate. Again, minimizing the dose and duration of NMBDs appears to be the best practice.

C. **Assurance of adequate sedation and amnesia** is paramount when NMBDs are used. The sensation of being paralyzed while awake is both terrifying and inhumane to the patient. Administration of benzodiazepines, narcotics, or anesthetic drugs such as propofol or barbiturates (see Chapter 5) should accompany the use of NMBDs.

V. **Reversal of neuromuscular blockade**

A. Recovery from succinylcholine occurs in 10 to 15 minutes and does not require antagonism. Patients with atypical or altered plasma cholinesterase have a greatly prolonged duration of blockade. Reversal with an anticholinesterase can be attempted if residual weakness remains 20 to 25 minutes after administering the succinylcholine. Earlier reversal could worsen the block.

B. Reversal of a nondepolarizing block can be accelerated by administering an **anticholinesterase,** which increases the amount of acetylcholine available to compete with the NMBD for its binding sites. Anticholinesterases have both muscarinic and nicotinic effects. Muscarinic stimulation leads to salivation, bradycardia, tearing, miosis, and bronchoconstriction. Administration of an antimuscarinic drug (e.g., atropine or glycopyrrolate) prior to the anticholinesterase minimizes muscarinic receptor stimulation.

C. **Neostigmine,** (0.44 mg/kg IV; 3 mg in a typical adult), in combination with **glycopyrrolate,** (0.0085 mg/kg IV; 0.6 mg in a typical adult) is most commonly used for reversal.

D. Factors influencing the reversibility of a nondepolarizing block include the relaxant used, the mode of administration (i.e., single bolus, repeated boluses, or infusion), depth of blockade, concomitant use of anesthetics, and the choice of reversal agent. Clinical evidence of adequate neuromuscular recovery includes adequate ventilation and oxygenation, sustained grip strength; the ability to sustain head lift or movement of an extremity without fade; and the absence of discoordinated muscle activity. Attempts to reverse a deep block with excessive doses of neostigmine can paradoxically increase the degree of residual weakness. Reversal should not be attempted unless at least one response to a train-of-four stimulus is present.

SELECTED REFERENCES

Ali HH, Savarese JJ. Monitoring of neuromuscular function. *Anesthesiology* 1976;45:216–249.

Beemer GH, Bjorksten AR, Crankshaw DP. Pharmacokinetics of atracurium during continuous infusion. *Br J Anaesth* 1990;65: 668–674.

Bishop MJ. Hemodynamic and gas exchange effects of pancuronium bromide in sedated patients with respiratory failure. *Anesthesiology* 1984;60:369–371.

Coursin DB, Klasek G, Goelzer SL. Increased requirements for continuously infused vecuronium in critically ill patients. *Anesth Analg* 1989;69:518–521.

Dasta JF. Drug use in a surgical intensive care unit. *Drug Intell Clin Pharm* 1986;20:752–756.

Donati F, Antzaka C, Bevan DR. Potency of pancuronium at the diaphragm and the adductor pollicus muscle in humans. *Anesthesiology* 1986;65:1–5.

Durbin Jr CG. Neuromuscular blocking agents and sedative drugs: clinical uses and toxic effects in the critical care unit. *Crit Care Clin* 1991;7:489–506.

Fiamengo SA, Savarese JJ. Use of muscle relaxants in intensive care units. *Crit Care Med* 1991;19:1457–1459.

Giostra E, Magistris MR, Pizzolato G, et al. Neuromuscular disorder in intensive care unit patients treated with pancuronium bromide. Occurrence in a cluster group of seven patients and two sporadic cases, with electrophysiologic and histologic examination. *Chest* 1994;106:10–20.

Gooch JL, Suchyta MR, Balbierz JM, et al. Prolonged paralysis after treatment with neuromuscular junction blocking agents. *Crit Care Med* 1991;19:1125–1131.

Griffin D, Fairman N, Coursin D, et al. Acute myopathy during treatment of status asthmaticus with corticosteroids and steroidal muscle relaxants. *Chest* 1992;102:510–514.

Hansen-Flaschen JH, Brazinsky S, Basile C, et al. Use of sedating drugs and neuromuscular blocking agents in patients requiring mechanical ventilation for respiratory failure: a national survey. *JAMA* 1991;266:2870–2875.

Hansen-Flashen J, Cowen J, Raps E. Neuromuscular blockade in the intensive care unit: more than we bargained for. *Am Rev Respir Dis* 1993;147:234–236.

Hsiang JK, Chesnut RM, Crisp CB, et al. Early, routine paralysis for intracranial pressure control in severe head injury: is it necessary? *Crit Care Med* 1994;22:1471–1476.

Khuenl-Brady KS, Reitstatter B, Schlager A, et al. Long-term administration of pancuronium and pipecuronium in the intensive care unit. *Anesth Analg* 1994;78:1082–1086.

Kim C, Hirose M, Martyn JAJ. d-Tubocurarine accentuates the burn-induced upregulation of nicotinic acetylcholine receptors at the muscle membrane. *Anesthesiology* 1995;83:237–240.

Klessig HT, Geiger HG, Murrary MJ, et al. A national survey on the practice patterns of anesthesiologist intensivists in the use of muscle relaxants. *Crit Care Med* 1992;20:1341–1345.

Kupfer Y, Namba T, Kaldawi E, et al. Prolonged weakness after long-term infusion of vecuronium bromide. *Ann Intern Med* 1992;117:484–486.

Lee C. Intensive care unit neuromuscular syndrome? *Anesthesiology* 1995;83:237–240.

Manthous CA, Chatila W. Prolonged weakness after the withdrawal of atracurium. *Am J Respir Crit Care Med* 1994;150:1441–1443.

Meyer KC, Prielipp RC, Grossman JE, et al. Prolonged weakness after infusion of atracurium in two intensive care unit patients. *Anesth Analg* 1994;78:772–774.

Op de Coul AAW, Lambregts PCLA, Koeman J, et al. Neuromuscular complications in patients given Pavulon (pancuronium bromide) during artificial ventilation. *Clin Neurol Neurosurg* 1985;87:17–22.

Peat SJ, Potter DR, Hunter JM. The prolonged use of atracurium in a patient with tetanus. *Anaesthesia* 1988;43:962–963.

Prielipp RC, Coursin DB, Scuderi PE, et al. Comparison of the infusion requirements and recovery profiles of vecuronium and *cis*-atracurium 51W89 in intensive care unit patients. *Anesth Analg* 1995;81:3–12.

Rudis MI, Sikora CA, Angus E, et al. A prospective, randomized, controlled evaluation of peripheral nerve stimulation versus standard clinical dosing of neuromuscular blocking agents in critically ill patients. *Crit Care Med* 1997;25:575–583.

Segredo V, Caldwell JE, Matthay MA, et al. Persistent paralysis in critically ill patients after long-term administration of vecuronium. *N Engl J Med* 1992;327:524–528.

Sitwell LD, Weinshenker BG, Monpetit V, et al. Complete ophthalmoplegia as a complication of acute corticosteroid—and pancuronium—associated myopathy. *Neurology* 1991;41:921–922.

Smith CL, Hunter JM, Jones RS. Vecuronium infusions in patients with renal failure in an ICU. *Anaesthesia* 1987;42:387–393.

Tobias JD, Lynch A, McDuffee A, et al. Pancuronium infusion for neuromuscular block in children in the pediatric intensive care unit. *Anesth Analg* 1995;81:13–16.

Topulos GP. Neuromuscular blockade in adult intensive care. *New Horizons* 1993;1:447–462.

Wadon AF, Dogra S, Anand S. Atracurium infusion in the intensive care unit. *Br J Anaesth* 1986;58:64S–67S.

Yate PM, Flynn PJ, Arnold RW, et al. Clinical experience and plasma laudanosine concentrations during the infusion of atracurium in the intensive therapy unit. *Br J Anaesth* 1987;59:211–217.

Nutrition

Ralph L. Warren

I. Introduction

A. The science of nutrition remains largely empiric. The nutritional requirements for healthy persons are uncertain—witness all the health, nutrition, and diet books and magazines written in the past few decades. Even Recommended Daily Allowances (RDAs) officially change every year or two. One thing that makes progress in nutritional science difficult is that the effects of nutrition are apparent only over weeks to months. Because so much happens to a critically ill patient during this time, it is difficult to determine the exact effect nutrition has on patient outcome. This chapter provides a practical guide for the critical care practitioner who may not have specialized knowledge in nutrition. Consultation with a nutritional support service can provide important additional information.

II. The basic, general principles for nutrition in the critically ill, which are outlined in **Section III,** can be summarized.

A. *Primum non nocere*

B. Adequate protein administration is probably more important than caloric intake. Try to feed at least 1 g/kg/d [e.g., if fluid restricted or intolerant, give a high nitrogen formula (70 g protein, 210 g CHO)], then increase the protein as tolerated up to 1.5 g/kg/d. Finally, increase caloric intake up to the resting energy expenditure (REE).

C. Feed enterally if possible, even at low rates. This may still supply substrate to the gut mucosa. Make up the additional protein and caloric needs with parenteral nutrition.

III. The basics—step by step

A. **Decide if the patient needs nutritional support:**
   1. No food intake (NPO) expected for more than 7 to 10 days.
   2. Earlier if hypermetabolic (e.g., sepsis, multitrauma).
   3. Pre-existing undernourishment: loss of ≥ 10% of usual body weight.

B. **Estimate basal energy expenditure (BEE) in kcal/day:**
   1. Harris-Benedict equations are often used:
      a. Male: BEE (kcal/d) = $66 + [13.7 \times W] + [5 \times H] - [6.8 \times A]$
      b. Female: BEE (kcal/d) = $665 + [9.6 \times W] + [1.7 \times H] - [4.7 \times A]$
      W, weight in kg; H, height in cm; A, age in years.
   2. Alternative estimates: 850 to 950 kcal/m²/d or 20 to 30 kcal/kg/d.

3. Simple approximations: Body weight = 50 kg → 1300 kcal/d; 60 kg → 1500 kcal/d; 70 kg → 1700 kcal/d; 80 kg → 1900 kcal/d.

C. Estimate REE in kcal/d (Table 8-1): REE = (BEE) × (stress factor)

D. Estimate caloric needs ≅ REE × (activity, fever factor):

1. Muscular work activity (e.g., out of bed, walking, combative, or agitated) increases needs 10% to 25%.
2. Fever increases needs 5% to 10%/°C/d.

E. Decide on enteral versus parenteral route of administration.

1. Enteral route *always* preferred because of trophic effects on gut mucosa.
2. Give *some* enteral feeding, if possible, even if unable to provide all nutritional requirements enterally. Make up the difference with parenteral nutrition.
3. For enteral feeding:
    a. Choose an appropriate enteral formula based on patient and diagnoses.
    b. Choose rate to meet caloric needs.
    c. Additives as desired: vitamins, glutamine, and so forth.

F. Determine protein needs.

1. One gram nitrogen = 6.25 g protein.
2. Normal ≅ 1 g/kg/d protein.
3. Multiply by stress factors as above, maximum ≈ 2.0 to 2.5 g/kg/d. In burns and open wounds, more protein is lost from wound itself ⇒ administer up to 3.5 g/kg/d maximum.
4. An alternative method: [caloric needs (kcal)]/150 = nitrogen needed, or 6.25 × (kcal/150) = protein needed.
    a. Most formulas are "1:150" (i.e., 1 g nitrogen for every 150 nonprotein kcal).
    b. A normal average diet is 1:300.
    c. A ratio of 1:350 during relative starvation will conserve protein.
    d. Some nutritionists advocate a ratio of 1:100.
5. The 1:150 diet has 25 kcal [(1 g) × (6.25 g protein/g nitrogen) × (4 kcal/g)] from protein for every 150

Table 8-1.   Stress factors

Stress factor	
Major operation, no complications	1.0–1.1
Moderate trauma; moderate peritonitis	1.25
Severe injury/infection/organ failure	1.3–1.6
Burn ≥40% of body surface area	2.0

nonprotein kcal, or 17% of total calories from protein.

G. **Determine nonprotein calories.**

    1. **Carbohydrate:** ~ 60% (maximal glucose in critically ill patients ≈ 400 to 500 g/d, or a maximal infusion rate of 4 to 5 mg/kg/min).

    2. **Fat:** ≥ 3% and ≤ 30% of total calories (up to 40% to 50% in septic patients).

    3. **Optimal ratio** of carbohydrate:fat *calories* is ~ 70:30.

H. **Insulin**

    1. Administered according to serum glucose levels and administered glucose concentration.

    2. Standard total parenteral nutrition (TPN) has 210 g glucose/L; fluid restricted formula has 250 g/L; renal formula has 280 g/L.

    3. Estimated initial insulin requirements:

        a. Serum glucose > 150 mg/dl ⇒ 10 U/250 g carbohydrate.

        b. Serum glucose > 200 mg/dl ⇒ 20 to 25 U/250 g carbohydrate.

        c. Serum glucose > 250 mg/dl ⇒ 30 to 50 U/250 g carbohydrate.

I. **Electrolytes**

    1. **Sodium (Na), potassium (K), calcium (Ca), magnesium (Mg), chlorine (Cl), acetate (Co_2), and phosphorus (PO_4)** are administered according to measured serum levels.

    2. **Sodium:** 60 to 150 mEq/d (usually 100–120; decrease for volume overload and severe malnutrition).

    3. **Potassium:** 30 to 100 mEq/d, maximal concentration 80 mEq/L.

    4. Start with equal amounts of chloride and acetate.

    5. **High Cl losses** (e.g., nasogastric suction): administer more Cl.

    6. **High bicarbonate losses (e.g., diarrhea), acidosis:** administer more acetate.

    7. **Amino acids** in TPN are administered as hydrochloric acid (HCl) salts. If hyperchloremic acidosis results, add more acetate.

    8. **Calcium** (as gluconate): 5 to 15 mmol/d.

    9. **Magnesium** (as SO_4): 8 to 20 mmol/d.

    10. **Phosphorus:** 12 to 24 mmol/d.

J. **Vitamins, minerals, and trace elements** are already in enteral formulas, but are added to parenteral nutrition. See Tables 8-2 and 8-3 for recommended amounts.

IV. **Further considerations**

A. **Assessment**

    1. No single measurement of body indices or blood chemistry is either sensitive or specific for identifying malnutrition. The history and physical examination remain the best indicators: Has there been an unintentional weight loss (5% in 1 month,

Table 8-2.   Vitamin supplementation for total parenteral nutrition

Vitamin	RDA	MGH TPN
A (retinol), IU	3,300	3,000
As β-carotene, mg (6 μg = 1 RE)	15	—
3.3 IU retinol = 1 μg RE = 10 IU β-carotene	—	—
D (ergocalciferol), IU	400	200
Cholecalciferol, μg, (40 IU = 1 μg)	10	—
E (α-tocopherol), IU (15 IU = 10 mg)	30	10
K, μg/kg	1	None
B_1 (thiamine), mg	1.5	3.0
B_2 (riboflavin), mg	1.7	3.6
B_6 (pyridoxine), mg	2	4.0
B_{12} (cobalamin), μg	2	5.0
Niacin, mg	20	40
Pantothenic acid, mg	10	15
Folate, μg	400	400
Biotin, μg	100	60
C, mg	60	600

RDA, recommended daily allowance; MGH, Massachusetts General Hospital; TPN, total parenteral nutrition; IU, international unit; RE, retinol equivalent.

Table 8-3.   Trace element additives

Trace elements (mg)	RDA (oral)	RDA (IV)	MGH TPN
Zinc	15	2.5–5	5
Copper	2.0	0.5–1.5	1
Manganese	2.5–5	0.15–0.8	0.5
Chromium	0.02	0.01–0.015	0.01
Iron	10–18	3.0	None
Iodine	0.15	0.075	—
Selenium	0.07	—	0.06
Fluorine	2.0	—	None
Molybdenum	0.2	—	None

RDA, recommended daily allowance; MGH, Massachusetts General Hospital; TPN, total parenteral nutrition.

7.5% in 3, 10% in 6 months)? Has there been pre-existing inadequate intake, absorption, or both, or increased losses? What is the anticipated length of time before sufficient intake will resume?

2. **Serum markers** have variable half-lives in the circulation:
   a. Albumin: $t_{1/2}$ = 20 days.
   b. Transferrin: $t_{1/2}$ = 8 days.
   c. Prealbumin: $t_{1/2}$ = 1 day.
   d. Retinol binding protein: $t_{1/2}$ = 1/2 day.

3. Major but uncomplicated elective surgery increases REE by less than 10%. If the patient is hypermetabolic (e.g., sepsis, head injury), err on the side of earlier nutritional support. Note that males have almost three times more variation in BEE with height, and more variation with both age and weight, than females.

B. **Protein**
   1. **Protein provides 4 kcal/g,** and is associated with a respiratory quotient (RQ) of 0.8. In general, 15% to 25% of calories should come from protein. We cannot eliminate hypercatabolism in a sick patient, but we can support anabolism. It takes 70 g protein to make the first day's acute phase reactants, and 30 g/d protein to sustain a white blood cell (WBC) count of $30 \times 10^3/mm^3$. Note also that cortisol's primary metabolic effect is to increase protein catabolism into amino acids.

   2. **Essential amino acids (AAs)** for humans are leucine, isoleucine, valine (the branched-chain AAs or BCAAs); lysine, threonine, tryptophan, histidine; methionine (metabolized to cysteine); phenylalanine (metabolized to tyrosine). Arginine and glutamine are considered by some experts to be conditionally essential, especially during times of stress. What is the optimal mix of AAs to administer? Many experts believe that it should be the same as that which is released by skeletal muscle during fasting or stress: one fourth to one third glutamine, one fourth to one third alanine (the principal precursor for hepatic gluconeogenesis), and one fourth essential AAs.

   3. **Nitrogen balance** can be calculated by the formula:

$$N \ loss(g/d) = 1.2 \times [UUN \ (mg/dl) \times UO(ml/d)$$
$$\times 1g/1000 \, mg \times 1dl/100 \, ml] + 2 \, g/d$$

N, nitrogen; UUN, urinary urea nitrogen; UO, urine output

Urea accounts for 80% of nitrogen lost in urine (the rest being NH_4 and NO_3). Nitrogen loss $\approx$ (UUN + 4). The extra 2 g/d are for stool and skin losses (2–4 g/d gastrointestinal, 0–4 g/d skin). Desired nitrogen balance is +2–4 g/d.

4. **Glutamine** is the primary fuel for gut mucosal enterocytes and perhaps for leukocytes. It also serves in nitrogen transport and excretion. Glutamine is unstable in solution beyond a day or two and, therefore, is not present in most TPN solutions or enteral feeds. Glutamine-enhanced TPN at the Massachusetts General Hospital has glutamine comprising 28% of the total AAs (11 g/L). Glutamine (10 gm) can be given enterally three times daily, easily and inexpensively.

5. **Arginine**, which is an immunomodulator that can enhance the depressed immune response in sick patients, is a component of many research TPN solutions. Its use is avoided in transplant patients.

C. **Carbohydrate**

1. **Anhydrous glucose** yields 4 kcal/g; hydrated carbohydrate (CHO) (dextrose = hydrated glucose) gives 3.4 kcal/g and an RQ of 1.0. For TPN, the optimal rate of glucose infusion is approximately 4 mg/kg/min (80 ml/h for 70 kg). Carbohydrate sufficient to meet 25% of BEE (in normal patients, or 50% of BEE in hypermetabolic or stressed patients) prevents the use of the patient's endogenous proteins for gluconeogenesis. The brain, red cells, renal medulla, and bone marrow, which are all obligate glucose users, require 125 g/d glucose. Manufacturing this amount of glucose via gluconeogenesis would require 250 g of protein.

2. **Excess carbohydrates** cause hyperosmolarity, hyperglycemia, water retention, hypercarbia, increased ventilatory drive, and increased difficulties weaning from the ventilator. Moreover, excess CHO is converted into fat and deposited in the liver, causing hepatic steatosis (triglycerides fill the hepatocyte vacuoles). A good rule is to keep glucose infusion less than 5 mg/kg/min (< 100 ml/h of standard TPN for a 70-kg adult), especially in cases of any glucose intolerance or difficulty in weaning from the ventilator. Standard TPN is 21% dextrose (21 g/100 ml).

3. Patients on dialysis absorb significant amounts of glucose from the dialysate. For peritoneal dialysis, assume that 50% of instilled glucose is absorbed, and check the effluent glucose level for a better estimate. For continuous venovenous hemofiltration or dialysis, if the replacement fluid is 1.5% glucose, assume that 80% to 90% is absorbed; again, check the outflow glucose level for a better estimate. Alternative replacement fluids such as citrate or bicarbonate solutions are available.

D. **Fat**

1. **Fat has a high caloric density.** Triglycerides (= 1 glycerol + 3 fatty acids) yield 9 kcal/g, and an RQ of 0.7. The only essential fatty acids are linoleic

(18:2 ω6) and linolenic (18:3 ω6) acids. Both are long-chain polyunsaturated fatty acids (PUFA). Essential fatty acid deficiency causes impaired wound healing and decreased immune function. To prevent deficiency, at least 3% of total kilocalories should be from fat (linoleic acid).

2. **Excess fat administration** causes hyperlipidemia, hypoxemia, immunosuppression, and increases susceptibility to infection secondary to reduced reticuloendothelial function. Administer ≥ 0.5 mg fat/kg/d to avoid too much CHO, but restrict fat to $\leq 30\%$ of total calories (or $\leq 50\%$ if renal failure or difficulty weaning). Measure the serum triglycerides twice a week. The amount of lipids administered may have to be decreased if the patient is intolerant.

3. **Propofol emulsion** contains 0.1 g fat (1.1 kcal)/ml.

E. **Vitamins and trace elements**

1. **The fat-soluble vitamins,** A, D, E, K, can produce toxicity because they are stored in adipose tissue and high concentrations can be accumulated. **The water-soluble vitamins** are C, B complex (B_1, B_2, B_6, B_{12}, niacin, pantothenic acid, biotin), and folate; do not give more than 10 times the RDA (except perhaps for vitamin C).

2. **Deficiencies of vitamins A, Bs, C, and Zn** can impair wound healing.

3. **Vitamin E** decreases the oxidation of fatty acids (especially polyunsaturated fatty acids).

   a. Greater than 800 mg/d may slightly increase the prothrombin time.

   b. **Deficiencies** of vitamin E are caused by malabsorption. Vitamin E deficiency can produce muscular dystrophy in animals and neuropathy and encephalopathy in children. In G6PD-deficient patients, anemia may occur.

   c. **Vitamin E** (400 to 600 mg/d) can be administered enterally in critically ill patients.

4. **Zinc** deficiency occurs in alcoholics; pancreatic insufficiency, malabsorption, short bowel syndrome, gastrointestinal fistulas, renal failure with dialysis; nephrosis, burns and, large wounds.

   a. **Symptoms of zinc deficiency** include impaired wound healing, dermatitis, alopecia, depressed immune function, diarrhea, depression, and hypogeusia.

   b. **Zinc toxicity** can occur if more than 300 mg/d are administered orally or 90 mg/d are administered intravenously. Signs and symptoms include flushing, sweating, blurred vision, and immunosuppression.

   c. Supplementation can be administered intravenously (50 mg/d for 5 days in critically ill adult patients) or enterally by administering zinc sulfate (220 mg three times daily is equivalent to 150 mg/d of zinc). An additional 12 mg per liter of small bowel drainage or 17 mg per liter of stool or ileostomy output can be administered.

5. **Iron** supplementation is rarely necessary for patients in the ICU. Total body iron stores are usually adequate.

6. **Selenium** is important for antioxidant activity. Deficiencies can occur with malabsorption syndromes and enteral fistulas. Symptoms include muscle weakness and cardiomyopathy. Selenium supplementation can be provided by administering 70 to 200 µg/d in a critically ill adult.

F. **Modified parenteral formulas**

1. **Renal failure** formulas include an increased concentration of carbohydrates, which can reduce protein breakdown in catabolic patients better than fat. Protein requirements are approximately 1 to 1.2 g/kg/d while on hemodialysis and 1.2 to 1.5 g/kg/d while on peritoneal dialysis. Supplement vitamins every other day.

2. **Fluid-restricted** formulas are higher in fat than renal failure formulas: 60% to 70% of kilocalories are from carbohydrates, 30% to 40% from fat.

3. **Hepatic failure** formulas include increased concentrations of branched chain amino acids and no aromatic amino acids.

V. **Indirect calorimetry**

A. **Goals** for performing indirect calorimetry include ensuring that adequate caloric intake is being provided, while avoiding overfeeding.

B. **Metabolic rate (kcal/h).**

$$= \dot{V}O_2(ml/min) \times 60\,min/h \times 1L/1000\,ml \times 4.83\,kcal/L$$

$$= 3.9 \times \dot{V}O_2(L/H) + 1.1 \times \dot{V}CO_2$$

C. **Oxygen consumption (VO_2):**

1. $\dot{V}O_2$ (ml/min) = CO (L/min) $\times$ [CaO_2 (ml/L) $-$ $C\bar{v}O_2$ (ml/L)]

2. Normal $\dot{V}O_2$ is approximately 250 ml/min (3.5 ml/kg/min).

3. Normal CO_2 production ($\dot{V}CO_2$) is approximately 200 ml/min (2.6 ml/kg/min).

D. **Requirements**

1. If intubated, $FIO_2 \le 0.6$. Breathing air if not intubated.

2. Measurements are most repeatable when the patient is resting and supine, fasting for more than 2 hours, or receiving nutrition by a constant infusion.

3. Sources of error include gas leaks (e.g., endotracheal tube cuff leak, bronchopleural fistula), vari-

able patient activity, and calibration errors of the equipment.

E. **Respiratory quotient (RQ)** = $\dot{V}co_2/\dot{V}o_2 = \dot{V}e(Feco_2)/[\dot{V}i(Fio_2) - \dot{V}e(Feo_2)]$

1. CHO 1.0.
2. Protein 0.82.
3. Fat 0.71.
4. Mixed diet 0.85.
5. Ketosis 0.67 to 0.70.
6. Lipogenesis 1.0 to 1.2.

VI. **Enteral feeding**

A. Most enteral formulas are 1 kcal/ml and lactose free. Carbohydrates are provided by oligosaccharides, polysaccharides, and maltodextrins; fat is supplied by medium and long-chain triglycerides, the protein provided is intact or partially hydrolyzed (Table 8-4).

1. **Elemental formulas** provide protein as crystalline amino acids. They generally include simple sugars (mono-, di-, oligosaccharides), provide essential fatty acids and medium-chain triglycerides, and are hypertonic (see Table 8-4).

2. **"Stress" formulas** (e.g., Impact) have increased concentrations of branched-chain amino acids (leucine, isoleucine, valine), which can be used directly by tissues. Other amino acids require hepatic deamination first.

3. **Hepatic formulas** (e.g., Hepatic-Aid) have increased concentrations of branched-chain amino acids, reduced methionine concentrations, and reduced concentrations of aromatic amino acids (phenylalanine, tyrosine, tryptophan), which are precursors of false neurotransmitters.

4. **Renal formulas** (e.g., Nepro) have decreased protein concentrations. They include only essential amino acids.

B. **Gastric feedings** buffer gastric pH. Sucralfate can be used for additional prophylaxis for gastric ulceration.

C. **For jejunal feedings,** start with one-half strength formulas, especially if the osmolality of the formula is greater than 300 mmol/kg.

D. **For diarrhea:**

1. Check for the presence of *Clostridium difficile* toxin. If present, treat with enteral flagyl or vancomycin or intravenous flagyl.

2. Decrease the rate of feeding or the osmolality (not both).

3. Check for the presence of sorbitol in medications, which can cause an osmotic diarrhea.

4. **Kaopectate** (30 ml orally every 4 hours) may provide symptomatic relief. Consider **Immodium** if other measures are ineffective and the stool is negative for *C. difficile*.

5. **Malabsorption** can be assessed by specialized testing.

Table 8-4.   Common enteral formulas

Formula	Calories/ml	Comments
Alitraq	1.0	Elemental; increased protein, high glutamine (14 g/L), arginine, 13% kcal fat; osmolality 575 mmol/kg
Ensure plus HN	1.5	Low residue; fluid-restricted formula
Glucerna	1.0	Reduced carbohydrates for diabetics with poor glucose tolerance
Impact	1.0	Includes ω-3 fatty acids, arginine, and glutamine
Jevity	1.06	17% of kcal as protein (44.4 g/l); 53% kcal as CHO, 30% kcal as fat; osmolality 310 mmol/kg; lactose-free polymeric, isosmolar, low residue
Lipisorb	1.35	Reduced fat; fat supplied as medium chain triglycerides, indicated for fat malabsorption
Nepro	2.0	High calorie, low electrolyte; high osmolality, fluid-restricted formula for dialysis patients
Osmolite	1.06	Low residue; reduced protein and potassium
Osmolite HN	1.06	Low residue; similar to Jevity, but without fiber
Promote	1.0	High protein (25% kcal); indicated in burns, open wounds
Suplena	2.0	High calorie, low electrolyte; reduced protein, fluid-restricted formula for patients with renal failure not on dialysis
Vital HN	1.0	Elemental; increased fat (10% kcal); osmolality 500 mmol/kg
Vivonex Plus	1.0	Elemental; 33% branched chain amino acids; increased carbohydrates, low fat; osmolality 650 mmol/kg

SELECTED REFERENCES

Marano MA, Lowry SF. Enteral and parenteral nutrition. In: Barie PS, Shires GT, eds. *Surgical intensive care.* Boston: Little, Brown and Company, 1993:907–923.

Moore FA, Feliciano DV, Andrassy RJ. Early enteral feeding, compared with parenteral, reduces postoperative septic complications. The results of a meta-analysis. *Ann Surg* 1992;216:172–183.

Souba WW. How should we evaluate the efficacy of nutritional support? *J Trauma* 1997;42:343–344.

Souba WW. Nutritional support. *N Engl J Med* 1997;336:41–48.

Hypotension and Shock

John L. Chow, Keith Baker, and
Luca M. Bigatello

I. **Hemodynamic instability** requires treatment in the intensive care unit (ICU), where patients can receive appropriate monitoring and resuscitative measures. Frequent causes of hemodynamic instability include hypotension, dysrhythmias, hypertension, myocardial ischemia, infarction and failure. The physiologic determinants of hemodynamic instability are outlined in Chapter 1 and its pharmacologic treatment in Chapter 10. This chapter outlines the pathophysiology and management of the most severe manifestation of hemodynamic instability, **circulatory shock.**

II. **Shock** is a syndrome of **hypotension and decreased tissue perfusion.** Initially, neurohumoral compensatory mechanisms maintain perfusion to vital organs. If appropriate treatment is not promptly instituted, these compensatory mechanisms are overwhelmed, producing ischemia, cellular damage, multiple organ failure, and death. Shock is classified on the basis of its cause and characteristic hemodynamic patterns (Table 9-1).

   A. **Hypovolemic shock** is caused by an acute loss of more than 20% to 25% of the circulating blood volume.

   B. **Cardiogenic shock** is caused by primary failure of the heart to generate an adequate cardiac output.

   C. **Distributive shock** is characterized by decreased vascular tone resulting in arterial vasodilation, venous pooling, and redistribution of blood flow. It may be caused by any of the following: live bacteria and their byproducts during **septic shock,** mediators of the **systemic inflammatory response syndrome (SIRS)** (see Chapter 27), vasoactive compounds during **anaphylactic shock,** or loss of vascular tone during **neurogenic shock.**

   D. **Obstructive shock** is associated with a mechanical impediment to venous return, arterial outflow of the heart, or both. Causes include tension pneumothorax, pulmonary embolism, pericardial tamponade, abdominal compartment syndrome, and, occasionally, positive-pressure ventilation (see Chapters 2, 17, and 33).

III. **Pathophysiology of shock**

   A. **Tissue hypoperfusion** secondary to prolonged hypotension or decreased O_2 delivery leads to tissue hypoxia, anaerobic metabolism, and disruption of cellular integrity. This cellular injury is the basis for the functional abnormalities of individual organs described

Table 9-1.   Hemodynamic parameters in shock

Type of shock	Systemic pressure	CVP	PAOP	CO/SV
Hypovolemic	↓	↓	↓	↓
Cardiogenic				
Left ventricular	↓	↔	↑	↓
Right ventricular	↓	↑	↔/↓	↓
Distributive				
Septic	↓	↔	↔	↑
Anaphylactic	↓	↓	↓	↔/↑
Neurogenic	↓	↓	↓	↔
Obstructive	↓	↑	↑[a]	↓

CVP, central venous pressure; PAOP, pulmonary artery occlusion pressure; CO, cardiac output; SV, stroke volume.

[a] In pulmonary embolism, pulmonary artery pressure is elevated, but PAOP can be low.

in section **III. D.** Paradoxically, cellular injury is worsened during tissue reperfusion, when excess O_2, local metabolites, and oxidative enzymes generate O_2 **free radicals** and other cytotoxic products.

B.   **Neurohumoral responses** to hypotension increase sympathetic discharge through carotid **baroreceptors,** which enhance myocardial contractility and peripheral vasoconstriction. Hypotension also induces release of **stress hormones** such as catecholamines, glucagon, aldosterone, adrenocorticotropic hormone, and antidiuretic hormone. The ultimate effect is to maintain perfusion pressure by vasoconstriction and enhanced myocardial contractility and to increase distal tubular reabsorption of sodium and water to preserve circulating volume.

C.   **Metabolic responses.** The effects of anti-insulin hormones (e.g., glucagon, epinephrine, and glucocorticoids) promote insulin resistance, hyperglycemia, and lipolysis. Inflammatory mediators and cellular hypoxia cause muscle proteolysis, which provides amino acids necessary to sustain liver protein synthesis essential for host defense and survival (e.g., acute phase reactants). This generalized **catabolic state** causes muscle wasting and weakness, poor wound healing, loss of gastrointestinal (GI) mucosal integrity, hypoalbuminemia, and anergy.

D.   **Effect of shock on specific organ systems**
1.   **Central nervous system (CNS).** Confusion and obtundation are indications of inadequate cerebral perfusion. Pituitary dysfunction can lead to diabetes insipidus (**DI**). Rarely, vasomotor and ventilatory control can fail because of decreased blood supply to centers within the brainstem.

2. **Cardiovascular system.** Hypoperfusion and hypoxemia predispose to myocardial ischemia, impaired contractility, and dysrhythmias. Myocardial dysfunction can also occur as a consequence of circulating myocardial depressant substances.

3. **Respiratory system. Acute respiratory failure** can manifest early in the course of circulatory shock. The anatomy of the lungs exposes them to all circulating toxins and mediators of cellular injury. Vasoconstrictor substances (e.g., thromboxane and prostaglandins of the lipo-oxygenase pathway) can cause bronchospasm and acute pulmonary hypertension with consequent ventilation–perfusion mismatch and pulmonary edema. This initial acute lung injury often evolves in the **acute respiratory distress syndrome** (see Chapter 20).

4. **Renal system.** Circulating catecholamines, vasoconstrictor prostaglandins, and angiotensin contribute to renal arteriolar vasoconstriction, decreased glomerular filtration, and redistribution of blood flow from the cortex to the medulla, an area at high risk for ischemia. **Nephrotoxic agents** [e.g., aminoglycoside antibiotics and intravenous (IV) contrast agents] can exacerbate the effects of these physiologic responses and cause **acute tubular necrosis.**

5. **GI system.** Splanchnic hypoperfusion can damage the GI mucosa and predispose to **translocation** of bacteria and their toxic byproducts from the gut lumen into the portal circulation. This can produce bacteremia, gram-negative sepsis, and, ultimately, **multiple organ dysfunction syndrome (MODS).** Splanchnic hypoperfusion also can cause GI hemorrhage, gastroparesis, ileus, acute pancreatitis, and hepatic failure. The onset of hepatic failure usually is an ominous sign, because of the multiple synthetic and clearance functions of the liver.

6. **Hematologic system.** In various shock states, platelets and clotting factors may be depleted by dilution, consumption [e.g., **disseminated intravascular coagulation (DIC)**], or adverse drug reactions [e.g., **heparin-induced thrombocytopenia (HIT)**]. Platelet dysfunction without thrombocytopenia can be caused by hypothermia, sepsis, and uremia (see Chapter 12).

IV. **Initial management of shock**

A. **General measures,** which are initiated along with treatment of the underlying cause of shock, include control of the airway, volume resuscitation, and treatment of hypotension and acidemia.

1. **The airway (see Chapter 3)** must be secured by endotracheal intubation if its patency is in jeopardy (e.g., in anaphylactic shock with airway

edema), if risk of aspiration exists (e.g., local trauma, altered mental status), or if long-term mechanical ventilation is required.

2. **Positive-pressure ventilation (see Chapter 4)** may be required to treat hypoxemia and ventilatory depression. Caution must be exercised when instituting positive-pressure ventilation in a hypovolemic patient, because the increase of intrathoracic pressure can impede venous return and reduce cardiac output.

3. **Peripheral IV access.** Short, large-bore catheters (e.g., percutaneous sheath introducers, peripheral venous rapid infusion catheters, 12-gauge double lumen hemodialysis catheters, and 14-gauge peripheral cannulas) permit rapid volume administration. Central venous access can be helpful for monitoring and for rapid drug administration.

4. **Standard monitoring** includes continuous electrocardiographic (ECG) monitoring, pulse oximetry, noninvasive measurement of systemic blood pressure, urinary output, and core temperature (see Chapters 1 and 2).

5. **Indications for invasive monitoring**
   a. **Intraarterial** pressure monitoring, which is the most reliable method to measure blood pressure, should be used in patients with unstable or rapidly changing hemodynamics.
   b. **Central venous pressure (CVP)** measurement is a useful reflection of systemic and central volume status when significant left ventricular dysfunction is absent.
   c. **Pulmonary artery (PA) pressure** measurement with a PA catheter allows measurement of cardiac output and assessment of left and right ventricular performance. Although the utility of PA catheters has been questioned, the physiologic information provided by a PA catheter is of unique utility when properly interpreted (see Chapter 1).
   d. **Monitoring for early signs of cellular and tissue injury** would be ideal. **Metabolic acidemia** is a sign of anaerobic metabolism, but is nonspecific and often occurs as a late sign of shock. Reversible signs of cellular injury can include a high serum **lactate** concentration and a low **mixed venous** Po_2. A low **gastric intramucosal pH (pH_i),** measured via a specially designed nasogastric tube, has been suggested to be an early sign of splanchnic hypoperfusion and a useful parameter to measure during resuscitation of patients in shock. None of these parameters has been proved to be specific, reliable, or of clinical utility in the care of patients with shock.

6. The **Trendelenburg position** reduces cerebral perfusion pressure, impedes ventilation, and has minimal benefit on cardiac output, compared with the supine position. Its use as a general resuscitative maneuver is not recommended.

V. **Hypovolemic shock**

A. **Etiology. Hemorrhage** can be external or concealed (e.g., long bone fractures, retroperitoneal bleeding, and hemothorax). *Nonhemorrhagic* causes include fluid losses through the GI tract (e.g., vomiting, diarrhea, gastric suctioning and fistulas), the urinary system (e.g., polyuria from diuretics, osmotic loads, and DI), the skin (e.g., burns), and through "leaky" capillaries during inflammation and sepsis.

B. **Pathophysiology.** The physiologic hallmark of hypovolemic shock is decreased venous return to the heart and, consequently, decreased stroke volume, cardiac output, and systemic blood pressure. Central venous pressure, PA pressure, and PA occlusion pressure (PAOP) are low.

C. **Clinical presentation.** The severity of hypovolemic shock is a function of the volume deficit, the rate of volume loss, and the patient's premorbid status. Physical examination reveals thready pulses, flat neck veins, and cold, clammy skin.

D. **Differential diagnosis.** Similar signs of peripheral hypoperfusion are present in **cardiogenic shock.** Diagnosis of cardiogenic shock derives from the clinical history, jugular veins distention (JVD), and pulmonary congestion. In **neurogenic** and **anaphylactic** shock, relative hypovolemia is caused by vasodilation. Thus, signs of peripheral hypoperfusion are less marked and volume administration alone often does not reverse hypotension. In **hypoglycemic coma,** symptoms are very similar; a history of diabetes mellitus and insulin therapy guides the diagnosis. Ischemia-reperfusion injuries associated with prolonged or severe hypovolemic shock can serve as a trigger for the **SIRS**, which can be heralded by hypotension that is refractory to volume repletion, disseminated intravascular coagulation, and end-organ failure.

E. **Management**

1. **Volume replacement** is the cornerstone of treatment (see Chapter 33 for additional details). Regardless of the cause of hypovolemia and of the type of fluid employed, volume resuscitation must be prompt to prevent organ hypoperfusion and damage. Side effects of massive volume replacement, namely **tissue edema,** generally are acceptable and reversible complications. In patients at risk for volume-related complications [i.e., those with a history of congestive heart failure (CHF)], invasive monitoring should guide volume resusci-

tation. Normal **body temperature** and **coagulation function** must be maintained. Hypothermia, in particular, is frequent in hypovolemic shock and predisposes to dysrhythmias, coagulopathies, and immunosuppression. Prevention and reversal of hypothermia is achieved by increasing ambient temperature, using fluid warmers, and warm forced air blankets.

a. Commonly used **crystalloid** solutions are **lactated Ringer's (LR)** and **normal saline solution.** Crystalloids rapidly leave the intravascular space. A volume equal to three to four times the intravascular deficit must be infused to restore circulating volume. The advantages of isotonic crystalloid solutions include low cost, easy storage, and availability. Dextrose-containing solutions should not be used in the initial phase of rapid volume resuscitation, because of difficulties adequately monitoring blood glucose levels and the dangers of hyperglycemia. **Hypertonic saline** (3% NaCl), which can replete intravascular volume without significantly increasing extravascular volume, may be useful in the resuscitation of patients with head injuries with cerebral edema. The use of hypertonic saline has not reached widespread acceptance for routine resuscitation.

b. **Colloid solutions** increase plasma oncotic pressure and maintain circulating volume longer than crystalloids.

(1) **Hydroxyethyl starch** is a synthetic polymer of amylopectin, available in 6% **(Hetastarch)** and 5% **(Pentastarch)** solutions. Volume expansion persists for variable periods (3–24 hours) because of the different molecular weights of the starch fragments in solution, which are eliminated by the kidney at various rates. Hetastarch particles have been observed in hepatic histiocytes weeks after administration, but have not been associated with any pathologic effect. Hetastarch doses greater than **20 ml/kg** (1–1.5 L in adults) can cause a decrease of Factor VIII levels and platelet function.

(2) **Dextran** is a solution of synthetic glucose polymers of either 40 kd (D-40) or 70 kd (D-70). The main disadvantage of dextran is a high incidence of anaphylactic reactions (1% to 5%) compared with hetastarch.

(3) **Human albumin** is available as 5% and 25% solutions in saline. Human albumin

is heat treated, which eliminates the risk of transmission of viral infections. In critically ill patients, albumin has no proven advantage over crystalloid solutions or synthetic colloids. Given its high cost, it should be reserved for specific indications, mainly as replacement for massive albumin losses.

(4) **Blood products,** such as packed **red cells** and **fresh frozen plasma,** are used to expand intravascular volume in patients experiencing blood loss. Blood products can transmit infectious diseases; they are expensive and in scarce supply. Components should be transfused to treat specific conditions (i.e., anemia with packed red cells and coagulopathy with plasma). (See Chapter 12 for further information concerning transfusion practices.)

(5) **Vasopressors and inotropes** have a role only as temporizing measures to maintain organ perfusion pressure until an intravascular volume deficit can be repleted.

VI. Cardiogenic shock

A. Etiology. Causes of cardiogenic shock include myocardial infarction and its acute complications (e.g., rupture of a papillary muscle, the interventricular septum, or the myocardial free wall), dysrhythmias, acute myocarditis, cardiac contusion, pharmacologic depressants, proximal aortic dissection, and pulmonary embolism.

B. Pathophysiology. The physiologic hallmark of cardiogenic shock is an acute **decrease of myocardial contractility** causing a decrease of stroke volume, cardiac output, and systemic blood pressure. Central venous pressure, PA pressure, and PAOP are increased.

C. Clinical presentation. Cardiogenic shock is the result of a severe primary event, such as massive myocardial infarction or pulmonary embolism. **The risk of mortality is very high.** Common features include hypotension with cutaneous vasoconstriction, cold and mottled extremities, cyanosis, and hypoxemia. Other signs can include JVD, a new heart murmur, an S_3 gallop, a pericardial rub, and pulmonary rales.

D. Differential diagnosis. The physical signs of hypervolemia are generally sufficient to rule out **hypovolemic shock.** The signs of peripheral hypoperfusion differentiate this clinical picture from the "warm shock" of **sepsis.** Invasive monitoring generally is diagnostic; the combination of systemic hypotension, low cardiac output, and high central pressures is characteristic.

E.   Management. The therapeutic objectives in cardiogenic shock include improving cardiac output, maintaining sinus rhythm, and restoring organ perfusion pressure.

1. **Inotropic agents** are used to improve cardiac output (see Chapter 10). When tolerated, the addition of a vasodilator to reduce ventricular "afterload" may improve peripheral perfusion.

   a. **Dobutamine** improves cardiac contractility and decreases vascular tone. The combination of these two effects makes dobutamine an excellent agent for the treatment of cardiogenic shock. Limitations to the use of dobutamine are its intrinsic vasodilator effect, which can cause systemic hypotension, and its mild chronotropic effect.

   b. **Dopamine** is a moderate inotrope at intermediate doses and has no significant vasoconstrictive effect until high doses are reached. Its predictable chronotropic and prodysrhythmic effects limit its use in patients with ongoing or underlying myocardial ischemia.

   c. **Dopexamine** has a similar hemodynamic profile to dopamine but lacks β activity, thus producing minimal chronotropic and prodysrhythmic effects. Experience with dopexamine in the United States is limited.

   d. **Norepinephrine** and **epinephrine** provide potent inotropic and vasoconstrictor effects.

   e. **Phosphodiesterase inhibitors. Amrinone** and **milrinone** have positive inotropic and vasodilator effects that are similar to those of dobutamine.

2. **Vasodilators** can be beneficial in the treatment of cardiogenic shock if systemic blood pressure is preserved (see Chapter 10). Various vasodilators can be used, including **nitrates, labetalol, or angiotensin converting enzyme (ACE) inhibitors** such as captopril or enalaprilat. Vasodilator therapy can be initiated alone or in combination with inotropic agents. Hemodynamics should be monitored continuously during this time.

3. **Intravenous sedatives and analgesics** such as **benzodiazepines** and **opioids** can reduce myocardial oxygen consumption by decreasing preload, vascular tone, and sympathetic discharge.

4. **Intraaortic balloon counterpulsation** augments diastolic coronary perfusion pressure and decreases afterload. It is effective in patients with acute CHF and unstable angina (see Chapter 13).

5. **Thrombolysis, percutaneous transluminal coronary angioplasty (PTCA),** and **cardiac surgical interventions** can also be considered in patients with cardiogenic shock secondary to

acute myocardial infarction (see Chapters 17, 18, and 36).

VII. Distributive shock
A. Septic shock
1. **Etiology.** Sepsis can produce refractory hypotension and organ failure (see Chapter 27).
2. **Pathophysiology.** Septic shock is characterized by systemic **hypotension** and, usually, a normal or increased stroke volume and cardiac output. Reversible acute myocardial dysfunction can occur from circulating myocardial depressant factors. Central venous pressure, PA pressure, and PAOP may be normal or variable, depending on the patient's volume status and degree of myocardial dysfunction. When fluid resuscitation is adequate, septic shock is characterized by a **hyperdynamic circulation,** with an increased cardiac output (6 to 12 L/min) and low systemic blood pressure. Acute pulmonary hypertension from circulating endotoxin and vasoconstrictive mediators may be present. These distributive abnormalities of systemic and pulmonary blood flow result in decreased tissue O_2 supply, hypoxemia, and acidemia.
3. **Clinical presentation** includes hypotension, fever or hypothermia, and other typical features of infection (see Chapter 27) associated with signs of organ dysfunction (e.g., oliguria, acidemia, hypoxemia, thrombocytopenia, and altered mental status).
4. **Differential diagnosis** with other forms of shock is fairly straightforward in the presence of a hyperdynamic circulation. Other conditions, however, can cause a hyperdynamic circulation (e.g., **cirrhosis, hyperthyroidism,** and **arteriovenous fistulas**).
5. **Management**
   a. **Circulatory support** is directed to improve organ perfusion and O_2 delivery.
      (1) **Volume resuscitation** as described in section **V.E.1.** is required to replace intravascular fluids lost to ongoing capillary leakage and to counter the increased volume of capacitance vessels. Invasive monitoring is helpful in cases of severe shock. Volume administration is titrated to the lowest filling pressures that produce the maximal stroke volume (see Chapter 1).
      (2) Once volume resuscitation is achieved, **vasopressors** are used to preserve an adequate mean arterial pressure (usually 65–70 mm Hg) and counter myocardial depression. The goal is not to target an

arbitrary value of cardiac output or oxygen delivery. **Catecholamines** maintain perfusion pressure through their combination of α and β adrenergic effects. **Dopamine** often is used because of its additional dopaminergic effects, which can increase urine output. **Dobutamine** is usually not indicated because of its vasodilator effects. Both drugs can cause an unacceptable tachycardia or dysrhythmias. **Norepinephrine** produces peripheral vasoconstriction and increased inotropy. Because of its weak β_2-adrenergic agonist effects, norepinephrine usually does not produce a significant tachycardia or dysrhythmias.

  (3) **Diagnosis and treatment of the underlying cause is critical to survival of the patient.** A relentless search for sources of infection or nonviable tissue is undertaken and appropriate treatment begun as soon as possible. Broad spectrum, empiric antibiotics are administered when a bacterial source is suspected (see Chapters 27 and 28).

B. **Neurogenic shock (see Chapter 30 for additional details)**
  1. **Etiology.** Neurogenic shock is caused by traumatic spinal cord injury. Pharmacologic neuraxial blockade by spinal and epidural anesthesia also can produce hypotension from sympathetic blockade. Intracranial injuries normally do not cause shock; thus, the presence of shock in a patient with head injury necessitates a search for other causes.
  2. **Pathophysiology.** The physiologic hallmark of neurogenic shock is **hypotension** caused by **loss of peripheral vasomotor tone,** which decreases venous return to the heart and cardiac output. Values for CVP, PA pressure, and cardiac output depend mainly on the patient's volume status, but they are expected to be low prior to resuscitation. If the cord injury is below the midthoracic level, activation of the adrenergic system above the level of the lesion results in increased heart rate and contractility. If the injury is above the cardiac accelerator nerves (T1–T5), **bradycardia** is prominent (see Chapter 30).
  3. **Clinical presentation** includes hypotension without cutaneous vasoconstriction and a peripheral neurologic deficit. Nausea, vomiting, and central apnea may be present. Signs of predominant parasympathetic outflow (e.g., bradycardia, bronchospasm, diarrhea, and priapism) are expected with severe cervical cord injury.

4. **Differential diagnosis** is generally not problematic because of the obvious cause. Other types of shock, however, may coexist, particularly **hypovolemic shock.**
5. **Management**
   a. **Supportive measures.** The **airway** should be secured in patients with altered mental status, apnea, or compromised respiratory muscle function. **Fluid resuscitation** is carried out as described in section **V.E.1.** When indicated, **surgery** is performed to stabilize the spine.
   b. **Pharmacologic support** is aimed at increasing vascular tone and preventing reflex bradycardia. An α_1-adrenergic agonist such as **phenylephrine** can increase vascular tone, but also can worsen bradycardia. The addition of **dopamine, ephedrine** or, if hypotension is severe, **norepinephrine,** may be helpful in hypotensive and bradycardic patients. Antimuscarinic agents (e.g., **atropine** and **glycopyrrolate**) can be used alone or in combination with vasoconstrictor agents in patients with symptomatic bradycardia. With bradycardia refractory to vagolytics, an infusion of isoproterenol or dopamine, or temporary cardiac pacing should be considered. Permanent pacemakers are rarely indicated.

C. **Anaphylactic shock**
   1. **Etiology. Anaphylaxis** is an acute, antibody-mediated reaction that occurs on re-exposure to a particular antigen in previously sensitized individuals. An **anaphylactoid reaction** is a clinically similar syndrome that is not mediated by antibodies and does not require prior exposure. The term "anaphylaxis" often is used conversationally to describe both syndromes. The many causes of anaphylaxis in critically ill patients include antibiotics (especially penicillins), other drugs, radiographic contrast agents, and exposure to latex-containing products.
   2. **Pathophysiology.** In anaphylactic reactions, the antigen and IgE antibodies bind to receptors of mast cells and basophils, triggering degranulation and release of toxic mediators such as histamine, prostaglandins, leukotrienes, thromboxanes, platelet activating factor, bradykinin, serotonin, and complement components. In anaphylactoid reactions, degranulation and mediator release occur by direct exposure to the antigen. These substances produce flushing, urticaria, increased capillary permeability, edema, bronchoconstriction, and vasodilation. Shock occurs from vasodilation and loss of plasma volume through increased capillary permeability. Central venous pressure, PA

pressure, and PAOP usually are low, but cardiac output may be normal or even increased, depending on the degree of peripheral vasodilation and the patient's volume status. Owing to the frequent occurrence of severe **bronchospasm** and air trapping, central pressures can be elevated (when referenced to atmospheric pressure) and cardiac output decreased because of an increase of intrathoracic pressure. This phenomenon must be correctly interpreted and not be confused with a picture of myocardial dysfunction.

3. **Clinical presentation.** The severity of the reaction is partly a function of the route of entry and dose of the antigen. Greater than 50% of the patients who die do so within the first hour after exposure. Most (75%) deaths are caused by asphyxia; the remaining deaths, from circulatory failure. These patients may manifest a **biphasic response** in which the symptoms are delayed or recur hours after the initial insult. Common signs and symptoms of anaphylaxis include:

   a. **Skin.** Flushing, erythema, urticaria, pruritus, and sometimes angioedema.

   b. **Respiratory system.** Edema of the tongue and glottis lead to **upper airway obstruction. Bronchoconstriction** produces dyspnea, wheezing, air trapping, and acute respiratory failure.

   c. **Cardiovascular system.** Tachycardia and hypotension.

   d. **Central nervous system.** Restlessness or obtundation.

   e. **GI system.** Nausea, vomiting, crampy abdominal pain, and diarrhea.

   f. **Renal system.** Hematuria secondary to hemolysis.

4. **Differential diagnosis.** The temporal relationship of the event to exposure to the triggering agent is the clue to diagnosis. Bronchospasm and hematuria are almost pathognomonic of this type of shock. Quantitative analysis of serum histamine, tryptase, and IgE levels retrospectively confirms an anaphylactic event.

5. **Management.** Initial interventions include **identification and discontinuation of the suspected allergen, airway management, volume** resuscitation, and administration of **epinephrine.**

   a. **Airway management.** The potential for the development of glottic edema and **upper airway obstruction** mandates experienced management of the airway. This can include supplemental oxygen administration, endotracheal intubation, positive-pressure ventilation, and readiness to perform an emergency tracheostomy in cases of severe airway edema (see Chapter 3).

b. **Volume resuscitation,** as described in section **V.E.1.,** is required because of massive capillary leakage.

c. **Epinephrine** is the drug of choice (see Chapter 10). Its α_1-adrenergic activity increases systemic blood pressure. Its β_1- and β_2-adrenergic actions increase cardiac output, promote bronchodilation, and block mast cell degranulation. In adults, IV administration of 0.1 to 0.5 mg (0.1–0.5 ml of a 1:1,000 solution) is a common initial dosage for a hypotensive patient, followed by a continuous infusion of 1 to 4 µg/min. If the initial reaction is localized, part of this dose can be administered near the site of the reaction. In addition to continued volume resuscitation and epinephrine administration, standard **Advanced Cardiac Life Support (ACLS) protocols** are followed in cases of cardiac arrest (see Chapter 15).

d. **Antihistamines** are a logical adjuvant therapy, although their benefit in severe anaphylaxis is controversial. For adults, the IV doses of these drugs are diphenhydramine 50 mg and cimetidine 300 mg (or ranitidine 50 mg).

e. **Corticosteroids** are also an adjuvant therapy. Their maximal effect may not be seen for 4 to 6 hours. Common adult regimens are hydrocortisone 200 mg or methylprednisolone 50 mg IV every 6 hours for 1 to 2 days.

VIII. **Obstructive shock**

A. **Etiology.** Obstructive shock can be produced by **increased intrathoracic pressure** [e.g., tension pneumothorax, abdominal compartment syndrome, positive-pressure ventilation, positive end-expiratory pressure (PEEP), and auto-PEEP], or **vascular outflow obstruction** (e.g., pulmonary embolism, air embolism, aortic dissection, pulmonary hypertension, pericardial tamponade, and constrictive pericarditis).

B. **Pathophysiology.** Obstructive shock is characterized by a **decreased cardiac output** in the presence of increased systemic venous pressure. Central venous pressure, PA pressure, and PAOP may all be increased, often to equal values (**equalization of central pressures**), and stroke volume is decreased.

C. **Clinical features.** Common to different causes of obstructive shock are hypotension, tachycardia, respiratory distress, cyanosis, and JVD. Pulsus paradoxus (≥ 10 mm Hg decrease of systolic blood pressure during spontaneous inspiration) and Kussmaul's sign (an increase in venous pressure with inspiration during spontaneous breathing) may be present.

D. Differential diagnosis. Cyanosis, JVD, unequal breath sounds, a recent precipitating event (e.g., trauma, myocardial infarction, and status asthmaticus) and an increase and equalization of central pressures are characteristic of obstructive shock.

E. Management

1. **Volume resuscitation** provides temporary support by improving ventricular filling. Central pressures are elevated and do not accurately reflect transmural pressure and systemic volume status. They can be used as a way to monitor treatment.

2. **Inotropic support,** as described in section **VI.E.1.,** supports cardiac output while diagnosis and treatment are pursued.

3. **Operative interventions** often are the only effective treatment of this type of shock. **Tension pneumothorax** (see Chapter 35) is treated by emergency needle aspiration, followed by tube thoracostomy; **abdominal compartment syndrome** (see Chapter 33) is treated with a decompressive laparotomy; **cardiac tamponade** (see Chapter 36) is treated by pericardiocentesis; and **pulmonary embolism** (see Chapter 22) may require thrombolysis or thrombectomy.

SELECTED REFERENCES

American College of Chest Physicians/Society of Critical Care Medicine Consensus Conference. Definitions for sepsis and organ failure and guidelines for the use of innovative therapies in sepsis. *Crit Care Med* 1992;20:864–874.

Beal AL, Cerra FB. Multiple organ failure in the 1990s. Systemic inflammatory response and organ dysfunction. *JAMA* 1994;271: 226–233.

Bochner BS, Lichtenstein LM. Anaphylaxis. *N Engl J Med* 1991;324: 1785–1790.

Califf RM, Bengtson JR. Cardiogenic shock. *N Engl J Med* 1994;330: 1724–1730.

Cochrane Injuries Group Albumin Reviewers. Human albumin administration in critically ill patients: systematic review of randomized controlled trials. *BMJ* 1998;317:235–240.

Parrillo JE. Pathogenetic mechanisms of septic shock. *N Engl J Med* 1993;328:1471–1477.

Wheeler AP, Bernard GR. Treating patients with severe sepsis. *N Engl J Med* 1999;340:207–214.

Hemodynamic Control

John L. Chow, Keith Baker, and
Luca M. Bigatello

I. This chapter reviews the principles of **pharmacologic control** of **hemodynamic instability** in critically ill patients. It is closely tied to Chapter 1, which outlines the physiologic determinants of hemodynamic instability, and Chapter 9, which outlines the pathophysiology and general treatment of hypotension and shock.

II. **Adrenergic receptors pharmacology**
   A. **Adrenergic receptor subtypes**
   1. **α-1 receptors** are located on the postsynaptic membrane of blood vessels, smooth muscle, myocardium, uterus, iris, and gastrointestinal (GI) and genitourinary (GU) sphincters. Stimulation of α_1 receptors causes **smooth muscle contraction,** a minor inotropic effect, and glycogenolysis. Intense stimulation is associated with reflex bradycardia.
   2. **α_2 receptors**
      a. **Presynaptic α_2 receptors** are located **in the central nervous system (CNS)** where they inhibit sympathetic outflow. Stimulation of these receptors causes hypotension and bradycardia.
      b. **Postsynaptic α_2 receptors** are located in vascular smooth muscle, adipose tissue, GI tract, pancreatic β cells, and the CNS. Stimulation of these receptors produces vasoconstriction, inhibition of insulin release, and lipolysis.
   3. **β_1 receptors** are located in the myocardium, sinoatrial (SA) node, ventricular conduction system, adipose tissue, and kidneys. Stimulation of β_1 receptors produces positive **inotropic** and **chronotropic** effects, increases conduction velocity, and decreases refractoriness of the atrioventricular (AV) node. They also stimulate lipolysis and renin release.
   4. **β_2 receptors** are located in vascular, bronchial, GU, and uterine smooth muscle. Stimulation of β_2 receptors produces **vasodilation, bronchodilation,** bladder and uterine relaxation, insulin release, gluconeogenesis, and intracellular potassium uptake.
   5. **β_3 receptors** are less well characterized. They are involved predominately in lipolysis and regulation of metabolic rate.
   6. **Dopaminergic-1 (D_1) receptors** mediate vasodilation in mesenteric, renal, coronary, and cerebral vessels.

7. **D$_2$ receptors** primarily are presynaptic and inhibit norepinephrine release.
8. **Additional dopamine receptor subtypes** (e.g., D$_3$, D$_4$) have been identified. Their precise physiologic roles remain to be fully characterized.

B. **Adrenergic receptor regulation**
1. **Upregulation.** Decreased stimulation of adrenergic receptors, such as during **chronic β-blockade** therapy, increases the number of receptors. Hence, abrupt discontinuation of β blockade can result in rebound tachycardia and hypertension.
2. **Downregulation.** Prolonged stimulation of adrenergic receptors, such as during **chronic β-agonist therapy,** decreases the number of receptors. Consequently, when an intravenous (IV) β agonist is infused, higher doses than anticipated may be required.
3. **Mode of action. Adrenergic agonists** can act directly, by activating their receptors and increasing intracellular concentrations of cyclic adenosine diphosphate (AMP), or indirectly, by releasing endogenous catecholamines, or both. **Indirect agents** lose their effectiveness in denervated organs (such as a transplanted heart), and when catecholamine stores are depleted (e.g., after prolonged hypotension and shock). They can produce an exaggerated hypertensive response whenever catecholamine stores are increased (e.g, during chronic therapy with monoamine oxidase (**MAO**) inhibitors). **Direct-acting agents** are more predictable in their response and generally are easier to titrate to effect.

III. **Sympathomimetic agents (Table 10-1): catecholamines**
A. Epinephrine is a potent sympathomimetic agent produced by the adrenal medulla that exerts agonist effects on adrenergic receptors α$_1$, α$_2$, β$_1$, and β$_2$.
1. **Indications for epinephrine** use include treatment for refractory severe hypotension, bronchospasm (status asthmaticus), anaphylaxis, and cardiac arrest.
2. **Physiologic effects.** Low doses (1–2 µg/min) preferentially stimulate β$_2$ receptors, leading to bronchodilation and skeletal muscle vasodilation. Activation of β$_1$ receptors increases heart rate, contractility, and cardiac output, but arterial blood pressure may not rise initially because of β$_2$-mediated vasodilation. At higher doses (≥ 10 µg/min), increasing stimulation of α receptors produces marked vasoconstriction, hypertension, and tachycardia. Other effects include inhibition of inflammatory mediator release by mast cells and basophils, hypokalemia, increased secretion of renin, and hyperglycemia because of inhibition of insulin release.

Table 10-1. Sympathomimetic drugs

Drug	Target adrenergic receptor	Clinical effects
Catecholamines		
Epinephrine	β_1, β_2, α_1	↑CO, ↑BP, ↑HR, bronchodilation
Norepinephrine	β_1, α_1	↑BP, ↑CO
Dopamine	D, β_1, α_1	↑CO, ↑BP, ↑HR, ↑renal perfusion?
Synthetic catecholamines		
Dobutamine	β_1, β_2	↑CO, ↑HR, ↔/↓BP
Isoproterenol	β_1, β_2	↑CO, ↑HR, ↔/↓BP, bronchodilation
Dopexamine	D, β_1, β_2	↑CO, ↑HR, ↑renal perfusion
Fenoldopam	D	↑Renal perfusion, ↓BP
Synthetic noncatecholamines		
Ephedrine	β_1, β_2, α_1	Like epinephrine, but weaker
Phenylephrine	α_1	↑BP, ↓HR, ↑/↓/↔CO

BP, blood pressure, CO, cardiac output; HR, heart rate; D, dopaminergic.

3. **Administration.** Intravenous administration is always preferable, although subcutaneous and intratracheal administration are alternative routes.

   a. The drug should be administered into the central circulation whenever possible, because extravasation can produce local tissue necrosis. Given its very short duration of action, epinephrine usually is administered by continuous infusion, which is titrated to effect. Low doses (0.5–1 μg/min) are effective in treating severe **bronchospasm** and are rarely associated with more than a mild to moderate tachycardia. At higher doses, β_1- and α-adrenergic effects predominate.

   b. For **severe hypotension** and treatment of **anaphylaxis,** an initial bolus of 100 to 500 μg is followed by a continuous IV infusion titrated to effect. Refer to Chapter 15 for use during **cardiopulmonary resuscitation.**

   c. In the absence of IV access, epinephrine can be administered subcutaneously in doses equivalent to an initial IV bolus (100–500 μg) and repeated according to the clinical response. When the airway is intubated, epinephrine can be administered **endotracheally,** at two to three times the IV dose (diluted in 10 ml of normal saline). Epinephrine is inactivated by alkaline solutions.

   d.   **Adverse effects.** The most frequent complications of epinephrine are **tachydysrhythmias,** related to potent β_1 stimulation. Dysrhythmias can be atrial or ventricular; most commonly, they are accelerated rhythms that can be worsened by common risk factors such as hypomagnesemia, hypokalemia, hypoxia, acidemia, and concomitant administration of other pro-dysrhythmic agents. Given the short duration of action of epinephrine, these complications usually can be rapidly reversed by **decreasing** or **temporarily discontinuing the infusion.** α_1-mediated side effects include excessive vasoconstriction, leading to decreased blood flow to the heart, kidneys, and skin. Myocardial ischemia and infarction can occur. Patients on β-blockers may have an exaggerated hypertensive response from epinephrine because of unopposed α stimulation.

B. **Norepinephrine** is a potent sympathomimetic agent produced by postganglionic sympathetic nerve endings, which exerts agonist effects on adrenergic receptors α_1, α_2, and β_1. Its β_1 effect is equipotent to epinephrine. Norepinephrine is used to treat **hypotension** caused by low peripheral vascular tone, myocardial depression, or both.

   1.   **Physiologic effects.** The combination of β_1 and α_1 stimulation increases systemic and pulmonary blood pressure, myocardial contractility, and cardiac output. Blood flow may be redistributed away from skeletal muscle, the GI tract, and kidneys toward the heart and CNS. Heart rate can decrease because of intense α_1-adrenergic stimulation or a baroreceptor-mediated reflex response to the increased blood pressure. Compared with epinephrine, norepinephrine **lacks β_2-adrenergic effects,** which increases the potency of its vasoconstrictive actions.

   2.   **Administration.** Norepinephrine should be administered through a central line. Because of the potency of the drug, boluses are not administered. Instead, a continuous infusion should be titrated to effect. Typical dosages range from 1 to 20 µg/min.

   3.   **Adverse effects** are related mostly to its potent α_1 agonist effect. **Intense peripheral vasoconstriction** can cause organ hypoperfusion and ischemia. **Maintaining euvolemia** during vasopressor infusion improves organ perfusion. **Pulmonary vasoconstriction** can reduce right

ventricular (RV) output in patients with pre-existing pulmonary hypertension, right ventricular dysfunction, or both. The use of selective pulmonary vasodilators, such as prostaglandins and inhaled nitric oxide (NO) may be helpful. Vasopressor effects can be potentiated by MAO inhibitors and tricyclic antidepressants. Dysrhythmias are rare.

C. **Dopamine** is the biologic precursor of norepinephrine. It exerts dose-dependent effects on dopaminergic, β_1, and α_1-adrenergic receptors.

1. **Indications** include the treatment of hypotension, mainly because of decreased myocardial contractility, and promotion of urine output.

2. **Physiologic effects.** When increasing doses of dopamine are administered, dopaminergic, β, and α receptors are progressively stimulated. The specific doses are extremely variable. Rather than selecting an arbitrary dose range, the rate of infusion should be titrated to achieve the desired effect. Starting doses are usually in the range of 100 to 200 $\mu g/min$ (2–3 $\mu g/kg/min$).

   a. **At low doses** (dopaminergic range), selective activation of renal, splanchnic, coronary, and cerebral dopamine receptors promotes blood flow to these regions. Dopamine also increases glomerular filtration rate and water and sodium excretion. The protective effect of "renal dose dopamine" is not substantiated. On the contrary, a low dose of dopamine can redistribute blood flow within the splanchnic circulation and result in splanchnic hypoperfusion. The routine use of low doses of dopamine does not prevent acute renal failure or alter its course.

   b. **At higher doses,** β stimulation increases myocardial contractility, heart rate, and systemic arterial blood pressure. The inotropic effect of dopamine is modest relative to the other catecholamines.

   c. **At the highest doses** (generally > 10 $\mu g/kg/min$), α effects predominate, causing arterial and venous vasoconstriction. The persistent stimulation of dopamine receptors at these doses may help maintain renal blood flow.

3. **Administration** via a central IV line is preferable, but not as critical as with epinephrine and norepinephrine, because of the less potent vasoconstrictive action of dopamine. It is inactivated by alkaline solutions.

4. **Adverse effects.** Tachycardia is predictable at higher doses (β-range). Dysrhythmias and myocardial ischemia can occur, but less frequently than with epinephrine. At high doses, α effects

predominate, but are less intense than with epinephrine and norepinephrine.

IV. Sympathomimetic agents: synthetic catecholamines

A. **Dobutamine** has β_1, β_2, and minimal α_1-adrenergic effects. Dobutamine is indicated for the treatment of **low cardiac output states**.

1. **Physiologic effects.** β_1 stimulation produces inotropic and chronotropic effects and enhances AV conduction. The β_2 effect of dobutamine on the peripheral vasculature counterbalances its weak α_1 effect and causes vasodilation. Consequently, cardiac output and stroke volume may increase. Dobutamine has no significant effect on bronchial β_2 receptors.

2. **Administration** via a central IV line is preferable but not critical, because of the lack of vasoconstrictive action of dobutamine. The usual dose range is 100 to 500 µg/min (2 to 8 µg/kg/min). It is inactivated in alkaline solutions.

3. **Adverse effects** include tachycardia and dysrhythmias, related to its predominant β_1 effect. They are less frequent and severe than with epinephrine, dopamine, or isoproterenol. β_1 stimulation can increase myocardial oxygen consumption and produce myocardial ischemia in susceptible patients. β_2-adrenergic stimulation can cause hypotension. Tolerance develops over a period of days.

B. **Dopexamine** is a synthetic analog of dobutamine with dopaminergic and β_2 agonist effects. Dopexamine exerts β_1 effects by inhibiting norepinephrine reuptake. Dopexamine is used to treat **low cardiac output states**, particularly with coexisting **renal hypoperfusion.** Dopexamine is limited to investigational use in the United States.

1. **Physiologic effects.** The β effects increase cardiac output and heart rate and promote vasodilation. Dopaminergic stimulation can increase renal and splanchnic blood flow. In clinical trials, dopexamine improved cardiac output and produced fewer tachydysrhythmias than dobutamine in patients with acute cardiac failure.

2. **Administration** is preferably by the central IV route. The suggested dose range is 30 to 400 µg/min.

3. **Adverse effects** include dose-dependent tachydysrhythmias and tachyphylaxis.

C. **Fenoldopam** is a recently approved selective dopamine D_1-adrenergic agonist. It is used to treat severe hypertension in the setting of renal hypoperfusion.

1. **Physiologic effects.** Fenoldopam is an arterial vasodilator in the renal, mesenteric, skeletal muscle, and coronary circulation. Despite a dose-dependent decrease in arterial pressure, it in-

creases renal blood flow. Additionally, it has diuretic and natriuretic properties.

2. **Administration** is via continuous peripheral IV infusion at dose range 5 to 10 μg/min. At this time, it has been recommended for short-term use (≤ 48 h).

3. **Adverse effects** include hypotension, tachycardia, flushing, dizziness, nausea, and increased intraocular pressure. Tolerance develops with infusions lasting more than 48 hours.

D. **Isoproterenol** is a potent, β-adrenergic receptor agonist.

1. **Indications**
   a. Hemodynamically unstable **bradycardia** or heart block.
   b. **Low cardiac output states** associated with bradycardias (i.e., patients after heart transplantation).
   c. **Severe bronchospasm**

2. **Physiologic effects.** The β effects of isoproterenol increase heart rate, cardiac output, and conduction velocity. They also promote systemic and pulmonary vasodilation and bronchodilation.

3. **Administration** through a peripheral IV is acceptable because the drug does not produce vasoconstriction. The usual dosage in adults is 2 to 20 μg/min.

4. **Adverse effects** reflect β-adrenergic agonist activity and include tachydysrhythmias, hypotension, hyperglycemia, and hypokalemia. Its hemodynamic effects can be pronounced, and are undesirable in patients at risk for coronary ischemia. For these reasons, isoproterenol is seldom used in adults, although it remains a frequent therapy in critically ill children.

V. **Sympathomimetic agents: Synthetic noncatecholamines**

A. **Ephedrine** is a mixed adrenergic agonist with a pharmacologic profile qualitatively similar to epinephrine. It is used to treat **moderate hypotension,** particularly when associated with bradycardia.

1. **Physiologic effects.** Its α and β effects increase heart rate, cardiac output, and blood pressure and similarly, but to a lesser extent than epinephrine, promote bronchodilation. Unlike other α_1 agonists, it does not decrease uterine blood flow.

2. **Administration** is generally by IV boluses of 5 to 10 mg every 5 to 20 minutes. Ephedrine has a slower onset and longer duration of action than the endogenous catecholamines (e.g., epinephrine), making it less suited for severe hemodynamic instability and for continuous infusion.

3. **Adverse effects** are minor, because of ephedrine's low potency. A mild tachycardia is predictable. Tachyphylaxis occurs secondary to depletion of

endogenous catecholamines or persistent adrenergic blockade. Central nervous system stimulation (e.g., agitation, nausea) and mydriasis can occur. Ephedrine should **not be used** in patients taking **MAO inhibitors** because of the potential for triggering a hypertensive response.

B.   **Phenylephrine** is a pure α_1-adrenergic receptor agonist used to treat hypotension resulting from peripheral vasodilation.

1.   **Physiologic effects.** Phenylephrine causes arterial and venous vasoconstriction. It increases blood pressure both by augmenting arteriolar and venous tone and by increasing venous return to the heart. In hypovolemic patients, the phenylephrine-induced increase in blood pressure is largely the result of vasoconstriction; thus, organ perfusion can suffer. The pure α_1-adrenergic effect also causes reflex bradycardia.

2.   **Administration** by a central IV line is preferable, but not necessary because the vasoconstrictive potency of phenylephrine is relatively mild. Phenylephrine has a fast onset and short duration of action, making it ideal for continuous infusion. A bolus dose of 40 to 80 µg IV, an infusion of 30 to 300 µg/min, or both are commonly used.

3.   **Adverse effects** are minor, because of the relative low potency and favorable pharmacokinetics of phenylephrine. Reflex bradycardia is common. MAO inhibitors can potentiate its vasopressor effect, but less markedly than with indirect-acting agents such as ephedrine or amphetamines. Extravasation can cause cutaneous necrosis. Systemic vasoconstriction limits its use in patients with left ventricular dysfunction, aortic insufficiency, or mitral regurgitation.

VI.   **Nonsympathomimetic agents: Phosphodiesterase (PDE) inhibitors**

A.   **Amrinone,** the prototype of type III PDE inhibitors, provides positive inotropic and vasodilator effects fully independent of adrenergic receptor activation. It is used to treat **low cardiac output states** caused by systolic dysfunction or pulmonary hypertension.

1.   **Physiologic effects.** The positive inotropic, lusitropic (ventricular relaxation) and vasodilator effects of amrinone result from stimulation of adenylate cyclase and increase in intracellular cyclic AMP concentrations. The combination of positive inotropy and vasodilation is ideal in patients with biventricular failure. Its effects are not altered by β blockade and are additive to those of adrenergic agonists such as dobutamine.

2.   **Administration** is by IV infusion. Its slow onset and long duration of action (half-life: 3–5 hours) make amrinone difficult to titrate. Administration is begun with a bolus of 50 to 100 mg over 15 min-

utes, followed by an infusion rate of 300 to 700 µg/min. Hepatic and renal dysfunction prolong its effect. Amrinone is degraded by light and dextrose. Furosemide can precipitate if admixed with amrinone.

   3. **Adverse effects** are minor. Tachycardia can occur, but dysrhythmias are rare. Significant hypotension can occur in hypovolemic patients. Nonimmunologic thrombocytopenia occurs in 2% to 3% of the patients after more than 24 hours of therapy, but resolves when drug is discontinued. Abnormalities in liver function tests have been associated with the use of amrinone.

B. **Milrinone** is a derivative of amrinone, with similar physiologic effects but a shorter duration of action (2–3 hours).

   1. **Administration** in critically ill patients is via a central IV line, but an oral formulation also is available. The loading dose is 3 to 5 mg over 10 minutes, which is followed by an infusion of 25 to 75 µg/min. The dose must be reduced in patients with renal dysfunction.

   2. **Adverse hemodynamic effects** are similar to amrinone, but thrombocytopenia does not occur.

VII. **Other nonsympathomimetic agents**

A. **Digoxin** is the only cardiac glycoside currently used in the United States. It has antidysrhythmic and inotropic effects, mediated largely through the inhibition of the sodium–potassium ATPase, which increases the intracellular calcium (Ca^{2+}) concentration. Besides its use to treat atrial dysrhythmias, it is used to treat **low cardiac output** resulting from myocardial dysfunction.

   1. **Physiologic effects.** Digoxin increases stroke volume and cardiac output by increasing myocardial contractility. It has a negative chronotropic effect on the SA node (mild) and the AV node (strong).

   2. **Administration** of digoxin in critically ill patients starts with an IV loading dose of 0.25 to 1 mg over a few hours and continues with an average maintenance dose of 0.25 mg/d. Renal insufficiency decreases digoxin elimination; thus, the interval between doses must be increased. If the GI tract is working properly, the maintenance dose can be administered orally. Adjusting the dosage of digoxin is complicated by its long half-life (1–2 days) and high toxicity. Serum digoxin levels are not reliable predictors of efficacy or toxicity in an individual patient. For this reason, and because its inotropic effects are weaker than the agents reviewed above, digoxin use as an inotrope in critically ill patients has become rare.

   3. **Adverse effects.** The effects of digoxin on the cardiac conduction system are complex and can

result in multiple dysrhythmias. It is often difficult to diagnose a digitalis-induced dysrhythmia because patients on digoxin have multiple potential causes for dysrhythmias. Most common digoxin-induced dysrhythmias include **SA block, AV blocks, paroxysmal atrial tachycardia (PAT) with block,** and **ventricular ectopic activity.** Factors that potentiate toxicity include hypokalemia, hypomagnesemia, acidemia, and concomitant administration of other antidysrhythmics, such as type IIa agents, β blockers, and calcium channel blockers. **Cardioversion** can precipitate ventricular dysrhythmias in patients receiving digoxin.

B. **Calcium** is an inorganic element important in the process of excitation-contraction coupling in skeletal and cardiac muscle. It is sometimes used to treat **severe hypotension.**

1. **Physiologic effects** of Ca^{2+} include increased myocardial contractility and vascular tone, which increase cardiac output and systemic blood pressure. These effects are extremely rapid and short-lived (minutes), accounting for the use of Ca^{2+} as a **"rescue"** drug to temporarily increase blood pressure.

2. **Administration. Calcium chloride** ($CaCl_2$) in 10% solution provides more elemental Ca^{2+} (270 mg, 13.5 mEq/g) than an equal volume of 10% **calcium gluconate** (90 mg, 4.5 mEq/g). Calcium chloride generally is preferred for emergency treatment of hypotension: 100 mg to 1 g through a central IV line increases systemic blood pressure within a few seconds. It precipitates if mixed with bicarbonate.

3. **Adverse effects,** which are related to the administration of excessive doses, can result in hypertension, tachycardia, and dysrhythmias. In susceptible patients, these can cause myocardial ischemia.

C. **Glucagon,** which is produced by the α cells of the pancreas, is the principal anti-insulin hormone. It activates adenylate cyclase and increases intracellular cyclic AMP levels, leading to an intracellular Ca^{2+} influx and a potent inotropic effect. It is used to treat **hypotension,** particularly when produced by excessive β blockade.

1. **Physiologic effects.** Glucagon increases myocardial contractility and automaticity of the SA and AV nodes, thus increasing cardiac output and heart rate.

2. **Administration.** An initial IV bolus of 1 to 5 mg is followed by an infusion of 2 to 10 mg/h, depending on the severity of the myocardial depression. Given its very short half-life (3–6 minutes), the infusion rate can be titrated easily to effect.

3. **Adverse effects** include hyperglycemia, hypokalemia, nausea, and vomiting. Anaphylaxis is possible. Paradoxical hypoglycemia in response to insulin release can occur in patients with insufficient glycogen stores.

VIII. **Treatment of hypertension.** Chronic treatment of hypertension is continued in the ICU in all hemodynamically stable patients, using, when possible, their pre-existing regimen. If the GI tract is compromised, IV antihypertensives are available. In this section, we focus on the pathophysiology and treatment of **uncontrolled hypertension** (see Chapter 1 for details concerning blood pressure monitoring).

A. **Etiology.** Hypertension can be **primary ("essential")**, which includes 90% to 95% of all hypertensive individuals, or **secondary,** from:
1. **Renal parenchymal** disease.
2. **Renovascular** disease.
3. **Endocrine** disorders such as pheochromocytoma, hyperaldosteronism, Cushing's syndrome, and thyrotoxicosis.
4. **Neurologic** disorders (e.g., dysautonomia) and increased intracranial pressure.
5. **Catecholamine** excess from pain, anxiety, and hypoxemia.
6. **Other** causes include pre-eclampsia, coarctation of the aorta, rebound hypertension, and drug interactions (e.g., cocaine and MAO inhibitors).

B. **Pathophysiology of hypertensive crisis.** Organ blood flow is normally kept constant by **autoregulation:** As the upstream blood pressure increases, flow remains constant through reflex vasodilation. Autoregulation is less efficient in organs with very high basal blood flow, which is less amenable to rapid modifications. For example, the kidneys, with a high blood flow per gram of tissue, are very susceptible to hypotensive and hypertensive injury. **Chronic hypertension** decreases the range of autoregulation and the risk of organ damage. In most patients with hypertensive crises, the combination of increased vascular tone and compromised autoregulation results in organ injury.

C. **General therapeutic considerations.** Appropriate IV access and hemodynamic monitoring must be rapidly established. History and physical examination focus on the patient's premorbid status, cause of hypertension, and signs of organ injury (e.g., headache, vomiting, seizures, visual disturbances, papilledema, angina, and oliguria). Laboratory studies include electrolytes, blood urea nitrogen and creatinine, blood count, urinalysis, electrocardiogram and chest radiograph. The objective of the initial therapy is to **limit ongoing organ damage.** Because autoregulation is likely to be impaired, rapid normalization of arterial pressure can compromise organ perfusion. A 20% to 25% reduction is a reasonable initial target. Antihypertensive therapy is started with an IV agent that is easy to titrate (e.g., nitroglycerin or nitroprusside). A combination of different agents may later facilitate control and decrease adverse effects.

IX. **Vasodilators**
  A. **α-adrenergic antagonists**
    1. **Phentolamine,** an imidazoline, is an α_1- and α_2-adrenergic receptor antagonist.
      a. **Indications**
        (1) **Severe hypertension,** especially that caused by pheochromocytoma (see Chapter 26).
        (2) **Extravasation** of vasopressors.
      b. **Physiologic effects.** The α_1-antagonist effect primarily causes arteriolar vasodilation. The α_2-antagonist effect can produce a positive inotropic effect.
      c. **Administration** is initially IV, in 2.5 to 5 mg boluses repeated, as needed, at 20 to 40 minute intervals. Given its rapid onset and short half-life (approximately 20 minutes), phentolamine is easy to titrate and can be administered as a continuous infusion of 0.5 to 1 mg/min. Oral therapy is cumbersome because of its short duration of action. For treatment of **local extravasation** of vasopressors, subcutaneously inject 5 to 10 mg of phentolamine diluted in 5 to 10 ml of normal saline.
      d. **Adverse effects.** Rapid infusion can cause reflex tachycardia, dysrhythmias, and severe hypotension. Abdominal pain, nausea, vomiting, hypoglycemia, and exacerbation of peptic ulcer disease can also occur.
    2. **Prazosin** is a selective α_1 antagonist used to treat hypertension.
      a. **Physiologic effects.** Prazosin dilates both arterioles and veins. Because of its selective α_1 blockade, compensatory tachycardia is minimal.
      b. **Administration.** An IV formulation is not available. The oral dose ranges from 1.0 mg two or three times a day, to a maximum of 20 mg/d.
      c. **Adverse effects.** Postural hypotension and syncope can occur with the initial doses. Tachyphylaxis and fluid retention can occur.
  B. **α_2-adrenergic agonists.**
    1. **Clonidine.**
      a. **Indications.**
        (1) **Hypertension.**
        (2) **Opioid or alcohol withdrawal.**
      b. **Physiologic effects.** Stimulation of α_2 receptors inhibits central sympathetic outflow and

decreases arterial blood pressure, heart rate, and cardiac output. A dose-dependent sedative effect also occurs, which can be utilized as an adjuvant in the treatment of opioid and alcohol withdrawal.

   c. **Administration.** An IV formulation is not currently available. For treatment of hypertension, normal oral doses are 0.05 to 0.1 mg two to three times daily. **Transdermal patches** can provide 0.1 to 0.3 mg daily for a week and take 2 to 3 days to achieve therapeutic effect.

   d. **Adverse effects.** Hypotension and bradycardia are common, but seldom severe. Rebound hypertension can occur on sudden withdrawal. Clonidine should be tapered over 2 to 4 days.

C. **Nitrates** cause direct vasodilation through the release of nitric oxide (NO) and consequent accumulation of cyclic guanosine monophosphate (cGMP) in the vascular endothelium.

   1. **Nitroglycerin (NTG)** is both a venous and arterial vasodilator.

      a. **Indications**

         (1) **Myocardial ischemia.**

         (2) **Hypertension.**

         (3) **Congestive heart failure (CHF).**

      b. **Physiologic effects.** Nitroglycerin decreases venous tone, ventricular end-diastolic pressure, and arterial tone. Overall, these effects improve systolic function. Nitroglycerin also dilates large coronary vessels, relieving coronary spasm and redistributing myocardial blood flow from the epicardium to the subendocardium. As with other nitrates, nitroglycerin inhibits platelet aggregation. This action may be partially responsible for its antianginal effects.

      c. **Intravenous administration** of NTG can be titrated easily, and is the preferred route for critically ill patients. Common IV rates range from 25 to 1000 µg/min. Because NTG is absorbed by polyvinyl chloride IV tubing, its apparent effective dosage can decrease after 30 to 60 minutes, once the IV tubing is fully saturated. Other NTG preparations (e.g., transdermal, sublingual) are well absorbed and as effective as intravenous NTG, but are more difficult to titrate quickly and should be reserved for chronic use.

      d. **Adverse effects. Hypotension, reflex tachycardia**, and **headache** are common. **Tachyphylaxis** is the rule, but it can be reduced by providing several hours of drug-free time daily. In critically ill patients, a common strategy is simply to increase the rate of administration, generally over a period of a few days, until a ceiling effect is noted (usually at doses of about 1,000 to 1,200 µg/min). Alternative vasodilators can be substituted, if needed, as the dose of NTG is escalated. **Methemoglobinemia** can occur during prolonged, high-dose infusions. Nitroglycerin administration can **worsen hypoxemia** during acute respiratory failure by increasing pulmonary blood flow to poorly ventilated areas of the lung, which can worsen ventilation–perfusion mismatch and shunt.

2. **Sodium nitroprusside (SNP)** is a more potent arterial rather than venous vasodilator. It is used to treat severe hypertension.

   a. **Physiologic effects** of SNP include a potent arteriolar vasodilation, which decreases systemic and pulmonary arterial blood pressure and cardiac filling pressures. Nitroprusside increases venous capacitance, but a reflex tachycardia often compensates for decreased venous return.

   b. **Central venous administration** is preferred. The normal dose range is 1 to 20 µg/min. The rapid onset and short duration of action of SNP make it ideal for continuous infusion. Because it is photodegradable, protection with foil wrapping is necessary.

   c. **Adverse effects.** Nitroprusside contains nitrosyl moieties that liberate free cyanide ions (CN^-), which bind to cytochrome oxidase and uncouple oxidative metabolism, causing tissue hypoxia. At low infusion rates, cyanide can be converted to thiocyanate (by thiosulfate and rhodanase), which is less toxic than CN^-. The risk of cyanide and thiocyanate toxicity is dose-dependent and increases with renal impairment. Signs of **cyanide toxicity** include tachyphylaxis, increased mixed venous PO_2, and metabolic acidosis. **Rebound hypertension** can occur when SNP is discontinued. Hypoxic pulmonary vasoconstriction is blunted by SNP and **hypoxemia** can occur.

3. **Inhaled nitric oxide (NO)** is a direct-acting vasodilator that has been used to treat **pulmonary hypertension** and **hypoxemia,** especially in the term and near-term newborn.

   a. **Physiologic effects.** Inhaled NO selectively decreases pulmonary artery pressure and diverts pulmonary blood away from poorly ventilated lung regions, thus improving PaO_2. Other potential beneficial effects under investigation include anti-inflammatory and O_2 free-radical scavenger actions.

   b. **Administration.** The usual dose is 1 to 20 parts per million (ppm). The decrease in pulmonary pressure, but not the increase in PaO_2, can sometimes be enhanced at higher doses (maximum: 40 ppm in adults and 80 ppm in neonates).

    c. **Adverse effects.** Pulmonary toxicity from inhaled NO and its reactive metabolites is a concern, but has not been documented at the doses used clinically. As with all nitrates, methemoglobinemia is also possible.

D. Hydralazine directly relaxes arteriolar smooth muscle by interfering with Ca^{2+} transport. It is used to treat hypertension, particularly when associated with bradycardia.

    1. Physiologic effects. By producing arterial vasodilation, hydralazine decreases systemic blood pressure, increases heart rate, and may increase cardiac output. Coronary, renal, splanchnic, uterine, and cerebral blood flow are maintained or increased. Because of its positive effect on uterine blood flow, it is used to treat hypertension associated with pre-eclampsia.

    2. Intravenous administration is preferred in critically ill patients. Because of its relatively long duration of action, hydralazine is seldom administered by continuous infusion. Doses of 2.5 to 20 mg IV every 4 to 6 hours are effective. Hydralazine can be administered orally (e.g., 10 mg every 6 hours) in hemodynamically stable patients.

    3. Adverse effects. Reflex tachycardia is common. If undesired, it can be minimized by concurrent administration of a β-adrenergic blocker. A lupus-like syndrome can occur after an extended oral administration.

E. Prostaglandin E₁ (PGE₁) and **prostacyclin (PGI₂, epoprostenol, flolan)** are metabolites of the arachidonic acid-cyclo-oxygenase pathway. Both drugs undergo significant first-pass metabolism within the lung and are especially well-suited to treat **pulmonary hypertension.** Both agents have relatively similar pharmacologic profiles, and are used to treat pulmonary hypertension, especially when associated with right ventricular failure. Prostacyclin generally is used for chronic treatment.

    1. Physiologic effects. Both PGE_1 and PGI_2 produce **systemic and pulmonary vasodilation,** decreasing blood pressure and increasing heart rate and cardiac output. They are partially selective for the pulmonary circulation.

    2. Administration is by central IV infusion. For PGE_1, a continuous infusion is started at 0.05 to 0.1 µg/kg/min and increased as tolerated. Prostacyclin initially is administered at 2 ng/kg/min and increased as tolerated. Chronic doses average 5 to 9 ng/kg/min, but must be titrated to the individual patient. With both drugs, tachyphylaxis can occur with chronic administration and the maximal tolerated dose usually is limited by nausea, vomiting, headache, or systemic hypotension. Both drugs have been experimentally administered by nebulization into the airway, which appears to enhance the selectivity of pulmonary vasodilation.

   3.   Adverse effects. Systemic hypotension and hypoxemia can occur and are dose-related. Platelet aggregation can be inhibited. Flushing, diarrhea, nausea, and vomiting can occur.

X.   β-adrenergic blocking agents are effective in the treatment of myocardial ischemia or infarction, hypertension, and tachydysrhythmias.

   A.   Mechanism of action. β blockers have negative chronotropic and inotropic properties. The latter is more evident in states of intense sympathetic stimulation (e.g., hypovolemia and shock). The mechanism of blood pressure reduction is not fully understood; it may be caused by inhibition of renin release, reduction of CNS sympathetic discharge, decreased cardiac output, and (for some compounds in this group) direct vasodilation. These effects lead to an overall **reduction in myocardial oxygen consumption,** which is probably the basis for the effectiveness of β blockade in patients with myocardial ischemia and infarction.

   B.   Choice of agent
   1.   Cardioselectivity. β_1 selective compounds tend to have less extracardiac effects, such as **bronchospasm,** peripheral **vasoconstriction, hypoglycemia,** and **hyperkalemia.** Cardioselectivity, however, diminishes when high doses are needed and seems to be associated with a less potent negative chronotropic effect.
   2.   Intrinsic sympathomimetic activity is present with some agents, which interact with β receptors to produce an agonist effect while blocking endogenous catecholamines. A higher resting heart rate and cardiac output and a lower systemic blood pressure are typical with these agents.
   3.   Duration of action. A fast onset and short duration of action are ideal for use in critically ill patients. The many compounds available in this class of drugs offer a wide choice.

   C.   Individual agents
   1.   Propranolol is a nonselective β blocker and the prototype of its class. Despite the great number of newer agents, it is still widely used because of its effectiveness, safety, and low cost. Propranolol is a frequent choice for the treatment of supraventricular tachycardia (SVT) in doses starting at 0.5 to 1 mg IV and titrated to effect up to 2 to 5 mg. Although the serum half-life of propranolol is relatively long (1–6 h), the duration of action of small IV doses is only 20 to 30 minutes. Continuous

infusion of propranolol at 1 to 10 mg/h is effective, simple to manage, and inexpensive compared with newer β blockers. Side effects are caused by its lack of selectivity.

2. **Metoprolol** is a β_1-selective blocker, but only at low doses. Acutely, it can be administered in repeated doses of 5 mg IV up to 15 to 25 mg to reach the desired effect on blood pressure and heart rate. Given its long half-life, it is not ideal for continuous infusions. Metoprolol can be continued enterally at doses of 25 to 100 mg two to three times daily.

3. **Labetalol** is a mixed α_1 and β antagonist with an α:β blockade ratio of 1 to 7 with IV administration. Because of this peculiar combination of effects, labetalol has very specific indications, such as treatment of hypertension and tachycardia. Initial IV doses of 5 to 10 mg can be increased to 15 to 20 mg in 5-minute intervals and followed by a continuous infusion of 1 to 5 mg/min.

4. **Esmolol** is a short acting, β_1-selective blocker that is hydrolyzed by red blood cell esterases. This accounts for its very **short half-life** (minutes), which makes it particularly suitable for continuous infusions. The adult starting dose is 10 to 40 mg IV, which can be increased every 3 to 5 minutes to a total 100 to 300 mg. Continuous infusions of 2.5 to 10 mg/min are effective in controlling SVT. The disadvantages of esmolol include its high cost and frequent onset of hypotension at high doses.

D. **Adverse effects**
1. **Bradycardia and heart block** occur frequently, especially in patients with known cardiac conduction defects, or in those taking other negative chronotropic agents (e.g., digoxin or calcium channel blockers).

2. **Bronchospasm** is uncommon, but is more likely to occur in patients with asthma or reactive airways. β_1-selective agents are less likely to increase airway reactivity.

3. **Heart failure** can occur in the setting of intense sympathetic stimulation (e.g., **hypovolemia, shock, or severe CHF**), where cardiac performance is maximally sustained by catecholamines.

4. **CNS effects** include depression, insomnia, and hallucinations.

5. **Rebound hypertension** and **tachycardia** can occur on abrupt discontinuation of β blockade.

XI. **Calcium channel blockers** are structurally diverse compounds used to treat hypertension, angina, SVT, and cerebral vasospasm.
A. **Classification**
1. **Dihydropyridines. Nifedipine** is the prototype of this group. They are potent arteriolar vasodila-

tors; they have mild to moderate negative inotropic activity and no bradycardic effect. The second generation agents (e.g., **amlodipine, nicardipine, and nimodipine**) have more vasodilator and less negative inotropic effect and prolonged durations of action.

2. **Non-dihydropyridines. Verapamil** and **diltiazem** are prototypes of this group. They have arterial vasodilator as well as substantial negative chronotropic and inotropic effects.

B. **Mechanism of action.** Calcium channel blockers inhibit the slow-inward Ca^{2+} channels, reducing the Ca^{2+} influx necessary for excitation–contraction coupling in cardiac and vascular smooth muscle. This also slows depolarization of SA and AV nodes. Hemodynamic effects include a **decrease in myocardial contractility, heart rate, AV nodal conduction, and systemic blood pressure.**

C. **Choice of the agent.** All calcium channel blockers cause vasodilation and effectively treat hypertension. Their varying effects on the heart rate determine the choice between the two main classes. All calcium channel blockers are negative inotropes, particularly the non-dihydropyridines **verapamil** and **diltiazem,** which should not be used in patients with significant myocardial dysfunction. Non-dihydropyridines are effective agents for treatment of SVT, except Wolf-Parkinson-White syndrome, in which verapamil can precipitate ventricular fibrillation. **Nimodipine** crosses the blood–brain barrier and is an effective cerebral vasodilator. Intravenous **nicardipine** is useful in treatment of hypertensive crises because of its potency, rapid onset of action, and minimal myocardial depression.

D. **Adverse effects**
1. **Bradycardia and heart block** can occur with verapamil and diltiazem, especially in combination with β blockers or digoxin.
2. **Heart failure** is particularly likely in patients with marginal myocardial function treated with verapamil or diltiazem.
3. **Peripheral edema** is associated with dihydropyridines (nifedipine).
4. **Hypotension** can occur, especially in hypovolemic patients, or during unmonitored sublingual nifedipine use.
5. **Reflex tachycardia** can occur with dihydropyridines.
6. **Other adverse effects** include flushing, dizziness, headache, constipation, rash, nausea, and vomiting.

XII. **Renin-angiotensin system inhibitors.** Angiotensin converting enzyme (**ACE**) inhibitors are used in the management of hypertension, myocardial infarction, CHF, and renal disease. A new class of inhibitors, angiotensin

II (**AT II**) receptor antagonists, are also effective in treating hypertension.

A. **Classification**
   1. **ACE inhibitors** (e.g., captopril, enalapril, lisinopril, fosinopril). The clinical differences among these drugs are their duration of action and the necessity for hepatic activation (prodrug).
   2. **AT II inhibitors** (e.g., losartan, valsartan, irbesartan, candesartan) block the binding of AT II to type-1 AT II receptors.

B. **Mechanism of action.** Sympathetic nervous system stimulation and reduction in renal perfusion pressure (e.g., renal artery stenosis, hypovolemia) stimulate the release of renin from the kidneys. Renin converts angiotensinogen to angiotensin I, which is hydrolyzed in the lung by ACE to a potent vasoconstrictor, angiotensin II. Circulating AT II constricts arterioles and stimulates aldosterone secretion, thereby enhancing reabsorption of sodium and water and excretion of potassium. The antihypertensive effect of ACE and AT II inhibitors is primarily through the prevention of AT II formation or action.

C. **Choice of the agent.** ACE inhibitors improve the outcome of acute, hemodynamically stable myocardial infarction, CHF, and the progression of diabetic nephropathy. ACE inhibitors are effective agents for the initial and chronic management of hypertension. The main practical differences among the several available agents are the **duration of action** and **availability of an IV formulation.**

D. **Administration. Enalaprilat** is the active form of enalapril; it is available for IV use in doses of 0.25 to 5 mg every 6 hours. **Captopril** also is used in IV doses of 6.25 to 25 mg every 6 to 8 hours.

E. **Adverse effects**
   1. **Hypotension** occurs, especially in patients who are hypovolemic or receiving diuretics.
   2. **Renal failure.** Patients with bilateral **renal artery stenosis** or high-grade stenosis in a solitary kidney can develop acute renal failure from a decrease in renal perfusion pressure. Functional renal insufficiency can develop in other patients; it responds to a dose reduction of the ACE inhibitor or a withholding of the medication until renal function improves. The ACE inhibitor then can be restarted at a lower dosage.
   3. **Angioedema** in its severe form can cause airway obstruction, which necessitates endotracheal intubation. Angioedema is rarely observed with AT II inhibitors.
   4. **Hyperkalemia.** Patients with impaired renal function or receiving potassium supplements or potassium-sparing diuretics are at greater risk.

XIII. **Diuretics** are useful in the treatment of CHF and fluid overload, but they have a limited role in hypertensive crises.

A. Diuretics are **classified** by their primary site of action on renal tubules and the mechanism by which they alter the excretion of solutes.

1. **Loop diuretics** (e.g., furosemide, bumetanide, ethacrynic acid) act on the ascending loop of Henle, inhibiting reabsorption of sodium and chloride and promoting urinary excretion of sodium, chloride, and water.

2. **Thiazide** (e.g., chlorothiazide, hydrochlorothiazide) and **related sulfonamide diuretics** (e.g., metolazone) act on the cortical portion of the ascending loop of Henle and, to a lesser extent, on the proximal and distal renal tubules.

3. **Carbonic anhydrase inhibitors** (e.g., acetazolamide) act on the proximal convoluted tubule, inhibiting bicarbonate reabsorption, which produces metabolic acidosis.

4. **Potassium-sparing diuretics** (e.g., spironolactone, triamterene, amiloride) act on the distal convoluted tubule and collecting duct, increasing urinary excretion of sodium and chloride.

5. **Osmotic diuretics** (e.g., mannitol) increase osmolarity of renal tubular fluid and prevent reabsorption of water.

B. **Choice of the agent. Loop diuretics** have a potent effect and fast onset. Acute renal failure and CHF are common indications. During **hypertensive crises,** the role of diuretics is limited to cases in which fluid overload is present. Combinations of diuretics that act on different parts of the renal tubules (e.g., furosemide and a thiazide) can enhance the natriuretic response. Because of its venodilator effect, furosemide is an effective adjunct in the treatment of CHF.

C. **Adverse effects** are mostly dose related.

1. **Hypokalemia** and **hypomagnesemia** can be induced by thiazide and loop diuretics and potentiate ventricular ectopic activity, especially when concomitant digoxin, β-adrenergic therapy, or preexisting myocardial irritability is present.

2. **Insulin resistance.** Thiazides and, to a lesser degree, loop diuretics can cause hyperglycemia secondary to insulin resistance.

3. **Metabolic alkalosis** can occur with thiazides and loop diuretics, secondary to loss of large amounts of fluids and potassium.

4. **Ototoxicity.** Transient or permanent deafness is a rare complication produced by large amounts of furosemide or ethacrynic acid.

SELECTED REFERENCES

Brater DC. Diuretic therapy. *N Engl J Med* 1998;339:387–395.

Chernow B. *Essentials of critical care pharmacology,* 2nd ed. Baltimore: Williams & Wilkins, 1994.

Hardman JG, Limbird LE. *Goodman & Gilman's the pharmacological basis of therapeutics,* 9th ed. New York: McGraw-Hill, 1996.

Joint National Committee on Prevention, Detection, Evaluation, and Treatment of High Blood Pressure. The sixth report of the Joint National Committee on Prevention, Detection, Evaluation, and Treatment of High Blood Pressure. *Arch Intern Med* 1997;157: 2413–2446.

Massie BM. The safety of calcium-channel blockers. *Clin Cardiol* 1998;21:II12–II17.

Stoelting RK. *Pharmacology and physiology in anesthetic practice,* 3rd ed. Philadelphia: Lippincott-Raven, 1999.

Neurocritical Care

Colin McDonald, Mustapha Ezzeddine,
and Lee H. Schwamm

I. **Neuroprotection** is the goal of neurocritical care.
   A. **Common presenting symptoms** that require neurocritical care intervention include weakness, cognitive dysfunction, reduced alertness with or without impaired airway reflexes, uncontrolled seizures, and respiratory muscle failure.
   B. **Diagnoses** likely to produce these symptoms include subarachnoid, subdural or intracerebral hemorrhage, ischemic stroke, brain tumor, infectious or inflammatory meningoencephalitis, traumatic brain or spinal cord injury, status epilepticus, toxic-metabolic encephalopathy, amyotrophic lateral sclerosis, myasthenia gravis, and acute myopathies or polyneuropathies.
   C. Because cerebral ischemia and hypoxemia are the most common mechanisms of secondary brain injury, a thorough understanding of the regulation of cerebral blood flow is necessary. In addition, familiarity with the neurologic examination of the critically ill patient is required for early recognition of secondary brain injury and subsequent evaluation of the efficacy of therapeutic interventions.
   D. Three aspects distinguish hemodynamic management in neurocritical care from that of other critically ill patients:
      1. Assessment of end-organ perfusion is at times more difficult to determine.
      2. Because of the lack of local energy reserves, the interval to end-organ failure under adverse conditions is more rapid.
      3. Unlike most other organs, injury to even small regions of brain can have devastating consequences.

II. **Intracranial hemodynamics**
   A. **Intracranial compliance.** The skull is a rigid box filled with incompressible brain parenchyma. When the volume inside the skull increases, evacuation of cerebrospinal fluid (CSF) into the extracranial subarachnoid space occurs, followed by a rapid rise in intracranial pressure (ICP) (Fig. 11-1). Intracranial pressure is normally less than 10 mm Hg; transient elevations up to 30 mm Hg are well tolerated. When ICP rises above 20 mm Hg [or cerebral perfusion pressure (CPP) falls below 60 mm Hg], cerebral blood flow (CBF) may be inadequate.
   B. **Cerebral blood flow** equals the CPP divided by the cerebrovascular resistance (CVR), according to Ohm's

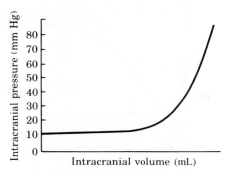

Fig. 11-1. Intracranial compliance curve. In the normal intracranial pressure (ICP) range, increases in intracranial volume produce minimal changes in ICP initially. Further small increases in intracranial volume at the "elbow" of the curve, however, can produce an abrupt increase in ICP.

Law. The CPP is the difference between the mean intracerebral artery pressure (difficult to measure) and mean ICP (easy to measure). The CVR (difficult to measure) is the ability of the precapillary arterioles to dilate and constrict in response to changes in pressure or metabolic factors. Because CBF is cumbersome to measure directly and CBF is held relatively constant over a mean arterial pressure (MAP) between 50 and 150 mm Hg in healthy, young individuals, a CPP of 60 to 90 mm Hg likely provides appropriate CBF (Fig. 11-2).

C. **Autoregulation of CBF is often impaired** in patients with acute cerebral injury. In this setting, reductions in CPP below 60 mm Hg may decrease CBF and cause cerebral ischemia. Increases in CPP above 80 mm Hg can increase CBF and cause vasogenic edema and increased ICP. An optimal CPP goal, therefore, should include both a minimal and maximal valve.

D. **Tissue oxygen delivery.** Because brain energy metabolism is dependent on continuous tissue oxygen influx, the primary focus should be optimal tissue oxygen delivery. Over a wide range of temperature and pH, oxygen delivery is proportional to the oxygen saturation, hemoglobin content, and cardiac output. Cardiac output can be compromised because of hypovolemia, sepsis, impaired myocardial contractility or cardiac dysrhythmia as a complicating factor of brain or spinal cord injury.

E. **Oxygen extraction.** The immense energy requirements of the brain demand a system for oxygen deliv-

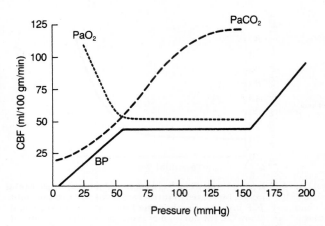

Fig. 11-2. Autoregulation maintains a constant level of cerebral blood flow (CBF) over a wide range of carotid artery mean blood pressures (BPs). Independent of this effect, CBF is elevated by hypercarbia ($PaCO_2$) and hypoxemia (PaO_2); hypocarbia diminishes CBF.

ery that can tolerate sudden increases in demand (e.g., seizures) or decreases in supply (e.g., hypotension and hypoxemia). Unlike other organs, a system of "oxygen reserve" exists in which the brain can vary its oxygen extraction from a baseline of approximately 30% to an extreme of 70% under conditions of oligemia (CBF 20–30 ml/100 g/min). It is only when CBF decreases below 20 ml/100 g/min that electrical and chemical cellular functions are interrupted and ischemic symptoms develop. Increased oxygen extraction can be demonstrated with radiolabeled oxygen species using positron emission tomography (PET) or single photon emission computed tomography (SPECT) imaging, (not practical in the management of most critically ill patients), or as a decrease in cerebral mixed venous oxygen saturation via cerebral venous jugular bulb sampling ($SjvO_2$). The latter has been used at the bedside as a measure of inadequate CBF in patients with traumatic brain injury or those undergoing cardiopulmonary bypass.

F. **Medications that influence ICP**
    1. **Vasodilators** (e.g, hydralazine, nitroprusside and nitroglycerin) can induce cerebral vasodilation. In patients with poor intracranial compliance, this can increase ICP.
    2. **Beta-adrenergic blockers** (e.g., labetolol or propranolol) have minimal direct effect on CBF or ICP and are easily titrated. Because labetolol also

blocks α-adrenergic tone, it may reduce sympathetically mediated large vessel vasoconstriction. This better simulates the endogenous mechanisms of lowering blood pressure (BP) and helps to prevent regional ischemia as BP is lowered pharmacologically.

3. **Barbiturates** (e.g., thiopental and pentobarbital), although typically administered to lower ICP, are also potent antihypertensive agents that decrease venous tone and cardiac contractility. These usually undesirable side effects may require the use of α, β, or both, adrenergic agonists (e.g., phenylephrine, norepinephrine) to maintain adequate CPP.

4. **Catecholamines** have an unpredictable potential to increase cerebral metabolic rate and CBF. These effects are likely to be more pronounced as BP is increased above normal and in the presence of blood–brain barrier disruption.

5. **Hypo-osmolar and iso-osmolar solutions** (e.g., lactated Ringer's solution, D5 1/2 NS) can exacerbate brain edema in the setting of osmotic diuretic therapy. **Glucose-containing solutions** can produce hyperglycemia, which increases cerebral metabolism and can lead to neurologic worsening after brain ischemia.

G. **Other factors that influence ICP**

1. Intracranial pressure is increased by many of the complications of **central venous access,** including pneumothorax, carotid puncture, painful stimulation, and body position (e.g., Trendelenberg, lateral head rotation, jugular compression). Patients should be kept in optimal position for ICP management until the last possible moment prior to puncture.

2. **Noxious stimuli** can increase ICP, CBF, and cerebral metabolic rate and should be prevented and treated aggressively.

III. **Extracranial hemodynamics.** The primary goal of systemic blood pressure management is defined by the type of central nervous system (CNS) or systemic injuries present. An optimal CPP must be maintained at all times. Because mean arterial blood pressure decreases to the same extent (< 20%) between the aortic root and the distal middle cerebral arteries or the radial arteries, conventionally measured systemic MAP is a reasonable surrogate for mean intracerebral artery pressure.

A. **Reduced CPP.** In the case of reduced CPP, the primary objective should be the lowering of ICP, but systemic MAP may need to be pharmacologically augmented while the ICP reduction strategies are initiated. The first choice in patients with adequate myocardial contractility should be a pure **α-adrenergic agonist** (e.g., phenylephrine), because it is well tolerated and causes minimal cerebrovascular vasoconstriction. If this does not produce sufficient blood pressure elevations or there is inadequate contractility to support the increased systemic vascular resistance, then additional inotropic support is required.

B. **Excessive CPP.** When evidence is seen of excessive CBF because of severe hypertension or impaired autoregulation or blood–brain barrier permeability (e.g., eclampsia, brain neoplasm), MAP should be reduced in a reliable and highly titratable manner. Hypertension alone, in the absence of excessive CBF or myocardial dysfunction, should not be treated, as it often reflects a homeostatic response to acute cerebral ischemia. Reductions in blood pressure can provoke cerebral ischemia in this setting.

1. **Sympathetic antagonists** (e.g., labetolol) reduce the systemic effects of the high catecholamine output states frequently associated with CNS injury, including arterial hypertension, tachycardia, cardiac irritability, neurogenic pulmonary vascular injury, and large vessel vasoconstriction.

2. Often, additional agents are necessary, and **sodium nitroprusside** can cause a reliable and titratable response.

3. **Avoid** sublingual administration of short-acting calcium channel blockers, which lower pressure unpredictably without reducing sympathetic output.

C. **Cardiac dysrhythmias**

1. In large strokes and subarachnoid hemorrhage, **ST segment changes** may be seen on the electrocardiogram (ECG), but these do not predict future cardiovascular morbidity. Electrocardiographic changes may be diffuse or confined to a cardiovascular territory. Myocardial ischemia should always be excluded.

2. **The sympathetic outflow** associated with brain injury less frequently provokes ventricular dysrhythmias in patients with coronary artery disease.

3. **Guillain Barré syndrome** can produce an autonomic cardioneuropathy.

4. **Cervical spine injury** can cause sympathetic cardiac denervation and unopposed vagal tone, leading to bradydysrhythmias.

IV. **Airway and ventilation**

A. **Indications for endotracheal intubation.** Impairment of airway reflexes occurs frequently in the brain-injured patient, which predisposes the patient to aspiration and poor clearance of secretions. **Neuromuscular respiratory failure** can be seen in amyotrophic lateral sclerosis, myasthenia gravis, acute inflammatory demyelinating polyneuritis (AIDP) and critical care myopathy or polyneuropathy. **Transient apnea** in the setting of a self-limited generalized convulsion is not an indication for intubation or assisted ventilation.

B. **Complications of endotracheal intubation** include hypotension, reduced CBF, and paradoxically increased ICP from increased transthoracic pressures. A physician skilled in airway management should be present at the intubation of a patient with intracranial hypertension or hemorrhage.

C. **Permissive hypercapnia** may be effective in reducing pulmonary morbidity and mortality in acute respiratory distress syndrome (ARDS) (see Chapters 4 and 20). Unfortunately, it also is associated with unacceptable elevations in ICP and is generally not tolerated by patients with intracranial hypertension or blood–brain barrier injuries.

D. **Spontaneous or induced hyperventilation** causes acute cerebral vasoconstriction in a brain in which CO_2 reactivity is preserved (Fig. 11-2). This decreases cerebral blood volume (CBV) and ICP. If pressure autoregulation is preserved, the increased CPP restores adequate CBF.

1. **The brain quickly equilibrates** to changes in P_{CO_2}. A new steady state is established within 3 to 4 hours in most patients. This is accomplished by carbonic anhydrase and other non-bicarbonate buffer systems.

2. **With excessive hypocapnia,** excessive vasoconstriction can produce regional or generalized cerebral ischemia.

3. **A rapid return to baseline P_{CO_2}** can produce cerebral vasodilation, causing increased CBV and a further deleterious rise in ICP. Therefore, hyperventilation should be used as a temporizing measure until more effective and durable measures can be initiated.

4. **Lack of response to hyperventilation** is a poor prognostic sign.

V. **Sodium and water homeostasis**

A. **Sodium balance.** The goal of fluid resuscitation in the brain-injured patient is to maintain **hyperosmolar euvolemia.** This is accomplished with the use of osmotic diuretics (e.g., mannitol, 3% saline) and hyperosmolar IV fluid replacement (e.g., normal saline). Brain injury can disturb sodium balance in several different ways, sometimes simultaneously. Rapid shifts in plasma sodium can produce demyelination or aggravate cerebral edema.

1. **Hyponatremia.** Cerebral injury can cause release of **naturetic factors,** leading to profound salt wasting that may require up to 200 ml/h of normal saline replacement. This is seen most often in vasospasm after subarachnoid hemorrhage.

a. **Syndrome of inappropriate antidiuretic hormone** release should be treated aggressively with normal or hypertonic saline and loop diuretics when intravascular volume repletion is essential and fluid restriction is contraindicated.

    b. High dose osmotic diuretic administration (mannitol 50 g IV every 4 hours) rarely demands renal solute excretion to such a degree that it causes paradoxical free water retention. This is easily treated with small doses of loop diuretic to degrade the renal concentrating ability.

    c. Intravascular volume depletion remains the most common cause of hyponatremia in the neurointensive care unit. Bladder catheterization and monitoring of central venous pressure (CVP) and plasma sodium are essential.

  2. Diabetes insipidus producing **hypernatremia** is seen after pituitary tumor resection, traumatic brain injury, and central herniation syndromes. Hypotonic fluids and vasopressin therapy may be indicated, and hourly monitoring of urine output and specific gravity are required.

B. Water balance

  1. Plasma osmolality = $(2 \times [Na^+]) + ([BUN]/18) + ([Glucose]/100)$ and is normally 280 to 290 mOsm/kg.

  2. When plasma osmolality is increased above normal for more than 48 hours, intracellular osmotic particles are generated and a new steady state is achieved to restore cell volume. Any rapid correction of plasma osmolality after this time will result in a shift of free water into the intracranial compartment. Therefore, once osmotic agents have been initiated with sustained osmolality, they must be withdrawn gradually to permit excretion of these **idiogenic osmoles.** This is true regardless of the osmotic agent.

  3. Mannitol should be given to attain the minimal osmolality sufficient to produce the desired effects, and this often results in a step-wise increase in osmolality targets (e.g., 300, 310, 320 mOsm/kg). Osmolality in excess of 320 mOsm/kg with mannitol does not produce incremental benefits and is associated with acute renal failure.

VI. Hypothesis-driven neurologic examination

  A. The neurologic examination of the critically ill patient should document cortical, brainstem, and spinal cord function in a simple and easily reproducible manner that can be recognized by a colleague at a later point in time.

    1. Avoid confusing eponyms and empty summaries (e.g., "MS nonfocal").

    2. Report the neurologic examination in the following order: cognitive functions (alertness, orientation, attention, language), cranial nerves, strength, sensation, deep tendon reflexes, other.

3. **Use the minimal stimulus** first, then escalate as needed (e.g., speak before yelling, yell before pinching).

4. **Coma** is produced by bilateral cortical or bilateral brainstem dysfunction.

B. **Cortical function. Language and attention** are lateralized in the human brain, and essentially all righthanders and 85% of lefthanders process language in the left hemisphere and attention in the right hemisphere. The **motor cortex** (precentral gyrus) controls the contralateral limbs and directs voluntary gaze (saccades) to the contralateral field. **Sensation** is processed in the postcentral gyrus of the contralateral hemispheres. **Inattention,** which is common in critically ill patients, often is caused by medication or metabolic insults. Lateralizing hemiparesis, sensory loss, or gaze deviation, however, should trigger urgent investigation. **Cortical injury** often produces face and arm weakness because of the large area they represent on the brain's surface.

C. **Brainstem function.** The brainstem controls involuntary eye movements, pupillary function, facial sensation, and vital functions. Knowledge of its functions is critical in the evaluation of the comatose patient and the posterior circulation acute stroke syndromes (see Table 11-1).

Table 11-1. Common findings in midbrain lesions

Lesion level	Common findings	Anatomic pathway
Midbrain	Midposition fixed pupils	Light reflex pathways
	Ophthalmoplegia	Oculomotor nuclei
	Hemiparesis, Babinski sign	Cerebral peduncles
High pons	Pinpoint, reactive pupils	Sympathetic fibers
	Internuclear ophthalmoplegia	Medial longitudinal fasciculus
	Facial weakness	Facial nerve
	Reduced corneal sensation	Trigeminal nerve
Low pons	Horizontal gaze paralysis	Abducens nerve, horizontal gaze center
	Hemiparesis, Babinski sign	Corticospinal, corticobulbar tracts
Medulla	Disordered breathing	Respiratory center
	Hypotension, hypertension, dysrhythmias	Vasomotor center

D. Spinal cord function. In contrast to brainstem and cortical injury, spinal cord injury often produces bilateral, symmetric impairment of the limbs but never facial weakness. Always distinguish anterior column function (strength, sensation of pain or temperature) from posterior column function (sensation of vibration, proprioception) and document sacral functions (anal sphincter tone, bulbocavernosus reflex). The **anterior spinal artery** receives contributions from the vertebral arteries in the cervical region and the artery of Adamkiewicz (a branch of the abdominal aorta) in the thoracolumbar region. This anatomy creates a "watershed" vascular territory, which is susceptible to hypoperfusion in the high thoracic cord.

1. **Brown-Sèquard syndrome** or hemisection is characterized by ipsilateral loss of motor and proprioceptive functions and contralateral loss of pain and temperature.

2. **Central cord syndrome** is characterized by weakness in arms more than legs and variable sensory, bladder, and bowel dysfunction. This predilection for arm involvement is caused by the medial lamination of arm fibers in the descending corticospinal tracts.

3. **Anterior spinal artery syndrome** is characterized by bilateral symmetric motor weakness and disassociated sensory loss, with impairments in pain and temperature sensation and preservation of proprioception and vibration.

4. **Cauda equina syndrome** is characterized by variable degrees of bilateral lower motor neuron weakness in the legs (sparing the arms), sensory loss of the lower extremities and sacrum, and dysfunction of bowel and bladder.

5. **Mixed tract syndromes** occur commonly in traumatic injury to the spinal cord. The aim of localization is to identify the highest level of injury (see Table 11-2 and Chapter 33).

VII. Neuroimaging. Recent advances in **computed tomography (CT)** and **magnetic resonance imaging (MRI)** now make it possible, noninvasively, to image neurovascular structures and identify sites of venous sinus thrombosis, arterial occlusion, nonocclusive dissection, focal tissue ischemia, and diffuse axonal injury (Figs. 11-3, 11-4, and 11-5). Areas of mismatch between tissue hypoperfusion (oligemia) and tissue ischemia can be identified to measure tissue at risk. Spinal cord compression or ischemia can also be evaluated rapidly. With appropriate planning, MRI can be performed in the presence of a halo vest or invasive monitoring. Extra lengths of rigid tubing can pass from the patient, through a small hole placed in the shielding wall, to monitoring equipment and infusion pumps located in the MRI control room. **Nuclear medicine blood flow imaging** is useful to assess cerebral perfusion in cases of suspected brain death, especially when factors that confound the clinical evaluation are present.

Table 11-2. Representative motor functions of spinal roots

Spinal root(s)	Representative motor function
C3–C4	Diaphragm function (phrenic nerve)
C5	Shoulder adduction
C5–C6	Elbow flexion (biceps, brachialis)
C7	Elbow extension (triceps)
C8–T1	Hand grip (finger flexors), finger adduction, oculosympathetics
T2–T12	Expiration (intercostal muscles)
L1–L2	Hip flexion (iliopsoas)
L2–L4	Knee extension (quadriceps)
L5–S1	Knee flexion (hamstrings)

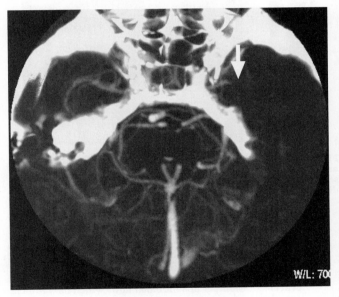

Fig. 11-3. Computed tomography angiogram in a patient with acute ischemic stroke. *Arrow* indicates abrupt cut-off at the left middle cerebral artery stem.

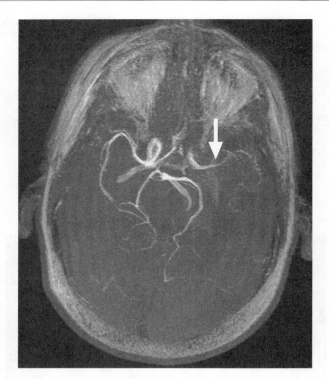

Fig. 11-4. Three-dimensional time of flight magnetic resonance angiography collapsed MIP image in a patient with left carotid dissection. The *arrow* indicates poor flow-related enhancement of the distal left middle cerebral artery.

Transcranial Doppler ultrasound imaging can identify regions of increased blood flow velocity consistent with focal arterial narrowing (e.g., atherosclerosis, vasospasm), retrograde flow (which provides information about collateral circulation), or absent blood flow (which may indicate complete occlusion).

VIII.   Coagulation disturbances. Because of the release of large quantities of brain tissue thromboplastin, massive brain injury can be associated with activation of the clotting cascade, disseminated intravascular coagulation, and subsequent clinical hemorrhage or clotting. Fresh frozen plasma can be administered to treat coagulopathies in the setting of intracerebral hemorrhage (see Chapter 12 for diagnosis and management of coagulopathies). Brain tumors, coma, and paraplegia place patients at high risk for deep vein thrombosis (see Chapter 22 for diagnosis and treatment).

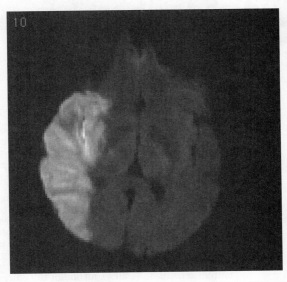

Fig. 11-5. Axial diffusion-weighted image in a patient with acute ischemic stroke. The region of hyperintensity represents a large area of early cytotoxic edema caused by ischemic cell injury.

SELECTED REFERENCES

Adams RD, Victor M. *Principles of neurology.* New York: McGraw-Hill, Inc., 1993.

Arieff AI, Kerian A, Massry SG, et al. Intracellular pH of brain: alterations in acute respiratory acidosis and alkalosis. *Am J Physiol* 1976; 230:804–812.

Fisher CM. The neurological examination of the comatose patient. *Acta Neurol Scand* 1969;45 (Suppl 36):1–56.

Guarantors of brain. *Aids to the examination of the peripheral nervous system.* London, England:Bailliere Tindall, 1986.

Paulson OB, Standgaard S, Edvinsson L. Cerebral autoregulation. *Cerebrovasc Brain Metabolism Reviews* 1990;2:161–192.

Plum F, Posner JB. *Diagnosis of stupor and coma,* 3rd ed. Philadelphia: FA Davis, 1982.

Ropper AH. *Neurological and neurosurgical intensive care,* 3rd ed. New York: Raven Press, 1993.

Schwamm LH, Koroshetz WJ, Sorensen AG, et al. Time course of lesion development in patients with acute stroke: serial diffusion- and hemodynamic-weighted magnetic resonance imaging. *Stroke* 1998;29:2268–2276.

Wijdicks EF. *The clinical practice of critical care neurology.* New York: Lippincott-Raven, 1997.

Hematology and Transfusion Therapy

Rae M. Allain and Richard M. Pino

I. **Indications for transfusion therapy.** Blood component transfusion is usually performed because of decreased production; increased utilization, destruction, or loss; or dysfunction of a specific blood component (red cells, platelets, or coagulation factors).

   A. **Anemia**

   1. **Hematocrit.** The main reason for transfusing red cells is to maintain oxygen-carrying capacity to the tissues. Healthy individuals or individuals with a chronic anemia can usually tolerate a hematocrit (Hct) of 20% to 25%, assuming normal intravascular volume. In patients with coronary artery disease, it is clinical practice to maintain higher hematocrits (28% to 30%), although the efficacy of this practice is unproved.

   2. If a patient is anemic, the cause should be clarified. It may be secondary to decreased production (marrow suppression), increased loss (hemorrhage), or destruction (hemolysis).

   3. Estimating the volume of blood to transfuse can be calculated as follows:

   $$\text{Volume to transfuse} = (\text{Hct}_{desired} - \text{Hct}_{present}) \times \text{BV}/\text{Hct}_{transfused\ blood}.$$

   The blood volume (BV) of an adult is approximately 7% of lean body mass or 70 mL of blood/kg of body weight.

   B. **Thrombocytopenia.** Spontaneous bleeding is unusual with platelet counts above 5,000 to 10,000/μL, but in the immediate postoperative period, counts above 50,000 are preferable. Thrombocytopenia is caused by either decreased bone marrow production (e.g., chemotherapy, tumor infiltration, alcoholism) or increased utilization or destruction (e.g., hypersplenism, idiopathic thrombocytopenia purpura, drug effects (e.g., heparin, H_2 blockers, ticarcillin). It is also seen with massive blood transfusion.

   C. **Coagulopathy.** Bleeding associated with documented factor deficiencies or prolonged clotting studies [prothrombin time, (PT) partial thromboplastin time (aPPT)] mandates replacement therapy to maintain normal coagulation function.

   1. **Coagulation studies.** The most important clue to a clinically significant bleeding disorder in an otherwise healthy patient remains the history.

Prior surgical bleeding, gingival bleeding, easy bruising, epistaxis, or menorrhagia should raise concern. Many tests are available to assess coagulation, but no single test measures the integrity of the entire coagulation system.

a. **Partial thromboplastin time (aPTT)** is performed by adding particulate matter to a blood sample to activate the intrinsic coagulation system. Normal values for the aPTT are between 25 and 37 seconds and depend on normal levels of clotting factors in the intrinsic coagulation system. The test is sensitive to decreased amounts of coagulation factors and is elevated in patients on heparin therapy. The aPTT will also be abnormal if a circulating anticoagulant is present (e.g., lupus anticoagulant, antibodies to Factor VIII). The clinician should remember that an abnormal aPTT does not necessarily correlate with clinical bleeding. Aggressive correction of an abnormal aPTT in surgical patients is not always indicated, unless the patient is actively bleeding.

b. **Prothrombin time,** a measure of the extrinsic coagulation system, is measured by adding a thromboplastin reagent to a blood sample. Although both PT and aPTT are affected by levels of Factors V and X, prothrombin, and fibrinogen, the PT is specifically sensitive to deficiencies of Factor VII. The PT is normal in deficiencies of Factors VIII, IX, XI, XII, prekallikrein, and high molecular-weight kininogen. The **INR** (International Normalized Ratio) standardizes PT values to permit comparisons of PT value among laboratories or within one laboratory but at different times. The INR is the ratio of patient PT to control PT that would be obtained if international reference reagents had been used to perform the test. Prior to the development of the INR, differences in thromboplastin reagent activity prevented meaningful comparisons of PT values. Oral anticoagulation therapy can be guided by a target INR value that is independent of laboratory variability. Use of the INR is limited to oral anticoagulation therapy; it has no role in the assessment of a prolonged PT unrelated to warfarin use.

c. **Activated clotting time (ACT)** is a modified whole blood clotting time in which diatomaceous earth is added to a blood sample to activate the intrinsic clotting system. The ACT is the time until clot formation. A normal ACT is between 90 and 130 seconds. The ACT, a relatively easy and expedient test to perform, is useful in monitoring heparin therapy when immediate results are required.

    d. **The bleeding time** was thought to be a crude assay of platelet function. Results are technician dependent, poorly reproducible, and do not correlate with clinical observations of hemostasis in the perioperative period. The bleeding time is no longer recommended for assessment of coagulation status.

    e. **Fibrinogen** can be depleted by excessive consumption, as in massive hemorrhage or disseminated intravascular coagulation (DIC). A normal fibrinogen level is 170 to 410 mg/dl. It is an acute phase reactant and is often elevated in postoperative patients or following trauma or inflammation. For extensive surgical procedures associated with bleeding or in cases of massive transfusion, it is prudent to maintain the fibrinogen level above 100 mg/dl.

    f. **Fibrin(ogen) degradation products (FDP)** are peptides produced from the action of plasmin on fibrinogen or fibrin monomer. They are measurable by serum assays and can aid in the diagnosis of primary fibrinolysis or DIC. FDPs modulate further clotting or lysis by interfering with fibrin monomer polymerization and by impairing platelet function. FDPs are often elevated in severe hepatic disease because of failed clearance from the circulation.

    g. **D-dimer** is a specific fragment produced when plasmin digests cross-linked fibrin (clot). It is measurable by serum assay and is elevated in pulmonary embolism, DIC, and in patients receiving surgery within the preceding 48 hours.

    h. **Factor assays** are specialized tests that quantitate the activity of individual coagulation factors. Most of these are performed in the setting of an unexplained coagulopathy that has not improved after attempted repletion of coagulation factors; they are usually obtained in concert with a clinical pathology or hematology consultation. Classically, factor assays are used to confirm the diagnosis of hemophilia A or B.

II. **Blood typing and cross-matching**

  A. **Donor and recipient blood** is typed in the red cell surface **ABO and Rh systems** and screened for antibodies to other cell antigens. Cross-matching involves directly mixing the patient's plasma with the donor's red cells to establish that hemolysis does not occur from any undetected antibodies. An individual's red cells have either A, B, AB, or no surface antigens. If the patient's red cells are lacking either surface antigen A or B, then antibodies will be produced against it. A person who is type B will have anti-A antibodies in the serum, and a type O individual (having neither

A nor B surface antigens) will have circulating anti-A and anti-B antibodies. Consequently, a person who is type AB will not have antibodies to either A or B and can receive red blood cells from any blood type. Type O blood has neither A nor B surface antigens and can donate blood cells to any other type (universal red cell donor).

B. Rh surface antigens are either present (Rh-positive) or absent (Rh-negative). Individuals who are Rh-negative will develop antibodies to the Rh factor when exposed to Rh-positive blood. This is not a problem with the initial exposure, but hemolysis will occur because of the circulating antibodies with subsequent exposures. This can be a particular problem during pregnancy. The anti-Rh antibodies are IgG and freely cross the placenta. In Rh-negative mothers who have developed Rh antibodies, these antibodies are transmitted to the fetus. If the fetus is Rh-positive, massive hemolysis will occur, termed "hemolytic disease of the newborn." **Rh-immune globulin,** an Rh blocking antibody, prevents the Rh-negative patient from developing anti-Rh antibodies. Rh-immune globulin is routinely administered to Rh-negative women pregnant with Rh-positive fetuses and should be given to Rh-negative individuals who receive Rh-positive blood, especially women of childbearing age. The recommendation is one dose (~ 300 μg/vial) for every 15 ml of Rh-positive blood transfused.

III. Blood component therapy

A. Whole blood

1. Whole blood has been largely replaced by component therapy because of storage impediments and no demonstrable superiority. The one exception may be children aged less than 2 years undergoing complicated cardiovascular surgery where whole blood may have an outcome benefit in reduced transfusions. Overall, component therapy is far more efficient and practical for transfusion.

2. Whole blood must be ABO and Rh identical.

B. Red blood cells (RBC)

1. One unit of packed RBC (hematocrit ~ 70%, volume about 250 ml) usually raises the hematocrit of a euvolemic adult by 2% to 3% once equilibration has taken place.

2. RBCs must be ABO compatible (see Table 12-1). If an emergency blood transfusion is needed, type-specific (ABO) red cells can usually be obtained within minutes if the patient's blood type is known. If type-specific blood is unavailable, type O Rh-negative red cells should be transfused. Type-specific blood should be substituted as soon as possible to minimize the amount of type O plasma (containing anti-A and anti-B antibodies) transfused.

C. Platelets

1. One unit of random donor platelets increases the platelet count by 5, 000 to 10,000/μL. If thrombo-

Table 12-1.   Transfusion compatibility^a

Recipient			Donor			
Red Blood Cells	A	B	O	AB	Rh+	Rh−
A	X		X			
B		X	X			
O			X			
AB	X	X	X	X		
Rh+					X	X
Rh−						X
Fresh frozen plasma						
A	X			X		
B		X		X		
O	X	X	X	X		
AB				X		
Rh+					X	X
Rh−					X	X

^a Compatible transfusions are marked by X.

cytopenia is caused by increased destruction (e.g., from development of antiplatelet antibodies), platelet transfusions will be less efficacious. A posttransfusion platelet count, drawn 10 minutes after completion of platelet transfusion, confirms platelet refractoriness if the count fails to increase by $5,000/\mu L$ per random donor unit transfused.

2. **ABO-compatible platelets** are not required for transfusion, although they may provide a better response as measured by the posttransfusion platelet count. **Single-donor platelets** are obtained from one individual by platelet pheresis; one unit is equivalent to approximately six random donor units. Single-donor platelets can be used to reduce exposure to multiple donors, or in cases of poor response to random donor platelets where destruction is suspected. In cases where alloimmunization causes platelet refractoriness, **HLA-matched platelets** may be required for effective platelet transfusion. **Rh-negative women** of childbearing age should receive Rh-negative platelets if possible because some RBCs are transfused with platelets. If this is impossible, Rh-immune globulin can be administered.

D. **Fresh-frozen plasma (FFP)** in a dose of 10 to 15 ml/kg will generally increase plasma coagulation factors to 30% of normal.

1. Factors V and VIII are most labile and quickly become depleted in thawed FFP. Fibrinogen levels increase by 1 mg/ml of plasma transfused. Acute

reversal of warfarin requires only 5 to 8 ml/kg of fresh-frozen plasma.

2. ABO-compatible FFP transfusion (Table 12-1) is required, but Rh-negative patients can receive Rh-positive FFP.

3. Six units of platelets contain the equivalent of one unit of fresh-frozen plasma.

4. Volume expansion in itself should not be an indication for FFP transfusion.

E. **Cryoprecipitate** is the material formed from thawing FFP at 1°C to 6°C.

1. Each unit of cryoprecipitate contains a minimum of 80 IU of Factor VIII and approximately 200 to 300 mg of fibrinogen. It also contains Factor XIII, von Willlebrand's factor, and fibronectin.

2. **Indications for cryoprecipitate** include hypo-fibrinogenemia, von Willebrand's disease, hemophilia A (when Factor VIII is unavailable), and preparation of fibrin glue. The dosage of cryoprecipitate is 1 U/7 to 10 kg, which raises the plasma fibrinogen by approximately 50 mg/dl in a patient without massive bleeding.

3. ABO-compatibility is not required for transfusion of cryoprecipitate, but it is preferred because of the presence of 10 to 20 ml of plasma per unit.

F. **Factor concentrates.** Individual coagulation factors are available for patients with discrete factor deficiencies. These can be derived from pooled human plasma or synthesized by recombinant gene technology. For an intractable coagulopathy with seemingly adequate factor replacement, some clinicians have used **Factor IX complex** (Konyne 80) (Bayer Corporation, Berkeley, CA), which contains Factors II, VII, IX, and X in a small volume. This product should be used extremely cautiously in patients with liver disease, because of the risk of widespread thrombosis occurring from impaired hepatic clearance of activated clotting factors from the circulation.

G. **Technical considerations**

1. Compatible infusions. Blood products should not be infused with 5% dextrose solutions, which will cause hemolysis, or with lactated Ringer's, which contains calcium and can induce clot formation. Sodium chloride (0.9%), albumin (5%), and fresh-frozen plasma are all compatible with red blood cells.

2. **Blood filters (80 μ)** should be used for all blood components, except platelets, to remove debris and microaggregates. **Leukocyte filters** can be used to remove white blood cells in order to prevent transmission of cytomegalovirus to the immunocompromised patient, to prevent alloim-munization to foreign leukocyte antigens, and to diminish the incidence of febrile reactions. **Platelets** should be transfused through a 170 μ blood filter.

IV. Plasma substitutes. Various colloid products are available commercially. Their main limitations are their cost and the dilution of red cells and coagulation factors that occurs with their administration.

   A. Albumin is available as either an isotonic 5% or a hypertonic 20% or 25% solution. Albumin has an intravascular half-life of 10 to 15 days.

   B. Hydroxyethyl starch is manufactured from amylopectin. After infusion, hydroxyethyl starch is stored in the reticuloendothelial cells of the liver for a prolonged time. The starch can increase the serum amylase for several days, which may confuse the diagnosis of pancreatitis. Whereas a decrease in Factor VIII levels and decreased platelet function can be seen, hydroxyethyl starch dosages up to 1 gm/kg have been used without adverse bleeding problems. Anaphylactoid reactions are rare.

V. Pharmacologic therapy

   A. Erythropoietin increases red cell mass by stimulating proliferation and development of the erythroid precursor cells. It has been used to correct anemia in patients with chronic renal failure and increase preoperative hematocrits and red cell mass prior to preoperative autologous donation. A less clear-cut use for erythropoietin may be in the severely anemic patient who refuses blood transfusion (**see XI.B**). Patients taking erythropoietin should also receive iron and folate. Side effects (hypertension and seizures) have been reported in renal failure patients. Initial recommended dosages in renal patients range from 50 to 100 IU/kg intravenously (IV) or subcutaneously (SQ) three times a week.

   B. Granulocyte colony-stimulating factor (GCSF) and granulocyte-macrophage colony-stimulating factor (GMCSF) are myeloid growth factors useful for shortening the duration of neutropenia induced by chemotherapy. GCSF is specific for neutrophils, whereas GMCSF increases production of granulocytes, macrophages, and eosinophils. Administration of these drugs not only enhances neutrophil counts but also killing by neutrophils. As such, they are frequently used in the treatment of febrile neutropenia. Treatment results in an initial brief decrement in the neutrophil count (because of endothelial adherence), then a rapid (usually after 24 hours) sustained leukocytosis that is dose-dependent. Recommended dosages are GCSF 5 µg/kg/d SQ or GMCSF 250 µg/ m²/d SQ until absolute neutrophil count is greater than 10,000/µL.

   C. Thrombopoietin is a hematopoietic growth factor for the megakaryocyte line. It is currently undergoing clinical testing as a means to increase the platelet count in thrombocytopenic patients.

   D. Desmopressin or 1-desamino-8-d-arginine vasopressin (DDAVP) is a vasopressin analog with a more potent and longer duration antidiuretic effect. Desmopressin increases endothelial cell release of von Willebrand's factor, Factor VIII, and plasminogen activator and, thus, has utility in certain bleeding disorders, including hemophilia A (Factor VIII deficiency), classic von Willebrand's disease, and uremic bleeding. The dosage is 0.3 μg/kg IV slowly, as rapid administration can cause hypotension. Repeat dosing at intervals of 12 to 24 hours may be necessary, but tachyphylaxis usually occurs after three or four doses.

E. **Conjugated estrogens** are useful for diminishing bleeding in patients who are uremic. The mechanism is unknown. Unlike desmopressin, the duration of hemostatic effect is long-lasting—usually 10 to 15 days. The onset of effect is delayed compared with the immediacy of desmopressin. Estrogen can be administered IV (0.6 mg/kg/d) or orally (50 mg/d) for a course of 4 to 7 days. Hormonal side effects (gynecomastia, hirsutism, menometrorrhagia) from this short course of therapy are unusual.

F. **Lysine analogues, aminocaproic acid** and **tranexamic acid** inhibit fibrinolysis, the endogenous process by which fibrin clot is broken down. They act by displacing plasminogen from fibrin, diminishing plasminogen conversion to plasmin, and preventing plasmin from binding to fibrinogen or fibrin monomers.

1. **Aminocaproic acid** is used to provide prophylaxis for dental surgery in hemophiliacs, to prevent bleeding in prostatic surgery (TURP), and to reduce hemorrhage in cases of excessive fibrinolysis (e.g., during orthotopic liver transplantation). Because cardiopulmonary bypass can initiate fibrinolysis, aminocaproic acid has been used during cardiac surgery to diminish postoperative bleeding, but its effects on transfusion requirements have been variable. The dosage is 5 g IV load over 1 hour followed by 1 to 2 g/h IV.

2. **Thrombotic risks** of aminocaproic acid have been suggested via case reports, but have not been substantiated by clinical trials. Nevertheless, because normal function of the coagulation cascade involves a balance between pro- and anticoagulant effects, using aminocaproic acid in circumstances where uninhibited clotting may be disastrous (e.g., DIC) is ill-advised and should be undertaken only with expert guidance.

G. **Aprotinin** is a serine protease inhibitor used to decrease blood loss from complicated cardiac procedures and perhaps major surgeries associated with massive hemorrhage, including orthotopic liver transplantation.

1. Aprotinin inhibits trypsin, plasmin, and kallikrein. In clinical practice, aprotinin helps prevent the platelet dysfunction seen with cardiopulmonary

bypass, but the mechanisms for this effect are poorly understood. One of these mechanisms involves protecting the glycoprotein Ib receptor on platelets, thereby preserving platelet adhesive capability.

2. **Complications of aprotinin treatment** include potential anaphylactic reaction. The incidence is approximately 0.1% and greatest in the first 6 months of repeat exposure. Toxicity is primarily renal because of extensive binding and metabolism in renal tubular cells; these effects appear to be reversible and dose-related. Just as with aminocaproic acid, thrombotic complications related to aprotinin use are feared. These fears have generally not been borne out by clinical evidence, but the risks make use of the drug for treatment of DIC very controversial.

3. **Because of the risk of allergy,** an initial IV test dose of 10,000 kallikrein inactivating units (KIU) is recommended. For cardiac surgery, a "high dose" aprotinin regimen (2 million KIU IV load, 2 million KIU cardiopulmonary bypass pump prime, and 500,000 KIU/h IV infusion) and a "low dose" regimen (one half of the preceding) have been described. Advantages to low dose therapy appear to be preserved blood conservation with potentially less renal toxicity. For orthotopic liver transplantation, similar regimens are employed without the pump prime.

4. Aprotinin appears to be more efficacious when it is used prophylactically as opposed to "hemostatic salvage" in the face of massive hemorrhage and coagulopathy. Continuous IV infusion at up to 500,000 KIU/h can be continued postoperatively until bleeding has stopped.

5. **Celite ACTs** are artificially prolonged following heparin administration to patients receiving aprotinin. Kaolin-activated ACTs remain accurate.

VI. **Blood conservation and salvage techniques**
   A. **Autologous donation** usually begins 4 to 5 weeks prior to surgery and can greatly reduce the need for homologous blood transfusion. The length of the predonation period is limited by the length of time that blood can be stored—currently 35 days. If the red cells are frozen, predonation time can be lengthened almost indefinitely. Current blood bank guidelines require a predonation hemoglobin of at least 11 gm/dl, donations no more frequently than every 3 days, and no donations in the 72 hours prior to surgery. Most patients tolerate autologous donation without complication. Because most fatal transfusion reactions are caused by clerical errors, autologous blood should not be transfused unless indicated. The availability of autologous blood should be checked prior to transfusing a patient admitted to the intensive care unit (ICU) following elective surgery.

B. **Intraoperative cell saver or autotransfusion** uses blood collected from the surgical field by a double-lumen suction device. Heparinized normal saline is infused through one lumen so that the blood is anticoagulated as it is suctioned from the surgical field. The aspirated and heparinized blood is filtered and collected in the reservoir. The blood is centrifuged to remove plasma and any debris, washed in normal saline, and then recentrifuged. The hematocrit of these processed units is approximately 50%. These units are deficient in plasma, clotting factors, and platelets. Patients who have received large volumes of autotransfused blood may have a prolonged aPTT because of incomplete removal of heparin from the washed RBCs. The aPTT usually normalizes within several hours or, if the patient is bleeding, the effect can be rapidly reversed with protamine.

C. **Chest tube salvage devices** allow the reinfusion of blood collected from thoracostomy drainage tubes. These are useful for reducing homologous transfusions in the immediate postoperative period. Use of these devices requires skilled nursing for proper administration and sterile technique. They are contraindicated in pleural or mediastinal infection. A potential danger is hyperkalemia from reinfusion of hemolyzed cells, which is occasionally life-threatening.

VII. **Complications of blood transfusion therapy**
   A. **Transfusion reactions**
      1. **Acute hemolytic transfusion reactions** are estimated to occur in 1 of 30,000 transfusions, usually because of clerical errors. Symptoms include anxiety, agitation, chest pain, flank pain, headache, dyspnea, and chills. Nonspecific signs include fever, hypotension, unexplained bleeding (DIC), and hemoglobinuria. If a transfusion reaction is suspected, the following steps should be taken:
         a. Stop transfusion.
         b. Send unused donor blood and a fresh patient sample to the blood bank to be re-cross-matched.
         c. Send blood samples for free hemoglobin, haptoglobin, Coombs' test, and DIC screening. Pink plasma in a spun sample indicates at least 20 mg/dl of free hemoglobin.
         d. Treat hypotension with fluids and vasopressors as indicated.
         e. Consider corticosteroids.
         f. Preserve renal function by increasing renal blood flow and maintaining brisk urine output (IV fluid, furosemide, mannitol).
         g. Be alert for DIC.
      2. **Nonhemolytic transfusion reactions** are usually caused by antibodies against donor white cells or plasma proteins. These patients may complain of anxiety, pruritus, or mild dyspnea. Signs include

fever, flushing, hives, tachycardia, and mild hypotension. The transfusion should be stopped and a hemolytic transfusion reaction ruled out (see above).

  a. If the reaction is only urticaria or hives, the transfusion should be slowed, and antihistamines (diphenhydramine, 25–50 mg IV) and glucocorticoids (hydrocortisone, 50–100 mg IV) can be administered.

  b. In patients with known febrile or allergic transfusion reactions, leukocyte-poor red cells (leukocytes removed by filtration or centrifugation) can be given and the patient pretreated with antipyretics (acetaminophen, 650 mg) and an antihistamine.

  c. **Anaphylactic reactions** occur rarely and may be more common in patients with an IgA deficiency. These reactions are usually caused by plasma protein reactions. Patients with a history of transfusion anaphylaxis should only be transfused with washed red cells (plasma-free).

B. Metabolic complications of blood transfusions

  1. **Potassium (K$^+$)** concentration changes are common with rapid blood transfusion, but seldom of clinical importance. With storage, red cells leak K$^+$ into the extracellular storage fluid. This is rapidly corrected with transfusion and replenishment of erythrocyte energy stores.

  2. **Calcium** is bound by citrate, which is used as an anticoagulant in stored blood products. Rapid transfusion (1 unit of packed RBCs in 5 minutes) may decrease the ionized calcium level. An equal volume of an FFP transfusion is more likely to cause citrate toxicity, compared with packed RBCs, because citrate tends to concentrate in plasma during blood processing. Usually, the decreased ionized calcium level is transient because the citrate is rapidly metabolized by the liver. Severe hypocalcemia, manifested as hypotension, QT segment prolongation on the electrocardiogram, and narrowed pulse pressure, can occur in patients who are hypothermic, have impaired liver function, or have decreased hepatic blood flow. Ionized calcium levels should be monitored during rapid transfu-sions, and calcium replaced intravenously with calcium gluconate (30 mg/kg) or calcium chloride (10 mg/kg) if signs or symptoms of hypocalcemia are present.

  3. **Acid-base status.** Although banked blood is acidic because of the citrate anticoagulant and accumulated red cell metabolites, the actual acid load to the patient is minimal. Acidosis in the face of severe blood loss more likely results from hypoperfusion and will improve with volume resuscita-

tion. Alkalosis (from metabolism of citrate to bicarbonate) is common following massive blood transfusion.

C. **Infectious complications of blood transfusions**
   1. **Hepatitis**
      a. **Hepatitis B** infections from blood transfusions have decreased since testing donated blood for hepatitis B antigen became routine in 1971. The current risk is estimated to be 1 case per 60,000 units transfused. Although most infections are asymptomatic, long-term morbidity can be significant.
      b. **Hepatitis C (HCV).** Institution of routine testing for antibody to HCV in 1990 has reduced the risk of transfusion-related HCV to approximately 1 case per 100,000 units transfused.
      c. **Pooled products** (e.g., cryoprecipitate) have an increased risk proportional to the number of donors.
   2. **Human immunodeficiency virus (HIV).** Because of improved screening and testing, the risk of transfusion-associated HIV has been estimated to be about 1 case per 450,000 units transfused in the United States.
   3. **Cytomegalovirus (CMV).** The prevalence of antibodies to CMV in the general adult population is approximately 70%. The incidence of transfusion-associated CMV infection in previously noninfected patients is quite high. Usually the infection is asymptomatic, but immunosuppressed patients and neonates can have severe reactions. CMV-negative blood may be available for these patients on request, or a leukocyte reduction filter can be used during transfusion.
   4. **Lymphotrophic viruses.** Retroviruses have been implicated as causative agents of some leukemias and lymphomas. **Human T-cell lymphotrophic virus-I** (HTLV-I) is associated with tropical spastic paraparesis, a chronic myelopathy, and with adult T-cell malignancies. This virus is transmitted by transfusion at a rate of 1 case per 640,000 units transfused. **HTLV-II** has also been associated with hairy-cell leukemia. Food and Drug Administration (FDA) requirements include routine testing of donated blood to detect HTLV-I and II. HTLV-III is synonymous with HIV (**see VII.C.2**).
   5. **Bacterial infections.** Exclusion of donors with evidence of infectious disease and the storage of blood at 4°C reduce the risk of transmitted bacterial infection. Occasional contamination by organisms that can grow at 4°C (e.g., *Yersinia enterocolitica* and *Pseudomonas aeruginosa*) rarely occurs, but transfusion-acquired sepsis carries a very high mortality rate. Bacterial contamination of warm blood is a concern; for this reason, blood

must be kept refrigerated prior to transfusion. Platelets are particularly problematic because they must be stored at room temperature. Organisms infecting platelet concentrates are typically *Staphylococcus aureus,* coagulase negative *Staphylococcus,* and diphtheroids. The impact of transfusion of bacterially infected blood on the individual patient depends on the size of the innoculum and the immunocompetence of the recipient.

   6. **Parasitic infections** are rare in the United States and Europe, but are commonly a concern elsewhere. Malaria, tick-borne babesiosis, filariasis, and trypanosomiasis (Chagas' disease) can be transmitted by transfusion in endemic areas. Toxoplasmosis has been transmitted by blood transfusion, but in immunocompetent adults, the infection is usually asymptomatic. To reduce the risk of parasitic infections, individuals who have recently traveled to endemic areas are asked not to donate blood.

   D. **Transfusion-induced immunosuppression** through impaired cell-mediated immunity and increased prostaglandin E production can occur but the clinical significance is uncertain.

VIII. **Coagulopathies**
   A. **Massive transfusion** is arbitrarily defined as the administration of at least 8 to 10 units of blood transfused within a 12-hour period.

   1. Following the administration of 1 to 1.5 blood volumes (assuming a blood volume = 75 ml/kg), **dilutional thrombocytopenia** can result in diffuse oozing and failure to form clot. Platelets should be readily available and transfused when clinical evidence of bleeding exists. In adults, the usual dose is 1 U/10 kg.

   2. The normal human body has tremendous reserves of clotting factors. Small amounts of the stable clotting factors also are present in the plasma of each unit of red cells transfused. Bleeding from factor deficiency during a massive transfusion usually results from diminished levels of fibrinogen and labile factors (V, VIII, and IX). Factor VIII levels can sometimes increase with massive transfusion, probably because of endothelial cell release. Bleeding from hypofibrinogenemia is unusual unless the fibrinogen level is below 75 mg/dl. Labile clotting factors are administered in the form of fresh-frozen plasma.

   3. **Additional complications of massive transfusion** include hypothermia from the rapid infusion of blood, citrate toxicity (**see VII.B.2**), and dysrhythmias (secondary to hypocalcemia or hypomagnesemia). If ongoing bleeding is present, hypotension secondary to hypovolemia and metabolic acidemia secondary to organ hypoperfusion

are to be expected. Hypotension can also result from ischemic- or septic-mediated myocardial depression.

4. In addition to transfusion of appropriate blood products, the strategy for massive transfusion includes maintaining intravascular volume, administering calcium as needed to offset the effects of citrate, and the use of vasopressors with inotropic properties as a temporizing measure to maintain systemic arterial pressure until euvolemia has been established. A pulmonary artery catheter can be useful to assess cardiac output and stroke volume. Ongoing surgical bleeding is an indication for operative correction. Antifibrinolytic agents can be considered and used if fibrinolysis is contributing to bleeding. Frequent laboratory measures of coagulation status are indicated because these parameters change rapidly in the setting of massive hemorrhage and transfusion. Finally, direct communication with the blood bank is important to expedite component preparation.

B. **Disseminated intravascular coagulation** refers to the abnormal, diffuse systemic activation of the clotting system. It occurs secondary to a primary underlying insult (Table 12-2). Its presentation can

Table 12-2. Causes of disseminated intravascular coagulation

Acute	Chronic
Sepsis	Malignancy
Shock	Liver disease
Trauma	Aortic dissection/aneurysm
Head injury	Retained dead fetus
Crush injuries	Peritoneovenous shunt (LeVeen shunt)
Pregnancy complications	Intraaortic balloon pump
Placental abruption	
Amniotic fluid embolism	
Septic abortion	
Hemolytic transfusion reaction	
Extensive burns	
Fat embolism	
Cholesterol emboli	
Acute respiratory distress syndrome	
Liver disease	
Obstructive jaundice	
Acute hepatic failure	
Extracorporeal circulation	

range from mild and asymptomatic to severe and marked by massive hemorrhage, thrombosis, and multiorgan failure.

1. **Causes of DIC** include infection, shock, trauma, complications of pregnancy (e.g., amniotic fluid embolism, placental abruption, septic abortion), burns, fat embolism, and cholesterol embolism. Endothelial cell damage with exposure of collagen may be the cause of DIC seen in shock and infections. DIC is common in extensive **head injury,** because of the high content of thromboplastin in brain tissue. **Chronic causes of DIC** include cirrhotic liver disease, aortic aneurysm (particularly with intramural thrombus), aortic dissection, and malignancies.

2. **The pathophysiology of DIC** involves excessive formation of thrombin resulting in fibrin formation throughout the vasculature, platelet activation, fibrinolysis, and consumption of coagulation factors.

3. **Clinical features** include petechiae, ecchymoses, bleeding from venipuncture sites, and hemorrhage from operative incisions. The bleeding manifestations of DIC are most obvious, but the diffuse microvascular and macrovascular thromboses are common, difficult to treat, and frequently life-threatening because of ischemia to vital organs. Bradykinin release during DIC can also cause hypotension.

4. **Laboratory features of DIC** include an **elevated D-dimer,** indicating fibrin degradation by plasmin, in all cases. The PT and aPTT are prolonged in most cases. FDPs are elevated, but this is not specific to DIC because FDPs may be present from the formation of fibrin by fibrinogen or from the degradation of fibrinogen by plasmin. **Serial measurements** demonstrating a falling fibrinogen level and decreasing platelet count are characteristic of DIC. Serial measurements are more useful than a single measurement because each can be abnormal at baseline in the critically ill patient. Examination of the peripheral blood smear in the patient with DIC reveals schistocytes in approximately 50% of cases; these are formed from the shearing of RBCs by intravascular fibrin strands.

5. **Treatment**
   a. The primary treatment of DIC involves treating the precipitating cause.
   b. **Transfusion** of appropriate blood components is indicated to correct bleeding. Fibrinogen levels should be maintained above 50 to 100 mg/dl by infusion of FFP (if also indicated for replacement of consumed coagulation factors) or cryoprecipitate.

c. **Pharmacologic treatment** of DIC is controversial. In cases associated with inappropriate
thrombosis rather than bleeding, **heparin
therapy** to decrease fibrin formation can be
considered, but cautious administration is
warranted because this treatment risks life-
threatening bleeding. Low dose heparin treatment has been effective for chronic DIC with
thrombosis. Clinical circumstances where heparin treatment of DIC may be beneficial include malignancy with thrombosis, ischemic
digits or skin, amniotic fluid embolus with ongoing passage of amniotic fluid into the vasculature, and stable aortic aneurysm scheduled
for elective repair. In cases of large vessel
thrombosis, full dose heparin therapy is indicated. The efficacy of heparin is defined by an
increase in fibrinogen levels without exogenous replacement.

d. **Inhibitors of fibrinolysis** administered
during DIC have some theoretic value but
are risky given the possibility of diffuse intravascular thrombosis. In this respect, aminocaproic acid and aprotinin are generally
contraindicated for DIC, although aprotinin
would likely be more appropriately considered because of its kallikrein-inhibiting and
platelet-sparing effects.

e. **Experimental, unproved treatments** for
DIC include antithrombin III concentrate, protein C and S concentrates, and direct thrombin
inhibitors (e.g., hirudin, argatroban).

C. **Chronic liver disease.** With the exception of Factor
VIII and von Willebrand's factor, which are manufactured by the endothelium, coagulation factors are
synthesized by the liver. Patients with hepatic dysfunction may have decreased production of coagulation factors and decreased clearance of activated
factors. Patients can have an ongoing consumptive
coagulopathy, similar to DIC, if circulating activated
clotting factors are increased. Because the liver is also
instrumental in removing the by-products of fibrinolysis, circulating FDPs may be increased. Patients
with liver disease frequently have a prolonged PT because of decreased synthesis of clotting factors. Many,
however, will respond to vitamin K (**see VIII.D**) and,
thus, should receive a trial of vitamin K therapy.
Failed response to vitamin K and the immediate need
to correct coagulopathy require FFP transfusions
until the PT has normalized or bleeding has stopped.
Thrombocytopenia, which also occurs frequently in
liver disease because of splenic sequestration of platelets, can be treated with platelet transfusion.

D.   Vitamin K deficiency. Vitamin K is required by the liver for production of Factors II, VII, IX, and X and proteins C and S. Because vitamin K cannot be synthesized by humans, interference with vitamin K absorption will cause a coagulopathy and a prolonged PT. This can be treated with vitamin K (2.5 to 25 mg SQ or 10 mg SQ once daily for 3 days). Intravenous administration of vitamin K can correct the PT slightly faster, but is accompanied by a rare risk of anaphylaxis. If used IV, vitamin K should be administered very slowly. If faster correction of PT is required, FFP (5–8 ml/kg) can be used.

IX.   Anticoagulation. Indications include the prevention or treatment of deep venous thrombosis (DVT), pulmonary embolus (PE), intracardiac thrombus in atrial fibrillation or severe ventricular dysfunction, and vascular graft thrombosis. Anticoagulation also may be required for renal replacement therapy (dialysis or hemofiltration), extracorporeal circulation (ECMO), or cardiac support (intraaortic balloon pump).

A.   Heparin is a naturally occurring anticoagulant produced from bovine lung or porcine intestine that acts by accelerating the effect of antithrombin III (AT III). Structurally, heparin is a heterogeneous mixture of glycosaminoglycans with molecular weights ranging from 3,000 to 30,000 d. A repetitive pentasaccharide glucosamine sequence that is present in only one third of the heparin molecules is necessary for AT III binding. The heparin-AT III complex inactivates several factors in the coagulation cascade, but most importantly thrombin (Factor II) and Factor X. Longer heparin chains are required for thrombin inhibition than for X inhibition.

1.   **For full anticoagulation,** as in the treatment of DVT or PE, heparin can be administered by a continuous IV infusion, sometimes after an initial bolus. Efficacy is measured by the aPTT, which is prolonged to 60 to 85 seconds. The aPTT is determined every 6 hours until the level of anticoagulation is stable. Heparin has a short half-life (~ 90 minutes). Stopping a heparin infusion for approximately 2 to 4 hours usually reverses the effect. If faster reversal is required, **protamine,** a natural antagonist, can be used. Protamine (1 mg for every 100 U of heparin remaining in the patient) should be given slowly, because adverse reactions (e.g., hypotension, pulmonary hypertension, hypersensitivity reactions) are common. Institution-wide heparin protocols facilitate adequate anticoagulation.

2.   **"Heparin resistance"** occurs frequently in critically ill patients because circulating acute phase reactants nonspecifically bind heparin and limit its anticoagulant effect. The resulting tachyphylaxis to heparin can usually be overcome with increas-

ing doses of the drug. Occasionally, **antithrombin III** levels may be depleted in critically ill patients, also contributing to heparin failure. If antithrombin III levels are low, AT III concentrate or, alternatively, FFP can be administered to replete AT III and restore heparin efficacy. Of note, **heparin-induced thrombocytopenia (see X.B.2.b.2)** should always be considered in the differential diagnosis of heparin tachyphylaxis.

3. **Heparin can be administered subcutaneously** in low dose for DVT prophylaxis. Usual dosage is 5,000 U SQ every 12 hours. This dose usually does not prolong the aPTT.

B. **Low molecular weight heparins (LMWH)** are commercially prepared by fractionating heparin into molecules of 2,000 to 10,000 d. Most of these lower weight molecules are incapable of crosslinking to both antithrombin and thrombin and, thus, exert their anticoagulant effect primarily by inhibiting Factor X. Treatment with LMWH generally does not prolong the aPTT and usually does not require laboratory monitoring of anticoagulation. The anticoagulant effect can be assessed by measuring anti-Xa levels, if desired.

1. **Advantages.** LMWH has been shown to be superior to standard heparin in DVT prophylaxis of certain high risk patients, including patients undergoing elective hip or knee replacement or hip replacement because of a fracture. Studies also support a therapeutic advantage in trauma and spinal cord injured patients. LMWH has a more predictable dose–response relationship for anticoagulation than unfractionated heparin. This occurs because LMWH has much less non-specific binding to acute phase reactants than unfractionated heparin. The more predictable effect of LMWH decreases or eliminates the need for laboratory monitoring of drug effect. LMWH anticoagulation can be associated with fewer bleeding complications than standard heparin. Finally, the incidence of heparin-induced thrombocytopenia (HIT) is less with LMWH compared with unfractionated heparin.

2. **Disadvantages** of LMWH include its long half-life (4 hours), incomplete reversal with protamine, renal clearance, and expense.

3. **Several commercial preparations of LMWH** are available with slightly different mean molecular weights and anti-Xa activity. LMWH can be administered intravenously but excellent bioavailability and long half-life permit convenient subcutaneous dosing. Dosage for DVT prophylaxis is 30 mg SQ every 12 hours for enoxaparin, 2,500 to 5,000 anti-Xa units SQ once daily for dalteparin. Dosage for DVT treatment is 1 mg/kg SQ

every 12 hours for enoxaparin, 100 U/kg SQ every 12 hours for dalteparin.

C. **Heparinoids** are the glycosaminoglycans heparan sulfate, chondroitin sulfate, and dermatan sulfate. They are by-products of heparin production. Anticoagulant activity is via inhibition of Factor Xa. **Danaparoid,** commercially available in the United States as Orgaran (Organon Inc. West Orange, NJ), is a LMW heparinoid that has been used as an alternative to heparin in patients with HIT. Anticoagulant activity can be measured by anti-Xa activity just as with LMWH. The drug has a half-life of 18 to 28 hours (longer in renal failure) and is not effectively reversed with protamine. Dosage is 750 anti-Xa SQ units every 12 hours for DVT prophylaxis. Intravenous dosing can also be done, guided by assay of anti-Xa.

D. **Warfarin** inhibits vitamin K epoxide reductase. This produces a deficiency of vitamin K, preventing the hepatic carboxylation of Factors II, VII, IX, and X, and proteins C and S to the active form. The half-life of warfarin is approximately 35 hours, requiring days for reversal. If quick reversal of warfarin is required, active factors can be given in the form of FFP (5–15 ml/kg). **Vitamin K** (2.5–25 mg IV or SQ) can also be given for warfarin reversal, but its effect requires 6 or more hours. Warfarin can be administered enterally or parenterally once daily. Anticoagulation does not occur for approximately 3 to 4 days and may require a week or more to achieve a stable level. Therapy is guided by measurement of the PT or, more usefully, the INR (**see I.C.1.b**). Cautious dosing should be undertaken in patients who are vitamin K-depleted to avoid over-anticoagulation and possible bleeding complications.

E. **Hirudin and argatroban** are specific, direct thrombin inhibitors that can used for the treatment of or as alternative anticoagulants in HIT. Hirudin was originally isolated from the salivary gland of leeches, but is now produced by recombinant genetic technology and marketed as Lepirudin. Argatroban is a small, synthetic molecule derived from L-arginine. Both agents act independently of cofactors (e.g., AT III) to inhibit both circulating thrombin and clot-bound thrombin, thereby inhibiting clot enlargement. Antithrombin agent dosage is guided by prolongation of the ACT or aPTT to therapeutic range. The short half-lives (30–45 minutes) of these agents allow relatively rapid reversal of anticoagulation by stopping the drug. Hirudin was approved in 1998 in the United States for treatment of HIT complicated by thrombosis. Dosage is based on measurement of ACT or aPTT and should be reduced in renal failure because of the drug's renal metabolism and excretion. Argatroban has a greater pharmacodynamic predictability than hirudin and may have a decreased risk of bleeding because it is reliably excreted even in moderate renal failure. In addition, argatroban crosses the blood–brain barrier and may serve a role in the treatment of ischemic or thrombotic stroke. Starting dosage of argatroban in HIT is 5 to 10 μg/kg/min IV and subsequently guided by the aPTT. Further information regarding the usage, dosing, and safety of the direct thrombin inhibitors will likely be gained as clinical experience accumulates.

F. **Thrombolytic agents** act by dissolving thrombi via conversion of plasminogen to plasmin, which lyses fibrin clot. They are intended to reverse thrombosis and recanalize blood vessels. These agents are used to treat acute occlusion of coronary, cerebral, pulmonary, and peripheral arteries, typically in combination with heparin to prevent reocclusion. Three thrombolytic agents—**tissue plasminogen activator (tPA), streptokinase,** and **urokinase**—are used commonly in clinical practice, each with slightly different pharmacodynamic and side effect profiles. Each of these drugs results in a hypofibrinogenemic state and carries a substantial risk of bleeding. They are generally contraindicated perioperatively. If emergent surgery is required following thrombolytic therapy, the effect can be reversed by administration of aminocaproic or tranexamic acid. Additionally, the fibrinogen level can be restored by transfusion of cryoprecipitate or FFP (**see III.D, III.E**).

G. **Platelet inhibitors** can be useful for reducing thromboembolic events in patients with arterial vascular disorders (e.g., carotid stenosis), prosthetic heart valves, or recent invasive arterial procedures (e.g., percutaneous coronary angioplasty or stenting). **Aspirin** and **nonsteroidal anti-inflammatory drugs** (NSAIDs) inhibit platelet aggregation by interfering with the cyclooxygenase pathway. Aspirin permanently inhibits the pathway for the lifespan of the platelet. Because the half-life of platelets in circulation is approximately 4 days, 10 days are required before platelet function returns to normal after aspirin ingestion. The other NSAIDs reversibly inhibit the cyclooxygenase pathway; their effects dissipate within 3 days of discontinuing the drug. **Dypyridamole** is a phosphodiesterase inhibitor that increases platelet cyclic adenosine monophosphate (cAMP), thereby inhibiting platelet aggregation. It can be used in combination with warfarin for thromboembolism prophylaxis in patients with prosthetic heart valves. **Ticlopidine** and **clopidogrel** are newer antiplatelet agents that inhibit adenosine diphosphate (ADP)-mediated platelet aggregation. Immediate reversal of platelet inhibitors can require platelet transfusion (**see III.C**).

X. **Abnormalities of hemostasis**
  A. **Bleeding disorders**
    1. **Classic hemophilia or hemophilia A** is caused by an abnormality of Factor VIII. The incidence

in the United States is 1 of 10,000. It is a sex-linked recessive trait, affecting males almost exclusively.

a. **Clinical features.** The diagnosis should be suggested in a patient with the appropriate history and an elevated aPTT but normal PT. Bleeding episodes are related to the level of Factor VIII activity (normal activity is 100%):

   (1) Less than 1% activity—spontaneous bleeding.

   (2) 1% to 5% activity—bleeding after minor trauma.

   (3) More than 5% activity—infrequent bleeding.

b. Because these patients have normal platelet function, they are able to form an initial clot, and they will have normal bleeding times. Because they are unable to stabilize the blood clot, however, bleeding will recur.

c. **Treatment** consists of lyophilized Factor VIII, cryoprecipitate, or desmopressin. A dose of 1 U/kg of Factor VIII will increase the activity of Factor VIII by approximately 2%. Activity levels of 20% to 40% are recommended prior to surgery. The half-life of Factor VIII is 8 to 12 hours. Because up to 20% of patients will eventually develop resistance because of antibodies against Factor VIII, Factor VIII activity levels should be measured before and after transfusion. Patients with resistance must then be treated with high dose Factor VIII, activated Factor IX, or plasmapheresis. Because many hemophiliacs have received multiple transfusions over their lifetimes, many are seropositive for the human immunodeficiency virus (HIV) and hepatitis.

2. **Hemophilia B, or Christmas disease,** is caused by a Factor IX abnormality. It also is sex-linked, occurring almost exclusively in males, and has an incidence of 1 of 100,000. These patients present similarly to patients with classic hemophilia; they have an abnormal aPTT and a normal PT. Therapy consists of Factor IX concentrates or FFP. For surgical hemostasis, activity levels of 50% to 80% are necessary (0.5–0.8 U/ml). A dose of 1 U/kg of Factor IX will increase its activity by about 1%. The half-life of Factor IX is approximately 24 hours.

3. **von Willebrand's disease** is associated with abnormalities of von Willebrand's factor. von Willebrand's factor is a glycoprotein manufactured by megakaryocytes and endothelial cells and has multiple functions. It serves as an anchor for platelet adhesion to collagen, it interlinks platelets

(aggregation) in clot formation, and it protects and stabilizes Factor VIII. von Willebrand's disease is most commonly inherited in an autosomal dominant pattern with variable penetrance.

a.   Clinical features. The bleeding tendency of these patients is quite variable. Most commonly, these patients have episodes of mucocutaneous bleeding (e.g., epistaxis).

b. The most common laboratory finding is a prolonged bleeding time, although the aPTT can also be prolonged.

c.   Treatment for these individuals includes desmopressin (**see V.D**), cryoprecipitate, or both. Plasma products may also be required for an actively bleeding patient. Cryoprecipitate is preferred; fresh-frozen plasma can be used if cryoprecipitate is unavailable. In patients with acquired von Willebrand's disease, high dose IV gamma globulin (1 gm/kg for 2 days) has been used successfully.

4.   Other rare factor deficiencies that predispose patients to bleeding have been described, including deficiencies of fibrinogen, Factor II (prothrombin), Factor V, Factor VII, Factor X, Factor XI, and Factor XIII. Treatment usually consists of factor concentrate or blood component replacement, and is best guided by expert hematology consultation.

B.   Clotting disorders

1.   Congenital hypercoagulability abnormalities, which predispose to clotting, can cause thrombosis and concurrent critical illness. Many specialized tests are available to diagnose these abnormalities and guide therapy, which usually consists of life-long anticoagulation. Test results can affect both the patient and family members because many of these disorders are genetically transmitted. For patients presenting with **venous thromboembolism,** consideration should be given to testing for Factor V Leiden (activated protein C resistance), antithrombin III defects, protein C and S deficiency, antiphospholipid antibodies, and hyperhomocysteinemia. The exact tests to be performed are best determined by patient and family history. Many of these tests are unreliable during an acute illness because of the presence of acute phase reactants. For these reasons, a clinical pathology or hematology consultation is advisable when a congenital hypercoagulable state is suspected.

2.   Acquired disorders

a.   Surgery, pregnancy, and trauma all predispose to thrombosis. The cause is multifactorial. In surgical patients, venous stasis during perioperative immobility is a contributory factor. In addition, surgery and trauma produce a systemic response marked by an increase in acute phase reactants, including increases in fibrinogen, Factor VIII, and α_1 antitrypsin. Fibrinolytic proteins and coagulation inhibitors are decreased. Platelet activation and aggregation are enhanced. All of the preceding events promote a hypercoagulable state in surgical and trauma patients and mandate aggressive prophylaxis for thromboembolism (see Chapter 22). Prophylaxis can include pneumatic compression boots, early ambulation, and treatment with heparin, LMWH, heparinoids, or warfarin (**see V**).

3. **Heparin-induced thrombocytopenia (HIT)** occurs in two forms:

   a. **HIT type I,** a common, nonimmune-mediated phenomenon, is a benign drop in platelet count within 5 days of institution of heparin therapy. Platelet counts rarely fall to less than 100,000 and recover to normal after approximately 5 days. HIT I does not require discontinuation of heparin or carry a risk of thrombosis.

   b. **HIT II** is an immune-mediated thrombocytopenia triggered by IgG antibodies, which can form against heparin-platelet factor 4 (PF 4) complexes. The heparin-PF 4 complexes are seen as "antigens"; they are bound to the Fc receptor on the platelet, activating the platelet and causing platelet aggregation and further PF 4 release. The result is thrombocytopenia, platelet aggregation, and the potential for arterial and venous thromboses. The incidence of HIT antibody formation is estimated at approximately 10% of patients exposed to unfractionated heparin; only 2% to 3% develop clinical HIT. The diagnosis is easy to make with enzyme-linked immunosorbent assay (ELISA) testing in the proper clinical setting. Confirmation with the platelet serotonin release assay, an expensive "gold standard" for diagnosis, may be required because the ELISA has an imperfect specificity. The onset of thrombocytopenia is usually 5 to 12 days after a first exposure to heparin or may be more rapid after re-exposure to the drug. The platelet count generally falls by more than 50% from baseline, with the median lowest count approximately 50,000. The degree of thrombocytopenia can be severe, but rarely falls to less than 20,000. **Thrombosis** from platelet activation and aggregation is the major complication, occurring in one third of patients with HIT II. Thrombosis caused by HIT II can result in DVT, PE, myocardial or mesenteric infarction, limb ischemia leading to amputation, or stroke. The thrombi largely consist of clumps of activated platelets obstructing the vasculature, giving rise to the term "white clot syndrome." Mortality is significant at 20% to 30%.

c. **The treatment of HIT II** is immediate discontinuation of all heparin, including subcutaneous heparin and small amounts of heparin in flush solutions. An increase in the platelet count should occur within a few days and return to normal after approximately 4 to 10 days. The patient should not be re-exposed to heparin, including LMWH. Heparin-free central venous catheters (including pulmonary artery catheters) should be used if required. Platelet transfusions should be avoided except in the case of frank bleeding.

d. **Alternative anticoagulation** for the patient with HIT II is problematic. The ideal alternative is warfarin, but frequently these patients are too unstable to receive a slowly reversible, poorly titratable anticoagulant. In addition, warfarin treatment during the acute phase of HIT is ill-advised, because a brief period of hypercoagulability occurs from protein C depletion during the institution of warfarin therapy. **Danaparoid (see IX. C.** above) may be an alternative. Of note, a 10% *in vitro* cross-reactivity with the HIT antibody to danaparoid has been reported, necessitating vigilant monitoring of the platelet count to detect a similar reaction to danaparoid. The **direct thrombin inhibitors** (hirudin and argatroban) are also acceptable anticoagulants for the patient with HIT and they carry no risk of cross-reactivity. Antiplatelet agents (aspirin, NSAIDs, clopidogrel) may be considered, but they are generally ineffective in preventing the platelet aggregation induced by HIT.

e. **Prevention of HIT** is not yet possible because any patient who receives heparin, even LMWH, is at risk. The development of the HIT antibody is greatest with unfractionated heparin, less with LMWH, and least with danaparoid.

XI. **Special considerations**

A. **Sickle cell (SC) disease** has a prevalence of approximately 1% in the African American population of the United States. Sickle cell disease is caused by the substitution of valine for glutamic acid at the sixth position on the β chain of hemoglobin. Homozygotes for this substitution (as well as double heterozygotes SC or β-thalassemia) have clinical sickle cell disease.

1. **Clinical features.** The abnormal hemoglobin polymerizes and causes a sickling deformity of the red cell under certain conditions (e.g., hypoxia, hypothermia, acidosis, and dehydration). Sickled cells cause microvascular occlusion with tissue ischemia and infarction. A sickle cell crisis typically presents with excruciating chest or abdominal pain, fever, tachycardia, leukocytosis, and hematuria. The red cells have a shortened survival time of 12 days (normal being 120 days), leading to anemia and extramedullary hematopoiesis. Neonates are usually protected from sickle crisis for the first few months of life because of persistent fetal hemoglobin (hemoglobin F). Patients with sickle cell trait are usually asymptomatic.

2. **The perioperative management** of these patients remains controversial. It had been common practice to give patients preoperative red cell transfusions to increase the hematocrit and decrease the relative proportion of hemoglobin S red blood cells. Past guidelines suggested transfusing to an end point of having 70% hemoglobin A and less than 30% hemoglobin S cells, as measured by hemoglobin electrophoresis, prior to major surgery. Recently, this practice has been questioned and routine preoperative transfusion of asymptomatic patients is not recommended. Perioperative care should be directed at reducing the risk of sickling. Because hypoxia is a known precipitant of sickling, these patients should be well oxygenated at all times. Acidosis should be avoided. Patients should be well hydrated to maintain intravascular volume and ensure adequate tissue perfusion (preventing systemic acidosis). Hypothermia should also be avoided, because it can precipitate sickle cell crises, probably from increased blood viscosity and stasis.

B. **Jehovah's Witness patients** generally may refuse to receive blood or blood products (e.g., fresh frozen plasma, platelets, cryoprecipitate, or albumin) based on their religious beliefs even when such refusal results in death. Some patients may accept autotransfused or chest tube salvaged autologous blood, especially if it remains in contiguous circulation with their vasculature.

1. Special considerations regarding homologous transfusion can apply when the patient is a minor, is incompetent, or has responsibilities for dependents, and in certain emergency circumstances. An ethical dilemma may present when unexpected hemorrhage is encountered in the operating room or critical care unit following a preoperative agreement not to transfuse. Careful documentation of preoperative discussions and informed con-

sent is mandatory. Legal precedent generally supports patient autonomy regarding the acceptance of transfusion.

2. **In the critically ill Jehovah's Witness** patient who refuses blood transfusion, blood conservation measures are extremely important. Efforts to minimize iatrogenic blood loss, including minimizing phlebotomies, should be employed. Erythropoietin (which contains a small amount of human albumin) is sometimes used in combination with iron to increase red cell mass perioperatively. In extreme circumstances of anemia, measures to diminish oxygen consumption via sedation, pharmacologic paralysis, and hypothermia can be attempted. Hypothermia, however, can contribute to coagulopathy and cause further bleeding. Finally, hyperbaric oxygen therapy has been used in these patients to increase tissue oxygenation, but improved outcome has not been demonstrated.

SELECTED REFERENCES

American Society of Anesthesiologists Task Force on Blood Component Therapy. Practice guidelines for blood component therapy. *Anesthesiology.* 1996;84:732–747.

Cooper JR. Perioperative considerations in Jehovah's Witnesses. *Int Anesthesiol Clin.* 1990;28:210–215.

Davis R, Whittington R. Aprotinin: a review of its pharmacology and therapeutic efficacy in reducing blood loss associated with cardiac surgery. *Drugs.* 1995;49:954–983.

Development Task Force of the College of American Pathologists. Practice parameters for the use of fresh-frozen plasma, cryoprecipitate, and platelets. *JAMA.* 1994;271:777–781.

Fareed J, Callas D, Hoppensteadt DA, et al. Antithrombin agents as anticoagulants and antithrombotics: implications in drug development. *Semin Hematol.* 1999;36(Suppl 1):42–56.

Geerts WH, Jay RM, Code KI, et al. A comparison of low-dose heparin with low-molecular weight heparin as prophylaxis against venous thromboembolism after major trauma. *N Engl J Med.* 1996;335: 701–707.

Greinacher A, Volpel H, Janssens U, et al. The clinical management of heparin-induced thrombocytopenia. *Semin Hematol.* 1999;36 (Suppl 1):17–21.

Lake CL, Moore RA, eds. *Blood: hemostasis, transfusion, and alternatives in the perioperative period.* New York: Raven; 1995.

de Moerloose P, Bounameaux HR, Mannucci PM. Screening tests for thrombophilic patients: which tests, for which patient, by whom, when, and why? *Semin Thromb Hemost.* 1998;24:321–327.

Mueller-Velten HG, Potzsch B. Recombinant hirudin (lepirudin) provides safe and effective anticoagulation in patients with heparin-induced thrombocytopenia: a prospective study. *Circulation.* 1999;99: 73–80.

Nee R, Doppenschmidt D, Donovan DJ, et al. Intravenous versus subcutaneous vitamin K_1 in reversing excessive oral anticoagulation. *Am J Cardiol.* 1999;83:286–288.

Riewald M, Riess H. Treatment options for clinically recognized disseminated intravascular coagulation. *Semin Thromb Hemost.* 1998; 24:53–59.

Royston D. Blood-sparing drugs: aprotinin, tranexamic acid, and aminocaproic acid. *Int Anesthesiol Clin.* 1995;33:155–179.

Schreiber GB, Busch MP, Kleinman SH, et al. The risk of transfusion-transmitted viral infections. *N Engl J Med.* 1996;334:1685–1690.

Smith RE. The INR: a perspective. *Semin Thromb Hemost.* 1997;23: 547–549.

Intraaortic Balloon Counterpulsation

Brian J. Poore

I. **Intraaortic balloon counterpulsation (IABC)** therapy is initiated by placing a flexible catheter with an elongated balloon mounted on its end into the descending thoracic aorta (Fig. 13-1). Most intraaortic balloon (IAB) catheters have two lumens: a central one for the measurement of proximal aortic pressure, and a second lumen for the passage of helium gas between console and balloon. The balloon, usually 40 ml in volume, is rapidly inflated with helium at the onset of diastole, and deflated at the onset of systole (ventricular isovolumic contraction). As it is inflated with an internal pressure of helium that is greater than intraaortic pressure, it will displace 40 ml of blood from the aorta. This added volume causes an increase in aortic pressure and diastolic blood flow (**diastolic augmentation**). The rapid deflation of the balloon leaves a 40-ml void, which effectively decreases aortic pressure and, thus, left ventricular (LV) afterload, during early systole. These beneficial hemodynamic changes—diastolic augmentation and systolic afterload reduction—can greatly increase coronary blood flow and decrease myocardial oxygen consumption.

II. **Indications.** Intraaortic balloon pumps (IABPs) are used to provide temporary circulatory support for several cardiovascular conditions.

   A. **Cardiogenic shock,** in which the heart itself, despite adequate preload, is unable to maintain cardiac output (CO) sufficient to provide adequate systemic perfusion. This condition can be treated with IABC to increase systemic perfusion and decrease myocardial work.

   B. **Unstable angina.** IABC therapy can improve the oxygen supply:demand ratio of the ischemic myocardium while other interventions (e.g., percutaneous transluminal coronary angioplasty) are being pursued.

   C. **Perioperative.** Preoperatively, the IABP can stabilize a hemodynamically compromised patient awaiting an operative intervention. Weaning from cardiopulmonary bypass in patients with poor LV function can be facilitated by IABC therapy. Patients with myocardial dysfunction after bypass can be supported in anticipation of gradual improvement over the next 24 to 48 hours.

   D. **Bridge to transplant.** Transplant candidates with severely depressed myocardial function can be supported until a donor heart is available. In several instances, IABPs have been used for months.

   E. **Prophylactic support.** Patients with severe cardiac disease may benefit from IABC therapy during noncardiac operations.

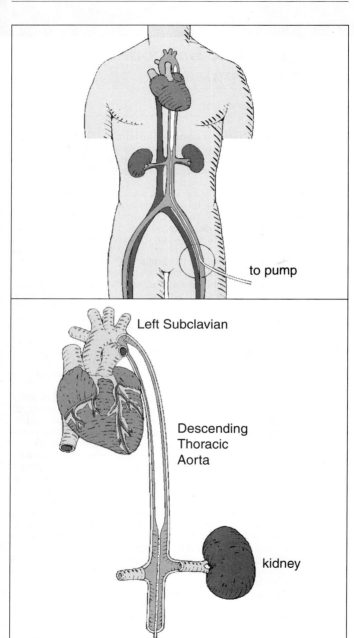

to pump

Left Subclavian

Descending
Thoracic
Aorta

kidney

III. Contraindications. IABC therapy requires an appropriate indication and an appropriate patient. Several patient characteristics preclude initiation of IABC.

A. Aortic valvular insufficiency. Depending on the severity of aortic valve regurgitation, the increased aortic diastolic pressure caused by the IABP will increase regurgitant flow into the left ventricle. This will increase LV end-diastolic volume and worsen the patient's hemodynamics.

B. Thoracic or abdominal aneurysm. Balloon counterpulsation against a diseased aortic wall may damage the aorta, causing dissection or rupture.

C. Severe atherosclerosis. Plaque-filled and tortuous femoral arteries may make IAB placement impossible by the transfemoral approach. A transthoracic IAB can sometimes be placed, if required, at the time of cardiac operation.

D. End-stage disease. IABC therapy is temporary. The high complication rate precludes permanent use. Intra-aortic balloon insertion should be reserved for patients with transient pathology, or for those awaiting definitive therapy.

IV. Placement. An important advantage of the IAB is the relative ease of placement. In experienced hands, a balloon catheter can be placed percutaneously in about 5 minutes. The procedure can be done in locations other than the operating suite [e.g., catheterization laboratory or intensive care unit (ICU)].

A. Approach. The most common site for IAB insertion is the femoral artery, which is cannulated via a percutaneous Seldinger technique or a surgical cut-down. The ascending aorta can be used, but this requires surgical placement and removal. The complication rates appear to be similar regardless of insertion site and method. The convenience of percutaneous insertion and removal make this approach the one most applicable to ICU patients.

B. Selection of an appropriately sized IAB is based on the patient's height and approximate aortic diameter. Ideally, the balloon should be 85% to 90% occlusive, and its proximal end should be positioned above (rather than covering) the origin of the renal arteries. Inflation volume can be decreased at the console, allowing more precise matching of balloon and aortic diameter.

1. For patient height less than 5'3" (167 cm), use a 30-ml balloon.

2. Patient height 5'4" to 6'0", use a 40-ml balloon.

3. For patient height more than 6'1" (183 cm), use a 50-ml balloon.

4. Pediatric balloon sizes are also available.

Fig. 13-1. Properly positioned intraaortic balloon catheter. Reprinted from Arrow: *Introduction to balloon pumping;* **with permission.**

C. **Technique.** Percutaneous insertion using a sheathed IAB, which is the method most commonly used, will be discussed here. These guidelines are an overview only; clinicians should refer to the manufacturers' specific insertion recommendations.

1. Preparation of the patient should emphasize sterile technique, including drapes and gowns. Prior to insertion, it is essential to examine the pedal pulses. Heparin (bolus and infusion to maintain the partial thromboplastin time at 50 to 60 seconds) should be administered.

2. Balloon preparation consists of ensuring that it is fully collapsed by aspirating the balloon port with a 60-ml syringe through a one-way valve. Flush the central lumen with sterile heparinized saline.

3. The femoral region should be prepared and draped and an appropriate amount of local anesthesia injected. The femoral artery is accessed using a long 18-gauge needle. Care should be taken to use a single anterior stick and not a transfixtion technique. The supplied J-tipped wire is placed through the needle into the femoral artery. The wire must advance easily; if any resistance is met during wire insertion, every effort must be made to ensure proper placement within the artery prior to dilating the puncture site. Fluoroscopy, if available, is useful to determine wire and balloon location. Alternatively, a small diameter catheter (18 gauge) can be inserted and the wire removed to verify arterial placement by transducing the catheter. Once an arterial pressure tracing is verified, the J-wire can be reinserted and the catheter removed.

4. Dilators are provided that are specific to the type and size of the balloon being used. A stab wound is made in the skin adjacent to the wire. Appropriate dilators are then advanced over the wire using a slight twisting motion. The final dilator is incorporated into the introducer sheath. The dilator is removed and the sheath and wire left in place.

5. As an estimate of the length of catheter required to place the tip of the balloon just below the left subclavian artery prior to insertion, the balloon or wire is held over the patient's body and the exact length needed to reach from the point of insertion to the sternal angle (angle of Louis) is measured. A clamp is placed on the drapes adjacent to the point on the thigh where the anchoring tabs will reside.

6. The balloon should remain within its protective cover until immediately prior to insertion. The fully collapsed balloon is threaded over the wire until the wire protrudes through the distal Luer-lock fitting. The IAB is now threaded through the sheath into the descending aorta. The final position of the balloon can be predicted by the prior mea-

surement, or verified using fluoroscopy. The tip of the catheter appears as an opaque rectangle on a chest radiograph, and it should be visible in the second or third intercostal space when properly placed. The wire is removed and the central lumen is aspirated. The arterial pressure monitoring line is connected to the central lumen and the one-way valve is removed from the balloon lumen. The balloon lumen connector is attached to the pump console tubing. The catheter's anchoring tabs can now be sutured to the patient's leg. Balloon counterpulsation can begin following the manufacturer's recommendations.

7. Recently, sheathless catheters have been developed in an attempt to decrease the cross section of the catheter and, thus, reduce the rate of vascular complications. See these catheters' special documentation for instructions.

V. Triggers and timing

A. **Triggers** are the physiologic signals from the patient that are used to time the inflation–deflation cycles of the IABP so that they occur at the proper points during the cardiac cycle. The two principal modes of triggering use either the electrocardiogram (ECG) or the arterial pressure waveform. These signals can be obtained directly from the patient or indirectly by "slaving" from a bedside monitor. The varieties of triggering modes allow selection of the most reliable trigger signal for a specific patient:

1. **ECG pattern** is the default setting on most pumps. The software may not be capable of recognizing widened QRS complexes or pacer spikes.

2. **ECG peak** is the mode of choice for wide complex rhythms (e.g., bundle branch blocks) or partially paced rhythms. It is also the preferred mode for tachycardias with heart rates greater than 140 bpm.

3. **Atrial fibrillation** is similar to peak mode. Deflation automatically occurs when an R wave is sensed; pacing spikes are ignored. This is the preferred mode for rhythms with varying R-R intervals.

4. **Ventricular pacing (V-pace)** uses the ventricular pacing spike as the trigger signal. The patient's rhythm must be 100% paced. This mode is also useful during atrioventricular pacing.

5. **Atrial pacing (A-pace)** uses the atrial pacing spike as the trigger. The rhythm must be 100% A paced.

6. **Arterial pressure** triggering is useful for situations where the ECG is distorted (e.g., patient transport, during cardiopulmonary resuscitation, or in the operating room where electrocautery can interfere with the ECG signal).

7. **Internal triggering** relies on the balloon console to cycle at a preset rate regardless of the patient's electrical or arterial activity. This mode can be used

initially during a cardiac arrest. When the patient's ECG or arterial waveform improves, the trigger mode should be changed.

B. **Timing** of the inflation and deflation of the IABP is crucial to maximize its beneficial effects. To properly adjust balloon timing, the characteristics of the unassisted and assisted arterial pressure waveform must be assessed. During adjustment of IAB timing, the assist ratio is set on 1:2 (one balloon inflation–deflation cycle during every other systole). Points to identify include the dicrotic notch, which coincides with the onset of diastole and the closure of the aortic valve, the peak diastolic pressure (diastolic augmentation), which reflects the increase in aortic pressure during balloon inflation, and the aortic end-diastolic pressure, which signifies aortic valve opening at the beginning of systole.

1. **Balloon inflation** should occur at the onset of diastole (i.e., just before the dicrotic notch on the arterial waveform). Improper inflation timing will decrease the magnitude of diastolic augmentation (Fig. 13-2).

2. **Balloon deflation** should begin just before systole (i.e., coincident with the end-diastolic pressure on the unassisted arterial pressure waveform). Improper deflation timing will fail to decrease afterload, and may increase myocardial work (Fig. 13-3).

VI. **Complications** of IABC occur in 20% to 30% of cases. Most are vascular complications, which can be categorized according to the time when they occur. The initial management of most IAB complications requires balloon removal and consultation with a vascular surgeon.

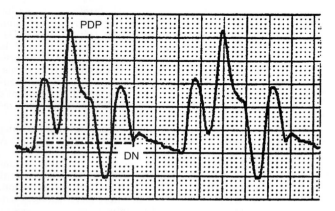

Fig. 13-2. Correct inflation timing. DN, dicrotic notch, which symbolizes beginning of diastole; PDP, peak diastolic pressure (also called diastolic augmentation). Courtesy of Arrow International, Inc., Reading, PA; with permission.

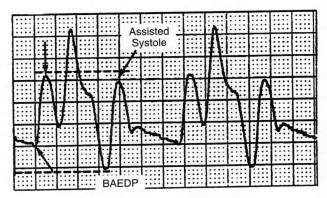

Fig. 13-3. **Correct deflation timing. BAEDP, Balloon aortic end-diastolic pressure. Fall in end diastolic pressure caused by balloon deflation. Assisted systole, the systole following a balloon inflate—deflate cycle (reduced peak systolic pressure). Courtesy of Arrow International Inc., Reading, PA; with permission.**

A. **During insertion**
   1. **Aortic dissection** occurs with a frequency of 1% during percutaneous femoral artery placement. It is important to be suspicious of any resistance when placing the wire or balloon. Always verify that blood can be aspirated from the central lumen prior to initiating counterpulsation.
   2. **Injury to the iliofemoral arteries** can present as catastrophic retroperitoneal hemorrhage, pseudoaneurysm formation, or local hematoma formation.

B. **During pumping**
   1. **Thromboembolism** to nearly any organ system, even those perfused by aortic branches proximal to location of the IAB, has been attributed to IABC therapy. Maintenance of anticoagulation may prevent these phenomena.
   2. **Loss of peripheral pulses** in the ipsilateral extremity occurs in as many as 25% of patients. This loss of pulse is most often asymptomatic, transient, and does not usually progress to limb ischemia.
   3. **Limb ischemia** occurs in about 10% of patients treated with IABC. Treatment includes balloon removal and thrombectomy. A small number of patients will require fasciotomy, vascular reconstructive surgery, or even amputation.
   4. **Infectious complications** of the IAB include fever, bacteremia, and superficial and deep wound infections. The frequency of infection is greater in emergency placements and with longer duration IAB support. Although not yet proved effective, most centers administer prophylactic antibiotics during IABC therapy.

   5. **Balloon rupture** is an infrequent complication of
     IABC therapy. Blood in the helium gas tubing is
     the most common sign of balloon rupture. Careful
     removal, watching for signs of balloon entrap-
     ment, is the treatment for IAB rupture; a new IAB
     can often be inserted.

 C. **During removal.** Serious vascular complications
   may not become apparent until IABP discontinuation.
   The patient should be observed closely for hypotension, decreasing hematocrit, and limb ischemia.

   1. **Dislodgement of atherosclerotic plaque** can
     cause distal embolism during balloon removal.

   2. **Balloon entrapment** can occur during removal.
     An entrapment must be suspected if undue resis-
     tance is encountered during IABC removal. Vas-
     cular surgery consultation and operative removal
     are likely to be necessary.

VII. **Discontinuation** of IABC therapy involves weaning of the
  support and removal of the catheter.

 A. **Weaning.** Patient characteristics and hemodynamic
   stability determine the timing and speed of IABC weaning. Patients requiring IABC therapy for poor ventricular function following cardiopulmonary bypass will likely wean earlier than those patients who needed IABC
   for cardiogenic shock after myocardial infarction.

   1. Weaning is usually done by changing the ratio of
     assisted to unassisted beats. The ratio is commonly
     changed from 1:1 (assistance on every beat), to 1:2
     (assistance every other beat), to 1:4, and 1:8, allow-
     ing a few hours at each support level to determine
     the patient's tolerance to reduced support. Some
     patients may not tolerate the assist ratio reduction
     method of weaning. An intermediate level of sup-
     port can be achieved by gradually reducing the in-
     flation volume of the balloon.

   2. When the assist ratio is 1:8 or the balloon volume
     is reduced by more than 20%, the risk of thrombus
     formation is increased. Follow the manufacturer's
     guidelines to prevent thrombus formation.

   3. Signs of intolerance to IABC weaning include:

     a. Decreased urine output.

     b. Cardiac output decreased by more than 20%.

     c. New dysrhythmias.

     d. Signs of systemic hypoperfusion.

 B. **Balloon removal.** The goals of balloon removal include the withdrawal of the balloon intact, minimizing
   bleeding, and preventing embolic events. The balloon
   manufacturer's specific recommendations should be
   followed. The percutaneous removal of a sheathed IAB
   is described.

   1. Remove the sutures and disconnect the balloon
     from the console.

   2. Aspirate the balloon with a 60-ml syringe to ensure
     that the balloon is fully collapsed. This is probably
     unnecessary but most clinicians still include this

step because it provides another opportunity to inspect the tubing for blood.

3. Remove the cuff from the sheath connector. Slowly withdraw the catheter through the sheath until resistance is met. This signals the entrance of balloon material into the end of the sheath.

4. Apply firm pressure to the femoral artery below the insertion site. Remove the balloon and sheath together as a unit. **Remember:** Should any undue resistance be met, surgical removal should be considered. **Do not** try to remove a balloon through a sheath.

5. Allow bleeding for 1 to 2 seconds to clear embolic material.

6. Apply firm pressure to the femoral artery above the insertion site and release the distal pressure. Allow back-bleeding for 1 to 2 seconds.

7. Apply firm pressure (for 30–40 minutes if the patient is anticoagulated) to the insertion site to provide hemostasis. Continue close observation for complications.

SELECTED REFERENCES

Anonymous. *Intraaortic balloon pumps.* Health Devices 1997;26: 184–216.

Quaal SJ. *Comprehensive intraaortic balloon counterpulsation,* 2nd ed. St. Louis: Mosby-Year Book; 1993.

Extracorporeal Membrane Oxygenation

William E. Hurford

I. **Extracorporeal support for acute respiratory failure**
   A. **Extracorporeal support** has been used to treat patients with acute respiratory failure since the early 1970s. Perfusion with a membrane lung can correct hypoxemia and hypercapnia while relieving the patient's lungs of their primary burden of respiratory gas exchange. During perfusion, the F_{IO_2} and ventilator pressures, possible sources of pulmonary injury, can be decreased, while continued access to the airway permits safe tracheal suctioning and pulmonary lavage. In addition, venoarterial perfusion provides hemodynamic support.
   B. **In neonates,** two randomized, controlled trials reported increased survival rates with extracorporal membrane oxygenation (ECMO) compared with conventional therapy. Since the mid to late 1980s, the number of centers capable of performing neonatal ECMO has increased rapidly.
   C. **Survival rates of neonates** vary according to the pathologic condition: meconium aspiration syndrome (93%), pulmonary hypertension (83%), sepsis or pneumonia (77%), hyaline membrane disease (84%), and other diagnoses (77%). Congenital diaphragmatic hernia (CDH) has the lowest survival rate of 59%.
   D. **In adults** with acute respiratory failure, randomized multicenter studies have reported no difference in survival between ECMO patients and those treated with conventional ventilation alone. Subgroups of patients or individual patients might benefit from ECMO. Currently, however, it remains unproven that extracorporeal support of adults with respiratory failure is justified by a lower mortality rate or shorter hospital stays.
II. **ECMO physiology**
   A. **Access** for ECMO can be performed by **venoarterial (VA)** or **venovenous (VV)** routes.
      1. **VA-ECMO** drains venous blood via a cannula placed into the right atrium and returns oxygenated blood into the arterial system via a cannula placed in the right common carotid artery. VA-ECMO oxygenates venous blood via a membrane lung and provides mechanical circulatory support (usually 80–150 ml/kg/min). All of the metabolically produced carbon dioxide is removed by the membrane lung. Disadvantages include ligation of the right carotid artery, systemic particulate and air embo-

lism, and increased "afterload" on the left ventricle, which can adversely affect cardiac performance.

2. **VV-ECMO** can be performed via cannulation of the jugular or femoral veins. This method preserves the right carotid artery, maintains normal pulsatile arterial flow, and perfuses the lung with oxygenated blood. Arterial oxygen saturation is usually less in patients treated with VV-ECMO compared with VA-ECMO.

3. **Extracorporeal CO_2 removal and low frequency positive-pressure ventilation or $ECCO_2$ R—LFPPV** uses the bypass circuit only to remove carbon dioxide. A low flow venovenous bypass circuit and large surface area membrane oxygenators are used. The goal of this form of extracorporeal gas exchange is to remove CO_2 with the membrane lung, while reducing the respiratory rate and mechanical ventilating pressures. Oxygenation is maintained using high levels of continuous positive airway pressure (CPAP) along with low frequency positive-pressure ventilation and intratracheal oxygen.

B. **Equipment for ECMO** includes an occlusive roller pump, pump base, venous return monitor, heating unit, coagulation timer, membrane mounting board, oxygen blender, carbon dioxide tank, O_2 and CO_2 flow meters, in-line temperature probes and in-line oxygen saturation monitor (Fig. 14-1). Blood is drained from the right atrium into a small distensible venous reservoir. This reservoir is designed to prevent a direct negative suction from the right atrium. If venous return is decreased, the reservoir collapses and stops the roller pump. Once the blood passes through this device, it proceeds into the pump that provides the driving force to deliver the blood into the membrane oxygenator. Gas diffuses across the membrane, increasing the oxygen tension and removing carbon dioxide from the blood. The blood is then heated to body temperature and delivered into the right atrium in VV-ECMO or into the aortic arch in VA-ECMO. A bridge exists between the arterial and venous cannulas to ensure continuous extracorporeal circulation when the cannulas are clamped.

C. **Vascular cannulation**
1. **Cannulation** of the internal jugular vein and common carotid artery is performed for VA-ECMO. A second venous drainage cannula is often placed cephalad into the jugular bulb. This cannula provides additional blood drainage and helps prevent venous hypertension within the brain.

2. **Neonatal venovenous (VV) ECMO** is performed by placing a 14 French double lumen catheter into the right atrium by way of the internal jugular vein. The "arterial" return portion of the cannula is positioned to encourage flow across the tricuspid valve and, thus, minimize recirculation within the

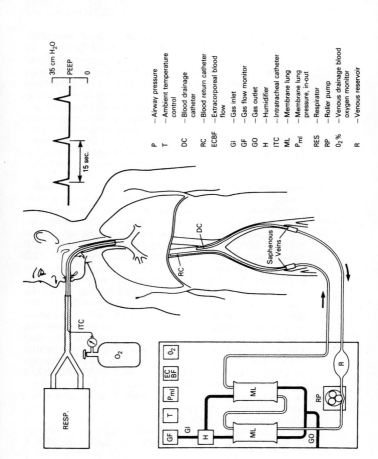

P — Airway pressure
T — Ambient temperature control
DC — Blood drainage catheter
RC — Blood return catheter
ECBF — Extracorporeal blood flow

GI — Gas inlet
GF — Gas flow monitor
GO — Gas outlet
H — Humidifier
ITC — Intratracheal catheter
ML — Membrane lung
P_{ml} — Membrane lung pressure, in-out
RES — Respirator
RP — Roller pump
$O_2\%$ — Venous drainage blood oxygen monitor
R — Venous reservoir

right atrium. A cephalad venous drainage cannula can be used in conjunction with the double lumen venovenous cannula.

3. **Cannulation for VA- and VV-ECMO in older children and adults** can be done in a similar fashion as for neonates. In adults, percutaneous cannulas can be placed using commercially available supplies. Depending on the size of the patient and the anticipated flow requirements, venovenous cannulation can be performed via the jugular and femoral routes, or via both femoral veins. When VA perfusion is needed in larger patients, the common femoral artery can be used instead of the carotid.

D. **Anticoagulation** with heparin is necessary to reduce both thrombosis formation within the circuit and the possibility of embolic events. Heparin-bonded circuits that reduce the need for systemic anticoagulation have been described.

E. **Thrombocytopenia** is common because of exposure of the blood to the bypass circuit. Platelet transfusions usually are indicated if the platelet count is below $100,000/mm^3$ or $150,000/mm^3$ if bleeding is evident.

F. **Maintenance and discontinuation of ECMO**

1. ECMO flow rates are usually begun at low levels to minimize rapid fluid shifts, disequilibrium syndrome, and hyperkalemia. Flow rates are gradually increased to 80 to 150 ml/kg/min. Venous oxygen saturation values are monitored continuously in the ECMO circuit and maintained above 65%.

G. **Weaning.** When it is appropriate to reduce the level of extracorporeal support during VA-ECMO, flow is decreased to 10 to 20 ml/kg/min, or 20% to 30% of the initial flow rate. After a successful trial off ECMO with the cannulas clamped, the patient can be decannulated. When VV-ECMO is used, only the gas flow rate over the membrane lung needs to be decreased during weaning.

H. **Complications** include coagulopathy, seizures, intracranial hemorrhage, and neuropsychological deficits.

III. **Neonatal ECMO**

A. **Indications** for ECMO include an oxygenation index OI = [FIO_2 × mean airway pressure (Cm H_2O) × 100]/ postductal PaO_2 equal to or greater than 40 over 4 hours or an OI greater than 25 for a period of 12 to 24 hours while on maximal conventional therapy, the presence of significant barotrauma, and the failure of conventional therapy. With the advent of new therapies such as high frequency oscillatory ventilation (HFOV) and inhaled nitric oxide, the criteria for ECMO are constantly changing.

B. **Current exclusion criteria** for ECMO include weight less than 2,000 g, gestational age less than 34 weeks,

---

Fig. 14-1. **Venovenous (VV) perfusion route with sapheno-saphenous percutaneous cannulation (From Zapol WM, Kolobow T. Extracorporeal membrane gas exchange. In: Crystal RG, West JB, et al., eds. The Lung: Scientific Foundations. New York: Raven Press, Ltd., 1991;2201.)**

greater than grade I intraventricular hemorrhage, severe neurologic impairment, and cyanotic congenital heart disease incompatible with survival.

IV. **Pediatric and adult ECMO**

A. **Indications** for ECMO in these patients are unclear, because of uncertainty regarding benefit. Classic "ECMO criteria" include a pulmonary venous admixture of greater than 30% or a PaO_2 less than 50 mmHg despite supplemental oxygen ($FIO_2 > 0.5$) and positive end-expiratory pressure (PEEP) greater than 5 cm H_2O.

B. **Exclusion criteria** include irreversible lethal diseases of other organ systems (e.g., disseminated cancer and severe immunosuppression). Active bleeding is a relative contraindication, but trauma patients have been successfully treated with ECMO.

REFERENCES

Anderson HL III, Delius RE, Sinard JM, et al. Early experience with adult extracorporeal membrane oxygenation in the modern era. *Ann Thorac Surg.* 1992;53:553–563.

Anderson HL III, Snedecor SM, Otsu T, et al. Multicenter comparison of conventional venoarterial access versus venovenous double-lumen catheter access in newborn infants undergoing extracorporeal membrane oxygenation. *J Pediatr Surg.* 1993;28:530–534.

Bartlett RH, Roloff DW, Cornell RG, et al. Extracorporeal circulation in neonatal respiratory failure: a prospective randomized study. *Pediatrics.* 1985;76:622–623.

Delius R, Anderson H III, Schumacher R, et al. Venovenous compares favorably with venoarterial access for extracorporeal membrane oxygenation in neonatal respiratory failure. *J Thorac Cardiovasc Surg.* 1993;106:329–338.

Delius RE, Bove EL, Meliones JN, et al. Use of extracorporeal life support in patients with congenital heart disease. *Crit Care Med.* 1992;20:1216–1222.

Fugate J, Ryan D. Extracorporeal membrane oxygenation. *Problems in Anesthesia.* 1989;3:271–287.

Gattinoni L, Pesenti A, Bombino M, et al. Role of extracorporeal circulation in adult respiratory distress syndrome management. *New Horizons.* 1993;1:603–612.

Gattinoni L, Pesentia A, Mascheroni D, et al. Low frequency pressure ventilation with extracorporeal CO_2 removal in severe acute respiratory failure. *JAMA.* 1986;256:881–885.

Hill JD, De Leval MR, Fallat RJ, et al. Acute respiratory insufficiency. Treatment with prolonged extracorporeal oxygenation. *J Thorac Cardiovasc Surg.* 1972;64:551–562.

Hirschl R, Schumacher R, Snedecor S, et al. The efficacy of extracorporeal life support in premature and low birth weight newborns. *J Pediatr Surg.* 1993;28:1336–1341.

Morris AH, Wallace CJ, Menlove RL, et al. Randomized clinical trial of pressure-controlled inverse ratio ventilation and extracorporeal CO_2 removal for adult respiratory distress syndrome. *Am J Respir Crit Care Med.* 1994;149:295–305.

O'Rourke PP, Crone RK, Vacanti JP, et al. Extracorporeal membrane oxygenation and conventional medical therapy in neonates with persistent pulmonary hypertension of the newborn: a prospective randomized study. *Pediatrics.* 1989;84:957–963.

Pranikoff T, Hirschl PB, Remenapp R, et al. Venovenous extracorporeal life support via percutaneous cannulation in 94 patients. *Chest.* 1999;115:818–822.

Stolar CJ, Snedecor SM, Bartlett RH. Extracorporeal membrane oxygenation and neonatal respiratory failure: experience from the extracorporeal life support organization. *J Pediatr Surg.* 1991;26: 563–571.

Zapol WM, Snider MT, Hill JD, et al. Extracorporeal membrane oxygenation in severe acute respiratory failure. A randomized prospective study. *JAMA.* 1979;242:2193–2196.

Adult and Pediatric Resuscitation

Richard M. Pino

I. **Overview.** The intensivist is frequently called on to assist with advanced cardiopulmonary resuscitation (CPR) throughout the hospital and to teach healthcare providers both basic and advanced life support techniques. This chapter provides basic information for adult and pediatric resuscitation. Formal training in these areas is encouraged and is often mandated by institutional policy. The protocols described below follow established guidelines with modifications for the clinician in a hospital setting. The algorithms serve as a useful starting point when confronted with a cardiac arrest. Central to any resuscitation effort is the delegation of responsibility and the maintenance of a sense of control and calmness.

II. **Cardiac arrest**
   A. **The diagnosis of cardiac arrest** is made swiftly in the intensive care unit (ICU) because of the low nurse: patient ratio, continuous monitoring of the electrocardiogram (ECG), routine use of arterial pressure monitoring, and the use of central monitoring stations. The ECG might reveal ventricular tachycardia, ventricular fibrillation, or asystole. Hypotension can occur with supraventricular tachycardias of multiple causes. In pulseless electrical activity, an organized ECG is present without a blood pressure. The absence of a palpable pulse in a major artery (e.g., carotid, femoral) in an unconscious, unmonitored patient is diagnostic of a cardiac arrest.

   B. **Etiology.** Cardiac arrest can be caused primarily by underlying cardiac and pulmonary disease or can result from metabolic and physical abnormalities such as:
      1. Hypoxemia.
      2. Acid-base disturbances.
      3. Derangements of electrolytes.
      4. Hypovolemia.
      5. Adverse drug events.
      6. Pericardial tamponade, tension pneumothorax.

   C. **Pathophysiology.** With the onset of cardiac arrest, effective blood flow ceases and tissue hypoxia, anaerobic metabolism, and accumulation of cellular wastes result. Organ function is compromised and permanent damage ensues unless the condition is reversed within minutes. Acidosis from anaerobic metabolism can cause systemic vasodilatation, pulmonary vasoconstriction, and a decreased responsiveness to the actions of endogenous and exogenous catecholamines. Following resuscitation, organ dysfunction may be exacerbated by reperfusion injury.

III. Adult resuscitation

A. Basic life support (BLS) is the foundation of resuscitation to maintain vital organ perfusion. The **ABCs** (**A**irway, **B**reathing, **C**irculation) of resuscitation should be evaluated for all patients in cardiac arrest. **Advanced cardiac life support (ACLS)** is the definitive treatment of a cardiac arrest with endotracheal intubation, electrical cardioversion and defibrillation, and pharmacologic intervention.

1. **Airway and breathing.** If the trachea is not already intubated, the airway should be evaluated for patency using the head tilt–chin lift or an oropharyngeal or nasopharyngeal airway as needed. Hemoglobin saturation can be readily monitored with pulse oximetry. If adequate spontaneous ventilation is still absent, bag-valve mask ventilation with 100% oxygen should be initiated until spontaneous ventilation returns. For example, a patient who has transient ventilatory depression shortly after the administration of a narcotic or a patient with hypotension related to a supraventricular tachycardia that resolves quickly with pharmacologic therapy or cardioversion might only require transient mask ventilation. If a definitive airway is needed, intubation is performed with minimal disruption of resuscitative measures by the most experienced person present (see Chapter 3). Correct placement of the endotracheal tube should be confirmed by auscultation and the presence of end-tidal CO_2. The latter can be monitored by capnography or via a colorimetric change in an indicator paper (e.g., the Easy Cap II, Nellcor Puritan Bennett, Inc., Pleasanton, CA). End-tidal CO_2 may not be detectable when pulmonary blood flow is absent or when cardiac compressions are inadequate. A self-inflating bulb (the esophageal detector) attached to the endotracheal tube or direct visualization by fiberoptic bronchoscopy has been suggested as alternative means of assessing proper placement of the endotracheal tube. **Epinephrine, lidocaine, naloxone,** and **atropine** can be administered by the endotracheal route if intravenous (IV) access has not been established. Dilution of these drugs in 5 to 10 ml of sterile saline ensures their more complete delivery. Higher doses (two- to threefold) may be warranted with endotracheal administration to achieve adequate peak concentrations.

2. **Circulation.** The circulation is assessed by feeling for a carotid artery pulse for 5 to 10 seconds. The presence of a pulse does not assure that an "adequate" mean arterial pressure is present. Although the ACLS protocols consider a systolic blood pressure of less than 90 mm Hg as unstable in a variety of scenarios, the precise value for an

individual patient must be considered with respect to coronary and cerebral perfusion pressures. Noninvasive blood pressure monitoring should be quickly employed in the absence of a preexisting arterial line. If the patient is pulseless or has an inadequate blood pressure, artificial circulation should be provided by external chest compressions. The patient must be on a firm surface (e.g., backboard or CPR position for a bed with an inflatable mattress) with the head at the same level as the thorax. The person doing chest compressions places the heel of one hand on the patient's sternum, two finger-breadths above the xiphoid process. The other hand can either sit on top of the first, interlocking the fingers, or it can grasp the wrist of the first hand. The shoulders should be directly over the patient, with the elbows locked for effective compressions. The sternum is depressed 1.5 to 2.0 inches in a normal-sized adult, with the compressions accounting for 50% of each compression–relaxation cycle, delivered at 80 to 100 per minute, and at a 5:1 ratio with ventilation. The return of spontaneous cardiopulmonary activity should be checked after the first four cycles and every several minutes thereafter.

3. **Cardioversion and defibrillation.** Cardiac arrest can result from ventricular tachycardia, ventricular fibrillation, asystole, and complete heart block. Symptomatic hypotension can result from bradycardia, multiple forms of supraventricular tachycardia, and ventricular tachycardia. As the duration of a harmful rhythm progresses, the rhythm tends to deteriorate into one that is more difficult to treat. Early attempts to treat dysrhythmias are crucial to a successful outcome. A solitary **precordial thump** is recommended for witnessed **ventricular fibrillation (VF)** when a defibrillator is not immediately available. **Pulseless ventricular tachycardia (VT)** is treated in the same fashion as ventricular fibrillation. Three asynchronous shocks are delivered in rapid succession to take advantage of the decrease in transthoracic impedance that occurs with each shock. The energy levels for the initial series of shocks are 200 J, 300 J, and 360 J, respectively, with subsequent shocks at 360 J that are repeated after each pharmacologic intervention. For recurrent episodes of VT, the lowest energy level that was successful for the last defibrillation is used. It is the responsibility of the person operating the defibrillator to ensure that all members of the resuscitation team are safe. Lower energies (e.g., 30 J) with synchronization are used to cardiovert supraventricular dysrhythmias such as **atrial flutter** and **paroxysmal supraventricular tachycardia (PSVT)** (Fig. 15-1). Hemodyanamically stable **VT** and

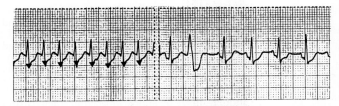

Fig. 15-1. Synchronous cardioversion of a supraventricular tachycardia. *Arrowheads (left)* indicate synchrony of the defibrillator with the patient's rate (300 bpm) prior to cardioversion (*right*) to a rate of 140 bpm that was followed with pharmacologic therapy.

        atrial fibrillation (AF) can be converted using 100 J as the starting point.

4. **Pacing (See Chapter 19).** If pharmacologic intervention is not successful in treating a significant bradycardia or a high-grade heart block, temporary cardiac pacing should be used. **Transcutaneous pacing** is the quickest method to increase the ventricular rate with the caveat that sedation will be required. **Transesophageal pacing** can be used if atrioventricular conduction has been maintained. **Transvenous pacing** is technically more difficult, but it can be used for more prolonged periods. Ventricular pacing is done with a single transvenous pacing wire. If the patient requires the insertion of a pulmonary artery catheter, one with pacing capabilities can be used to pace the atrium, ventricle, or both.

5. **Intravenous access.** An adequate means to deliver medications and fluid is imperative for successful resuscitation. The most desirable route for drug administration is into the central circulation. Many patients in the ICU will have some form of central access in place. Internal or external jugular, subclavian, femoral, or long peripheral lines can be used. The internal jugular and femoral veins are desirable because of the relative ease of insertion, fewer complications, and minimal interruption of resuscitative efforts during insertion. The antecubital veins are the next most desirable; they are fairly effective if the extremity is elevated and a large volume of IV fluid is used to flush the medication toward the central circulation. Do not overlook the utility of existing subcutaneous central venous ports or dialysis catheters. Peripherally inserted central catheters (PICC lines) are usually not suitable for extended resuscitation because of the high resistance to flow. Fluid replacement with crystalloids or blood products is indicated for patients with known or suspected intravascular

volume depletion. In the usual cardiac arrest scenario, fluids are used only to keep IV lines open and
to flush drugs toward the central circulation.

6. **Drugs.** Discussed below are drugs commonly used
to support the circulation. It is crucial to know
what drugs are infusing into a patient at the time
of an arrest. For example, stopping a dopamine
infusion in a hemodynamically stable patient with
a sudden onset of supraventricular tachycardia
might be the best therapeutic option. Similarly,
trying to revive a hypotensive patient with ventricular tachycardia would be difficult if a continuing infusion of nitroglycerin is not recognized.

   a. **Oxygen.** Because of profound tissue hypoxemia, 100% O_2 should be provided by positive-
   pressure ventilation to all cardiac arrest
   victims. For hemodynamically stable patients
   with dysrhythmias, oxygen can be provided
   via a face mask. The benefit of providing oxygen to a patient with chronic obstructive pulmonary disease in the latter situation clearly
   outweighs the theoretical suppression of ventilation.

   b. **Epinephrine.** No method of CPR tested to
   date, with the possible exception of open chest
   CPR, can sustain organ blood flow sufficiently
   to prevent ischemic injury. The addition of
   adrenergic agents to CPR greatly improves
   outcome. Epinephrine is the mainstay of pharmacologic therapy in cardiac arrest. The beneficial effect of epinephrine in this setting is
   thought to be a result of its α-adrenergic action. Epinephrine causes profound vasoconstriction in the noncerebral and noncoronary
   vascular beds. Although this vasoconstriction
   can actually decrease cardiac output, cerebral
   and myocardial blood flow can be increased at
   the same time. The current recommended dose
   of epinephrine for cardiac arrest is 1.0 mg IV,
   repeated every 3 to 5 minutes. Higher doses
   (up to 0.1 mg/kg every 3–5 min) have been considered as alternatives if the initial dose is
   ineffective; however higher doses do not significantly affect outcome.

   c. **Lidocaine** is the drug of choice for ventricular dysrhythmias. It is used for ventricular
   fibrillation, ventricular tachycardia, and premature ventricular complexes that are frequent (more than six complexes per minute),
   closely coupled, occur in runs of two or more, or
   are multifocal in configuration. The initial dose
   of lidocaine for a cardiac arrest is 1.5 mg/kg IV,
   which can be repeated as a 0.5 mg/kg bolus
   every 8 minutes to a total dose of 3 mg/kg. A
   continuous infusion of lidocaine at a rate of

2 to 4 mg/min is instituted after a successful conversion. Lidocaine is metabolized in the liver and is a myocardial depressant at high blood levels. The dosage of lidocaine should be reduced in patients with a low cardiac output, hepatic dysfunction, or advanced age.

d. **Bretylium** is indicated for the treatment of ventricular dysrhythmias resistant to other therapies. Caution must be exercised because it can produce hypotension through postganglionic adrenergic blockade. Bretylium is given as an initial 5 mg/kg bolus, followed by doses of 10 mg/kg every 15 minutes if needed, to a total dose of 30 mg/kg. If successful, bretylium should be continued as an infusion of 1 to 2 mg/min.

e. **Procainamide** is used to suppress ventricular dysrhythmias when lidocaine is contraindicated or has failed. It is also used to convert atrial fibrillation into a sinus rhythm. Boluses of 50 mg every 5 minutes or a continuous infusion of 20 to 30 mg/min to a total dose of 17 mg/kg are used. The initial loading phase of procainamide administration should be terminated when the dysrhythmia is suppressed, hypotension occurs, the patient become nauseated (if not obtunded), or the QRS complex is widened by 50% of its original size. When the dysrhythmia is suppressed, a maintenance infusion of 1 to 4 mg/min should be started. The procainamide dosage should be reduced in patients with renal failure. The ECG should be examined at least daily for QRS widening. The total effective blood concentration of procainamide is the sum of the native drug's concentration and that of N-acetylprocainamide (NAPA), its active metabolite.

f. **Amiodarone** is the one of the newest of the commonly used antidysrhythmics. It should not to be confused with the phosphodiesterase inhibitor, amrinone. Although it primarily has class III characteristics (i.e., lengthening the cardiac action potential), it has properties of all four classes of antidysrhythmics (i.e., sodium channel blockade at high frequencies of stimulation, noncompetitive antisynaptic actions, and negative chronotropism). It is indicated for the treatment and prophylaxis of recurrent VT and VF. As for procainamide, amiodarone can be used to suppress supraventricular tachycardias and convert atrial fibrillation into a sinus rhythm. The recommended initial dosing is 150 mg over 10 minutes (15 mg/min), 360 mg over the next 6 hours (1 mg/min), then 540 mg over the next 18 hours (0.5 mg/min). Side effects include bradycardias that are not dose related, hypothyroidism secondary to the inhibition of the peripheral conversion of thyroxine to triiodothyronine, and increases in the levels of enzymes associated with hepatic function. Alveolar pneumonitis and pulmonary fibrosis are a concern for patients chronically receiving amiodarone.

g. **Magnesium sulfate** is a cofactor in many enzyme reactions including Na^+K^+-adenosine triphosphatase (ATPase). Hypomagnesemia has been associated with dysrhythmias, including the precipitation of refractory VF and sudden death. Magnesium administration can reduce dysrhythmias after a myocardial infarction and is the agent of choice for the treatment of torsades de pointes. The dose is 1 to 2 g in 10 ml 5% dextrose in water (D_5W) over 1 to 2 minutes, but it can be given as an IV push for VF. For torsades, 5 to 10 g can be administered. Hypotension and bradycardia are side effects with rapid administration.

h. **Atropine** is useful in the treatment of hemodynamically significant bradycardia or atrioventricular (AV) block occurring at the nodal level. Atropine increases the rate of sinus node discharge and enhances AV nodal conduction by its vagolytic activity. For bradycardia or AV block, it should be administered as a bolus (0.5 mg) and repeated, if necessary, every 5 minutes to a total dose of 2 mg. In the case of asystole, atropine is given as a 1 mg bolus and repeated in 5 minutes if needed.

i. **Dopamine** has dopaminergic (at < 2 µg/kg/min), β-adrenergic (2–5 µg/kg/min), and α-adrenergic (5–10 µg/kg/min) activities. These dose ranges are traditional and approximate values. In reality, because significant α and β effects can be evident at very low concentrations, the drug should be started at 50 to 100 µg/min and titrated until the desired effect (e.g., increased urine output, increased heart rate or inotropy, increased blood pressure) is seen or undesired side effects (e.g., tachycardia) occur.

j. **Isoproterenol** is a $β_1$- and $β_2$-adrenergic agonist. Because its $β_2$-adrenergic activity can cause hypotension, it is a second-line drug used to treat hemodynamically significant bradycardia that is unresponsive to atropine. Isoproterenol can be used temporarily while awaiting pacemaker insertion. An infusion of 2 to 10 µg/min is titrated to achieve the desired heart rate.

k. Verapamil and diltiazem are calcium channel antagonists that depress AV nodal conduction. They are useful for the treatment of hemodynamically stable PSVTs that have AV nodal pathways of conduction and that do not respond to vagal maneuvers. The initial dose of verapamil is 2.5 to 5 mg IV. Subsequent doses of 5 to 10 mg can be administered every 15 to 30 minutes. Diltiazem is given as an initial bolus of 20 mg with a second dose of 25 mg, if needed, and an infusion of 5 to 15 mg/h. Both drugs are vasodilators and negative inotropes that can cause hypotension, exacerbation of congestive heart failure, bradycardia, and enhancement of accessory conduction in patients with Wolff-Parkinson-White syndrome. The hypotension can be reversed with 0.5 to 1.0 g of calcium chloride.

l. Propanolol and metoprolol are used in the treatment of hemodynamically stable PSVT and atrial fibrillation and flutter with high rates of ventricular response. Propanolol is a β_1- and β_2-adrenergic antagonist. The initial dose is 0.25 to 0.5 mg IV. Subsequent doses can be increased to 1 mg or higher and given every 5 minutes until the rhythm is controlled. Propanolol, in contrast to verapamil and diltiazem, is not a direct negative inotrope, does not cause vasodilatation, and is less likely to cause hypotension. It can cause bronchospasm in a subset of patients with chronic obstructive pulmonary disease because of β_2-adrenergic inhibition. Metoprolol blocks β_1-adrenergic receptors more selectively. Because of the absence of β_2 activity at normal doses, it is often used in patients with reactive airways. The initial dose is 5 mg every 10 to 15 minutes for a total dose of 15 mg.

m. Calcium. Multiple studies have failed to demonstrate a beneficial effect of calcium administration during CPR. Some evidence exists that high levels of calcium can worsen neurologic outcome following a cardiac arrest. It should be used only when hyperkalemia, hypermagnesemia, hypocalcemia, or toxicity from calcium channel blockers is present. Calcium chloride (2 to 4 mg/kg IV) is given into a central vein in these situations and repeated as necessary.

n. Sodium bicarbonate is used in the treatment of cardiac arrest only in the setting of a preexisting metabolic acidosis or hyperkalemia, and then only when standard ACLS protocols have been unsuccessful. The initial dose of bicarbonate should be 1 mEq/kg IV.

Subsequent doses of 0.5 mEq/kg can be given every 10 minutes (as guided by measurements of arterial pH and P_{CO_2}). Because sodium bicarbonate administration can cause a paradoxical intracellular acidosis, its indiscriminate use during cardiopulmonary resuscitation is discouraged.

o. **Adenosine** is an endogenous purine nucleotide with a half-life of 5 seconds. By virtue of slowing AV nodal conduction and interruption of AV node reentry pathways, it can convert a PSVT to a sinus rhythm. It is also used to assist with the diagnosis of supraventricular tachycardias (e.g., atrial flutter with a rapid ventricular response versus PSVT) (Fig. 15-2). The initial dose (6 mg) is a rapid IV bolus. A brief asystole ensues that is followed by P waves, flutter waves, or fibrillations that are initially without a ventricular response. PSVT is sometimes converted to a sinus rhythm with an initial dose of 6 mg. A second injection of 12 mg might terminate PSVT if the first dose is unsuccessful. Recurrent PSVT, AF, and atrial flutter require longer-acting drugs for definitive treatment. The doses of adenosine

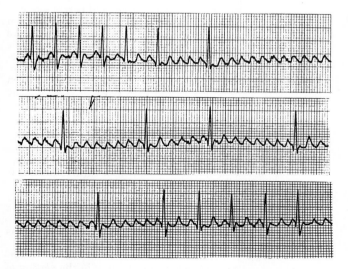

Fig. 15-2. Diagnosis of a rhythm with adenosine. The initial ventricular response of 180 bpm disappears after atrioventricular conduction is inhibited by adenosine, revealing an underlying rhythm of atrial flutter (300 bpm, *top*), followed by a 6 to 8:1 block (*middle*), then a 2 to 3:1 block of atrial flutter with a ventricular rate of 120 bpm.

should be increased in the presence of methylxanthines (because of competitive inhibition) or decreased if dipyridamole (from potentiation via blockage of nucleoside transport) has been administered.

7. **Specific ACLS protocols**

    a. Ventricular fibrillation (Fig. 15-3).

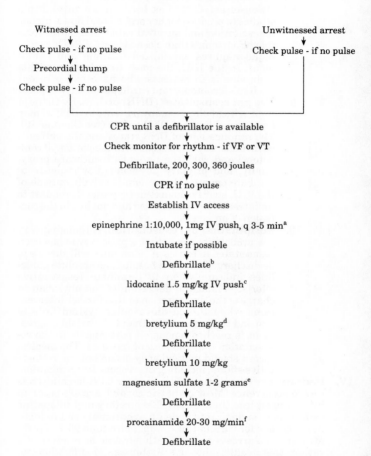

Fig. 15-3. AHA ACLS protocol for ventricular fibrillation. [a]Up to 0.1 mg/kg may be used. [b]Defibrillate after each epinephrine administration; use the lowest energy that was successful with initial defibrillation. [c]If successful, infusion of 1 to 4 mg/min. [d]If successful, infusion of 1 to 2 mg/min. [e]If intravenous access is present, give earlier when indicated. [f]Maximal dose of 17 mg/kg or termination with dysrhythmia suppression, hypotension, or QRS width of 50%; if successful, infusion of 2 mg/kg/h. VF, ventricular fibrillation; VT, ventricular tachycardia; CPR, cardiopulmonary resuscitation; IV, intravenous(ly).

b. Ventricular tachycardia and wide-complex tachycardia of uncertain types (Fig. 15-4).

c. Asystole (Fig. 15-5).

d. Pulseless electrical activity (Fig. 15-6).

e. Paroxysmal supraventricular tachycardia (Fig. 15-7).

f. Bradycardia (Fig. 15-8).

g. Ventricular ectopy (Fig. 15-9).

8. **Open-chest CPR** has been shown in multiple studies to produce higher organ blood flows, higher resuscitation and survival rates, and better neurologic outcomes than closed-chest CPR. This technique requires specialized training and equipment. In the ICU, the most frequent use of this technique is in patients who have had a recent median sternotomy and cardiopulmonary bypass.

9. **"Do not resuscitate" (DNR) orders.** By virtue of their critical illness, many patients in the ICU may have varied types of DNR orders (see Chapter 16). The ramifications of DNR status and the patient's wishes should be discussed with the patient, if competent, and with the patient's healthcare proxy, family, and primary physician. For requests to intubate emergently or semi-electively outside of the ICU, swiftly ensure that a patient's request to limit treatment is respected and not lost in the confusion of an arrest.

10. **Termination of resuscitation.** Although a very low probability exists that a patient who has been resuscitated in excess of 30 minutes will survive to be discharged from the hospital, no absolute guidelines indicate when to terminate resuscitative efforts. It is at the discretion of the physician in charge of the resuscitation to stop further interventions when the cardiovascular system fails to respond to adequate treatment. Invariably, agreement is reached among all participants in the resuscitation that the patient has died. The medical record should meticulously document the resuscitative efforts, including the reasons for termination.

IV. **Pediatric resuscitation.** The need for CPR in children is a rare occurrence. Most pediatric cardiac arrests occur in infants aged less than 1 year. Respiratory and idiopathic causes (e.g., sudden infant death syndrome) are predominant reasons for CPR in this group. More than 90% of pediatric cardiac arrests present with asystole or bradycardia rather than ventricular dysrhythmias. Modifications of adult resuscitation algorithms include age-related changes in the rate, magnitude, and position of chest compressions, and weight-based defibrillator settings and drug doses.

A. **Airway and breathing.** Airway establishment is the same as in the adult with two important exceptions. Hyperextension of an infant's neck for the head tilt–chin lift maneuver can lead to airway obstruction because of the small diameter and ease of compression of the

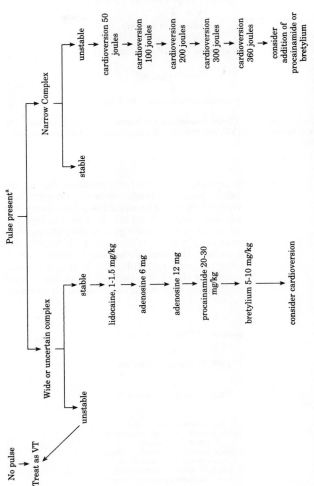

Fig. 15-4. American Heart Association Advance Cardiac Life Support protocol for ventricular tachycardia (VT) and wide complex tachycardia of uncertain type. [a]Administration of oxygen and intravenous access.

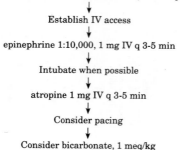

If rhythm is unclear and possible ventricular
fibrillation, defibrillate as for VF. If asystole is present
↓
Establish IV access
↓
epinephrine 1:10,000, 1 mg IV q 3-5 min
↓
Intubate when possible
↓
atropine 1 mg IV q 3-5 min
↓
Consider pacing
↓
Consider bicarbonate, 1 meq/kg

Fig. 15-5. American Heart Association Advance Cardiac Life Support protocol for asystole. VF, ventricular fibrillation; IV, intravenous(ly); q, every.

immature airway. Submental compression during the chin lift might push the tongue into the pharynx and obstruct ventilation. Breaths should be given slowly and with sufficient volume to cause the chest to rise, but with low airway pressures to avoid gastric distention. Ventilation rates vary with age (Table 15-1). If a definitive airway is needed, the size of the endotracheal tube is based on the patient's age [tube size in millimeters of internal diameter (ID) = 4 + (age/4)] for children aged more than 2 years. For younger children, an endotra-

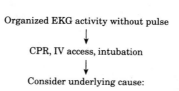

Organized EKG activity without pulse
↓
CPR, IV access, intubation
↓
Consider underlying cause:

hypovolemia (give volume)
tension pneumothorax (relieve pressure)
hypoxemia (oxygen)
cardiac tamponade (pericardiocentesis)
hypokalemia (give potassium)
metabolic acidosis (bicarbonate)
drug overdose (treatment appropriate to substance)
massive myocardial infarction
(heparin, thrombolysis, intraaortic balloon pump, etc.)
↓
epinephrine 1:10,000 IV q 3-5 min

Fig. 15-6. American Heart Association Advance Cardiac Life Support protocol for pulseless electrical activity. EKG, electrocardiogram; CPR, cardiopulmonary resuscitation; IV, intravenous; q, every.

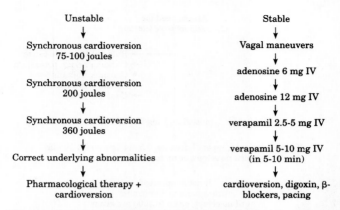

Fig. 15-7. American Heart Association Advance Cardiac Life Support protocol for paroxysmal supraventricular tachycardia. IV, intravenous.

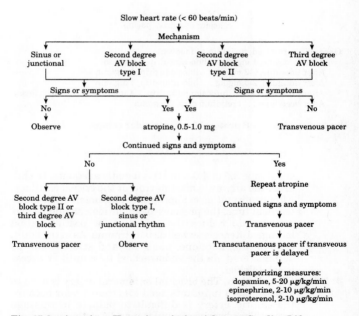

Fig. 15-8. American Heart Association Advance Cardiac Life Support protocol for bradycardia. AV, atrioventricular.

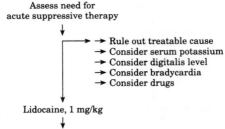

Assess need for
acute suppressive therapy

→ Rule out treatable cause
→ Consider serum potassium
→ Consider digitalis level
→ Consider bradycardia
→ Consider drugs

Lidocaine, 1 mg/kg

If not suppressed, repeat lidocaine, 0.5 mg/kg every 2-10 min
until no ectopy, or up to 3 mg/kg given

If not suppressed,
procainamide 20 mg/min
until no ectopy, or up to 1000 mg given

If not suppressed,
and not contraindicated,
bretylium, 5-10 mg/kg over 8-10 min

If not suppressed,
consider overdrive pacing

Once ectopy resolved, maintain as follows:
    After lidocaine, 1 mg/kg . . . lidocaine drip, 2 mg/min
    After lidocaine, 1-2 mg/kg . . . lidocaine drip, 3 mg/min
    After lidocaine, 2-3 mg/kg . . . lidocaine drip, 4 mg/min
    After procainamide . . . procainamide drip, 1-4 mg/min (check blood level)
    After bretylium . . . bretylium drip, 2 mg/min

Fig. 15-9.   AHA ACLS protocol for ventricular ectopy.

cheal tube 3.5 or 4.0 mm ID is usually adequate. In children, the airway is most narrow at the cricoid cartilage. After confirmation of appropriate placement of the endotracheal tube, the presence of an air leak should be documented to reduce the potential for postintubation laryngeal stenosis as well as barotrauma. As in the adult, epinephrine, lidocaine, naloxone, and atropine can be administered via the endotracheal tube until IV access is established.

B. Circulation. The brachial or femoral artery is used to assess pulses in infants aged less than 1 year because the carotid artery is difficult to palpate in this age group. The absence of a pulse mandates the immediate need for chest compressions. The rate and depth of sternal compressions are age-related (Table 15-1). Chest compressions in infants are delivered at a point 1 cm below the intermammary line. Compressions are performed with two fingertips applied to the sternum or by encircling the chest with both hands and using the

Table 15-1. Pediatric cardiopulmonary resuscitation

Age	Ventilations/min	Compression/min	Ventilation-compression ratio	Depth (inches)
Infant	20–24	100–120	1:5	0.5–1.0
Young child (1–4 years)	20	100	1:5	1.0–1.5
Older child (>4 years)	16	80	1:5	1.5–2.0

From Pino RM. Adult, pediatric, and newborn resuscitation. In: Hurford WE, Bailin MT, Davison JK, Haspel KL, Rosow C, eds. *Clinical anesthesia procedures of the Massachusetts General Hospital*, 5th ed. Philadelphia: Lippincott-Raven, 1998:653.

Table 15-2. Drugs used in pediatric advanced life support

Drug	Dose	How supplied	Remarks
Atropine sulfate	0.02 mg/kg/dose	0.1 mg/ml	Minimum dose of 0.1 mg (1.0 ml)
Calcium chloride	20/mg/kg/dose	100 mg/ml (10%)	Give slowly
Dopamine hydrochloride	2–20 µg/kg/min	40 mg/ml	α-Adrenergic action dominates at 15–20 µg/kg/min
Dobutamine hydrochloride	5–20 µg/kg/min	250 mg/vial lyophilized	Titrate to desired effect
Epinephrine hydrochloride	0.1 ml/kg (0.01 mg/kg)	1:10,000 (0.1 mg/ml)	1:1000 must be diluted
Epinephrine infusion	Start at 0.1 µg/kg/min	1:1000 (1 mg/ml)	Titrate to desired effect (0.1–1.0 µg/kg/min)
Isoproterenol hydrochloride	Start at 0.1 µg/kg/min	1 mg/5 ml	Titrate to desired effect (0.1–1.0 µg/kg/min)
Lidocaine	1 mg/kg/dose	10 mg/ml (1%) 20 mg/ml (2%)	
Lidocaine infusion	20–50 µg/kg/min	40 mg/ml (4%)	
Norepinephrine infusion	Start at 0.1 µg/kg/min	1 mg/ml	Titrate to desired effect (0.1–1.0 µg/kg/min)
Sodium bicarbonate	1 mEq/kg/dose or 0.3 × kg × base deficit	1 mEq/ml (8.4%)	Infuse slowly and only if ventilation is adequate

From Pino RM. Adult, pediatric, and newborn resuscitation. In: Hurford WE, Bailin MT, Davison JK, Haspel KL, Rosow C, eds. *Clinical anesthesia procedures of the Massachusetts General Hospital*, 5th ed. Philadelphia: Lippincott-Raven, 1998:655.

thumbs to depress the sternum. In older children, compressions are applied at the same point as in adults, but only one hand is used to depress the sternum. As for any resuscitation, the return of spontaneous cardiopulmonary activity is reassessed on a periodic basis.

C. **Defibrillation.** Defibrillator paddles 4.5 cm in diameter are used for infants and 8 cm in diameter for older children. The pediatric defibrillator paddles are built in beneath the adult paddles in most modern defibrillators; they are exposed by sliding the adult paddles off the handles. The energy level for the initial shock is 2 J/kg. If this energy level is unsuccessful, subsequent shocks are delivered at 4 J/kg and repeated as necessary. A treatable cause for the arrest, such as hypoxemia, hypercarbia, acidosis or hypothermia, should be sought. Defibrillation at the lowest effective energy level is repeated after each pharmacologic intervention, as for the adult patient. For cardioversion, the initial energy is 0.2 J/kg and escalated to 1.0 J/kg as needed.

D. **Pacing.** Symptomatic bradycardia and complete heart block are initially treated with atropine, dopamine, or isoproterenol titrated to effect. If the pharmacologic treatment is unsuccessful, transcutaneous pacing, with sedation if needed, is used until transvenous pacing is established.

E. **IV access.** The principles of IV access are the same as for the adult: use peripheral IV or endotracheal routes until central venous access is available. The **intraosseous** route can also be used in children. For this, a bone marrow or spinal needle is inserted into the tibial shaft away from the epiphyseal plates to gain access to the large venous sinuses of the bone marrow.

F. **Medications.** The drugs described in the adult resuscitation section apply to children, with dosages adjusted for weight (Table 15-2). Epinephrine doses (100 to 200 µg/kg) can be effective in children if the initial 10 µg/kg dose is not.

G. **Resuscitation algorithms.** The protocols for adult resuscitation described above also apply to children, with the appropriate reduction of drug dosages and defibrillator energy.

V. **Newborn resuscitation.** Resuscitation of the newborn usually is performed by a pediatrician with advanced training in neonatology or by an anesthesiologist at delivery. Care of the neonate is outlined in Chapter 39.

SELECTED REFERENCES

Anonymous. *Basic life support heartsaver guide.* Dallas: American Heart Association; 1993.

Chameides L, Hazinsk MF. *Textbook of pediatric advanced life support.* Dallas: American Heart Association; 1994.

Cummins RO, ed. *Textbook of advanced cardiac life support.* Dallas: American Heart Association; 1994.

Emergency Cardiac Care Committee and Subcommittee, American Heart Association: guidelines for cardiopulmonary resuscitation and emergency cardiac care. *JAMA* 1992;268:2171–2288.

Ethical and End-of-Life Issues

Rae M. Allain and William E. Hurford

I. **Introduction.** Care of the critically ill patient necessarily involves acknowledgment that some patients will die despite best medical therapy. Mortality rates in intensive care units (ICUs) vary widely depending on practice type and patient population, but a minimal 10% mortality rate is typical. Observational studies reveal that most deaths in ICUs today are preceded by decisions to withhold or withdraw some form of therapy. Thus, imminent death is usually a predictable event that has been discussed among the critical care team, patient's family, and patient, if possible. In this setting, ethical and end-of-life issues come to the forefront and sometimes provoke conflict. This chapter explores the ethical and end-of-life issues that frequently arise in the ICU and offers suggestions for avoiding and resolving conflicts. Customs, laws, ethical beliefs, and religious practices differ considerably in different cultures and societies. This chapter describes the prevailing practice at the Massachusetts General Hospital in Boston, Massachusetts and is meant to be thoughtful, rather than definitive.

II. **Treatment decisions**

A. Society in the United States highly values patient **autonomy** (i.e., respect for an individual's preferences) as a guiding ethical principle in medicine. Competent adult patients can and may choose to accept or refuse medical therapies offered. If a patient's competence is questionable, a psychiatrist should evaluate the patient to determine if he or she has decision-making capacity. This requires an ability to receive and understand medical information, to discern the various options presented, and to choose a course based on the information offered and one's values.

B. Autonomy is best preserved by obtaining the patient's **informed consent** for procedures (e.g., endotracheal intubation) and therapies [e.g., intravenous (IV) vasopressors] whenever possible. Very frequently, however, critically ill patients are incompetent to make medical decisions because of the gravity of their illness or because of sedative or analgesic medications used to diminish suffering.

1. **An advance directive,** a document specifying the types of treatment that the patient wishes to receive or reject should future need arise, is very useful in this circumstance. (An advance directive can be referred to as a **"living will."**)

2. In addition to or in the absence of an advance directive, a patient can designate a **surrogate** (healthcare proxy, healthcare power of attorney)

who is charged with executing the patient's wishes should he or she become incompetent. The surrogate must offer **substituted judgment** for the patient, providing decisions that the patient would make if competent. If the patient has not designated a surrogate prior to becoming incompetent, the next of kin may become the *de facto* surrogate. In some circumstances where no family is living or available, a trusted friend can act as the patient's surrogate.

3. A court-appointed legal **guardian** may be necessary in rare instances where no family member or friend is able to make decisions in the best interest of the patient.

C. **Communication with family**
1. **Discussions** with family members regarding treatment of the incompetent patient are best conducted in a quiet, private environment, in an unhurried fashion. Physicians should refrain from such discussions in the ICU itself or in hospital corridors, because real or apparent distractions and breaches of confidentiality will threaten to destroy the family's confidence in the critical care team. A comfortable conference room near the ICU is the ideal setting.

2. **Attendants** to the family meeting should include:
   a. The patient's close family, including the **healthcare proxy** or person who will serve as **surrogate.**
   b. The patient's **primary care physician** or alternate physician with whom the patient has had a long-term, trusting relationship.
   c. The ICU **attending physician and ICU nurse.** Occasionally, it is helpful to have adjuvant team members (e.g., respiratory therapist, physical therapist, or occupational therapist) present.
   d. Consulting **specialists,** if needed to present information regarding the patient's condition, therapeutic options, or prognosis.
   e. Ancillary support staff, including **social worker** and **chaplain,** when appropriate.

3. **The goals of ICU therapy** should be confirmed with the family. For many patients, the obvious goals will include preventing imminent death, "curing" the acute disease, discharging the patient from the ICU, and eventually returning the patient to his or her premorbid level of function. Some patients hope only to delay the disease process sufficiently to gain a few more months or years of meaningful living. Occasionally, ICU care is requested to sufficiently prolong a patient's life for close relatives to arrive to pay last respects or to consent for organ donation.

a. **The prognosis** of the patient is very important to setting realistic therapeutic goals. For example, a family may consent to a brief trial of dialysis for a patient who had previously been opposed to chronic dialysis if the prognosis for recovery of renal function is good. Alternatively, a grim prognosis can allow family members to abandon insistent demands for continued aggressive care. It is important for the healthcare team to discuss the patient's prognosis and arrive at a consensus before meeting with the family. Variant opinions about a patient's prognosis only serve to confuse the family, often resulting in delayed decisions, additional anguish, and sometimes hostility toward the care team. If opinions of consulting specialists differ, the intensivist or trusted primary physician should assume responsibility for summarizing the patient's overall condition for the family. Presenting a poor prognosis can be devastating to the family; care should be taken to express compassion and empathy. Time should be allowed for the family to contemplate what has been said and to ask questions. Often the first response is denial of the loved one's condition. The intensivist should gently reaffirm what has been presented and allow family members to express their grief. Acceptance of a poor prognosis may require several discussions over days or even a few weeks.

b. Once the prognosis has been discussed, the family may request or the physician may suggest a **"do not resuscitate" (DNR)** status for the patient. A DNR status seeks to clarify what therapies will be offered to the patient in case of acute, life-threatening instability that requires immediate treatment to prevent death. Clear instructions should be given and documented in the chart regarding preferences for specific interventions [e.g., cardiopulmonary resuscitation (CPR), endotracheal intubation, electrical therapy, and medical therapy] in case of sudden cardiac or respiratory failure. The simple phrase "DNR" in the physician's orders is insufficient because the meaning will vary to different caregivers. When discussing DNR status with the family, physicians should use their best clinical judgment to describe each therapy, including the potential risks and benefits, and the expected outcome or prognosis for recovery. This step is important because one study of the elderly has shown that individuals revise their decisions regarding CPR once the procedure is described to them with outcome data. Many of those who would have requested to receive CPR will forgo this treatment when presented with information about odds for full recovery. Notably, a DNR status does not signify that a patient's condition is hopeless or that therapies other than those specifically discussed will be withheld. Families need to be reassured that current therapies intended to improve the patient's health will be continued unless a further decision to withdraw or withhold therapy has been made (see below).

c.   Eventually, a **decision to withdraw or withhold** therapies may be made. Most critically ill patients are incompetent to make this decision and, thus, a surrogate is involved. As in deciding the DNR status, the patient's surrogate should approach this decision using substituted judgment, or determining what type of care the patient would have wanted for himself or herself. The surrogate should refer to written indications of the patient's preferences or to past conversations concerning end-of-life wishes. Surrogates should refrain from incorporating their own preferences or values into decision-making. If the patient's wishes regarding end-of-life care are unknown, the principle of relative **benefit versus burden** may be used. In this process, the potential helpful versus harmful effects of each therapy are weighed, resulting in a choice to accept or reject each therapy. Thus, a surrogate can choose, for example, to accept antibiotics for the patient in the hope of curing a pneumonia, but to reject a lung biopsy because of the pain associated with the procedure. Neither an ethical nor legal distinction exists between withdrawing and withholding therapies, but some families may see a psychological advantage to withholding rather than withdrawing life-sustaining measures.

(1)   If the ICU team determines that ongoing care is **futile** (i.e., useless), they may advise that therapies be withdrawn to reduce the suffering of the dying patient. Determining futility can be problematic, because technology can prolong the survival of patients with multiorgan failure and because few physicians are able to judge with unequivocal certainty that a patient will die in the ICU. All members of the ICU team should agree that further treatment of the patient is futile before meeting with the family. Again,

patience and compassion are paramount to the family's acceptance of this determination.

> **(2)** Once a decision has been made to withdraw or withhold life-sustaining measures, maintaining the patient's **comfort** becomes the primary goal of therapy. This may include discontinuing endotracheal suctioning, daily chest radiographs, and routine laboratory tests while adjusting the dosages of sedative or analgesic medications to a desirable level.

d. Therapeutic goals need to be reevaluated as the patient's condition changes. Communication with the family should be ongoing throughout a patient's ICU course. **Conflict** is best resolved via ongoing discussion with individuals involved. ICU physicians must recognize and respect cultural differences that influence end-of-life decisions. Unresolvable conflict between family members, healthcare team members, or between the family and the medical care team is best addressed by the institutional ethics committee (see below).

D. The **pediatric** patient deserves special consideration when ethical and end-of-life issues are confronted. Legally, end-of-life decisions are deferred to the parents. Ethically, however, the child can participate in these decisions depending on his or her developmental level and decision-making capacity. If the child is too immature to participate in decisions, parents are relied on to make decisions in the child's best interest by weighing the benefit versus burden of each therapy. Pediatric intensivists must be sensitive to individual family dynamics and parenting styles when approaching end-of-life discussions for the pediatric ICU patient.

E. The **institutional ethics committee** is generally composed of a group of healthcare professionals trained in medical ethics.

1. **The purpose** of the ethics committee is to educate and advise clinicians regarding ethical dilemmas and to enable resolution of ethical conflicts. The ethics committee offers an objective analysis of the patient's case and can draw on basic ethical principles to guide the patient, physician, and family to a consensus about the therapeutic course. Ideally, the ethics committee should be accessible to all members of the healthcare team and to the patient and family. This diminishes inequalities of power present in the hospital environment and promotes a climate of respect for all viewpoints.

2. When the ethics committee is requested to consult on a case, the question to be answered or the nature of the conflict should be clearly stated. The patient's condition and prognosis should be documented. An ethics committee consultation is never a substitute for communication with the family regarding end-of-life issues. Rather, the ethics committee serves to elucidate pertinent ethical issues and thereby aid conflict resolution. Members of the ethics committee can help organize or attend a family meeting in order to facilitate decision-making.

3. The ethics committee uses guiding ethical principles to make recommendations to the healthcare team, the patient, and the family. The role is one of expert consultant, not arbiter in a dispute. In rare situations where irreconcilable differences exist between the physician and the patient or family, care of the patient can be transferred to another accepting attending physician. It is even more extraordinary for ethical conflicts to reach resolution by judicial intervention.

III. **Guidelines for withdrawing care**
  A. **Goals** for withdrawal of care include:
    1. Promoting comfort and respecting the wishes of the patient.
    2. Promoting comfort of the family.
    3. Maintaining or achieving the patient's ability to communicate.
    4. Withdrawing burdensome therapies.
    5. Allowing death to occur.
  B. All physician orders should be reexamined with a goal toward **palliative** and **comfort care.** Therapies that increase patient comfort or relieve pain, anxiety, or agitation should be continued or added (Table 16-1). Therapies directed toward supporting physiologic homeostasis or treating the underlying disease process are no longer indicated and may be discontinued. These include many of the "routine" procedures and interventions associated with being an ICU patient

---

Table 16-1. Examples of comfort and palliative measures

Clearance of oral secretions
Continuation of general nursing care and cleanliness
Offering of food/water to alert patients
Antiseizure or antiepileptic regimens
Narcotics
Sedatives
Antipyretics
Nonsteroidal anti-inflammatory drugs
Prophylaxis for gastrointestinal bleeding
Antiemetics

(Table 16-2). The benefit: burden ratio of each intervention should be used to determine which interventions should be eliminated. The precise order of discontinuation is often determined by patient or family preference, or the patient's individual situation (e.g., the patient with an external ventricular assist device). Most commonly, a stepwise approach is followed with mechanical ventilation discontinued only after the withdrawal of vasopressors, antibiotics, or enteral feedings. No substitute exists for the continual presence of a concerned and caring medical staff, especially including the experienced physician, at the bedside. Clear plans for monitoring the patient's level of discomfort and intervening with additional medications should be made and shared with the family in attendance. The decision to withdraw life-sustaining treatment should be accompanied by an increase of vigilance and bedside attention, not withdrawal of the medical staff.

C. A large variability of **individual situations** should be anticipated. Each situation is unique, making "cookbook" solutions for the discontinuation of life-sustaining therapies problematic. Paramount during the process are the wishes of the patient or the patient's surrogate. Patient autonomy must be respected. Immediately secondary to this is assurance of patient comfort and the comfort of the patient's family. Cultural practices and beliefs of the patient and the family should be identified and respected. In each situation, the process of withdrawal should be clearly explained. Practical wishes of the patient and family concerning the desirability of extubation can usually be easily accommodated. The anticipated rapidity of the dying process or realities of the patient's medical condition, however, may dictate specific choices concerning therapies to be withdrawn, the rate of withdrawal, and the ability to accommodate the requests of families. Such situations should be clearly explained to the family. When a rapid death is anticipated, such as with the removal of extracorporeal circulatory support, it may not be possible to accommodate requests to extubate and communicate with the patient or hold prolonged vigils.

Table 16-2.   Examples of routine measures that may be withdrawn at the end of life

Frequent phlebotomy for laboratory tests
Frequent vital sign determinations
Placement of intravenous and central lines
Radiographic examinations
Aggressive chest physiotherapy and endotracheal suctioning
Wound debridement

D. Specific life-sustaining therapies that may be withdrawn include:

1. **Vasopressor** and **inotropic** medications. Continuous chemical circulatory support can be discontinued without weaning. The gradual withdrawal of circulatory support appears to offer no benefit for patient comfort.

2. **Extracorporeal support.** Such therapies are usually considered quite invasive by the patient and family. They require maintenance of vascular cannulas and the presence of additional equipment and personnel at the bedside. Intermittent extracorporeal support (e.g., intermittent hemodialysis) may simply not be restarted. Continuous renal support [e.g., continuous venovenous hemodialysis (CVVH), and so forth] can be discontinued. Death is usually not immediate following the discontinuation of dialysis. Studies have reported mean survival to be 8 to 9 days following the discontinuation of dialysis. Continuous circulatory support (e.g., ventricular assist, extracorporal membrane oxygenation, intraaortic balloon counter pulsation) can be discontinued and death anticipated soon after termination of support.

3. **Antibiotics** and other curative pharmacotherapy. Once the decision to terminate life-sustaining treatments is made, it is no longer consistent to consider therapies directed toward "curing" the patient. Such therapies include cancer chemotherapy, radiation therapy, steroids, and antibiotics. It is reasonable, however, to continue treatments such as topical antifungal agents used for oral hygiene or antibiotics aimed at treating painful lesions.

4. **Supplemental oxygen.** Because the avoidance of hypoxemia is no longer a therapeutic goal, supplemental oxygen can be discontinued and the patient returned to breathing room air. This is reasonable even if it is decided that mechanical ventilation will be continued. If the patient is removed from the ventilator but continues to have an artificial airway in place (e.g., endotracheal tube or tracheostomy), humidified air or oxygen can be administered to avoid the irritation of drying of the airway and tracheal secretions.

5. **Mechanical ventilation.** Several studies have suggested that mechanical ventilation is the most common therapy withdrawn when life-sustaining therapies are discontinued. Some physicians, however, prefer to withdraw therapies other than mechanical ventilation (such as vasopressors) with the expectation that the patient will die while still receiving mechanical ventilation. Similarly, during a prolonged illness, the patient's family may have become comfortable with the surroundings

of the ICU, the monitors, the artificial airway, and the mechanical ventilator. They may voice fears that the patient will suffer if mechanical ventilation or airway support is withdrawn. In such cases, it is reasonable to continue mechanical ventilation and airway support while discontinuing other life-sustaining therapies. Nevertheless, mechanical ventilation does not differ morally from other life-sustaining treatments such as dialysis, and can be discontinued if the patient or his or her proxy believes that it represents unwanted therapy.

a. **Mechanical ventilation can be gradually withdrawn** by decreasing the FIO_2 to room air, decreasing positive end-expiratory pressure, and then slowly decreasing ventilatory rate. The rate of decrease is quite variable among practitioners. A relatively slow weaning process can prolong the dying process and may provide the family with a misleading hope for survival.

b. **Mechanical ventilation can be discontinued** and humidified air administered via a T-piece or the patient can simply be removed from the ventilator and the trachea extubated. Extubation can more quickly result in death compared with gradually decreasing the intensity of mechanical ventilation. Importantly, extubation appears not to be objectively associated with greater discomfort or with the administration of greater doses of opioids. Each technique is applicable in certain situations. The ability of the patient to maintain a patent airway, the presence of secretions, the perceptions of the patient and family, and the confounding presence of anesthetic drugs and neuromuscular blocking agents all may dictate a particular method of discontinuing mechanical ventilation. Invasive monitoring and analysis of arterial blood gas tensions or oxygen saturation are unnecessary during withdrawal of mechanical ventilation.

c. The **timing of death** after the withdrawal of mechanical ventilation is uncertain and dependent on the cause and severity of respiratory failure. Usually death occurs within a few hours to 1 day. In some studies, however, a small proportion of patients with chronic lung disease did well and were discharged alive from the hospital after deciding to forego mechanical ventilation.

6. **Nutrition** (enteral or parenteral), fluid resuscitation, blood replacement, and IV hydration are all therapies that have the goal of returning the patient to health and can be discontinued. Naso-

gastric and orogastric tubes can be discontinued. Case reports and controlled studies suggest that little, if any, discomfort accompanies the withdrawal of enteral nutrition and IV hydration.

E. Indications for pharmacologic intervention

1. Presumption for **comfort measures.** Clinicians should not withhold comfort measures for fear of hastening death. Patients given large doses of opioids to treat discomfort during the withdrawal of life-sustaining treatments, on average, live as long as patients not given opioids, suggesting that it is the underlying disease process, not the use of palliative medications, that usually determines the time of death.

2. **Standard of care.** The administration of sedatives and analgesics during the withholding or withdrawal of life-sustaining treatments is consistent with the standard of care for critically ill patients. Most patients in the ICU do receive these medications during the withholding or withdrawal of support. Certainly, competent patients can refuse pharmacologic intervention to preserve lucidness. Drugs may not be indicated for patients who will gain no benefit (e.g., comatose patients). Sedatives and analgesics are not indicated in patients who have been declared brain dead.

F. Specific indications

1. **Pain.** The patient's report of pain or discomfort is certainly the best guide of treatment. Frequently, the patient is unable to communicate effectively. Other signs and symptoms of pain such as vocalizations, diaphoresis, agitation, tachypnea, and tachycardia may be valuable.

2. **Air hunger (dyspnea).** Especially with the withdrawal of supplemental oxygen and mechanical ventilatory support, discomfort should be expected and anticipatory doses of anxiolytics and opioids should be administered. Additional doses should be immediately available and opioids continued as a continuous infusion. Clinicians must be immediately and continuously available to assess the patient's level of comfort and provide additional medication as necessary.

3. **Death rattle.** Noisy, gargling breathing may occur in patients who are close to death, particularly in extubated patients. Although these sounds can be accompanied by dyspneic symptoms in the patient, they are usually more distressing to family members present. Treatment can include repositioning, gentle oropharyngeal suctioning, and anticholinergics to diminish oral and respiratory secretions.

4. **Anxiety.** Alert patients may display varying levels of anxiety at the prospect of termination of life-support. Whereas nonpharmacologic means

of allaying anxiety can be extremely effective, sometimes patients request to be deeply sedated or unconscious prior to the discontinuation of life-sustaining therapies such as mechanical ventilation. Although death can be hastened by deep sedation, such requests should be honored.

5. **Agitation or excessive motor activity.** Non-specific motor activity can occur in some patients. Such activity is often interpreted as discomfort or distress by those attending the patient. It is reasonable that the level of sedation be increased in such situations. Neuromuscular blockade is never indicated because it does not treat the presumed underlying distress of the patient.

6. **Avoidance of drug withdrawal.** Often, patients are already receiving high doses of opioids or sedatives during the course of their illness. The patient's individual dose ranges can be used as a guide to provide increased amounts of opioids and sedatives during the discontinuation of support. Certainly, little reason is seen to decrease therapeutic dosages of sedatives or opioids prior to the discontinuation of support for fear that the patient will not breathe adequately once the ventilator is discontinued.

IV. **Pharmacologic choices**

A. **Opioids** are the first line of treatment for pain, dyspnea, or tachypnea during the discontinuation of life-sustaining measures. It is imperative that the route, dosage, and schedule be individualized. Intravenous administration is by far the most common route used. Bolus administration is the fastest route for providing relief. Time to peak effect is determined by the lipid solubility of the drug. Onset time ranges from 1 to 5 minutes with fentanyl and 10 to 15 minutes with morphine. An initial bolus dose may be followed by a continuous infusion with additional bolus doses available as needed. Commonly used opioids and their doses are summarized in Table 16-3. Additional details are available in Chapters 5 and 6.

Table 16-3.   **Examples of initial opioid doses**

Generic name	Trade name	Bolus dose	Infusion
Dihydromorphone	Dilaudid	0.02 mg/kg	—
Fentanyl	Sublimaze	0.5–1.5 µg/kg	2–4 µg/kg/h
Methadone	Dolophine	0.1 mg/kg	—
Meperidine	Demerol	0.5–1.0 µg/kg	0.5 mg/kg/h
Morphine	—	0.05–0.1 mg/kg	0.1–0.5 mg/kg/h

Note: These represent typical initial doses for a patient without tolerance. Doses should be titrated to effect without regard to a maximal dose.

1. **Morphine** is most commonly used. In a recent prospective study of critically ill adults by Faber-Langendoen et al., the mean morphine dose was 13.9 mg/h following the discontinuation of mechanical ventilation. The morphine doses were similar in extubated and "terminally weaned" patients. In rare circumstances, drugs other than morphine should be considered, mostly because of troublesome side effects or tolerance to morphine administration.

2. **Dihydromorphone** is the second drug of choice. It is more potent than morphine and is often tolerated in patients who have side effects from morphine.

3. **Meperidine** continues to be widely used for acute treatment and is useful in some patients. Its use is complicated by its well-known toxicities, including accumulation of the epileptogenic metabolite normeperidine. This can be particularly problematic in those with renal dysfunction, and in patients taking monoamine oxidase inhibitors.

4. **Fentanyl** is often used in bolus doses for short-term analgesia or for continuous infusion in patients receiving mechanical ventilation. Accompanying side effects, such as chest wall rigidity and nausea, can limit its usefulness. As a continuous infusion, little advantage is seen to fentanyl over morphine or dihydromorphone.

5. Opioid dosages for **children** are not as well established as for adults. For babies and infants, continuous morphine infusions (10–25 μg/kg/h) can be administered after an initial bolus (0.1 to 0.2 mg/kg IV as a starting point). Doses can be increased as necessary. Sometimes very large doses may be necessary to assure the absence of discomfort.

6. **Alternative routes of administration.** When an IV route of administration is not available, oral, intramuscular, subcutaneous, transdermal, or rectal routes can be used. The oral route is convenient and achieves steady blood levels. For patients who have difficulty swallowing, many opioids are available as elixirs. Others can be easily crushed and put into concentrated emulsions. With the exception of sustained release formulations, most of the oral opioids reach peak effect within 30 to 60 minutes. Although commonly used, painful intramuscular injections are rarely indicated. Subcutaneous infusions of opioids can be substituted. Transdermal fentanyl has been used for chronic pain and is extremely convenient as steady blood levels are attained. A patch (25 μg/h) is equivalent to 10 mg of IV morphine every 8 hours. Given the lag to peak effect (24–72 hours), however, this method of drug delivery is not usually suitable in

the acute setting. Rectal administration, although not commonly used, permits rapid absorption of opioids and is an alternative to the oral or IV route in patients with no other access available.

B.   Benzodiazepines are the drugs of choice for the treatment of anxiety (see Chapter 5 for details.). **Diazepam** produces rapid and reliable sedation with relatively little cardiovascular or respiratory depression. An initial oral (PO) or IV dose of 5 to 10 mg usually suffices and can be repeated as necessary. Diazepam should not be given intramuscularly because injection is painful and absorption unpredictable. Alternatively, **lorazepam** (1–2 mg IV or PO in the adult; 0.015–0.03 mg/kg) or **midazolam** (1–3 mg IV in the adult; 0.015–0.045 mg/kg) may be used.

C.   Haloperidol may be indicated in the presence of delirium (acute confusional states) or agitation not controlled with benzodiazepines and opioids. In one survey of practitioners, haloperidol was used at least occasionally as an adjunct to the discontinuation of life-sustaining measures by 24% of physicians. Haloperidol does not affect the respiratory drive.

D.   Propofol (2, 6-diisopropylphenol) can be used for sedation or for the induction or maintenance of general anesthesia. Doses of 2.0 to 2.5 mg/kg IV rapidly produce unconsciousness (approximately 30–45 seconds), whereas lower doses produce conscious sedation. Propofol has no analgesic properties. Decreases of arterial blood pressure and cardiac output, as well as respiratory rate and tidal volume and the ventilatory response to hypercarbia, are dose-dependent. An infusion of 25 to 75 µg/kg/min is often sufficient to produce sedation, but much higher doses may be necessary in tolerant patients (100–150 µg/kg/min or greater, titrated to effect).

E.   Barbiturates, such as thiopental, thiamylal, and methohexital, are useful for induction of general anesthesia and are rarely indicated for sedation. The drugs rapidly produce unconsciousness. Repeated doses or infusions can produce prolonged sedation or unconsciousness. The drugs decrease arterial blood pressure, cardiac output, respiratory rate, and tidal volume in a dose-dependent manner. Barbiturates can reliably and painlessly cause death and have been used to execute prisoners and perform euthanasia and assisted suicide. Barbiturates are not analgesic. Subhypnotic doses produce hyperalgesia and are generally not useful. In general, barbiturates should be used only when the goal is to produce deep sedation or unconsciousness. Barbiturate infusions may be indicated to relieve anxiety and suffering when all other alternatives have failed (e.g., extreme tolerance to opioids), to produce unconsciousness before tracheal extubation (e.g., a patient who requests to be "asleep" when the ventilator is withdrawn), and to relieve nonphysical suffering (e.g., fear of pain during discontinuation of life-sustaining measures). They may be best viewed as an adjunct to the use of opioids and benzodiazepines. When titrated levels of sedation are required, a propofol infusion may be more easily controlled, more pleasant for the patient, and produce minimal unintended side effects. Usual doses for achieving unconsciousness in healthy individuals for thiopental and thiamylal are 3 to 5 mg/kg IV, for pentobarbital 2 to 3 mg/kg IV, and for methohexital 1 to 2 mg/kg IV. For continued effect, these drugs can be administered by IV infusion. Because tolerance rapidly develops, progressively increasing doses are often necessary.

F. **Anticholinergic medications** (e.g., atropine, ipratropium bromide, and glycopyrrolate) can be used to diminish copious oral and respiratory secretions that can produce death rattle. In general, atropine should be avoided because of its potential central nervous system side effects. Glycopyrrolate is a potent antisialogogue that can be administered IV or nebulized (5–10 μg/kg every 4 hours via either route).

G. **The chemically paralyzed patient.** Neuromuscular blocking agents are sometimes administered to deliberately eliminate the respiratory efforts of the patient so that nonphysiologic patterns of mechanical ventilation can be imposed. The clinical rationale for continuing neuromuscular blocking agents is lost once the decision to forgo life-sustaining treatments is made. Additional paralytic agents do not contribute to patient comfort. They have no analgesic or sedative properties, and relieve suffering only to the extent that they cause death. Paralyzed patients are unable to express discomfort by attempting to communicate, move, or become tachypneic. The precise doses of opioids and anxiolytics necessary to avoid discomfort are then difficult to determine. Although it may be preferable to permit reversal of neuromuscular blockade prior to the withdrawal of mechanical ventilation, sometimes prolonged drug effect that precludes adequate reversal or profound weakness is present. Many clinicians are uncomfortable with extubating a patient with no capability of maintaining spontaneous ventilation or a patent airway. In such cases, physicians may decide to forgo the withdrawal of mechanical ventilation or proceed only after administering high doses of sedatives and opioids to assure the absence of patient awareness. It is not clear, however, that the effects of all previously administered drugs must be eliminated prior to the discontinuation of life-sustaining treatments. The right of the patient's surrogate to refuse unwanted therapy may be a stronger mandate.

H. **Euthanasia.** Drugs should not be administered with the sole and express purpose of causing death. Such interventions include the administration of neuromuscular blocking agents to produce apnea or the administration of potassium chloride to produce asystole.

V.   Indications for altering dose

A.   Absence of a maximal dose. Typically, patients will already be receiving sedative, hypnotic, or analgesic medications. The amount of additional medication necessary can be judged based on past clinical responses. No predetermined or maximal dose for these drugs can be uniformly applied. Ceiling doses should be established only by the occurrence of troublesome side effects such as excessive sedation, hypotension, or respiratory depression. Many patients may have developed tolerance to these medications because of prior repeated or continual exposures. In case of tolerance to a specific drug class (e.g., narcotics), the addition of a different drug class targeted to achieving sedation is reasonable (e.g., beginning a propofol infusion for a patient already receiving large doses of narcotics).

B.   Anticipatory dosing. Prior to withdrawal, assess the patient's level of awareness and discomfort. Anticipatory dosing of opioids and sedatives may be necessary prior to a sudden discontinuation of life support. A review of the medication record is useful in determining the starting point for dosages of opioids and sedatives to be administered in anticipation of discomfort created by the withdrawal of support. The variation of adequate dose requirements for sedatives and opioids is extremely wide.

C.   Reactive dosing. Dosages of opioids and sedatives can be increased according to perceptual criteria (e.g., reports of pain and sedation by patient, providers, family, and other observers). Physiologic criteria can be used as additional surrogate endpoints. Such criteria include increases of respiratory rate and alteration of breathing pattern; changes of heart rate, blood pressure, and sympathetic responses (e.g., pupillary changes and diaphoresis).

VI.   Brain death

A.   "Brain death" is a term used to connote that death has been determined via evaluation of brain function and as such is distinct from cardiac death. Ethically and legally, however, no difference exists with respect to death. Practically, the diagnosis of brain death means that a patient can potentially become an organ donor on the conditions of consent (premorbidly by the patient or postmortem by the family) and medical acceptability.

B.   Locally accepted guidelines are used to establish the diagnosis of brain death (see Chapter 29 for details).

VII.   Organ donation. Often, critically ill patients are unable to become organ donors because of the nature of illness (e.g. sepsis) or failure of the vital organs. Some patients, however, usually those suffering from traumatic head injury or devastating intracranial event, may be eligible for tissue or organ donation.

A. **Approaching the family** regarding organ donation must be done tactfully and in consultation with trained professionals from the regional organ procurement agency. Ideally, the discussion should be coordinated by a physician with whom the family has developed a rapport. The topic can be introduced by asking the family if the deceased had ever expressed an opinion regarding use of his or her organs after death. Many families are consoled by the thought that their loved one's body parts may be life-saving to another individual and may in some sense carry on the life that has been lost.

B. **Early contact** with the organ procurement agency is important in cases of potential organ donors. Agency preferences regarding medications (e.g., vasopressors, diuretics), mechanical ventilator settings, and laboratory blood work after death should be known to the ICU team.

C. **Care of the patient** for organ donation is challenging. Problems frequently encountered include hypotension, dysrhythmias, hypoxemia, and diabetes insipidus. If a successful donation is to occur, the vigilant attendance of the ICU team, in concert with direction from the organ procurement agency, is necessary.

D. If the institutional transplant team will participate in harvesting or transplanting organs, it is prudent to establish contact with the team and immediately apprise them of any change in the donor's condition that might warrant expedited harvest.

VIII. **Supporting survivors**

A. **Support** of the patient's survivors during and following death begins with honest, frequent, and compassionate communication from physicians and nurses in the ICU. Families appreciate the guidance of experienced practitioners to prepare them for what to expect during the dying process, especially when life-sustaining therapies have been withdrawn. Reassurance should be given that measures will be taken to ensure the patient's comfort and that some sights (e.g., gasps) and sounds (e.g., gurgling) are normal during dying and may not be completely obliterated.

B. **The environment** where death occurs should accommodate the wishes of the patient and family as much as possible.

1. **Privacy** is important for a dignified death. This can be achieved by closing ICU cubicles and shielding the dying patient and family from the routine commotion of a busy ICU. Alternatively, the patient or family may request to be moved to a private room on a hospital ward or to an in-

hospital hospice unit to die. If the condition of the patient allows transfer before death will occur, these requests should be granted.

2. **Cultural background and individual values** will affect who is at the bedside of a dying patient. For some patients, one or two close family members may attend; for others, a vigil is maintained by a large extended family. The ICU staff should strive for flexibility when presented with each situation.

   a. The medical social worker may be an important source in understanding the family's religious and cultural background and communicating family wishes to the medical care team.

   b. Many patients and families find solace in the presence of clergy at death. If so, arrangements should be made for the patient's own religious representative or a hospital-based chaplain to attend the death.

IX. **Legal considerations.** Physicians who follow the process outlined above regarding honest, open communication with patients and their families about ethics and end-of-life care should rarely find themselves resolving such issues in a court of law. Nevertheless, several recent judicial rulings have implications that may prove useful to the clinician when confronted with ethical and end-of-life issues.

A. **Patient autonomy is primary in decision-making.** That patients may refuse life-sustaining or other therapies has been repeatedly affirmed. Wishes of the patient may be expressed via advance directives or, lacking this, via prior voiced opinion. The role of a surrogate in providing substituted judgment has been supported.

B. **Human life has qualification beyond mere biologic existence.** Thus, a surrogate's decision to withdraw care may be based on the potential for meaningful existence (**"quality of life"**).

C. **Care once rendered can be withdrawn.** The idea that a life-sustaining therapy that has been implemented can never be stopped is not valid.

D. **End-of-life decisions are best addressed by the physician, the patient, and family** with help from institutional facilitators (e.g., ethics committee) as needed. Permission to withdraw therapies does not require a "court order."

E. **Withdrawal of hydration or nutritional support is not legally different from withdrawal of other life support.** In addition to legal decisions, this stance has been supported by numerous medical societies, including the American Medical Association and the American Academy of Neurology.

F. **Physicians are not bound to provide care that they deem futile.** Although still somewhat controversial, the latter was supported by a jury decision involving a patient at the Massachusetts General Hospital from whom ventilatory support was withdrawn despite the objection of one family member. It is advisable for a physician, however, to pursue every avenue of conflict resolution, including removing oneself from the care of a patient, before exercising this dictum against a family's wishes.

G.   **For unusual or questionable cases,** it is appropriate to seek the advice of the institutional legal counsel before acting on decisions.

SELECTED REFERENCES

Asch DA, Hansen-Flachen J, Lanken PH. Decisions to limit or continue life-sustaining treatment by critical care physicians in the United States: conflicts between physicians' practices and patients' wishes. *Am J Respir Crit Care Med* 1995;151:288–292.

Brody H, Campbell ML, Faber-Langendoen KF, et al. Withdrawing intensive life-sustaining treatment—recommendations for compassionate clinical management. *N Engl J Med* 1997;336:652–656.

Faber-Langendoen K. The clinical management of dying patients receiving mechanical ventilation: a survey of physician practice. *Chest* 1994;106:880–888.

Hurford W. Practical guidelines for the withdrawal of life-sustaining therapies. In: Braunwald E, Fauci AS, Isselbacher KJ, Kasper DL, Hauser SL, Longo DL, Jameson JL, eds. *Harrison's online,* 14th ed. http://www.harrisononline.com.

Luce JM. Physicians do not have a responsibility to provide futile or unreasonable care if a patient or family insists. *Crit Care Med* 1995;23:760–766.

Luce JM. Withholding and withdrawal of life support: ethical, legal, and clinical aspects. *New Horizons* 1997;5:30–37.

Meisel A. Legal myths about terminating life support. *Arch Intern Med* 1991;151:1497–1502.

Murphy DJ, Burrows D, Santilli S, et al. The influence of the probability of survival on patients' preferences regarding cardiopulmonary resuscitation. *N Engl J Med* 1994;330:545–549.

Prendergast TJ. Resolving conflicts surrounding end-of-life care. *New Horizons* 1997;5:62–71.

Schneiderman LJ, Jecker NS, Jonsen AR. Medical futility: its meaning and ethical implications. *Ann Intern Med* 1990;112:949–954.

Todres ID, Armstrong A, Lally P, et al. Negotiating end-of-life issues. *New Horizons* 1998;6:374–382.

Wilson WC, Smedira NG, Fink C, et al. Ordering and administration of sedatives and analgesics during the withholding and withdrawal of life support from critically ill patients. *JAMA* 1992;267:949–953.

Medical Considerations

Coronary Artery Disease

John L. Chow

I. **Introduction.** Despite our understanding of the pathophysiology of coronary artery disease (CAD) and the recent advancements in reperfusion therapy for treatment of acute myocardial infarction (AMI), CAD remains the leading cause of morbidity and mortality among adults in the United States. Although approximately one third of patients with AMI die, most deaths are caused by fatal dysrhythmia early in the prehospital course. Identifying patients at risk and preventing heart disease through risk modification and medical therapy should be the primary medical objectives. The major **risk factors** of CAD include hypertension, diabetes mellitus, smoking, dyslipidemia, obesity, elevated homocysteine levels, and a family history of CAD.

   A. **Definitions.** Although chest discomfort is the most common complaint of patients with ischemia, electrocardiographic (ECG) changes without accompanying typical anginal symptoms ("silent" ischemia) are common, especially in diabetic and elderly patients.

      1. **Angina pectoris** is chest discomfort (tightness, pressure, pain) that is generally retrosternal; it occurs at rest or is precipitated by physical or emotional stress; and it lasts approximately 10 minutes or less. Associated symptoms include nausea, vomiting, diaphoresis, and shortness of breath. Pain or paresthesia may be referred to the jaw, throat, arms, or back. Angina is a manifestation of myocardial ischemia without myocardial necrosis.

      2. **Stable angina** is a predictable form of angina pectoris that has not changed in frequency, duration, precipitating factors, or ease of relief within recent months. It is commonly caused by a fixed coronary artery atherosclerosis.

      3. **Unstable (crescendo) angina** refers to angina of recent onset (within 2 months) occurring with increasing frequency, intensity, progressively less effort, or at rest. Prognosis is poor because approximately 10% of these patients have left main CAD and up to 20% of patients will progress to AMI within 3 months. Plaque rupture, platelet aggregation, coronary arterial thrombosis, and vasospasm are the underlying causes.

      4. **Prinzmetal's (variant) angina** is characterized by resting angina that generally is worse in the morning; it lasts for several minutes and is accompanied by transient ST-segment elevation, ventricular dysrhythmias, or both. This form of angina can also be induced by exercise. It is caused by coronary vasospasm usually occurring within an atherosclerotic artery.

B. **Pathophysiology**
1. **Myocardial oxygen supply-demand balance.** At rest, the myocardium extracts oxygen maximally such that during exertion or hemodynamic stress, oxygen delivery must be increased to meet the demand. Myocardial ischemia and infarction occur when oxygen demand exceeds delivery.
   a. **Myocardial oxygen supply** is determined by:
      (1) **Coronary blood flow,** which occurs mainly during diastole and is a function of the pressure gradient from aortic root to downstream coronary pressure. In normal coronary arteries, exercise or stress can increase coronary blood flow four- to fivefold. Stenoses in these arteries can reduce oxygen supply.
      (2) **Oxygen content,** which is determined by hemoglobin concentration, oxygen saturation (SaO_2), and dissolved oxygen concentration. Oxygen content can be augmented mainly by increasing hemoglobin and SaO_2, because the contribution from dissolved oxygen is small.
   b. **Myocardial oxygen demand** is determined by:
      (1) **Ventricular wall tension,** which is the product of transmural pressure and ventricular radius divided by two times ventricular wall thickness. Changes in any of these parameters can affect oxygen demand.
      (2) **Heart rate,** which can promote an increased oxygen consumption through associated increases in myocardial contractility. Tachycardia also decreases the duration of maximal coronary perfusion in the atherosclerotic vessels, thus limiting oxygen supply.
      (3) **Contractility,** which is directly proportional to oxygen demand.
2. **Causes of myocardial oxygen supply-demand imbalance.** The most common (90%) cause of myocardial ischemia and infarction is coronary atherosclerotic narrowing. Other causes include vasospasm, vasculitis, trauma, thromboembolism of the coronary artery, valvular heart disease (i.e., aortic stenosis), hypertrophic or dilated cardiomyopathies, and thyrotoxicosis.

II. **Myocardial ischemia.** The principal objectives of diagnosing myocardial ischemia are to identify the cause, assess the severity of CAD, guide therapeutic options, and minimize any future ischemic insult or MI.
A. **Diagnosis**
1. **History.** Risk factors of CAD should be noted. Determine the character, location, duration, radia-

tion, exacerbating (physical or emotional stress, eating, or cold weather) and alleviating (rest or medications) factors; accompanying symptoms; and change in pattern over the past few weeks. The type of angina should be identified, based on the history. Chest discomfort exceeding 20 to 30 minutes is highly suspicious of AMI.

2. **Physical examination.** Although the physical examination can be normal or nonspecific, physical distress, anxiety, tachycardia, hypertension, an S_4 gallop, pulmonary rales, xanthomas, or evidence of peripheral atherosclerosis may be evident.

3. **Noninvasive studies**

   a. **Resting electrocardiogram (ECG)** is normal in approximately one half of patients with ischemia. Transient ST-segment depression (≥ 1 mm) or T-wave inversion occurring during angina strengthens the diagnosis. Ischemia secondary to coronary vasospasm can result in ST-segment elevation. Isolated J-point elevation can occur as a normal variant in young, healthy adults. Significant Q waves suggest prior MI. Bundle branch block (BBB) or artificial pacer rhythms on ECG increases the difficulty of detecting ST-segment or T-wave abnormalities. In general, reversibility of ECG changes after therapeutic interventions is highly suggestive of ischemia. Table 17-1 outlines the ECG changes associated with specific regions of ischemic myocardium.

   b. **Exercise ECG.** Exercise ECG's sensitivity to detect obstructive CAD is dependent on the severity of stenosis and the extent of disease. The sensitivity is 86% and specificity is 53% for three-vessel or left main CAD. Patients with a positive stress test should be considered for cardiac catheterization to explore the potential

Table 17-1. Location of ischemia or infarct by electrocardiographic criteria

Region	Leads	Vessel
Anterior	V_1–V_4	Left anterior descending
Anteroseptal	V_1–V_2	Left anterior descending
Anterolateral	I, aVL, V_1–V_6	Left anterior descending
Lateral	I, aVL, V_5–V_6	Circumflex
Inferior	II, III, aVF	Right coronary artery
Posterior	Large R wave in V_1, V_2, or V_3 with ST depression	Right coronary artery
Right ventricular	V_3R, V_4R	Right coronary artery

of revascularization. Contraindications to exercise stress testing include recent AMI (a submaximal or symptom-limited study still can be performed), resting angina, severe aortic stenosis, uncompensated CHF, advanced atrioventricular (AV) block, hypertension [blood pressure (BP) > 170/100], or rapid ventricular or atrial dysrhythmias.

   c. **Myocardial injury enzymes.** Patients with unstable angina or those in whom evolving MI is suggested should have myocardial injury enzyme levels followed as part of their diagnostic evaluation. **Creatine phosphokinase (CPK), troponin,** and **lactate dehydrogenase (LDH)** are released during myocardial injury and necrosis. Subfractions specific to cardiac muscle are the CPK-MB band, troponin I and T, and LDH_1 isoenzyme. Changes in the serum concentration of these enzymes over time are important for the diagnosis of MI.

     (1) **CPK.** An elevation of CPK levels by itself is not diagnostic. Increases in the concentration of CPK-MB or CPK-MB/CPK index provide greater sensitivity and specificity. The time course of CPK-MB increase is between 4 and 6 hours with a two- to tenfold peak in 18 to 24 hours and a return to normal within 2 to 3 days from the initial onset of symptoms, if no further myocardial injury occurs. Other major causes of increased CPK-MB include muscle trauma, rhabdomyolysis, myopathies, or polymyositis. Generally, CPK with MB isoenzyme should be determined at intervals of 8 to 12 hours for at least 24 hours or until the diagnosis is established.

     (2) **Troponin** is more sensitive and specific than CPK-MB to indicate myocardial cell damage. Up to 30% to 40% of patients with unstable angina have elevated troponin levels, although CPK-MB levels are often normal. These patients generally have a less favorable prognosis. The time course of troponin I and troponin T increase is between 3 and 12 hours, peaks in 1 to 2 days, and returns to normal within 4 to 14 days. Troponin levels are of special value to rule out MI in the immediate postoperative period (when CPK-MB may be elevated because of skeletal muscle injury), in patients with normal CPK-MB but in whom a high clinical suspicion of having an AMI exists, or in patients with symptoms occurring days prior to presentation. Clinically, troponin levels should be measured at baseline and repeated 12 to 24 hours later.

(3) **LDH.** In general, LDH_1 is a nonspecific isoenzyme that can be elevated because of acute renal infarction, AMI, hemolysis, hemolytic anemia, or megaloblastic anemia. The specific isoenzyme $LDH_1 : LDH_2$ ratio in excess of 1 is suggestive of MI. In uncomplicated MI, the $LDH_1 : LDH_2$ ratio increases at 8 to 12 hours, peaks at 24 to 72 hours, and remains elevated for 7 to 12 days. Because of its low specificity, the test is not commonly used to diagnose MI.

d. **Radionuclide perfusion imaging** provides a safe and effective method of assessing myocardial perfusion and function.

(1) **Exercise myocardial perfusion imaging.** Thallium-201 (^{201}Tl) is a radioactive tracer that is injected intravenously (IV) during peak treadmill exercise and avidly extracted as a potassium analog by viable myocardium in proportion to regional myocardial blood flow. Regions of perfusion defect correlate with the severity of coronary artery stenosis supplying the regions. On delayed imaging, a fixed defect devoid of tracer represents an area of prior infarct, whereas a region with thallium redistribution is considered to be myocardium at risk of ischemia. The test has a sensitivity of 85% and specificity of 90%.

(2) **Exercise radionuclide ventriculography.** Technetium-99m (^{99m}Tc) sestamibi is injected intravenously and accumulated in myocardium in proportion to blood flow. Using a first pass technique, multiple ventricular images synchronized to the cardiac cycle are acquired at rest and during exercise. The occurrence of regional wall motion abnormalities and the inability to increase left ventricular (LV) ejection fraction (EF) during exercise are suggestive of myocardial ischemia.

(3) **Pharmacologic stress perfusion imaging.** Intravenous coronary vasodilators (e.g., dipyridamole or adenosine) can produce relative hypoperfusion in myocardium served by stenotic coronary arteries. These heterogeneities can be imaged with either ^{201}Tl or ^{99m}Tc sestamibi. The tests are useful in patients who are unable to exercise adequately.

e. **Echocardiography** with Doppler capability can evaluate ventricular function, ventricular size, pericardial effusions, anatomic abnormalities [e.g., ventricular septal defect (VSD), ventricular free wall rupture], valvular defects (e.g., mitral regurgitation), and ventricular thrombus and aneurysm. The finding of regional wall motion abnormalities is more than 90% sensitive and specific for detecting ischemia. Transesophageal echocardiography (TEE) provides better visualization of valvular function, the left atrial appendage, ascending aorta, mural or atrial thrombi, and aortic aneurysms than does transthoracic echocardiography. Exercise and pharmacologic (e.g., dobutamine) stress echocardiography has similar sensitivity and specificity as a radionuclide imaging study for the detection of CAD.

   4. **Invasive study. Coronary angiography** remains the standard to detect the presence and to quantify the extent of CAD. Hemodynamic parameters, anatomy of the heart and coronary vessels, and wall motion abnormalities can be obtained. A coronary obstruction is considered clinically significant when more than 70% of the coronary artery luminal diameter is narrowed.

B. **Differential diagnosis of CAD** includes MI, aortic dissection, pulmonary embolism, pneumothorax, costochondritis, pericarditis, anxiety disorder, peptic ulcer disease, gastroesophageal reflux disease, and acute cholecystitis.

C. **Management**

   1. **General approach.** The initial goals are to reduce myocardial oxygen consumption, improve oxygen supply, relieve pain, stabilize hemodynamics, and prevent coronary thrombosis. Supplemental oxygen should be provided. Routine vital signs should be monitored. Potential precipitating conditions (e.g., tachycardia, dysrhythmias, hypertension, anemia, thyrotoxicosis) should be identified and rectified. Patients with unstable angina should be placed on bedrest and possibly anxiolytic medication; intense antianginal pharmacologic therapy should be initiated; serial ECGs and cardiac enzyme determinations performed; and referral made for coronary catheterization.

   2. **Medications.** See Chapter 10 for details of pharmacology and adverse effects of most of these agents.

      a. **β-adrenergic antagonists** decrease exertional angina symptoms and total mortality. They reduce myocardial oxygen demand and relieve angina by lowering heart rate, blood pressure, and contractility. Generally, β_1 selective agents without intrinsic sympathomimetic activity (ISA) (e.g., metoprolol, atenolol, esmolol) are more effective in slowing resting heart rate and are better tolerated in patients with reactive airway diseases (asthma, chronic obstructive pulmonary disease). Low doses (e.g., atenolol, 25–50 mg, orally once daily; metoprolol, 50–100 mg, orally twice daily) initially are administered and titrated upward until a resting heart rate of 50 to 60 bpm and an exercise heart rate less than 100 bpm is achieved or adverse effects are observed.

b. **Nitrates** provide relief of angina primarily by decreasing venous return and ventricular wall tension. Other effects include coronary vasodilation, relief of coronary vasospasm, redistribution of coronary blood flow, and antiplatelet activity. The net effect is a reduction in myocardial oxygen demand and anginal symptoms. For acute anginal attacks, a rapidly acting sublingual preparation is preferred. The usual sublingual dose is 0.3 to 0.4 mg every 5 minutes, repeated up to three times if systolic blood pressure is more than 90 mm Hg or heart rate is more than 50 or less than 100 bpm. **Long-acting nitrate formulations,** either as monotherapy or in combination with beta-blockers, are effective in chronic management of exertional angina symptoms. The titratability of **IV nitroglycerin** is useful in the acute management of ischemia or unstable angina in combination with administration of beta-blockers, heparin, and aspirin. The usual starting dose is 10 to 20 μg/min and titrated upward by dosage increments of 10 to 20 μg/min at intervals of 5 to 15 minutes, until symptoms resolve or adverse effects occur.

c. **Calcium channel antagonists** alleviate angina and improve the myocardial oxygen supply-demand ratio by inhibiting coronary vasospasm, dilating coronary arteries, reducing heart rate, and reducing peripheral vascular resistance. This class of agent is most effective in vasospastic angina, but is also useful in stable and unstable angina, especially when beta-blockers or nitrate therapy is not well tolerated. Therapy begins with modest doses and is advanced gradually over intervals of 2 to 3 days until symptoms improve or limiting side effects occur.

d. **Antiplatelet and antithrombin therapy. Aspirin** prevents acute coronary syndromes (i.e., AMI, unstable angina, sudden cardiac death) and improves mortality primarily by its antiplatelet action. The usual dose is 160 to 325 mg daily. Patients with unstable angina should receive aspirin in similar doses (chewed to speed absorption) and IV heparin for 48 hours or until the time of coronary catheterization. The loading dose of heparin is 75 U/kg followed by an infusion of 15 to 18 U/kg/h, titrated to keep activated partial thromboplastin time (aPTT) 1.5 to 2 times normal (50–75 seconds). The aPTT must be monitored every 4 to 6 hours after initiation of therapy or each dose adjustment to avoid bleeding complications and assure adequate anticoagulation. Complications of heparin therapy are discussed in Chapter 12.

   e. **Opioids.** Pain not adequately responding to antianginal medications should be controlled by opioids such as morphine sulfate (2.5–5 mg IV every 5–10 minutes) titrated to effect. Adverse effects of morphine in the patient with CAD include hypotension, which can be treated with supine positioning and fluid repletion; vagally mediated bradycardia, which can be treated with atropine (0.5–1 mg IV) if severe or when associated with hypotension, nausea, and vomiting, which may be difficult to distinguish from the symptoms of evolving MI; and respiratory depression, which may require treatment with naloxone.

3. **Invasive approaches.** Revascularization procedures are palliative, not curative. They are indicated to manage patients who have incapacitating angina refractory to medical therapy and to improve survival in selected populations.

   a. **Percutaneous transluminal coronary angioplasty (PTCA).** Patients with normal ventricular function and one- or two-vessel CAD refractory to medical therapy may benefit from PTCA. Patients who are not candidates for PTCA include those with minimal coronary stenosis (< 60% narrowing), left main CAD, and severe diffuse multiple vessel disease. Procedure-related complications include death (1%), MI (4% to 5%), and necessity for emergency bypass surgery (4% to 5%). Restenosis occurs in 25% to 30% of patients, usually within the first 6 months following the procedure. **Intracoronary stenting** in conjunction with **antiplatelet agents** (abciximab or ticlopidine) have substantially reduced the restenosis rate.

   b. **Coronary artery bypass grafting (CABG)** improves survival compared with medical management in patients with more than 50% stenosis of the left main coronary artery, three-vessel disease, depressed ventricular function (left ventricular EF < 40%), residual angina following MI, and those with multivessel disease and proximal left anterior descending (LAD) artery involvement. Anginal symptoms improve in approximately 95% of patients after CABG and up to 75% patients will remain symptom free for 5 years following CABG. The use of the internal mammary artery provides a 90% patency rate over 10 years. Perioperative mortality is about 1% to 3%, and perioperative MI is approximately 5% to 10%. Mortality risk decreases in centers with higher operative volume.

  c. **Intraaortic balloon pump (IABP) counterpulsation** temporarily assists a failing or ischemic myocardium until definitive therapy becomes effective or left ventricular function improves. **Intraaortic balloon counterpulsation** is discussed in Chapter 13.

  d. **Nonstandard therapies,** such as transmyocardial laser revascularization or long-term intermittent urokinase therapy, may be of benefit to selected patients with refractory angina pectoris.

III. **Myocardial infarction.** Causes of acute MI are listed in section **I.B.2.** A common feature of acute coronary syndrome is the instability of atherosclerotic plaques with intramural hemorrhage, fissuring, or plaque rupture that results in acute coronary obstruction. **Q-wave (transmural) infarction** results from persistent occlusive thrombi, whereas **non–Q-wave (subendocardial) infarcts** generally are secondary to incomplete or spontaneously recanalized thrombotic occlusions sufficient to cause myocardial necrosis. Non–Q-wave infarcts generally have less extensive infarction; however, they carry a greater risk of recurrent MI. Patients with concomitant cardiogenic shock have a poor prognosis, with mortality rates as high as 80%.

  A. **Diagnosis.** Two or more of the following features are required for the diagnosis of MI: (a) clinical history and physical examination suggestive of MI, (b) ECG evidence of myocardial injury, and (c) cardiac injury enzyme markers consistent with necrosis. The primary objective is the **rapid identification of patients who are candidates for thrombolysis** because survival benefit is lost after 12 hours from the initial onset of angina. The ideal time from arrival at the emergency room to time of thrombolysis should be less than 30 minutes. Patients with ECG ST-segment elevations (≥ 1 mm) in at least two contiguous leads or new left BBB with symptoms for less than 12 hours should be referred for thrombolysis or PTCA therapy at once.

  1. The **history** of patients with AMI is similar to those with ischemia.

  2. **Physical examination** findings resemble those found in patients with angina. In addition, signs of complications from MI may be found, including new murmur (VSD, mitral regurgitation), S_3 or S_4 gallop (noncompliant ventricle), pulmonary rales (left ventricular failure), jugular venous distention without pulmonary rales (right ventricular failure), pericardial rub (pericarditis), or dysrhythmias.

3. Noninvasive studies

a. Electrocardiogram.
Serial ECGs should be acquired on admission (within 10 minutes) and followed daily to assess response to therapy and detect any evidence of reinfarction or dysrhythmias. ST-segment elevations ≥ 1 mm imply injury to the epicardium. Symmetrically peaked T-waves or inverted T-waves are suggestive of ischemia or infarction. New BBB, dysrhythmias, or AV blocks may be seen. Evolution of pathologic Q-waves is indicative of myocardial necrosis. In patients with inferior wall MI, a right-sided ECG may be necessary to rule out right ventricular infarction. A new ST-segment elevation has a sensitivity of 46% and a specificity of 91% for diagnosing AMI. Previous infarction decreases the sensitivity of ECG to detect MI, whereas electrolyte derangements and pericarditis decrease the specificity.

b. Myocardial injury enzymes
(see section **II.A.3.c**)

c. Chest radiography
may help to detect some complications resulting from MI. Pulmonary vascular redistribution, pulmonary edema, and pleural effusions are indicative of CHF. An enlarged cardiac silhouette implies a dilated heart or pericardial effusions.

d. Radionuclide perfusion imaging
(section **II.A.3.d**). These tests are useful adjuncts in patients in whom clinical history, ECG, and enzyme pattern are nondiagnostic for MI. In general, ^{201}Tl scintigrams lack specificity for AMI because reduced uptake may result from ischemia, or previous or present MI. Exercise perfusion studies should not be used to evaluate patients with AMI.

e. Echocardiography
is helpful in patients with an equivocal diagnosis using the standard criteria. It identifies regional wall motion abnormalities as well as features caused by complications of MI (e.g., mitral regurgitation, VSD, ventricular free wall rupture, papillary muscle dysfunction). A limitation of echocardiography is its inability to differentiate between old or new infarctions. Compensatory hyperdynamic regions may be seen adjacent to the infarct zone (see section **II.A.3.e.**)

4. Invasive studies (see section **II.A.4**)

B. Management of acute myocardial infarction

1. General approach.
In addition to the goals described above for myocardial ischemia, minimizing infarct size, preventing recurrent ischemia and MI, and the early recognition and management of life-threatening complications are critical.

2. **Supportive measures.** Supplemental oxygen, IV access, routine vital signs, and continuous ECG monitoring should be established. Unless CHF or hypoxemia ($SpO_2 < 90\%$) occurs, supplemental oxygen generally is required only in the initial 2 to 3 hours after an uncomplicated MI. Patients with severe CHF or cardiogenic shock may require endotracheal intubation and mechanical ventilation. A pulmonary artery catheter should be used in the management of patients with complicated MI, severe or progressive CHF, cardiogenic shock, and significant hypotension. Laboratory studies include electrolytes with magnesium, lipid profile, complete blood count to assess anemia, and pulse oximetry to evaluate oxygenation, especially in patients with CHF or those in cardiogenic shock.

3. **Medications.** See Chapter 10 for details of pharmacology and adverse effects of most of these agents.

   a. **Aspirin** alone or in combination with certain thrombolytic therapies (e.g., streptokinase) improves survival. A dose of 160 to 325 mg should be given immediately and continued daily indefinitely. Chewable tablets provide quicker absorption, whereas the suppository form can be used in patients with nausea and vomiting. **Ticlopidine** can be used in patients who are intolerant to aspirin. Reversible neutropenia is the most serious adverse effect when ticlopidine is used for more than 2 weeks.

   b. **β-adrenergic antagonists** (see section **II.C.2.a**). Beta-blockers reduce infarct size, MI associated complications, and overall mortality during the initial and subsequent infarct course. Patients without contraindications, especially in those with persistent or recurrent angina or tachydysrhythmias, should be placed on beta-blockers within the first 12 hours of symptoms. Initially, **metoprolol** (5 mg IV every 5 minutes to a total of 15 mg) can be given, if tolerated; then, metoprolol (50 mg orally every 6–12 hours) can be administered for 2 days and then increased to 100 mg orally twice daily. Alternatively, **atenolol** can be administered on a similarly graded-dose schedule. Relative contraindications include heart rate (HR) less than 60 bpm, systolic blood pressure (BP) less than 100 mm Hg, severe LV failure, second- or third-AV block, and significant reactive airway diseases.

   c. **Nitrates** (see section **II.C.2.b**). Clinical evidence does not support the routine long-term use of nitrate therapy in uncomplicated MI. Those patients with AMI and CHF, large anterior infarction, persistent ischemia, or hypertension, however, may benefit from IV nitroglycerin for the first 24 to 48 hours. Those with continuing pulmonary edema or recurrent ischemia may benefit from more prolonged use of nitroglycerin.

d. **Heparin** (see section **II.C.2.d**). Prior to the widespread use of thrombolytic therapy, heparin was shown to reduce mortality and reinfarction in patients with AMI. Currently, the only additional survival benefit from heparin is when it is used in combination with **alteplase** (tissue plasminogen activator). Intravenous heparin should be titrated to keep the aPTT 1.5 to 2 times the normal range for 48 hours for patients receiving alteplase. Patients at high risk for developing thromboembolism (e.g., large or anterior MI, atrial fibrillation, previous embolus, or presence of LV thrombus) will require IV heparin for prophylaxis against thrombotic complications (Chapter 22). In patients with uncomplicated MI, subcutaneous heparin (7,500 U twice daily for 24 to 48 hours or until ambulatory) is recommended. Heparin also is indicated in patients undergoing PTCA or CABG.

e. **Angiotensin converting enzyme (ACE) inhibitor** administration can improve mortality after AMI, with the greatest benefit occurring among those with anterior infarction or a history of MI, CHF, or tachycardia. Given no contraindications, ACE inhibitors should be administered within the first 24 hours to patients with a suspected or documented MI, and those with CHF without hypotension (systolic BP > 100 mm Hg). One graded-dose schedule recommended is to administer **captopril** 6.25 mg orally followed by 12.5 mg 2 hours later, then 25 mg 10–12 hours later, and then 50 mg twice daily. Alternative agents (e.g., lisinopril, enalapril, quinapril, ramipril) can be used. In patients with uncomplicated MI and preserved LV function, ACE inhibitor can be discontinued after 4 to 6 weeks.

f. **Calcium-channel antagonists** have not been shown to improve survival after MI or prevent secondary ischemia or infarction. When beta-blockers are contraindicated or ineffective, verapamil or diltiazem can be used to treat atrial fibrillation with rapid ventricular response or persistent ischemia. **Immediate-release nifedipine** can be potentially harmful to patients with MI and hypotension.

g. **Opioids** (see section **II.C.2.e**).

h. **Magnesium** might reduce mortality in high-risk patients, if given early (< 6 hours) after the initial symptoms, but the results of clinical studies are conflicting. Magnesium produces coronary vasodilation, antiplatelet activity, and suppression of automaticity, and it may provide protection against reperfusion injury. Supplemental magnesium is currently recommended to correct hypomagnesemia and to treat torsade de pointes. Hypomagnesemia should be corrected with magnesium sulfate 2 g IV over 30 to 60 minutes, whereas torsade de pointes should be treated with 1 to 2 g IV over 5 minutes.

4. **Reperfusion therapy,** either pharmacologic or mechanical, reduces infarct size and mortality, and improves LV function. Restoration of perfusion is possible even after a prolonged period. Temporary myocardial impairment ("stunned myocardium") may exist after the injury is reversed.

   a. **Thrombolysis** produces greatest benefit when it is initiated within 6 hours of the onset of symptoms, although definite benefits still exist if administered within 12 hours. Response to therapy can manifest as improvement in ST-segment elevation and resolution of chest discomfort. Persistent symptoms and ST-segment elevation at 60 to 90 minutes after thrombolysis should be considered indications for urgent coronary angiography and possible PTCA. Thrombolytic treatment offers no clinical benefit to patients without ST-segment elevation or new BBB, or to those with MI complicated by heart failure or cardiogenic shock. Table 17-2 compares the commonly used thrombolytic agents. **Absolute contraindications** are suspected aortic dissection, active internal bleeding,

Table 17-2. **Comparison of thrombolytic drugs**

	tPA	Streptokinase	APSAC
Half-life	6 min	20 min	100 min
Dosage	100 mg[a]	1.5 million units	30 units
Administration	90 min	30–60 min	5 min
Fibrin-selective	Yes	No	Partial
Artery patency rate[b]	79%	40%	63%
ICH	0.6%	0.3%	0.6%
Lives saved/1000 treated	35	25	25
Antigenic	No	Yes	Yes
Hypotension	No	Yes	Yes
Heparin required	Yes	No	No
Cost per dose	$2750	$537	$2368

tPA, tissue plasminogen activator; APSAC, anisoylated plasminogen streptokinase activator complex; ICH, intracranial hemorrhage.
[a] 15-mg bolus, then 0.75 mg/kg over 30 minutes (maximum 50 mg), then 0.5 mg/kg over 60 minutes (maximum 35 mg) to provide total of 100 mg over 90 minutes.
[b] Artery patency rate at 90 minutes after treatment.

known intracranial neoplasm, and any prior hemorrhagic stroke or cerebrovascular accident within 1 year. **Relative contraindications** include known bleeding diathesis or concurrent use of anticoagulants, recent trauma (within 2–4 weeks), prolonged cardiopulmonary resuscitation (> 10 minutes), recent major surgery (< 3 weeks), recent internal bleeding (within 2–4 weeks), severe hypertension (BP > 180/110 mm Hg), other intracranial pathology, noncompressible vascular puncture sites, pregnancy, active peptic ulcer disease, or prior exposure (within 5 days to 2 years) to streptokinase or anisoylated plasminogen streptokinase activator complex (APSAC) treatment. **Patients requiring retreatment** who failed either streptokinase or APSAC should be managed with tissue plasminogen activator. Those who have contraindications to thrombolytic treatment should be considered for PTCA.

(1) **Tissue plasminogen activator (tPA)** is a natural protein produced by recombinant DNA technology. By increasing plasmin binding to fibrin, it provides relative clot-selective fibrinolysis without inducing a systemic lytic state. When coadministered with heparin, it has an early reperfusion rate that is slightly better than other agents. Compared with streptokinase and APSAC, it is less likely to cause hemorrhage requiring transfusion, and has the greatest survival benefit (10 additional lives of 1,000 patients treated). It also has a modest increase in the incidence of hemorrhagic stroke; however, it is more expensive than streptokinase and APSAC.

(2) **Streptokinase** is a bacterial protein that induces activation of free plasminogen and clot-associated plasminogen, eliciting a nonspecific systemic fibrinolytic state. It can induce hypotension and allergic-type reactions, but is relatively inexpensive.

(3) **APSAC** (Eminase or anistreplase) has clinical characteristics that fall between those of tPA and streptokinase (Table 17-2).

b. **PTCA.** The primary constraint of PTCA is the availability of personnel and supportive facilities. It is only available in about 20% of hospitals in the United States. Primary (direct) PTCA has a 90% success rate in restoring antegrade flow in the occluded infarct-related artery. Generally, PTCA is reserved for patients who have contraindications to thrombolysis or for those who have persistent symptoms, ST-segment elevations, or cardiogenic shock after thrombolysis. Several adjuncts to PTCA that reduce coronary reocclusion include **IV heparin** (section **III.B.3.d.**), **intracoronary stenting** (section **II.C.3.a**), and **antiplatelet agents** such as aspirin, ticlopidine, and abciximab (sections **II.C.3.a** and **III.B.3.a**).

c. **CABG** may be indicated on an emergency basis for (a) patients with operable coronary anatomy who have failed medical management but are not candidates for PTCA; (b) patients who failed PTCA and have persistent ischemia or hemodynamic instability; (c) those in cardiogenic shock; or (d) patients with surgically correctable mechanical complications (e.g., severe mitral regurgitation or VSD) from the AMI (section **II.C.3.b**).

5. **Intraaortic balloon counterpulsation** may be indicated for patients awaiting PTCA or CABG who are in cardiogenic shock or hemodynamically unstable despite medical therapy (section **II.C.3.c** and Chapter 13).

C. **Complications of myocardial infarction**

1. **Recurrent ischemia and infarction.** The most common causes of chest pain after MI are pericarditis (section **III.C.2.e**), ischemia, or reinfarction. After successful reperfusion, up to 58% of patients will exhibit early recurrent angina. Reinfarction occurs in approximately 3% to 4% of patients during the first 10 days after treatment with thrombolysis and aspirin. Patients with reinfarction are at increased risk of developing cardiogenic shock, fatal dysrhythmias, or cardiac arrest. The initial approach should be optimizing medical therapies while considering either repeat thrombolysis or PTCA, if not already performed. Emergency CABG may be considered for those who are refractory to both medical treatment and PTCA. Patients with active ischemia unresponsive to medical therapies can be placed on an IABP while awaiting coronary angiography.

2. **Mechanical complications**

a. **Mitral regurgitation** generally is secondary to papillary muscle rupture, which usually occurs between 3 and 5 days after MI, and is commonly associated with inferoposterior MI. A new apical systolic murmur and abrupt LV failure are the usual findings. The pulmonary artery occlusion pressure (PAOP) waveform may exhibit large V waves. Echocardiography will show the ruptured papillary muscle and mitral regurgitation. Treatment includes afterload reduction, inotropic agents, and, if ineffective, IABP while arranging for emergency surgical repair. Mortality with medical management is approximately 75% within the first 24 hours and is improved with prompt surgical correction.

b. **VSD** most commonly occurs between 3 and 5 days after anterior infarction. Clinical signs include new onset of a holosystolic murmur, systolic thrill, and cardiogenic shock. Echocardiography demonstrates an interventricular septal defect with left to right shunt. An increase or "step-up" of oxygen saturation between blood sampled from the right atrium and right ventricle can be confirmatory. Treatment is as outlined above for acute mitral regurgitation (section **III.C.2.a**). Hemodynamically stable patients may not require immediate surgical repair, but mortality in patients with cardiogenic shock is up to 90% without surgical intervention.

c. **Ventricular free wall rupture** accounts for about 10% of peri-infarct death. Risk factors include sustained hypertension after MI, a large transmural MI, late use of thrombolytics, female gender, advanced age, and exposure to steroids or nonsteroidal antiinflammatory agents. It occurs in the first 2 weeks after the first MI, with a peak incidence between 3 and 6 days after infarction. Recurrent chest pain and acute onset of heart failure and cardiovascular collapse suggest free wall rupture. Death can occur rapidly. Diagnosis is by echocardiography. Volume expansion, pericardiocentesis to decompress tamponade, and IABP are temporizing measures while transferring the patient to the operating room for definitive emergency surgical repair. Overall mortality is high.

d. **Ventricular aneurysm** is characterized by a protrusion of the ventricular scar and is associated with CHF, malignant dysrhythmias, and systemic embolism. It is generally caused by a thinning of the infarcted ventricular wall. Persistent ST-segment elevation may be evident on ECG; echocardiography confirms the diagnosis. Anticoagulation is required, especially in patients with documented mural thrombus. Surgical repair of ventricular geometry may be necessary.

e. **Pericarditis** is caused by the extension of myocardial necrosis to the epicardium; it occurs in approximately 25% of patients within several weeks after infarction. Pleuritic chest pain or positional discomfort, radiation to the left shoulder or scapula, a pericardial rub, ECG evidence of diffuse J-point elevation, concave ST-segment elevation, and reciprocal PR interval depression, and echocardiographic signs of pericardial effusion may be evident. The treatment of choice is **aspirin**, 160–325 mg daily, and increased to

650 mg every 4 to 6 hours, if necessary. Indomethacin, ibuprofen, and corticosteroids should be avoided because of the potential for wall thinning within the zone of myocardial necrosis, which may predispose to ventricular wall rupture.

3. **Dysrhythmias,** which are common, have multiple causes, including CHF, ischemia, reentrant rhythms, reperfusion, acidosis, electrolyte derangements (e.g., hypokalemia, hypomagnesemia, intracellular hypercalcemia), hypoxemia, hypotension, drug effects, and heightened reflex sympathoadrenal and vagal activity. Treatment of any correctable precipitating factors is prudent. Chapter 15 discusses emergency treatment of dysrhythmias.

    a. **Ventricular fibrillation (VF)** is defined as a pulseless, chaotic, disorganized rhythm of irregular pattern, size, and shape. Primary VF is an important cause of mortality within the first 24 hours of an AMI. It occurs in approximately 3% to 5% of patients within 4 hours of infarction. Prophylactic treatment with lidocaine may reduce the incidence of VF, but because it increases the mortality rate, it is not recommended. Beta-blockers are associated with a reduction in early VF and should be used if no contraindications exist. Maintaining normal potassium (>4 mEq/L) and magnesium (>2 mEq/L) levels may reduce dysrhythmogenic causes of VF. Specific therapies are discussed in Chapter 15. Initial treatment by **unsynchronized defibrillation** at 200 J should begin immediately. If no clinical response, a second shock at 200 to 300 J should be delivered, and, if indicated, a third shock at 360 J should be given. In the adult, adjunct IV pharmacotherapy should be given in the following order, with defibrillation at 360 J in between medications: epinephrine (1 mg), lidocaine (1–1.5 mg/kg), and bretylium (5–10 mg/kg). Epinephrine can be repeated every 3 minutes.

    b. **Ventricular tachycardia (VT). Premature ventricular contractions** (PVCs) are common after MI. Prophylactic therapy is not recommended. Treatment includes correction of abnormal electrolyte levels and continued beta-blocker therapy. **Nonsustained VT** is a run of PVCs lasting more than 30 seconds. **Sustained VT** lasts more than 30 seconds, is associated with hemodynamic instability, or both. **Sustained polymorphic VT** should be treated as VF. **Sustained monomorphic VT** with angina, CHF, or hypotension should be treated with synchronized cardioversion at 50 J initially and with subsequent incremental energy

(100 J→ 300 J→ 360 J) if not successful. Patients with hemodynamically stable, sustained monomorphic VT should be treated with either **lidocaine** (1–1.5 mg/kg IV initially and repeated at 0.5–0.75 mg/kg IV every 5–10 minutes to a maximum of 3 mg/kg, followed by an infusion of 1–4 mg/min), **procainamide** (20–30 mg/min IV infusion initially up to 17 mg/kg, followed by an infusion of 1–4 mg/min), or **amiodarone** (150 mg over 10 minutes, 360 mg over the next 6 hours, then 540 mg over the next 18 hours). **Synchronized cardioversion,** beginning at 50 J, can be performed if the rhythm is refractory to medical therapy. **Implantable cardioverter defibrillators** can be considered for patients who have survived episodes of sudden death from VT or VF or who have refractory dysrhythmias (Chapter 19).

c. **Accelerated idioventricular rhythm** occurs in approximately 10% to 20% of patients after MI. It can be caused by an ectopic ventricular pacer, enhanced automaticity, or variable exit block. It is generally self-limiting within 48 hours and treatment is not recommended unless the rhythm is associated with cardiovascular instability or precipitates VT or VF. In these cases, suppression with lidocaine, atropine, or overdrive atrial pacing is indicated.

d. **Atrial fibrillation (AF).** Up to 10% to 16% of patients will develop transient AF within 24 hours of an acute infarction. Risk factors include anterior and inferior MI, advanced age, large infarcts, or complications of infarct (e.g., CHF, advanced heart block, pericarditis, or ventricular dysrhythmias). Other precipitating factors include hypoxia, electrolyte derangements, chronic lung disease, sinus nodal ischemia, or increased sympathetic activity. In patients without hemodynamic instability, **β-adrenergic blockers** (e.g., atenolol 2.5–5 mg IV every 2–5 minutes to a total of 10 mg over 10–15 minutes or metoprolol on a similar schedule) are effective if no contraindications exist. Alternatively, **verapamil** (5–10 mg IV in 2 minutes, may repeat in 30 minutes) or **diltiazem** (20 mg IV in 2 minutes, may repeat in 15 minutes with 25 mg IV) may be used if beta-blockers are contraindicated or ineffective. Given their negative inotropic effects, these agents should not be considered as the first line of therapy. **Digoxin** (0.6–1 mg IV loading dose; half the dose initially and the remaining dose given in two equal doses every 4 hours) has been traditionally administered, but is not as effective as β-adrenergic blocking agents. In hemodynamically unstable patients,

synchronized cardioversion (beginning with 100 J, and, if no clinical response, followed by 200–300 J, then 360 J if needed) can be performed. Anticoagulation should be strongly considered for persistent atrial fibrillation.

e. **Bradycardia and AV blocks.** Sinus bradycardia is common after MI. It is frequently associated with increased vagal tone, inferior wall infarct, and right coronary artery reperfusion. Patients complicated by heart block after MI have increased in-hospital mortality. **Atropine** (0.5 mg IV increments to a maximum of 2 mg) is indicated in patients with symptomatic sinus bradycardia, ventricular asystole, or symptomatic AV block at the AV nodal level (second-degree type 1 or third-degree with a narrow complex escape rhythm). Patients with advanced AV block or bilateral BBB are at risk of developing complete heart block or asystole. **Pacing** (Chapter 19) should be instituted in patients with symptomatic sinus bradycardia (HR < 50 bpm), second-degree type 2 AV block, third-degree AV block, bilateral BBB, and right or left BBB with a first-degree AV block.

4. **Heart failure and cardiogenic shock** (Chapter 9)

5. **Hypertension** increases myocardial oxygen demand and can worsen myocardial ischemia. Causes of hypertension include premorbid hypertension, CHF, and elevated catecholamines as a result of pain and anxiety. Treatment includes adequate antianginal therapy and analgesia, anxiolytic therapy (if indicated), and IV nitroglycerin, beta-blockers, and ACE inhibitors. Calcium channel blockers (verapamil or diltiazem) may be indicated in patients who have contraindications to other agents. Nitroprusside may be required if hypertension is severe. See Chapter 10 for details of hypertensive treatment.

SELECTED REFERENCES

Bypass Angioplasty Revascularization Investigation (BARI) Investigators. Comparison of coronary bypass surgery with angioplasty in patients with multivessels disease. *N Engl J Med* 1996;335: 217–225.

Dries DL, Solomon AJ, Gersh BJ. Adjunctive therapy after reperfusion therapy in acute myocardial infarction. *Clin Cardiol* 1998;21: 379–386.

Fibrinolytic Therapy Trialists' (FTT) Collaborative Group. Indications for fibrinolytic therapy in suspected acute myocardial infarction: collaborative overview of early mortality and major morbidity results from all randomised trials of more than 1000 patients. *Lancet* 1994; 343:311–322.

Gottlieb SS, McCarter RJ, Vogel RA. Effect of beta-blockade on mortality among high-risk and low risk patients after myocardial infarction. *N Engl J Med* 1998;339:489–497.

Hennekens CH. Update on aspirin in the treatment and prevention of cardiovascular disease. *Am Heart J* 1999;137:S9–S13.

ISIS-1 (First International Study of Infarct Survival) Collaborative Group. Randomized trial of intravenous atenolol among 16,027 cases of suspected acute myocardial infarction. *Lancet* 1986;2:57–66.

Ryan TJ, Anderson JL, Antman EM, et al. ACC/AHA guidelines for the management of patients with acute myocardial infarction: a report of the American College of Cardiology/American Heart Association Task Force on Practice Guidelines (Committee on Management of Acute Myocardial Infarction). *J Am Coll Cardiol* 1996;28:1328–1428.

Schoebel FC, Frazier OH, Jessurun GA, et al. Refractory angina pectoris in end-stage coronary artery disease: evolving therapeutic concepts. *Am Heart J* 1997;134:587–602.

Valvular Heart Disease

Thomas Suarez and James G. Cain

Management of patients with valvular heart disease requires a broad understanding of the pathophysiology of each lesion and the physiologic compensatory mechanisms.

I. **Aortic stenosis**
   A. Three types of aortic stenosis (AS) are seen: **valvular** (most common), **supravalvular,** and **subvalvular.** Although the incidence of rheumatic aortic stenosis is decreasing, it, along with congenitally bicuspid valves (1% of the population) and senile degeneration, remain the primary causes of aortic stenosis.
   B. **Pathophysiology**
      1. As the valve orifice decreases, the heart maintains a normal stroke volume through increased pressure generation (> 250 mm Hg). This results in a **concentric hypertrophy** of the left ventricle (LV) chamber. Long-standing critical AS eventually results in cardiac dysfunction with pulmonary edema, myocardial ischemia, or sudden death from lethal dysrhythmias.
      2. Morbiditiy in the patient with AS results from a number of factors.
         a. The extreme intracavitary pressures (even during diastole) compress the subendocardium, such that ischemia can result. **It is vitally important to maintain adequate aortic root pressure to maintain adequate coronary perfusion. Ischemia can be very difficult to treat.**
         b. The increased LV systolic and diastolic pressures increase wall tension, which, in turn, increases myocardial oxygen demand.
         c. The high pressure required to create flow past the stenotic valve can create a Venturi effect and decrease pressure at the coronary ostia.
         d. Tachycardia or supraventricular dysrhythmias may decrease stroke volume to the point of causing ischemia. In the normal patient, the atrial contraction contributes 20% to 25% of the total stroke volume. In the patient with AS, this is increased to 30% to 40%. Thus, normal atrial contraction is essential for optimal function in the patient with AS.
   C. **Signs and symptoms**
      1. Aortic stenosis can be asymptomatic for many years. The onset of symptoms often indicates severe disease. The classic triad of angina pectoris,

syncope, and congestive heart failure (CHF) indicates a life expectancy of less than 5 years in patients with untreated AS.

2. **Anginal symptoms** can be from either existing coronary artery disease or AS in isolation.

3. Once LV failure has occurred, life expectancy is only 1 to 2 years.

4. **The physical examination** can aid in the diagnosis of AS. Some general physical findings that are indicative of AS include:

   a. A loud systolic, diamond-shaped murmur that is best heard at the base of the heart and which radiates to the neck.

   b. A strong apical pulse.

   c. A slow-rising carotid upstroke.

   d. A narrow pulse pressure and the absence of the sound of aortic closure are late and ominous signs.

5. **The degree of AS** can be measured by echocardiography or by cardiac catheterization. When using echocardiographic methods, it is important that the valve area be measured at the level of the greatest stenosis. The simplified **Gorlin equation** can be used to calculate the area if the mean pressure gradient has been measured via catheterization:

$$\text{Aortic valve area}\,(\text{cm}^2) = \frac{\text{cardiac output}\,(\text{L/min})}{\sqrt{(\text{mean pressure gradient}}}$$

   Stenosis can be graded as trace, mild, moderate, or severe. **The normal adult aortic valve area** measures 2.5 to 3.5 cm². Severe stenosis occurs when the valvular area is less then 0.7 cm², or the peak systolic pressure gradient is more than 50 mm Hg.

D. Hemodynamic changes

1. **The systemic arterial pressure wave** increases more slowly and can have a slanted upstroke. The anacrotic notch occurs lower in the pressure wave and the dicrotic notch is often absent.

2. **The pulmonary artery occlusion pressure (PAOP)** is increased in AS because of the elevated left ventricular end diastolic pressure (LVEDP). As the disease progresses, the mitral valvular annulus may become wider and atrial hypertrophy ensues, resulting in a prominent v wave.

E. Management

1. **Hypotension** must be treated immediately. An alpha-adrenergic agonist should be available immediately. Ischemia resulting from the aortic root pressure falling below the subendocardial pressure can begin a downward spiral of further ischemia, dysrhythmias, and hemodynamic instability that can be difficult to treat. Secondary to

the thickened myocardium and the small valvular area, cardiopulmonary resuscitation often is ineffective in these patients.

2. **Supraventricular and ventricular dysrhythmias** should be treated expeditiously. Supraventricular and ventricular ectopy can quickly result in an unstable situation that may be refractory to pharmacologic treatment.

3. **Both tachycardia and bradycardia** are tolerated poorly. Tachycardia may not allow enough time for proper diastolic filling, in addition to increasing myocardial oxygen requirements. Extreme bradycardia can overdistend the heart or not provide sufficient flow for proper perfusion. Changes should be made slowly unless an unstable situation exists. Cardiac depressive drugs (beta-blockers, calcium channel blockers) and cardiac stimulating drugs (atropine, dopamine) should be used judiciously.

4. **Nitroglycerin,** if needed, should be administered cautiously, because patients with AS are dependent on adequate venous return to maintain stroke volume.

5. **Pulmonary artery catheters** can help to guide fluid balance and monitor cardiac performance. Insertion of a pulmonary artery (PA) catheter, however, can precipitate dysrhythmias. If dysrhythmias occur during placement of the PA catheter, the position of the catheter should be immediately changed (withdrawn or advanced) to reduce further irritation to the endocardium. If a PA catheter is desired for hemodynamic monitoring, consider placing a PA catheter with **pacing** capabilities.

6. **Nodal rhythms** are poorly tolerated. A small amount of atropine (0.4 mg) can place the patient into a normal sinus rhythm. If ineffective, atrial pacing may be needed.

7. **Inotropic support** may be needed in cases of severe AS. Starting with small amounts of norepinephrine (1–4 μg/min) can be helpful. Phosphodiesterase inhibitors (amrinone, milrinone) can also be useful, but they decrease systemic vascular resistance (SVR). Likewise, dobutamine can decrease the aortic root pressure more than is desired. When using dopamine, dobutamine, or epinephrine, care must be taken to avoid tachydysrhythmias.

F. **Postoperative care after aortic valve replacement or commissurotomy**

1. Although stroke volume increases and LVEDP decreases following aortic valve replacement or repair, the left ventricle remains **hypertrophied** for many months. Maintaining adequate coronary artery perfusion is essential. After the hypertrophied myocardium has returned to a near normal

state, increased subendocardial pressures are less concerning.

2. Repaired or prosthetic valves can become incompetent or have perivalvular leaks on rare occasions.

3. Because of the nature of the incision required for aortic valve surgery, sudden loss of blood pressure, massive bleeding in the chest tubes, or hemothorax may indicate a myocardial rupture.

G. **Idiopathic hypertrophic subaortic stenosis.** Unlike valvular AS, patients with idiopathic hypertrophic subaortic stenosis have a dynamic obstruction to the forward flow of blood from the left ventricle. The myocardium may undergo a concentric hypertrophy. The main pathology lies in the large muscle mass of the subaortic region, which can cause total obstruction. These patients tend toward dynamic obstruction of the outflow tract during times of tachycardia and low filling volumes. Management includes maintenance of a slow heart rate to allow for a longer diastolic filling period and adequate intravascular volume repletion. These patients also are susceptible to lethal ventricular dysrhythmias.

II. **Aortic regurgitation (AR).** Aortic regurgitation occurs when the aortic valve becomes incompetent such that a portion of the ejected blood flows retrograde across the valve. Aortic regurgitation can be either acute or chronic, and has many causes, including rheumatic fever, syphilitic aortitis, bacterial endocarditis, aortic dissection, acute trauma (often blunt chest trauma), and congenital abnormalities.

A. **Pathophysiology**

1. **Acute AR** results from the sudden flow of blood back into the left ventricle during diastole. The compensatory response is increased sympathetic tone, resulting in tachycardia and increased inotropy. Often, this response is inadequate, and congestive heart failure ensues. In acute AR, the LV has not had time to remodel through eccentric hypertrophy (an increase in both size of the ventricular cavity and the thickness of the LV myocardium). Both left ventricular end-diastolic volume (LVEDV) and LVEDP increase acutely. In addition, a reduction in systemic arterial diastolic pressure can decrease coronary perfusion pressure, thus resulting in ischemia.

2. **Chronic aortic regurgitation** occurs more slowly, often over many years. In this case, the increase in LVEDV results in an eccentric hypertrophy of the myocardium (see above). Although the LVEDV increases, little change occurs in LVEDP because of compensatory changes in LV size and muscle mass. Thus, the heart may function normally for many years. In general, function usually remains near normal if the regurgitant fraction remains less then 40%. Symptoms often result when the regurgitant fraction exceeds 60%.

An LVEDP of greater then 20 mm Hg is a sign of poor compensation.

B. Signs and symptoms

1. **Acute AR** often presents with sudden congestive heart failure, angina, and tachycardia. Chronic aortic regurgitation, however, can be asymptomatic for years. When symptoms (shortness of breath, palpitations, fatigue, or angina) develop, the average survival rate, if untreated, is approximately 5 years.

2. **The physical examination** can aid in the diagnosis of AR. Some general physical findings that are indicative of AR include:

   a. A widened arterial pulse pressure.

   b. Bounding or "water hammer" peripheral pulses.

   c. Quincke's pulses (visible capillary pulsations with compression of the nail bed).

   d. A decrescendo diastolic murmur along the left sternal border.

   e. An Austin-Flint murmur (an apical diastolic rumble caused by regurgitant flow impinging on the anterior mitral leaflet).

   f. Maximal cardiac impulse shifted downward and to the left.

C. The degree of aortic regurgitation is graded in different manners, depending on the method used to measure it. The amount of AR will change, depending on the hemodynamic state (i.e., afterload, heart rate, inotropy). When evaluating AR with transesophageal echocardiography (TEE), many physicians use the grading system of *severe, moderate, mild,* and *trace,* depending on the width and height of the regurgitant jet. When grading AR using angiocardiographic methods, a more standardized system has been accepted that is based on the rate of dye clearance:

1. 1+: Small amount of dye in LV that is totally cleared during the next contraction.

2. 2+: Moderate amount of dye in LV that is not completely cleared during the next contraction.

3. 3+: Complete opacification of the LV from the regurgitant jet that does not clear for many cycles.

4. 4+: Similar to 3+, but the density of the dye is greater in the LV than in the aorta and it clears very slowly from the LV.

D. Hemodynamic changes

1. The systemic arterial pulse pressure often is widened, with a very rapid upstroke because of the large stroke volume.

2. A rapid downstroke of the arterial pressure waveform results from the rapid flow of blood back into the LV. Sometimes a double-peaked wave can be seen.

3. The PAOP may demonstrate prominent *v* waves, because of LV volume overload and accompany-

ing mitral regurgitation. The PAOP may underestimate the LVEDP because the aortic regurgitant jet causes premature closure of the mitral valve.

E.   **Management**

1.   **Afterload reduction,** an **increased heart rate** (to decrease filling time and thus decrease LVEDV), and **inotropic support** are keys to acute management. Acute surgical intervention may be necessary.

2.   A TEE can be useful in guiding therapy. The TEE can visualize changes in the regurgitant jet, inotropic state, and LV filling.

3.   **Dobutamine** often is the inotrope of choice for patients with AR. It increases contractility, reduces peripheral resistance, and maintains a relatively rapid heart rate. Milrinone and amrinone also provide inotropic support and afterload reduction, but with less increase in heart rate.

F.   **Postoperative care after aortic valve repair or replacement for AR**

1.   Because of persistent cardiomegaly, adequate ventricular filling remains essential for good cardiac function.

2.   Inotropic support may be required postoperatively.

3.   Although an intraaortic balloon pump is contraindicated in patients with AR prior to repair, as it augments diastole and therefore worsens regurgitant flow, such support often is safe and may be necessary after valve replacement or repair.

III. **Mitral stenosis (MS)**

A.   **Pathophysiology. Rheumatic fever** can result in the scarring, fibrosis, and calcification of the edges of the valve with eventual fibrosis of the commissures. Patients who have rheumatic heart disease often remain asymptomatic for more than 20 years. When symptoms appear, there is a 20% chance of death within the first year. **Senile calcification** can begin with calcification of the valvular annulus.

B.   **Signs and symptoms**

1.   **Symptoms** usually first present during exercise or other high output states. In many inactive patients, the onset of atrial fibrillation or flutter from atrial stretching causes the first symptoms.

2.   Patients often complain of dyspnea, palpitations, fatigue, chest pain, and paroxysmal nocturnal dyspnea. Some patients also complain of hoarseness because of compression of the left recurrent laryngeal nerve by the dilated left pulmonary artery or left atrium (LA). Some patients present with mild hemoptysis.

3.   **Dysrhythmias** such as atrial fibrillation can present with signs of CHF because of decreased diastolic filling time and increased left atrial pressure (LAP).

4. An **echocardiogram** can confirm the diagnosis of MS.
5. **The physical examination** can aid in the diagnosis of MS. Some general physical findings that are indicative of MS include:
   a. A loud S_1 heart sound.
   b. A presystolic or mid-diastolic rumble.
   c. A prominent jugular a wave.
C. **The degree of MS** can be assessed by echocardiography or angiography. As with AS, a modification of the Gorlin formula can be used to determine the mitral valve (MV) area.
   1. The area of the normal mitral valve is 4 to 6 cm^2.
   2. Patients with **moderate MR** (1.5–2.5 cm^2) often only show symptoms with increased cardiac demand. Symptoms (dyspnea, fatigue) are related to increased LAP.
   3. **Critical MS** is defined as a valve area less than 1.0 cm^2. Patients with critical MS are often symptomatic at rest and tolerate exercise poorly. Increased pulmonary vascular pressures can produce pulmonary edema. Chronic pulmonary hypertension ultimately may cause right ventricular (RV) failure.
D. **Hemodynamic changes**
   1. The PAOP is increased and may not accurately reflect LVEDP.
   2. The PAOP waveform can exhibit a large a wave, if normal sinus rhythm is present. Because MS often is associated with some degree of mitral regurgitation, large v waves can also be present.
   3. **Pulmonary hypertension** is common. The pulmonary arteries often are dilated and, thus, PA catheters may need to be inserted further than usual. Because of the increased PA pressures and decreased PA compliance, inflation of the balloon on the PA catheter has an increased risk of rupturing the PA.
E. **Management**
   1. **Adequate preload** is essential for good cardiac function. Although atrial pressures tend to be increased in MS, flow across the MV is partially based on maintaining atrial filling. This must be balanced with the tendency towards CHF in these patients. No particular value of PAOP is considered correct; rather, signs and symptoms of organ perfusion, oxygenation, and CHF must be followed.
   2. **A slow heart rate** is essential for proper LV filling. Blood flow across the MV occurs during diastole. A heart rate that is too fast does not allow sufficient time for proper filling. Too slow a heart rate will reduce cardiac output. Adequate organ perfusion in the absence of congestive heart failure indicates a proper rate.

3. In the event that AV pacing is required, a long PR interval (0.2 second) allows more time for blood to flow across the mitral valve. A PR interval that is too short will not allow sufficient time for the atrium to empty.

4. Patients with MS may need **inotropic support.** Digoxin commonly is used in these patients because of its negative chronotropic and positive inotropic effects. In the event that more aggressive inotropic support is needed, drugs that do not significantly increase heart rate (e.g., milrinone and amrinone) may be useful.

5. **Supraventricular dysrhythmias** that are hemodynamically significant (i.e., cause a decrease in blood pressure) must be treated aggressively, usually with direct current cardioversion. Many clinicians suggest starting with increased power (i.e., 200 J).

F. **Postoperative care after mitral valve replacement or commissurotomy**

1. **Mitral commissurotomy** is being performed more commonly. Although this operation does not totally relieve the stenosis, it greatly reduces it. One important advantage of this procedure is that the patient does not require postoperative anticoagulation.

2. **Preload augmentation** often is needed in the postoperative period. Stroke volume, PAOP, and TEE can be used to guide proper fluid replacement.

3. **Afterload reduction** can improve hemodynamics postoperatively, although preoperatively it has little effect because of the fixed stenosis.

4. **Inotropic support** may be required following valve repair or replacement, because of an underlying decrease in LV function caused by chronic underfilling of the ventricle.

5. **Chronic atrial fibrillation** is common in patients with long-standing MS. The use of amiodarone, procainamide, or overdrive pacing may be necessary (Chapter 17).

6. In the event of a sudden decrease in blood pressure following MV repair or replacement, consider the very rare possibilities of atrioventricular disruption or (in the case of valve replacement) a valve that is stuck in the closed position. Both atrioventricular disruption and a stuck valve are emergencies that often require surgery at the bedside.

IV. **Mitral regurgitation (MR)**

A. **Pathophysiology.** The cause of MR often is classified as rheumatic or nonrheumatic.

1. **Rheumatic MR** often occurs concomitantly with MS. As with MS, the asymptomatic period can last many years.

2. **Nonrheumatic MR** can be caused by papillary muscle dysfunction (often seen in patients with

posterior septal or anterior septal ischemia or infarction), bacterial endocarditis, or ruptured cordae.

3. **Acute MR** occurs with a sudden back flow of blood across the mitral valve back into the LA. This results in a sudden volume overload of the atrium, leading to increased pulmonary vascular pressures and, often, CHF. The compensatory response is one of increased sympathetic output, resulting in tachycardia, and increased inotropy. Annular dilation of the MV can occur secondary to increased LV volume, thus worsening the amount of regurgitation. **Myocardial ischemia** can occur because of increased myocardial oxygen demand (because of increased sympathetic output) and increased LVEDP.

4. **Chronic MR** is different from acute MR in that sufficient time exists for the LV to compensate for the increased volume load. Adaptations include eccentric hypertrophy of the LV, which causes the heart to dilate, allowing a relatively constant LVEDP despite a greatly increased LVEDV. The LA enlarges and can maintain a normal pressure. In the latter stages of the compensatory process, the dilation of the LV can lead to dilation of the mitral annulus and, thus, increased MR. The LV ejection fraction often remains normal, but forward flow may decrease. When the regurgitant fraction exceeds 60%, the likelihood of CHF increases dramatically. A decreasing ejection fraction (< 50%) indicates failing left ventricular function. In the final stages of chronic MR, the increased pulmonary pressures can precipitate RV failure.

B. **Signs and symptoms**

1. **Acute MR** often presents as sudden dyspnea, fatigue, or acute CHF. Patients often complain of palpitations secondary to atrial fibrillation; some also complain of chest pain. **Chronic MR** can remain asymptomatic for years, but the onset of symptoms often indicates a rapid downward course. Patients may present with dyspnea, fatigue, CHF, or atrial fibrillation.

2. **The physical examination** can aid in the diagnosis of MR. Some general physical findings that are indicative of MR include:

   a. A hyperdynamic apex with or without an apical lift or thrill.

   b. A holosystolic murmur best heard at the apex (that may radiate to the left axilla).

   c. Rarely, a midsystolic rumble.

C. **The degree of MR** is graded in different manners depending on the method of evaluation. Importantly, the amount of MR depends on the hemodynamic state (i.e., afterload, heart rate, and inotropy). When evaluating MR with TEE, many physicians use the grading system of *severe, moderate, mild,* and *trace,* depending on the width and height of the regurgitant jet. When grading MR using angiocardiographic methods, the degree of regurgitation is based on the amount of dye clearance:

1. 1+: Small amount of dye in the LA that is totally cleared during the next contraction.
2. 2+: Moderate amount of dye in the LA that is not completely cleared during the next contraction.
3. 3+: Complete opacification of the LA from the regurgitant jet that does not clear for many cycles.
4. 4+: Similar to 3+, clearing the LA more slowly.

D. **Hemodynamic changes**
1. The PAOP waveform is characterized by giant *v* waves. The size of the *v* wave does not necessarily correlate with the amount of the regurgitation. The size and morphology of the wave is more dependent on the compliance of the LA and the pulmonary vascular beds.
2. It can be difficult to differentiate between the PAOP and the pulmonary artery pressure (PAP) waveform in patients with MR because of the giant *v* waves. A helpful sign is that the peak of the PA pressure waveform shifts to the right, compared with the systemic arterial waveform, when the PA balloon is inflated and a PAOP tracing is obtained.

E. **Management**
1. **The heart rate** should be kept in a normal to high normal range. A slow heart rate can cause volume overload of the LV. Patients with MR can develop atrial fibrillation secondary to stretching of the atrium. Although this rhythm is often tolerated, the preference is to maintain normal sinus rhythm.
2. **Maintenance of adequate LV preload** must be weighed against the possibility that excess LV volume will dilate the mitral annulus and make the degree of the regurgitation worse.
3. **Afterload reduction** is often necessary. A decreased peripheral resistance increases the forward ejection of the stroke volume. It is important not to lower systemic blood pressure too much, especially in patients with concomitant coronary artery disease. In patients with coronary artery disease and MR, nitroglycerin can be a reasonable intervention, achieving coronary vasodilatation and some afterload reduction. Calcium channel blockers also have been used for this purpose.
4. **Inotropic agents** can increase forward flow. The use of an agent that both increases contractility and decreases afterload may be preferable. Dobutamine (2–20 μg/kg/min), milrinone, and amrinone are useful in this situation.

5. **Pulmonary hypertension** develops in severe cases of MR. Right ventricle failure may ensue. In these most fragile patients, care must be taken to avoid further increasing PA pressures (i.e., avoid hypoxia, hypercarbia, and acidosis). In the event of right ventricle failure, the use of prostaglandin E_1, prostacyclin, or inhaled nitric oxide (NO) may be beneficial. Intraaortic balloon counterpulsation may be lifesaving (Chapter 13).

F. **Postoperative care after mitral valve repair or replacement for mitral regurgitation**
   1. After repair of MR, the entire stroke volume is ejected into the aorta. The LV can fail secondary to this increased afterload.
   2. **Inotropic support** is often needed. In severe cases, intraaortic balloon counterpulsation may be necessary to augment forward flow and coronary perfusion.
   3. **Atrial fibrillation** is not well tolerated postoperatively. Every attempt should be made to maintain normal sinus rhythm. Procainamide, amiodarone, or overdrive atrial pacing may be necessary (Chapters 15, 17, and 36).
   4. **Transesophageal echocardiography** can be useful for determining valvular function and LV performance.

V. **Tricuspid stenosis (TS)**
A. **Pathophysiology.** Tricuspid stenosis occurs rarely compared with the aforementioned valvular lesions. Patients with TS often have associated MS. Tricuspid stenosis is most often caused by rheumatic fever, carcinoid syndrome, systemic lupus erythematosus, or endomyocardial fibroelastosis. Often, a very long asymptomatic period (> 20 years) occurs. As TS worsens, flow across the valve decreases, which can increase right atrial size and pressures. Atrial tachydysrhythmias are common. The cardiac output may be reduced because of decreased flow to the right ventricle.

B. **Signs and symptoms**
   1. The signs and symptoms of TS depend on whether the stenosis is isolated or exists in conjunction with other valvular lesions. In general, if it exists in isolation, signs of increased right-sided pressures (e.g., peripheral edema, jugular venous distention, ascites, hepatomegaly, and hepatic dysfunction) may be present. As is the case with MS and AS, symptoms of fatigue with exercise may be the presenting complaint. In addition, patients may first present with complaints of palpitations caused by supraventricular dysrhythmias. When TS is present in conjunction with MS, it is the severity of the dominant lesion that often presents first.

2. The physical examination can aid in the diagnosis of TS. Some general physical findings that are indicative of TS include:
    a. A holosystolic murmur that is best heard at the left sternal border. The murmur often becomes louder with inspiration.
    b. A right ventricular heave.
    c. Associated murmurs of other valvular abnormalities can be present.
    d. Hepatic pulsations, ascites, and peripheral cyanosis in severe cases.
3. The normal area of the tricuspid valve is 7 to 9 cm^2. Tricuspid stenosis is considered significant when the valve area decreases to 1.5 cm^2. The normal tricuspid gradient is 1 mm Hg. A gradient as small as 3 mm Hg indicates a moderate stenosis, whereas a gradient of 5 mm Hg is considered severe.

C. **Hemodynamic changes**
    1. A giant a wave is evident on the central venous pressure (CVP) waveform. This corresponds to the right atrium contracting against a high resistance orifice.
    2. CVP can be increased because of systemic volume overload.

D. **Management**
    1. **A slow normal heart rate** is essential to allow sufficient diastolic filling of the RV.
    2. **Tachydysrhythmias** can decrease cardiac output and increase CVP.
    3. **Adequate preload** is essential. It is important not to overfill the right atrium, because this will stretch it and predispose to supraventricular tachydysrhythmias.
    4. Although reducing RV afterload and increasing RV contractility will not directly affect the degree of TS, these maneuvers may help maintain cardiac output.

E. **Postoperative care after tricuspid valve replacement or repair for TS**
    1. These patients may have right-sided dysfunction secondary to a chronically underfilled RV. Right ventricular afterload reduction and inotropic support may be needed.
    2. Avoiding increased pulmonary artery pressures is essential. Prostacyclin, PGE$_1$, or inhaled NO may help reduce PA pressure and reduce RV afterload.
    3. **Supraventricular tachydysrhythmias** should be avoided. Procainamide or amiodarone may be necessary (Chapters 15, 17, and 36).
    4. Because of the new valve, these patients most often are managed with a central venous catheter. If a pulmon-ary artery catheter is deemed necessary, then it must be placed surgically, directly

cannulating the PA. Alternatively, a surgically placed LA catheter may be used.

VI. Tricuspid regurgitation (TR)

A. Pathophysiology

1. Tricuspid regurgitation usually accompanies other valvular lesions such as mitral stenosis or severe AS. Rarely, isolated TR is caused by endocarditis, chest trauma, and carcinoid syndrome.

2. TR occurs with a sudden back flow of blood across the tricuspid valve from the RV and into the right atrium. This results in a sudden volume overload of the atrium and increased pressure within the systemic venous system. Isolated TR is well tolerated. When pulmonary hypertension from valvular abnormalities or LV dysfunction causes TR, the ability to compensate is very poor.

B. Signs and symptoms

1. The increased volume load in the RA can cause distention of the atrium and associated **atrial fibrillation.** Atrial fibrillation or palpitations may be the presenting complaint.

2. **The physical examination** can aid in the diagnosis of TR. Some general physical findings that are indicative of TR include:
   a. An S_3 gallop (accentuated by inspiration).
   b. A systolic murmur that increases during inspiration.
   c. An accentuated P2 heart sound.

C. Hemodynamic changes

1. The **central venous pressure** may be normal or increased in TR.

2. The CVP waveform may exhibit giant v **waves,** corresponding to the large regurgitant jet during right ventricular systole. The size of the v wave depends on the compliance of the right atrium and does not necessarily correspond to the degree of the regurgitant volume.

D. Management

1. **A high heart rate** helps minimize peripheral congestion and RV volume overload, and increases forward flow from the RV.

2. **Atrial fibrillation** is common. Hemodynamic parameters nearly always improve if a sinus rhythm can be achieved.

3. **Adequate preload** is essential for forward flow. Decreased RV filling can severely limit cardiac output.

4. **Minimizing pulmonary vascular resistance** (i.e., avoiding hypoxemia, hypertension, and acidosis) can aid forward flow.

5. **Inotropic support** of the failing RV can be useful in TR. Drugs that provide increased inotropy and yet do not greatly increase PA pressures should be used. Dobutamine, amrinone, and milrinone are useful in this setting. Agents that will decrease PA pressures (e.g., prostaglandin E_1, prostacyclin, and

inhaled NO) may be helpful when used in conjunction with inotropic medications.
   E. **Postoperative care after tricuspid valve replacement or repair for tricuspid regurgitation**
      1. Because the TR is no longer present to provide a "pop off" and limit RV pressure, the pressure load of the RV can be acutely increased after tricuspid valve repair. Right ventricular dysfunction can occur and inotropic support may be necessary.
      2. If a tricuspid valve replacement is required, the new valve often is smaller, and may create a pressure gradient that would require increased venous return to ensure adequate forward flow.
VII. **Pulmonic valve disease**
   A. **Congenital pulmonic stenosis** occurs in infancy and childhood and presents as right ventricle failure. **Acquired pulmonic stenosis** is exceedingly rare.
   B. **Pulmonic regurgitation** is well tolerated hemodynamically, regardless of cause as long as right ventricular function is adequate. Acquired pulmonic regurgitation can result from infective endocarditis or rheumatic heart disease. Operative intervention in pulmonic regurgitation caused by endocarditis generally consists of excision of the affected valve without replacement by a prosthetic device.
VIII. **Prophylaxis for bacterial endocarditis.** Transient bacteremia following invasive procedures, surgery, and dental procedures can cause endocarditis. Blood-borne bacteria can lodge on damaged or abnormal tissues. Antibiotic prophylaxis is recommended for patients with prosthetic cardiac valves, a previous history of endocarditis, most congenital malformations, rheumatic valvular disease, hypertrophic cardiomyopathy, and mitral regurgitation. Prophylaxis is not recommended for patients with permanent pacemakers, implantable defibrillators, and mitral valve prolapse without regurgitation. Most institutions, as well as the American Heart Association (Dajani et al.), have specific recommendations concerning regimens for antibiotic prophylaxis.

SELECTED REFERENCES

Abrams J. *Mitral stenosis, essentials of cardiac physical diagnosis.* Philadelphia: Lea & Febiger, 1987:275–306.

Braunwald E, Turi ZG. Pathophysiology of mitral valve disease. In: *Mitral valve disease: diagnosis and treatment.* London: Butterworths, 1985.

Danjani AS, Bisno AL, Chung KJ, et al. Prevention of bacterial endocarditis. Recommendations by the American Heart Association. *JAMA* 1990;264:2919–2922.

Levinson GE. Aortic stenosis. In: Dalen JE, Alpert JS, eds. *Valvular heart disease.* Boston: Little Brown and Co, 1987.

Jackson JM, Thomas SJ, Lowenstein E. Anesthetic management of patients with valvular heart disease. *Semin Anesth* 1982;1:239–252.

Olson LJ, Subramanian R, Ackerman, DM, et al. Surgical pathophysiology of the mitral valve: a study of 172 cases spanning 21 years. *Mayo Clin Proc* 1987;62:22–34.

Pacemakers and Implantable Defibrillators

Thomas Suarez and James G. Cain

I. **Pacemaker definitions, generic codes and modes of pacing**
   A. **Pacemakers** and implantable defibrillators are becoming more common as the population in the United States ages. It is estimated that more than 500,000 patients have implanted or permanent pacemakers. Additionally, the number of **implantable cardioverter defibrillators** (ICDs) continues to grow. Knowledge about the issues surrounding pacemakers and ICDs is essential for the intensive care unit (ICU) physician. Patients who have a pacemaker or ICD also often have concomitant diseases such as coronary artery disease.
   B. **Pacemaker identification codes.** A five-letter code system has been adopted by both the North American Society of Pacing and Electrophysiology and the British Pacing and Electrophysiology Group. The letter in each of five positions describes the setting of any specific pacemaker (Table 19-1). Most modern pacemakers can be interrogated and programmed to adjust to the changing needs of the patient's disease process.
   C. **Definitions**
      1. **Unipolar pacing** occurs when a negative lead is placed within a cardiac chamber and a positive lead is placed outside the heart.
      2. **Bipolar pacing** requires that both leads (negative and positive) be placed within the chamber paced or sensed.
      3. **Asynchronous pacing.** A pacing current is generated at a specific timed interval (i.e., no sensing of the patient's underlying heart rate exists) and, thus, heart rate is fixed. Examples of asynchronous pacing include **AOO, VOO,** and **DOO.** The disadvantage of this mode of pacing is that the paced rate can compete with the intrinsic heart rate, which can produce dysrhythmias, including ventricular tachycardia (VT) and ventricular fibrillation (VF).
      4. **Synchronous pacing.** Current generation depends on whether a previous current has been generated either by the heart or by the pacemaker and sensed by the pacemaker.
      5. **Pacing rate and magnetic rate.** The **pacing rate** is simply the rate at which the pacemaker generates impulses. Generation of impulses does not ensure that the impulses are conducted by the heart, or result in cardiac contraction. Electrocardiographic (ECG) monitoring and evaluation of vital signs are

Table 19-1. Pacemaker codes

Position I Chamber paced	Position II Chamber sensed	Position III Response	Position IV Program	Position V Antitachydysrhythmia function
O = none	O = none	O = none	O = none	O = none
A = atrium	A = atrium	T = triggered	S = simple	P = pacing
V = ventricle	V = ventricle	I = inhibited	M = multiple	S = shock
D = dual (A + V)	D = dual (A + V)	D = dual (T + I)	C = communicating	D = dual (P + S)
		R = rate modulation		

necessary for confirmation of cardiac activity. **Magnetic rate** is a preset pacing mode that results when a magnet is placed over the generator. The magnet closes a switch within the pacemaker that places it in a preset asynchronous mode.

6. **Demand pacing** is also known as **synchronous pacing.** The pacemaker can either generate (**trigger**) or withhold (**inhibit**) an impulse when a spontaneous current is sensed. Demand pacemaker can be a single-chamber demand or synchronous (**AAI, VVI, AAT, VVT**) or dual-chamber demand (**VDD, VAT, DDD, DVI**).

7. **Universal pacemakers (DDD)** can function in a number of ways, depending on the patient's underlying atrial or ventricular rate: **DVI** mode during sinus bradycardia with abnormal atrioventricular (AV) conduction, **VDD** sensing normal sinus rhythm with abnormal AV conduction, and **AAI** during sinus bradycardia with normal conduction.

8. **Rate modulation.** In pacemakers with a R (rate) programmed mode, the pacing rate varies in accordance with the patient's level of activity. This is accomplished through different sensing mechanisms, including respiratory rate, transthoracic impedance, or venous blood temperature. Because of false sensing, rate modulation should be disabled during surgery.

II. **Temporary pacing**

A. **Temporary pacing** may be indicated in patients with sinus node dysfunction, hemodynamically significant bradycardia, drug-induced bradycardia, and hyperkalemia-induced bradycardia. Temporary pacing is often used in the postcardiac surgical patient. Pacing also can be used in a burst mode (rapid short pacing) to terminate certain tachydysrhythmias such as atrial flutter (but not atrial fibrillation or ventricular fibrillation) and torsades de pointes. Pacing can be used to treat bradycardias associated with prolonged QT intervals.

B. **Temporary pacing** is done by transvenous, transcutaneous, transesophageal, or epicardial routes.

1. **Transvenous pacing** is most often done by placing a pacing catheter or wire within the right atrium, using an internal jugular or subclavian vein approach. AV pacing requires that two wires (leads) be placed. This is done by placing specialized pacing pulmonary artery catheters. One type has leads incorporated into the catheter. Another allows placement of atrial, ventricular wires, or both through ports in the catheter.

2. **Transesophageal pacing** is a simple technique for atrial pacing. It is unreliable for ventricular pacing.

3. **Transcutaneous pacing** is used most often in emergencies (e.g., hemodynamically significant bradycardias or asystole). For transcutaneous pacing, large electrodes are placed on the anterior and

posterior chest walls. Subsequently, a current of 50–100 mA is applied. As in all pacing modes, constant monitoring of the ECG is necessary to detect capture and effective pacing. Transcutaneous pacing can fail because of improper placement of the electrodes or severe metabolic disturbances. Many patients find the skeletal muscle stimulation that accompanies transcutaneous pacing to be quite painful. Sedation or analgesia is often required once hemodynamic stability has been achieved.

4. **Epicardial pacing** requires that pacemaker wires be placed directly on the myocardium. Most frequently, these are applied during open-chest cardiac operations (Chapter 36).

C. **Permanent pacing.** Generally accepted indications for permanent pacing include:

1. **After myocardial infarction** that results in:
   a. Second degree or complete AV blocks in the His–Purkinje system.
   b. Persistent block at the AV node for longer than 16 days.

2. **Sick sinus syndrome** with symptomatic bradycardia.

3. **Acquired AV block in adults:**
   a. Permanent or intermittent complete AV block that is irreversible.
   b. Symptomatic bradycardia with type II second degree AV block (irreversible).
   c. Symptomatic or asymptomatic type I second degree AV block.
   d. Exercise-induced second degree or complete AV block without reversible ischemia.
   e. Symptomatic first degree AV block that is improved by temporary pacing.

4. **Chronic intraventricular blocks:**
   a. Symptomatic bundle branch block with second degree or complete AV block.
   b. Symptomatic bifascicular block with complete AV block.
   c. Exercise-induced second degree or complete AV block without ischemia as a demonstrable cause.
   d. Trifascicular block during 1:1 AV conduction.

5. **Malignant vasovagal syndromes.** Recurrent syncopal events associated with carotid sinus stimulation in the absence of medications that slow AV conduction.

D. **Atrial versus ventricular pacing.** Advantages of atrial pacing include:

1. Maintains atrial contraction, which is especially important in patients with decreased left ventricular compliance.
2. Improves mitral and tricuspid valve function.
3. Preserves normal sequence of electromechanical activation.
4. Suppresses atrial and ventricular ectopy.

III. Management of patients with pacemakers

A. Pacemaker location and evaluation. Defining the underlying disease process by taking a thorough history is the most essential part of evaluating a patient who presents with a pacemaker. The mode in which a pacemaker is functioning can be discerned several ways.

1. Bedside **telemetric interrogation** of the pacemaker by a qualified cardiologist can reveal the specific settings, programmable functions, and the patient's dependence on pacemaker function. The pacemaker also can be reprogrammed telemetrically on a temporary or permanent basis.

2. If such information is not readily available, **evaluation of the ECG** may indicate the mode in which the pacemaker is functioning.

3. **A chest radiograph** can provide information such as the manufacturer, model, and serial number of the implanted unit. The information visible and the pacemaker's appearance on the radiograph can be referenced to text or computer databases containing specific information on various pacemaker models.

4. **Capture** (i.e., when each paced beat results in ejection) is determined by monitoring the ECG and gently palpating the carotid pulse. Asynchronous pacing (placement of a magnet) may be required to determine if the pacemaker is functioning.

5. **Random reprogramming can occur** as a result of electromagnetic interference. If this is suspected, the pacemaker should be interrogated in a timely fashion.

B. Pulmonary artery (PA) and central venous catheters should generally be avoided during the first 4 to 6 weeks after a transvenous pacemaker has been placed. Most permanent pacemakers are placed in the pectoralis major muscle and are connected to transvenous pacing leads. Until the epicardial attachment sites of the leads are secured by local fibrotic reactions, the leads could be dislodged by placement of a central venous or PA catheter. If such a catheter is required, it may be prudent to place it under fluoroscopic guidance. Abdominally placed pacemakers often have epicardial leads that are not in danger of being dislodged during placement of a PA or central venous catheter.

C. Sedation and anesthesia. Etomidate can produce myoclonus that may inhibit a demand pacemaker. The depolarizing neuromuscular blocking drug succinylcholine produces muscle fasciculations that also can inhibit synchronous pacing. Interference from muscle activity under anesthesia can be eliminated by administering a small dose of a nondepolarizing muscle relaxant. Other commonly used sedatives and anesthetics are considered safe in patients with pacemakers.

D. Microshock, or the unintended direct delivery of electrical current to the heart, is most likely to occur with external temporary pacemakers. Microshock can induce ventricular fibrillation with as little as 50 µA of current. Pacer wires should be properly insulated and kept away from external electrical sources. It has also been suggested to avoid touching pacing wires with bare hands as this also can induce microshock.

E. **Loss of pacing and pacemaker-induced fibrillation. Acute hypokalemia and alkalosis** can increase membrane potentials and result in loss of pacemaker impulse capture. Conversely, **acidosis and hyperkalemia** can cause a decrease in the membrane potential and, thus, lead to ventricular fibrillation. Recent **myocardial infarction** in the area where the leads contact the endocardium or epicardium can increase the membrane potential and also result in loss of capture.

F. **Defibrillating pacemaker patients.** Although insulation of modern pacemakers has improved, both external and internal defibrillation can seriously damage the pacemaker. External defibrillator paddles should not be placed directly over the pacing box.

G. **Magnetic resonance imaging (MRI).** Serious, unpredictable malfunctions of the pacemaker can occur during MRI. Pacemaker output or rate can increase or decrease unpredictably. Permanent damage to pacemaker components can occur. If MRI is considered essential, consider turning the pacemaker off temporarily, if tolerated by the patient.

IV. **Implantable cardioverter defibrillator (ICD)**

A. ICDs are used to treat patients who are at high risk for sudden death due to VT or VF. In all cases, these patients have survived an episode of VF or VT and have been resuscitated. Implantable cardioverter defibrillators greatly reduce the risk of sudden death in this high-risk group. Additionally, these patients usually have irreversible causes of their underlying dysrhythmia. These units are growing in their technologic sophistication. Some combine defibrillator functions with pacing functions. These units may include VVI pacing for bradycardia, antitachycardia pacing, and defibrillation. Although most older units used epicardial patches for defibrillation, newer units use transvenous leads and the unit itself can be one of the leads in the circuit (i.e., active can). The units are often placed subcutaneously over the pectoralis muscle or the anterior abdominal wall.

B. **An ICD unit senses ventricular fibrillation** by monitoring the rate of the intrinsic R wave. A 15 to 30 J countershock is delivered if a sustained tachycardia is detected. Most units will deliver approximately five contiguous shocks before they stop functioning.

C. **Management of patients with an ICD.** As with patients with pacemakers, a clear history of the underlying cardiac pathology and concomitant diseases is essential. Cardiomyopathies, valvular dysfunction, and coronary artery disease are common. These patients are susceptible to dysrhythmias. A bedside external defibrillator

should be present. As with pacemakers, external defibrillating pads should never be placed directly over the
ICD. Although concern exists that contact with a patient
whose ICD is discharging can cause VF in the bystander,
this particular complication has not been reported.

D. **Temporarily suspending VT and VF detection.**
With most units, the application of a magnet to the ICD
temporarily suspends VT and VF detection. With some
CPI brand (Guidant Cardiac Rhythm Management
Group, St. Paul, MN) units, however, the first application of a magnet will produce audible tones that correspond to the R wave, followed by a continuous tone,
which indicates that the unit is deactivated. Conversely,
when a magnet is applied to a deactivated CPI unit, a
continuous tone will be heard for 30 seconds, after
which tones that correspond to the R wave are heard, indicating that the unit is reactivated. Commonly, ICDs
are deactivated prior to surgical procedures, because
high-frequency interference from electrocautery units
can be interpreted as VT or VF by the ICD. The ICD
should be reactivated following surgery.

E. **MRI** can cause ICDs to malfunction. Because patients
with ICDs remain dependent on them to ensure detection and treatment of malignant dysrhythmias, they
should not enter a room with an MR magnet.

SELECTED REFERENCES

Atlee JL. *Cardiac pacemakers in perioperative cardiac dysrhythmias:
mechanism, recognition and management.* Chicago: Year Book
Medical Publishers, 1985.

Bartecchi CE, Mann DE. *Temporary cardiac pacing.* Chicago: Precept
Press, 1990.

Braunwald E, ed. *Heart disease, a textbook of cardiovascular medicine,* 5th ed. Philadelphia: WB Saunders, 1996:705–736.

Dreifus LS, Fisch C, Griffin JC, et al. Guidelines for implantation of
cardiac pacemakers and antiarrhythmia devices: a report of the
American College of Cardiology/American Heart Association Task
Force on Assessment of Diagnostic and Therapeutic Procedures. *J
Am Coll Cardiol* 1991;18:1–13.

Fitzpatrick A, Sutton R. A guide to temporary pacing. *BMJ* 1992;304:
365–369.

Simon AB. Perioperative management of the pacemaker patient.
Anesthesiology 1997;46:127–131.

The Acute Respiratory Distress Syndrome (ARDS)

Luca M. Bigatello

I. **The acute respiratory distress syndrome (ARDS)** remains a tremendous challenge to the intensivist. Although great progress has been made in understanding its pathophysiology, treatment remains largely supportive. Over the past 10 years, however, the mortality rate from ARDS has declined, possibly because of the overall progress of intensive care practice and novel treatments of acute respiratory failure.

II. **Epidemiology**

   A. **Definition** (Table 20-1). "ARDS" defines a syndrome of acute respiratory failure of diverse etiology, characterized by noncardiogenic pulmonary edema, hypoxemia, and diffuse lung parenchymal consolidations. Recently, the term **acute lung injury** has been added to ARDS to define an early stage of alveolar injury that may or may not subsequently evolve into acute respiratory distress syndrome.

   B. **Etiology.** Table 20-2 lists the most common causes of ARDS from both within and outside the lung. Infectious pneumonia, aspiration pneumonitis, and lung contusion are frequent **pulmonary causes.** Abdominal sepsis, acute pancreatitis, and trauma are common **extrapulmonary causes.** Given the protean clinical presentations of these causes, patients with ARDS can differ greatly from one another. Most patients with ARDS treated in a medical intensive care unit (ICU) suffer from underlying pneumonia, exacerbation of a respiratory disease, or a systemic infection. Surgical ICUs treat ARDS from trauma, lung contusion, burns, and abdominal sepsis. Recent work suggests that different "types" of ARDS (i.e., surgical vs. medical or pulmonary vs. extrapulmonary) exist, based on differences in the mechanical properties of the respiratory system, which can lead to different clinical courses.

   C. The **incidence** of ARDS in the United States has been estimated to be 150,000 cases per year (75/100,000 population). Recent studies worldwide suggest a lower annual incidence of 3 to 5/100,000 population. Despite this relatively small occurrence, the impact of ARDS on resource utilization in tertiary care referral centers can be significant, because these patients suffer from multiple acute medical problems and may receive intensive care and subsequent rehabilitation for prolonged periods of time.

   D. **Prognosis.** Survival from ARDS depends on a number of factors such as its cause, the patient's age, and co-

Table 20-1.   Definition of acute lung injury (ALI) and acute respiratory distress syndrome (ARDS), according to the American-European Consensus Conference on ARDS, 1994

1. Acute onset of respiratory distress
2. Hypoxemia: ALI: $PaO_2/FIO_2 \leq 300$ mm Hg
   ARDS: $PaO_2/FIO_2 \leq 200$ mm Hg
3. Bilateral consolidations on chest radiograph
4. Absence of clinical findings of cardiogenic pulmonary edema

morbid factors. Young, previously healthy trauma victims with isolated ARDS have a more than 90% chance of survival. ARDS in elderly patients with chronic disease, multiple organ dysfunction syndrome (MODS), and sepsis has a significantly poorer prognosis, with mortality rates greater than 50%.

E.   **Recovery.** The same categories of patients who enjoy higher survival rates from ARDS (young patients with low comorbidity) also have a meaningful recovery. Over the first 3 to 6 months following discharge from the ICU, lung function steadily improves, reaching a level of approximately 70% of normal, and allowing these patients to lead a productive life.

III.   **Pathogenesis.** ARDS is primarily an inflammatory phenomenon. Regardless of its site of origin within the body, the cause of ARDS triggers a systemic inflammatory response that can injure the lungs and other organs. Activated leukocytes release mediators that further amplify local and systemic inflammation. Many fundamental homeostatic systems of the body may be variably activated or inhibited in ARDS. These include the complement system, the coagulation cascade, the cyclooxygenase and leukotriene pathways, cytokines and chemokines, and the nitric oxide (NO): cyclic guanosine monophosphate (cGMP) pathway. Alveolar injury occurs

Table 20-2.   Common causes of the acute respiratory distress syndrome (ARDS)

1. **Direct lung injury:**
   Aspiration and other chemical pneumonitis
   Infectious pneumonia
   Trauma: lung contusion, penetrating chest injury
   Near drowning
   Fat embolism

2. **Distant injury:**
   Inflammation, necrosis, infection (sepsis syndrome)
   Multiple trauma, burns
   Shock, hypoperfusion
   Acute pancreatitis

from the toxic action of O_2 free radicals, proteolytic enzymes, thrombin, and adhesion molecules. **Mechanical ventilation** with large tidal volumes and high pressures can worsen alveolar injury by direct mechanical damage as well as by triggering the release of inflammatory mediators.

IV. **Anatomy**

A. Despite the many causes of ARDS, the lung tends to respond to acute injuries in a reproducible manner, generating an anatomic picture known as **diffuse alveolar damage (DAD).** The main characteristics of DAD are:

1. **Acute alveolar injury.** The initial injury involves both the endothelial and the epithelial side of the alveolocapillary membrane, which is an important factor in understanding the evolution of ARDS as a syndrome of both the airways and the pulmonary vasculature.

2. **Exudative phase.** Interstitial and alveolar edema develop from endothelial damage rather than from hydrostatic forces. The exudate, which contains plasma proteins, white and red cells, platelets, and coagulation factors, eventually lines the alveolar walls with hyaline membranes. Inactivation of the existent surfactant and production of abnormal surfactant can occur. Alveolar consolidation and collapse produce hypoxemia and reduce compliance, which are the early physiologic hallmarks of ARDS.

3. **Pulmonary vascular lesions.** Tissue injury and activation of the coagulation cascade result both in alveolar hemorrhage and in thrombosis of small arteries. Remodeling may later obliterate sections of the pulmonary vasculature. Vascular cross-sectional area loss, vasoconstrictor mediators, and **hypoxic pulmonary vasoconstriction (HPV)** may contribute to the onset of moderate **pulmonary artery hypertension,** which fosters the formation of pulmonary edema and can cause right ventricular overload.

4. **Proliferative phase.** Within approximately 7 to 10 days, the inflammatory infiltrate acquires chronic characteristics, with a predominance of macrophages, monocytes, and, eventually fibroblasts. The initial lesions heal by collagen deposition, leading to obliteration of air spaces and interstitial fibrosis. At times, fibroproliferative phenomena are particularly intense (**honeycomb lung**) and can limit recovery of respiratory function.

B. **Anatomic diagnosis.** The time course of injury varies among adjacent areas of the lung and among patients. Infection, either as a cause or a result of ARDS, complicates the anatomic and pathologic appearance. The efficacy of various therapeutic options can vary with the anatomic stage of ARDS. For example, alveolar recruitment with positive pressure may be effective on the initial, inhomogeneous pattern of injury, whereas corticosteroid therapy may be indicated later, when fibrotic changes occur. Estimating the stage of ARDS and ruling out infection may be impossible on clinical grounds and **open lung biopsy** is occasionally indicated.

V. Physiology. Hypoxemia and low lung compliance are hallmarks of ARDS.

A. Hypoxemia in ARDS is caused by alveolar consolidation and collapse. As ventilation decreases or completely ceases in different areas of the lung, partially or fully desaturated blood mixes with oxygenated blood. When true shunt (i.e., no ventilation) rather than ventilation-perfusion ($\dot{V}/\dot{Q}$) mismatch (i.e., low ventilation) is the main determinant of hypoxemia, as it is in ARDS, PaO_2 can be increased only through the recruitment of nonventilated alveoli. The degree of mixing of deoxygenated blood with arterial blood (**venous admixture**) can be measured with the **shunt equation** (Chapter 2). Hypoxemia in ARDS, in part, is attenuated by the physiologic response of **HPV,** which diverts pulmonary blood flow away from hypoventilated alveoli. HPV can be inhibited by local production of vasodilator substances (e.g., prostanoids and NO) during inflammation. It can also be blunted by the administration of vasodilators such as nitroglycerin and sodium nitroprusside. Such drugs should be used carefully in ARDS patients because they can worsen hypoxemia.

B. Vascular occlusion, airways overdistention, hypovolemia, and administration of bronchodilators can create areas of high $\dot{V}/\dot{Q}$ and true **dead space** (i.e., $\dot{V}/\dot{Q} = \infty$). An increased dead space to tidal volume ratio (V_D/V_T) hinders CO_2 elimination, increases ventilatory requirements and, with that, the possibility of alveolar injury from mechanical ventilation.

C. Low lung compliance. In the early phase of ARDS, diffuse alveolar edema, consolidation, and collapse decrease lung compliance. Because this injury is not homogeneous, the low compliance of early ARDS is really the average of the various mechanical characteristics of individual lung regions. Subsequently, remodeling of the injured lung parenchyma by collagen deposition and fibrosis results in a generalized decrease of compliance.

1. Low chest wall compliance occasionally occurs as a result of abdominal distension, massive trunk edema, circumferential burns, or tight chest bandages. In these cases, intrathoracic pressure can be estimated by means of an esophageal balloon, and lung and chest wall mechanics can be separated.

2. Measurement of respiratory compliance may be helpful in following the evolution of the syndrome and in testing the effect of changes of ventilatory settings (sections **VI.C.** and Chapter 2). Methods to assess static respiratory compliance deliver small incremental volumes to a sedated and fully relaxed patient. A series of inflations are used to compute a **pressure-volume (P-V) curve,** the slope of which

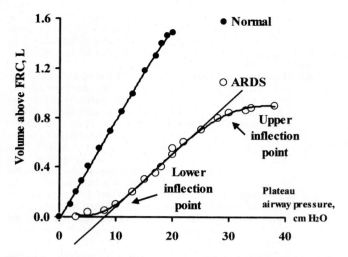

Fig. 20-1. Idealized compliance curves of the respiratory system. On the left, normal. On the right, in acute respiratory distress syndrome (ARDS), demonstrating the low compliance (reduced slope), a lower "inflection point" (suggested level above which to set positive end-expiratory pressure), and an upper "inflection point" (suggested level below which to set end-inspiratory pressure). (From Bigatello, LM and Zapol, WM, *Br J Anaesth* 1996;77:99–1096, with permission.)

is the compliance. Figure 20-1 shows compliance curves of a normal subject and an ARDS patient.

VI. Treatment of ARDS

    A. General measures. ARDS must be viewed as part of a systemic inflammatory injury, commonly associated with failure of other vital organs.

        1. Diagnosis and treatment of the underlying condition must be sought, even in times when the syndrome of respiratory failure dominates the clinical picture. Common etiologic factors are listed in Table 20-2.

        2. The hemodynamic management of patients with severe acute respiratory failure is controversial. The use of "supranormal" hemodynamics to enhance tissue O_2 delivery has not been proved to be efficacious. After adequate volume resuscitation, many clinicians prefer to restrict fluid administration to limit pulmonary edema. In general, it seems reasonable to base hemodynamic management on each patient's physiology, which can be complex and require invasive monitoring.

        3. Hemodynamic monitoring should be dictated by the patient's physiology and the clinician's expertise. An arterial catheter to measure systemic blood pressure and monitor arterial blood gas tensions is commonly used in severe acute respiratory failure. A pulmonary artery catheter may be useful to manage hemodynamic instability. Transthoracic or transesophageal echocardiography can complement the data of a pulmonary artery catheter and diagnose extrapulmonary shunts.

4. **Early treatment** of sources of inflammation and sepsis decreases later infection and hastens recovery. Early interventions include the drainage of abscesses, debridement of devitalized tissue, fixation of fractures, and grafting of burned tissue.

5. **Treatment of infections.** Appropriate antimicrobial therapy should be initially targeted to specific suspected organisms, and tailored as soon as possible to the results of pertinent cultures and antibiotic sensitivities. The appeal of broad-spectrum antibiotic coverage must be weighed against the potential for selecting resistant microbial flora.

   a. **Nosocomial pneumonia** occurs frequently in patients with acute respiratory failure (Chapter 28). Skillful airway management and measures to reduce the risks of aspiration (e.g., head-up position, adequate oral hygiene) may decrease the incidence of nosocomial pneumonia.

   b. Proper management of **intravascular catheters** includes the use of strict aseptic techniques and line removal when a blood-borne infection is suspected. Routine line changes, however, are not recommended.

6. **Nutrition** should be started early, because a prolonged stay in the ICU is likely. Enteral feeding is preferred (Chapter 8).

7. **Avoidance of iatrogenic complications.** All diagnostic and therapeutic decisions must be weighed in terms of benefits and risks. Iatrogenic complications during acute respiratory failure include O_2 toxicity, ventilator-induced lung injury, fluid overload, induction of bacterial resistance, and fungal overgrowth through the indiscriminate use of antimicrobial agents.

8. **Support of other organ systems function** is an integral part of the treatment of acute respiratory failure. Measures specific to ARDS patients include:

   a. **Hemodynamics** may need support because of preexisting cardiac disease or acute dysfunction from inflammation and sepsis. Right ventricular failure can occur as a result of myocardial depression or acute pulmonary hypertension (section **IV.A.3.**)

   b. **Renal function** can be supported by **continuous venovenous hemofiltration** even in the absence of overt renal failure (Chapter 23). Hemofiltration decreases total body fluid load and pulmonary edema while maintaining hemodynamic stability.

c. **Skeletal muscle** dysfunction occurs frequently during prolonged critical illness and mechanical ventilation and may be enhanced by neuromuscular blockade and corticosteroids. Adequate nutrition, physical therapy, and the proper use of neuromuscular blocking agents might avoid prolonged muscle weakness (Chapter 7).

d. **The gastrointestinal tract** is a reservoir of bacteria that may contribute to the evolution of MODS in critically ill patients. Adequate splanchnic perfusion and enteral feeding help protect the gastrointestinal mucosa and can decrease translocation of toxic microbial byproducts into the bloodstream.

B. Specific therapies

1. Antiinflammatory therapy

a. **Corticosteroids.** Several clinical trials of ARDS from all causes have found no benefit from early high-dose, short-term corticosteroid treatment. Recent clinical experience suggests that prolonged corticosteroid treatment can be efficacious in slowing the progression of the **late fibroproliferative phase** of ARDS. The main risk of this therapy is immunosuppression. Infection must be thoroughly ruled out before and during corticosteroid therapy.

b. **Immunotherapy.** A number of agents designed to block inflammation have been studied with disappointing results in critically ill patients. These include antiendotoxin and anticytokine antibodies, cytokine-receptor antagonists, and cyclooxygenase inhibitors (Chapter 27). Most trials included subgroup analysis on the development and the clinical course of acute respiratory failure and none proved efficacious against ARDS.

C. Mechanical ventilation

1. Ventilator-induced acute lung injury

a. The traditional approach to mechanical ventilation of ARDS included:

(1) Delivering large V_T (10–15 ml/kg) and positive end-expiratory pressure (PEEP) (10–20 cm H_2O) to recruit collapsed alveoli.

(2) Limiting the FIO_2 to minimize O_2 toxicity.

(3) Aiming for normal arterial blood gas tensions.

b. **This traditional philosophy has been challenged** because:

(1) Mechanical ventilation with high airway pressure and volume can severely damage the lung (**barotrauma**), particularly in the presence of alveolar injury. Trauma also may occur when the ventilating pres-

sure at end-expiration is too low and alveolar units must cyclically collapse and re-open during tidal ventilation.

    (2) Early ARDS is characterized by diffuse but **inhomogeneous lung injury** (Fig. 20-2), where alveoli with normal mechanical characteristics coexist with collapsed or consolidated alveoli. Recruitment with positive pressure or changes in body position (to redistribute positive pressure) converts collapsed alveoli into units suitable for gas exchange, but can also overdistend and damage normal alveoli.

  c. The ideal method of mechanical ventilation for these patients is still controversial, and **general recommendations are summarized in Table 20-3.**

2. **Limit transpulmonary pressure to 30 cm H_2O or less** when possible. This limit is the transpulmonary pressure at which alveolar overdistension occurs in normal lungs. In reality, it varies substantially from patient to patient and from time to time within the same patient. Limiting alveolar pressure may significantly decrease alveolar ventilation and it has become widespread practice to ac-

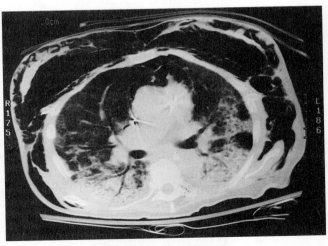

Fig. 20-2. High resolution chest computed tomography of a patient with early acute respiratory distress syndrome (ARDS). Note the inhomogeneous areas of consolidation, preferentially located in the dependent regions of the lungs, coexisting with normally aerated areas. Also note the massive subcutaneous emphysema, the peribronchial and pericardial air, and the subpleural loculated pneumothoraces, all consequences of barotrauma from mechanical ventilation.

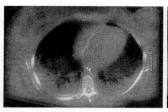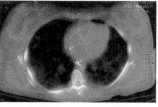

Fig. 20-3.   Portable chest computed tomography of a patient with severe acute respiratory distress syndrome (ARDS). On the left, the patient is ventilated on 20 cm H_2O positive end-expiratory pressure (PEEP). On the right, the patient is on 25 cm H_2O PEEP after a recruitment maneuver consisting of PEEP 40 cm H_2O, pressure control 20 cm H_2O, respiratory rate 10/min, inspiratory to expiratory (I:E) ratio 1:1 for 2 minutes. (Courtesy of Dr. Benjamin Medoff, Massachusetts General Hospital.)

cept an abnormally high $PaCO_2$ in patients with severe ARDS. This approach of **"permissive hypercapnia"** consists in allowing the $PaCO_2$ to rise slowly, as the arterial pH remains within reasonable limits through renal compensation or infusion of buffers such as sodium bicarbonate or tromethamine. Contraindications to permissive hypercapnia include increased intracranial pressure, right ventricular failure, and ongoing acidemia.

a.   Limiting airway pressure has not been uniformly shown to improve the course of ARDS. Hypoventilation can lead to alveolar derecruitment, and this strategy should be used in combination with **adequate lung expansion.**

b.   **Ideally,** an appropriate level of both end-expiratory and end-inspiratory airway pressure can be determined by performing a **static P-V curve** of the respiratory system (section **V.C.** and Fig. 20-1). The two "knees" of the sigmoid-shaped P-V curve may guide the choice of the necessary level of PEEP (above the "lower inflection point") and the safe level of end-inspiratory pressure (below the "upper inflection point"). If abnormal compliance of the chest wall is suspected, transpulmonary pressure can be estimated with the aid of an esophageal balloon.

c.   **In practice,** the correct performance of a static P-V curve is cumbersome because it requires a fully relaxed patient, precise measuring equipment, and considerable experience on the part of the operator. A simple and useful way to assess the appropriateness of a change in ventilator settings consists of assessing the effect of this change on the **semi-static compliance** of the respiratory system. Pressure-limited ventilation is ideal for this maneuver, because in this mode the flow at end-inspiration is zero or close to it and end-inspiratory pressure and volume are measured in nearly static conditions. For example, if increasing PEEP during pressure-limited ventilation increases V_T, then tidal ventilation is occurring on a steeper and more efficient portion of the compliance curve. When a further increase of PEEP decreases V_T, then ventilation probably is taking place on the more shallow upper portion of the compliance curve, and overdistention may be occurring. Aim to ventilate all patients on the steep and most efficient portion of the compliance curve.

3. **Recruitment maneuvers.** In patients with ARDS and severe hypoxemia, the application of a high level of continuous positive airway pressure (CPAP) for a short time (40 cm H_2O for 30 seconds) can expand areas of the lung that otherwise would remain collapsed and improve oxygenation (Fig. 20-3). High alveolar pressure, however, has the potential to cause **hemodynamic instability** and **lung damage.** Hence, these maneuvers should not be implemented in patients with normal lung compliance or in patients at increased risk for barotrauma because of bullae, air leaks, or tenuous suture lines within the lung parenchyma. Increasing levels of CPAP can be applied incrementally while observing their hemodynamic effects.

4. **Pressure-limited ventilation** often is recommended over volume-limited ventilation in ARDS. Although no controlled trial has shown a significant difference in outcome, pressure-limited ventilation has potential advantages:

   a. **The initial inspiratory flow rate is high and variable;** it depends on the capability of the ventilator, the patient's effort, and mechanical characteristics of the respiratory system. This inspiratory flow pattern mimics spontaneous ventilation and can allow more efficient ventilation.

   b. **The maximal airway pressure is reached early in inspiration** and then maintained throughout inspiration. This results in a decelerating inspiratory flow pattern, in contrast to the "square wave" flow pattern commonly used with volume-limited ventilation, in which the highest airway pressure is reached at the end of inspiration. Generally, the mean airway pressure during pressure-controlled ventilation is higher compared with a similar level of traditional volume-controlled ventilation. The higher mean pressure can improve alveolar recruitment and PaO_2.

D. **Ancillary ventilatory strategies.** Several additional therapeutic modalities are available to complement traditional mechanical ventilation. Although none has been proved universally effective, they can be considered for individual patients.

1. **Extracorporeal membrane oxygenation (ECMO)** provides a temporary "substitute" for transpulmonary respiration while severely injured lungs are allowed to rest and recover. Extracorporeal gas exchange techniques in adults remain confined to a few, highly specialized centers, for limited indications (Chapter 14).

2. **Exogenous surfactant.** Pulmonary surfactant often is dysfunctional in experimental models of aspiration pneumonitis and ARDS. Despite successful use of exogenous surfactant replacement therapy in newborns with respiratory distress, no clinical trials support the use of surfactant replacement in ARDS.

3. **High frequency ventilation (HFV)** delivers small V_T (2–3 ml/kg), at high rates (60–120 breaths/min) and at increased mean airway pressure. Proponents claim that HFV substantially limits barotrauma, but no controlled studies have confirmed this hypothesis.

4. **Inhaled NO** reduces pulmonary hypertension and increases PaO_2 in most patients with ARDS. Among its many functions, NO regulates vascular tone, neurotransmission, and immunomodulation. Small doses of NO administered by inhalation produce local selective vasodilation, decrease pulmonary hypertension, and improve $\dot{V}/\dot{Q}$ matching, with little acute toxicity. Inhaled NO reduces the necessity for ECMO in infants with acute respiratory failure. Controlled clinical trials in adults, however, have been unable to demonstrate a beneficial effect on outcome.

5. **Prone ventilation.** Delivering mechanical ventilation to patients placed in the prone position significantly increases PaO_2 in most ARDS patients. Generally, the PaO_2 improvement is maintained throughout the period of prone ventilation and fades at variable rates as the supine position is resumed. In centers experienced with this practice, patients are kept in the prone position for extended periods of time (e.g., 8 hours) and only temporarily turned supine for nursing care, physical examination, relief of skin pressure, and so on. How the prone position benefits gas exchange in ARDS is not fully understood. Although gravitational factors must play a role in redistributing ventilation to the previously collapsed dorsal areas of the lung, they do not fully explain the persistence of this effect as the prone position is maintained for pro-

Table 20-3.   Suggested algorithm for mechanical ventilation in patients with ARDS and other forms of severe respiratory failure

- Secure the airway and deliver positive-pressure ventilation with 5–10 cm H_2O PEEP
    - Obtain hemodynamic stability and patient comfort
    - Pursue diagnosis and therapy of the cause
        ↓
- Set FIO_2 to keep $SpO_2 > 90\%$ or $PaO_2 > 60$ mm Hg
        ↓
- With the ventilator in pressure-limited assist control mode, set pressure control and PEEP:
    - A. *Empiric* way (fast):
        - Set pressure control ≤ 20–25 cm H_2O ($V_T \approx 500$–600 ml) and respiratory rate aiming for a $PaCO_2$ and pH close to normal or mild respiratory acidemia.
        - Increase PEEP by 2.5 cm H_2O steps every 20–30 min, as long as SpO_2 and V_T increase or stay the same. Consider decreasing pressure control and increasing rate if the sum of PEEP and pressure control settings is ≥ 35 cm H_2O.
    - B. *Physiologic* way (slow):
        - Perform a static P–V curve of the respiratory system, and set PEEP and pressure control just above and below the lower and upper inflection points, respectively.
        - Reassess pressure control and PEEP settings daily.
        ↓
- If high ventilatory requirements persist (e.g., $FIO_2 > 0.6$, PEEP > 10 cm H_2O), consider:
    - A. Increasing sedation, considering neuromuscular blockade.
    - B. Recruitment maneuver.
    - C. Permissive hypercapnia.
    - D. Increasing inspiratory time.
    - E. Prone ventilation.
    - F. Inhaled NO.
    - G. If beyond 7 days of ARDS and no evidence of infection, consider corticosteroids.
        ↓
- If ventilatory requirements decrease and the patient is generally stable, consider:
    - A. Decreasing FIO_2 by 0.05–0.1 steps every 2–4 h, keeping $SpO_2 > 90\%$.
    - B. Discontinuing neuromuscular blockade, decrease sedation.
    - C. Decreasing I:E ratio toward $\approx 1:3$ (inspiratory time 1.0–1.5 s).
    - D. Decreasing respiratory rate to allow spontaneous ventilation.
    - E. Setting ventilator mode to PSV.

ARDS, acute respiratory distress syndrome; PEEP, positive end-expiratory pressure; PSV, pressure support ventilation.

longed periods of time. Other possible explanations include the triangular geometry of the human thorax, which would provide more effective ventilation in the prone position, and changes in chest wall compliance that limit overdistension of ventral areas of the lung and enhance ventilation of collapsed dorsal areas.

6. **Partial liquid ventilation.** In this somewhat futuristic modality of ventilatory support, the lungs are ventilated with perfluorocarbon, a fluid with high density and low surface tension that enhances recruitment of dependent lung regions, improves lung compliance, and favors the removal of airway secretions. Encouraging data have been reported in a small number of infants and children, and clinical studies are ongoing in adults.

SELECTED REFERENCES

American Thoracic Society. Round table conference. Acute lung injury. *Am J Respir Crit Care Med* 1998;158:675–679.

Artigas A, Bernard G, Claret J, et al. The American-European consensus conference on ARDS, Part 2. *Am J Respir Crit Care Med* 1998;157:1332–1347.

Ashbaugh DG, Bigelow DB, Petty TL, et al. Acute respiratory distress in adults. *Lancet* 1967;2:319–323.

Bigatello LM, Zapol WM. New approaches to acute lung injury. *Br J Anaesth* 1996;77:99–109.

Dreyfuss D, Saumon G. Should the lung be rested or recruited? *Am J Respir Crit Care Med* 1994;149:1066–1068.

Dreyfuss D, Saumon G. Ventilator-induced lung injury. *Am J Respir Crit Care Med* 1998;157:294–323.

Hall JB. Respiratory system mechanics in adult respiratory distress syndrome. *Am J Respir Crit Care Med* 1998;158:1–2.

Katzenstein A, Asken FB. Acute lung injury patterns: diffuse alveolar damage, acute interstitial pneumonia, bronchiolitis obliterans-organizing pneumonia. In: Katzenstein A, Asken FB, eds. *Surgical pathology of the non neoplastic lung diseases,* 2nd ed. Philadelphia: WB Saunders, 1990:9–56.

West JB, ed. Ventilation-perfusion relationships. In: *Respiratory physiology—the essentials,* 5th ed. Baltimore: Williams & Wilkins, 1995:51–69.

Chronic Obstructive Pulmonary Disease and Asthma

Kenneth E. Shepherd

I. **Introduction.** Patients with chronic obstructive pulmonary disease (COPD) and asthma have a wide spectrum of disease severity, which makes it impossible to give a detailed approach to the care of individual patients. This chapter discusses patients having moderate to severe stable or unstable obstructive lung disease requiring care in an intensive care unit (ICU). This chapter also provides a clinical guide to those patients with less severe lung dysfunction.

II. **Definitions.** The definitions below consider each disease process as an isolated entity. Although relatively pure forms of these processes occur, some degree of overlap is generally seen. Thus, many of the clinical findings and treatment modalities are similar. Nonetheless, the individual processes often differ in certain respects (e.g., cellular and inflammatory mediators, degree of reversibility) to warrant individual discussion.

    A. **COPD** is defined by the American Thoracic Society as a disease characterized by airflow obstruction caused by either emphysema or chronic bronchitis. The airflow obstruction is most often caused by cigarette smoking; it can be accompanied by airway hyperresponsiveness and may be partially reversible.

        1. **Emphysema** is anatomically defined as abnormal, permanent enlargement of the airspaces distal to the terminal bronchioles with accompanying destruction of the airspace walls.

        2. **Chronic bronchitis** is clinically defined as the presence of productive cough for at least 3 months in each successive year in a patient in whom other causes of chronic cough have been ruled out.

    B. **Asthma** is an inflammatory condition in which complex cellular, chemical, and nervous system (sympathetic, cholinergic, and nonadrenergic-noncholinergic) mediators lead to heightened bronchial responsiveness and episodic, variable, and reversible airway obstruction.

III. **ICU evaluation**

    A. **History**

        1. The general respiratory history should elicit specific symptoms about cough, sputum, hemoptysis, dyspnea, chest tightness or pain, wheezing, and exercise tolerance. Information on cigarette, occupational, environmental, and infectious exposures; previous diagnostic tests and diagnoses; symptoms of sleep disordered breathing; current medications; allergies (e.g., drug, environmental, food); and stability of clinical status should be obtained.

2.   The most important historical information to obtain from patients with COPD is exposure to cigarette smoke and environmental or occupational pollutants. The most important symptoms to elicit are coughing, sputum production, and wheezing.

3.   The most important background information in patients with asthma is cough, sputum, and wheezing. Additionally important are the presence of nocturnal or exercise-induced dyspnea, cough, or wheezing; diurnal or seasonal variability of symptoms; and hospitalizations (and treatments) for asthma.

B.   **Physical examination and vital signs**

1.   **Inspection.** Especially in patients with asthma, the upper respiratory tract should be assessed for **nasal polyps.** Polyps suggest that aspirin and other nonsteroidal antiinflammatory drugs may induce bronchospasm in the patient. Nasal polyps can complicate nasal intubation. Inflammation of the pharynx is suggestive of aspiration, postnasal drainage, or infection. Assess the mobility of the trachea and the skin for evidence of a previous tracheostomy that could cause upper airway obstruction or difficulty with translaryngeal intubation. The neck veins and use of accessory respiratory muscles should be assessed. In COPD, neck vein distention combined with upper extremity venous distention suggests superior vena cava obstruction (e.g., from lung cancer). The chest should be inspected for signs of previous or current surgery or trauma, kyphoscoliosis, and increased anteriorposterior diameter ("barrel-chest"). The extremities should be assessed for clubbing, cyanosis, and edema.

2.   **Palpation.** When the chest is hyperinflated, the cardiac apical impulse (normally in the left midclavicular line) can be displaced toward the xiphoid process. Simultaneous palpation of the chest and abdomen reveals the presence of thoracoabdominal dyssynchrony that can occur with respiratory failure.

3.   **Percussion.** Bilateral hyperresonance may indicate the presence of hyperinflation. Unilateral hyperresonance suggests pneumothorax.

4.   **Auscultation.** Compare breath sounds bilaterally for uniformity, intensity, and presence or absence of adventitious sounds. **Rhonchi** in the spontaneously breathing patient suggest large airway secretions, a frequent finding in chronic bronchitis. **Crackles** that begin in early inspiration, **a forced expiratory time greater than 4 seconds,** and **wheezing** during expiration suggest airway obstruction, bronchospasm, or both. **Inspiratory stridor** suggests upper airway obstruction.

5.   **Vital signs.** Tachypnea and **pulsus paradoxus** (i.e., a difference in systolic blood pressure between

expiration and inspiration) greater than 15 mm Hg suggests bronchospasm.

C. **Laboratory studies suggestive of COPD or asthma**
   1. **Chest x-ray**
      a. Hyperinflation of the lungs (flattened diaphragms with increased retrosternal air) with decreased vascular markings is characteristic of emphysema. With asthma, the chest x-ray film may show hyperinflation with normal or increased vascularity.
      b. Blebs and bullae are consistent with COPD.
      c. Other findings, such as tracheal narrowing, pulmonary edema, pneumothorax, or pleural effusions can be present, and, although not necessarily caused by asthma or COPD, can complicate these diseases in the ICU.
   2. **Electrocardiogram**
      a. Hyperinflation can cause low-voltage and poor R-wave progression.
      b. **Cor pulmonale** can manifest as right axis deviation, right ventricular hypertrophy, or right bundle branch block.
   3. **Arterial blood gas tensions** can be helpful to assess clinical status and guide respiratory therapies.
      a. A **partial pressure of oxygen (Pao$_2$)** less than 60 mm Hg while breathing room air indicates significant pulmonary dysfunction and the need for supplemental oxygen therapy. The Pao$_2$ may be normal in stable asthmatics but is often low in acute asthma. The Pao$_2$ is usually low in COPD.
      b. The **partial pressure of carbon dioxide (Paco$_2$)** is often lower than normal (< 40 mm Hg) during mild asthma attacks, normal in controlled asthma and emphysema, elevated in chronic bronchitis, and elevated in acute exacerbations.
      c. **Measurement of pH** in conjunction with the Paco$_2$ allows the assessment of the acuteness and severity of the acid-base status.
   4. **Pulmonary function tests (PFTs) measure pulmonary mechanics.** PFTs give an indication of functional reserve and airway responsiveness and may help guide management. **Peak expiratory flow,** measured with an inexpensive peak flowmeter, is commonly used to guide the management of asthma. A peak flow less than 50% of predicted indicates severe asthma.

IV. **ICU management**
   A. Individual factors that act in variable combinations to produce respiratory failure in COPD and asthma are listed below. In asthma, the primary focus is often on increased airway inflammation and tone.
      1. **Increased resistive and lung elastic loads**
         a. Upper airway obstruction from tracheal stenosis or edema.

   b. Bronchospasm.
   c. Airway edema and secretions.
   d. Increased functional residual capacity and dynamic airway collapse.
   e. **Intrinsic positive end-expiratory pressure (PEEP)** or **auto-PEEP** that leads to dynamic hyperinflation. In patients with expiratory airflow obstruction, expiratory airflow can continue until the beginning of the next inspiration. Alveolar pressure fails to return to zero at the end of expiration (intrinsic PEEP) and lung volume fails to return to its normal functional residual capacity (dynamic hyperinflation). The increased lung volume places an excessive demand on the inspiratory muscles that are already at a mechanical disadvantage from COPD.
   f. Infiltrative processes in the lung parenchyma such as edema and pneumonia.
2. **Increased chest wall load**
   a. Preexisting kyphoscoliosis or obesity.
   b. Splinting caused by surgical pain.
3. **Decreased respiratory muscle strength and endurance**
   a. COPD places the diaphragm at a mechanical disadvantage.
   b. Preexisting (e.g., myasthenia gravis) or acquired (e.g., critical illness polyneuropathy) neuromuscular disease.
   c. Neuromuscular blockade from drugs.
   d. Decreased substrate delivery (e.g., shock, anemia).
   e. Respiratory muscle metabolic abnormalities resulting from decreased levels of magnesium, potassium, phosphate, calcium, and malnutrition.
   f. Acute hypoxemia, hypercarbia, and acidosis with depressant actions on the diaphragm and heart.
4. **Depressed respiratory drive**
   a. Narcotics.
   b. Anesthetic agents.
B. **Hypoxemia**
1. Unless an untoward event occurs, the primary gas exchange abnormality in patients with COPD is ventilation-perfusion ($\dot{V}/\dot{Q}$) mismatching. The hypoxemia caused by $\dot{V}/\dot{Q}$ inequality responds well to supplemental oxygen. Careful oxygen administration seldom leads to loss of respiratory drive, and oxygen is essential to prevent end-organ dysfunction. Reversal of hypoxemia can improve respiratory muscle function and reverse pulmonary hypertension that could otherwise cause right ventricular failure.
2. **Oxygen** can be administered by nasal cannula or air entrainment mask. Most commonly, oxygen is

administered by nasal cannula at 1 to 2 L/min. The response to oxygen administration is evaluated by arterial blood gas analysis. Although pulse oximetry is useful, it must be remembered that it provides little information about carbon dioxide retention. The target PaO_2 is 55 to 60 mm Hg, which usually has little effect on carbon dioxide retention.

C. **Wheezing**
  1. **Some patients with COPD** gain dramatic improvements by treatment of airway obstruction. Because even small improvements in airway resistance can be of significant benefit, many patients with COPD and wheezing are treated with bronchodilators, antibiotics, and corticosteroids. Chest physiotherapy is also commonly used, although its role is limited to those patients who have difficulty with secretion clearance. Chest physiotherapy has a very limited role in the management of asthma.
      a. **Anticholinergics.** Parasympatholytics have a direct bronchodilating effect by blocking formation of cyclic guanosine monophosphate. As the site of bronchospasm in COPD is often in central airways, corresponding to parasympathetic innervation, these drugs, when administered by inhalation, are often effective in patients with COPD. Specific agents include ipratropium bromide and glycopyrrolate (Table 21-1).
      b. **Sympathomimetics.** Beta$_2$-adrenergic receptor agonists cause bronchodilation via cyclic adenosine monophosphate (cAMP)-mediated relaxation of bronchial smooth muscle. Only short-acting agents (e.g., albuterol) are indicated in the acute situation (Table 21-2). Long-acting drugs in this class (e.g., salmeterol) are never indicated for acute bronchospasm. The beta agonists are generally administered by inhalation but can be given intravenously. For example, epinephrine (0.25–2 μg/min by continuous infusion in the adult) is used when other measures have failed. Epinephrine can be used safely in these doses by the parenteral (intravenous) route, but the clinician should recognize the greater likelihood of dysrhythmias and other undesirable side effects in older patients.
      c. **Corticosteroids.** These drugs act via complex and incompletely understood mechanisms to reduce airway inflammation, airway responsiveness, mucus secretions, and edema. They enhance beta-adrenergic responsiveness and relax bronchial smooth muscle. Their use in the ICU has not been adequately studied. Inhaled corticosteroids (e.g., beclomethasone, budesonide, flunisolide, and triamcinolone) may be useful to control airway inflammation

Table 21-1. Common inhaled anticholinergic drugs

Drug	Brand name	Administration	Initial adult dose[a]	Interval (h)
Glycopyrrolate methylbromide	Robinul	Nebulizer (0.2 mg/ml)	2–4 ml	4–6
Ipratropium bromide	Atrovent	MDI (18 µg)	2–3 puffs	4–6
		Nebulizer (0.2 mg/ml)		

MDI, metered dose inhaler.

[a] Initial adult doses are for spontaneously breathing adults. Increased doses are required for patients who are tracheally intubated.

Table 21-2. Some common inhaled beta-$_2$-adrenergic drugs

Drug	Brand name	Administration	Initial adult dose[a]	Interval (h)
Albuterol	Proventil Ventolin	MDI (90 μg) Nebulizer (5 mg/ml) powder inhaler (200 μg)	2 puffs 0.5 ml 1–2 caps	4–6
Isoetharine mesylate	Bronkosol	MDI (340 μg) Nebulizer (10 mg/ml)	1–2 puffs 0.25–0.5 ml	4–6
Metaproterenol	Alupent, Metaprel	MDI (650 μg) Nebulizer (50 mg/ml)	2–3 puffs 0.2–0.3 ml	3–4
Racemic epinephrine	VapoNefrin, MicroNefrin	Nebulizer (22.5 mg/ml)	0.25–0.5 ml	1–2
Salmeterol	Serevent	MDI DPI (50 μg)	2 puffs 1 inhalation	12 12
Terbutaline	Brethaire	MDI (200 μg)	2–3 puffs	4–6

MDI, metered dose inhaler; DPI, dry powder inhaler.
[a] Initial adult doses are for spontaneously breathing adults. Increased doses are required for patients who are tracheally intubated.

and responsiveness in asthmatics to prevent exacerbation (Table 21-3). The inhaled route avoids some untoward metabolic, wound healing, and infectious events that are possible with systemic administration. A single prospective trial in patients with COPD in exacerbation provides support for their use (methylprednisolone, 0.5 mg/kg every 6 hours) in the ICU when bronchospasm is difficult to control. Whether this is the optimal dose for either COPD or asthma in the ICU patient is unstudied. Corticosteroid use should be based on individual clinical circumstances. Of note, replacement corticosteroid therapy may be needed in patients with a history of recent corticosteroid use who are not currently receiving intravenous methylprednisolone in sufficient doses to prevent acute adrenal insufficiency. The need for replacement therapy can be guided by laboratory tests (e.g., cosyntropin stimulation testing) and is influenced by patient characteristics, preoperative dosage, duration and route of therapy, type of surgical procedure, and the presence or absence of postoperative complications.

d. **Nebulizer versus inhaler.** The use of nebulizer or inhaler for delivery of inhaled medications is controversial. Both methods have been used effectively. During acute exacerbations, many patients have difficulty using the inhaler correctly and effectively. It is also difficult to deliver high doses with the inhaler. For severe asthma, continuous nebulization of beta-agonists may be required. The use of a holding chamber improves the performance of the inhaler in patients with poor hand-breath coordination. The holding chamber also decreases pharyngeal deposition, which is important when inhaled steroids are used. The use of inhaler or nebulizer during mechanical ventilation is also controversial and the choice of method is often determined by clinician or institutional preference.

e. **Methylxanthines** are weak bronchodilators; among them are theophylline and aminophylline (80% theophylline by weight). They can improve respiratory drive and muscle function, but this is controversial and their effect is slight. Their mechanisms of action are complex, multiple, and incompletely understood. These include nonspecific inhibition of phosphodiesterase to increase intracellular cAMP, blockade of adenosine, and release of endogenous catecholamines. They are administered intravenously (with or without a loading bolus) in the ICU and have a half-life of 3 to 4 hours

Table 21-3. Common inhaled steroids

Drug	Brand name	Administration	Initial adult dose[a]	Interval (h)
Beclomethasone	Beclovent, Vanceril	MDI (42 µg)	2 puffs	6–8
Budesonide	Pulmicort	DPI (200 µg)	1–2 inhalations	12
Dexamethasone	Decadron respihaler	MDI (84 µg)	3 puffs	6–8
Flunisolide	Aerobid	MDI (250 µg)	2 puffs	12
Fluticasone	Flovent	MDI (44, 110, 220 µg)	2–4 puffs	12
		DPI (50, 100, 250 µg)	1–2 inhalations	12
Triamcinolone	Azmacort	MDI (100 µg)	2 puffs	6–8

MDI, metered dose inhaler; DPI, dry powder inhaler.
[a] Initial adult doses are for spontaneously breathing adults. Increased doses are required for patients who are tracheally intubated.

(that is prolonged unpredictably in patients with right ventricular failure and with certain concomitant drugs). They can cause gastrointestinal symptoms such as nausea and more serious toxic reactions such as dysrhythmias and seizures. Thus, they have limited use. The clinical effectiveness of intravenous epinephrine is greater and the toxicity less than theophylline. Given the shorter half-life of epinephrine, we favor the careful infusion of epinephrine. When methylxanthines are used, clinical findings and serum levels should be followed closely with dosage adjusted accordingly, always keeping serum theophylline levels less than 20 µg/dl.

f. **Mucolytics** such as nebulized acetylcysteine or hypertonic saline may be indicated in selected patients to decrease the viscosity of mucus. Because they induce bronchospasm, they should be administered with inhaled beta$_2$-adrenergic agonists.

g. **Leukotriene receptor antagonists (zafirlukast) and synthesis inhibitors (zileuton)** are modestly effective for maintenance treatment of chronic asthma, but are inadequately studied in patients with either COPD or asthma in the ICU.

h. **Cromolyn and nedocromil** stabilize mast cells and can modulate the nonadrenergic noncholinergic nervous system. Neither is indicated in acute bronchospasm and, thus, is not indicated in the ICU.

i. Most patients with asthma or COPD with bronchospastic components to their disease can have their disease controlled with the medications outlined above with tolerable side effects. However, some cannot easily achieve this control (or have intolerable side effects). Such patients may have chronic inflammation accompanied by tissue injury and airway-wall remodeling. Medications such as **magnesium, cyclosporin,** and **methotrexate** are occasionally used in such patients. On occasion, **helium-oxygen ('heliox')** is used successfully to decrease airway obstruction caused by postextubation edema in patients with COPD or asthma. Heliox is also effective in reducing the work of breathing in some patients with acute exacerbation of asthma.

j. **Anesthetic agents** (e.g., intravenous propofol or ketamine) and inhaled volatile anesthetics (e.g., sevoflurane) are used on occasion as bronchodilators and to facilitate patient–ventilator interactions when the patient is intubated. Sedatives must be used cautiously when the patient is breathing spontaneously.

2. The approach to the treatment of **patients with asthma** in the ICU is as described for patients with COPD and wheezing. Some specific differences include the greater effectiveness of beta$_2$-adrenergic agonists and the reduced effectiveness of anticholinergics. Higher doses of corticosteroids to control exacerbations are used in asthmatics than in COPD patients. Inhaled corticosteroids seem to be more effective in decreasing airway inflammation and responsiveness in asthma than in COPD, possibly because of the differences in inflammatory cell and cytokine profiles in the two groups of patients.

D. **Infectious processes**

1. The airways of patients with COPD are often colonized with potential pathogens. In the ICU, these patients are at increased risk of acute respiratory failure from worsening of airway colonization, which can lead to more severe purulent bronchitis and possibly pneumonia. It sometimes may be appropriate to treat patients with acute COPD with antibiotics, despite having no evidence of parenchymal lung infection. Unless acute respiratory failure is clearly caused by the worsening bacterial colonization (e.g., excessive mucus secretions), the patient is often not treated with antibiotics. Attention is more properly directed to aspects of care such as pain relief and secretion clearance. The presence of a parenchymal infiltrate represents a different problem. The diagnosis of pneumonia versus bronchitis (often with edema or atelectasis) in the intubated, mechanically ventilated patient with COPD is not straightforward. Nonetheless, pneumonia is poorly tolerated in patients with advanced COPD. Early or preemptive antibiotic therapy is often the most prudent course for the critically ill patient with COPD.

2. Patients with asthma generally do not have chronic bacterial colonization of their airway. The approach to diagnosis and therapy is as outlined above. In the asthmatic patient with bronchospasm and mucus production, but without infiltrates on chest radiography, performing both a Gram's and a Wright's stain of sputum may differentiate acute infection from a noninfectious exacerbation of asthma.

E. **Pulmonary embolism**

1. Patients with COPD often have a hypercoagulopathy from bedrest and are at risk of pulmonary embolism. History, physical findings, laboratory findings (e.g., D-dimers), arterial blood gas measurements, electrocardiogram, chest radiograph, and ventilation–perfusion scintigraphy may help exclude or rule in this diagnosis. If the findings are nondiagnostic, pulmonary angiography may be indicated. Therapy must be highly individualized (Chapter 22).

   F.   Other causes of respiratory failure include cardiac disease (e.g., ischemia, infarction, failure, dysrhythmia), pneumothorax, pleural effusion, and upper airway obstruction (e.g., edema, inflammation, infection, tracheal stenosis). Cause-specific measures should be instituted promptly.

V.   Mechanical ventilation (Chapter 4)
   A.   Specific conditions sometimes requiring mechanical ventilation include respiratory acidosis, severe hypoxemia, retained secretions, atelectasis, pneumonia, laryngospasm, and upper airway edema. A suggested approach to mechanical ventilation of the patient with obstructive lung disease is shown in Figure 21-1.
   B.   Noninvasive positive-pressure ventilation (NPPV)
      1.   Compared with conventional therapy, controlled studies have reported reduced tracheal intubation rates and increased survival with NPPV. The greatest benefit for NPPV has been shown in patients with acute exacerbations of COPD.

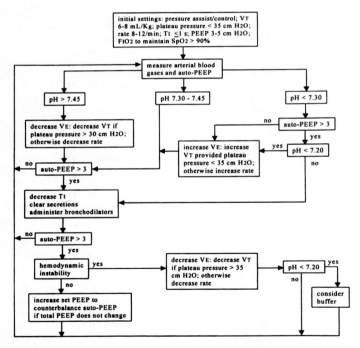

Fig. 21-1.   Suggested approach to mechanical ventilation of the patient with obstructive lung disease. (Adapted from Hess D, Medoff BD. Mechanical ventilation of the patient with chronic obstructive pulmonary disease. *Respir Care Clin N Am* 1998;4:439–473, with permission.)

2. NPPV should not be used if the patient requires an artificial airway for airway protection or secretion clearance.

3. Either **nasal or oronasal masks** can be used, but oronasal masks are preferred to avoid problems with mouth leak during acute respiratory failure.

4. Either critical care ventilators or portable pressure ventilators can be used to provide NPPV. Carbon dioxide rebreathing and supplemental oxygen administration are potential problems with portable pressure ventilators.

C. **Pressure versus volume ventilation**

1. **Volume ventilation** maintains a constant tidal volume during changes in airways resistance and lung compliance. The fixed inspiratory flow rate during volume ventilation can produce patient–ventilator dyssynchrony. The fixed tidal volume during volume ventilation can produce hyperinflation if auto-PEEP is present.

2. **Pressure ventilation** can improve patient–ventilator synchrony because flow varies with patient demand. Pressure ventilation also prevents hyperinflation if auto-PEEP occurs. The tidal volume will change with changes in airways resistance, respiratory system compliance, and patient effort.

3. **Inspiratory pressure–support ventilation** can produce an excessive inspiratory time in the patient with COPD, because a low inspiratory flow rate is required to cycle the ventilator to the expiratory phase. The patient may have to exhale actively against the ventilator breath to reduce the inspiratory flow rate and cycle the ventilator to exhalation. A simple way to correct this problem is to use pressure assist–control ventilation with a defined inspiratory time setting (e.g., 0.8–1.2 seconds).

D. **Mode**

1. **Synchronized intermittent mandatory ventilation (SIMV)** fails to completely relieve the patient's inspiratory efforts during both the mandatory breaths and the intervening unsupported breaths. This can produce fatigue and, therefore, this mode is not preferred.

2. **Assist–control ventilation** is preferred when respiratory muscle unloading is desired.

E. **Auto-PEEP**

1. **Auto-PEEP** is common during mechanical ventilation of patients with COPD and asthma.

2. **Auto-PEEP** is corrected by decreasing airways resistance (e.g., bronchodilator administration) or decreasing minute ventilation (e.g., permissive hypercapnia).

3. In patients with COPD, the addition of PEEP can counterbalance auto-PEEP and improve the patient's ability to trigger the ventilator. When this approach is used, care must be exercised to avoid further hyperinflation. PEEP often counterbalances

auto-PEEP in patients with dynamic airway closure (e.g., COPD). The effects of PEEP on other causes of auto-PEEP (e.g., asthma, high minute ventilation) are less predictable and more likely to exacerbate hyperinflation.

F. Weaning (Chapter 4)

1. Patients with COPD who fail a weaning trial quickly develop a pattern of **rapid and shallow breathing.** The most reliable weaning parameter is the **rapid shallow breathing index** [respiratory frequency (breaths/minute) divided by tidal volume in liters]. Weaning is more likely to be successful if the rapid, shallow breathing index is less than 100.

2. Several controlled studies have reported lower rates of successful weaning using SIMV compared with gradually tapering pressure–support ventilation or simply performing periodic trials of spontaneous breathing while otherwise providing assisted ventilation.

3. Patients should be regularly screened for weaning readiness: oxygenation, minute ventilation, hemodynamic stability, need for sedation, and rapid shallow breathing index.

4. If screening deems the patient ready for weaning, a trial of spontaneous breathing should be initiated. This can be performed with a T-piece, setting the ventilator to continuous positive airway pressure (CPAP) mode, or by using a low level of pressure support (5 cm H_2O).

5. If the patient tolerates 30 to 60 minutes of spontaneous breathing without signs of fatigue (e.g., tachypnea, tachycardia, increased accessory muscle use, diaphoresis), extubation should be considered.

SELECTED REFERENCES

Albert RK, Martin TR, Lewis SW. Controlled trial of methylprednisolone in patients with chronic bronchitis and acute respiratory insufficiency. *Ann Intern Med* 1980;92:753–758.

Alessandri C, Basili S, Violi F, et al. Hypercoagulability state in patients with chronic obstructive pulmonary disease. *Thromb Haemostasis* 1994;72:343–346.

American Thoracic Society. Hospital-acquired pneumonia in adults. *Am J Respir Crit Care Med* 1995;153:1711–1725.

American Thoracic Society. Standards for the diagnosis and care of patients with chronic obstructive pulmonary disease. *Am J Respir Crit Care Med* 1995;152:S77–S120.

Barnes PJ, Adcock I. Anti-inflammatory actions of steroids: molecular mechanisms. *Trends Pharmacol Sci* 1993;14:436–441.

Celli BR. What is the value of preoperative pulmonary function testing? *Med Clin North Am* 1993;77:309–325.

Corbridge TC, Hall JB. The assessment and management of adults with status asthmaticus. *Am J Respir Crit Care Med* 1995;151:1296–1316.

Crossley DJ, McGuire GP, Barrow PM, et al. Influence of inspired oxygen concentration on deadspace, respiratory drive, and $PaCO_2$ in intubated patients with chronic obstructive pulmonary disease. *Crit Care Med* 1997;25:1522–1526.

DeSouza G, deLisser EA, Turry P, et al. Comparison of propofol with isoflurane for maintenance of anesthesia in patients with chronic obstructive pulmonary disease: use of pulmonary mechanics, peak flow rates, and blood gases. *J Cardiothorac Vasc Anesth* 1995;9: 24–28.

Diaz O, Iglesia R, Ferrer M, et al. Effects of noninvasive ventilation on pulmonary gas exchange and hemodynamics during acute hypercapnic exacerbations of chronic pulmonary disease. *Am J Respir Crit Care Med* 1997;156:1840–1845.

Drazen JM, Israel E, O'Byrne P. Treatment of asthma with drugs modifying the leukotriene pathway. *N Engl J Med* 1999;340:197–206.

Falliers CJ, Tinkelman DG. Alternative drug therapy for asthma. *Clin Chest Med* 1986;7:383–391.

Fink JB, Tobin MJ, Dhand R. Bronchodilator therapy in mechanically ventilated patients. *Respir Care* 1999;44:53–72.

George RB, Light RW, Matthay MA. *Chest medicine,* 2nd ed. Baltimore: Williams & Wilkins, 1990.

Gladwin MT, Pierson DJ. Mechanical ventilation of the patient with severe chronic obstructive pulmonary disease. *Intensive Care Med* 1998;24:898–910.

Hess D, Medoff BD. Mechanical ventilation of the patient with chronic obstructive pulmonary disease. *Respir Clin North Am* 1998;4: 439–473.

Holleman DR, Simel DL. Does the clinical examination predict airflow obstruction? *JAMA* 1995;273:313–319.

Kass JE, Castriotta RJ. Heliox therapy in acute severe asthma. *Chest* 1995;107:757–760.

Keenan SP, Brake D. An evidence-based approach to noninvasive ventilation in acute respiratory failure. *Crit Care Clin* 1998;14:359–372.

Keenan SP, Kernerman PD, Cook DJ. Effect of noninvasive positive pressure ventilation on mortality in patients admitted with acute respiratory failure: a meta-analysis. *Crit Care Med* 1997;25:1685–1692.

Leatherman JW. Mechanical ventilation in obstructive lung disease. *Clin Chest Med* 1996;17:577–590.

Lesser BA, Leeper Jr KV, Stein PD, et al. The diagnosis of pulmonary embolism in patients with chronic obstructive pulmonary disease. *Chest* 1992;102:17–22.

Mansel JK, Stogner SW, Petrini MF, et al. Mechanical ventilation in patients with acute severe asthma. *Am J Med* 1990;89:42–48.

Manthous CA. Management of severe exacerbations of asthma. *Am J Med* 1995;99:298–308.

Manthous CA, Hall JB, Schmidt G, et al. The effect of heliox on pulsus paradoxus and peak flows in patients with severe asthma. *Am J Respir Crit Care Med* 1995;151:310–314.

Manthous CA, Schmidt GA, Pohlman A, et al. Heliox in the treatment of airflow obstruction: a critical review of the literature. *Respir Care* 1997;42:1034–1042.

Meduri GU, Mauldin GL, Wunderink RG, et al. Causes of fever and pulmonary densities in patients with clinical manifestations of ventilator-associated pneumonia. *Chest* 1994;106:221–235.

Rooke GA, Choi JH, Bishop MJ. The effect of isoflurane, halothane, sevoflurane and thiopental/nitrous oxide on respiratory system resistance after tracheal intubation. *Anesthesiology* 1997;86:1294–1299.

Schmidt GA, Hall JB. Acute or chronic respiratory failure. Assessment and management of patients with COPD in the emergency setting. *JAMA* 1989;261:3444–3453.

Shepherd KE, Hurford WE. Preoperative evaluation of the patient with pulmonary disease. In:Sweitzer BJ, ed. *Preoperative evaluation and management.* Philadelphia: Lippincott Williams & Wilkins, 2000:97–125.

Shepherd KE. Specific considerations with pulmonary disease. In: Hurford WE, Bailin MT, Davison JK, Haspel KL, Rosow C, eds. *Clinical anesthesia procedures of the Massachusetts General Hospital,* 5th ed. New York: Lippincott-Raven Publishers, 1997:35–46.

Warner DO, Warner MA, Barnes RD, et al. Perioperative respiratory complications in patients with asthma. *Anesthesiology* 1996;85: 460–467.

Williams TJ, Tuxen DV, Scheinskestel CD, et al. Risk factors for morbidity in mechanically ventilated patients with acute severe asthma. *Am Rev Respir Dis* 1992;146:607–615.

Pulmonary Embolism and Deep Venous Thrombosis

B. Taylor Thompson

I. **Overview.** Embolization of thrombus from the deep venous system to the pulmonary vascular bed results in a nonspecific clinical presentation that is frequently unrecognized. The estimated incidence of pulmonary embolism in the United States is 500,000 and the prevalence for nonfatal pulmonary embolism approaches 20/1,000 inpatients. Treatment with anticoagulants reduces mortality from 30% to 40% to 2% to 8%, primarily by preventing further emboli.

II. **Natural history**

A. **Deep venous thrombosis (DVT)** usually begins in the lower extremities, although occasional thrombi form in pelvic veins, renal veins, upper extremity veins, and the right ventricle. Most thrombi originate in the soleal veins of the calf near valve cusps or bifurcations. Calf thrombi can resolve spontaneously, and embolization to the lung is uncommon. Approximately 20% to 30% of clots propagate to the popliteal, femoral, or iliac veins (so-called proximal DVT), and an additional 10% to 20% of all DVTs begin in the thigh without prior calf involvement.

B. **Pulmonary emboli (PE).** Once in the pulmonary circulation, large emboli may lodge at the bifurcation of the pulmonary and lobar arteries, causing hemodynamic instability. Smaller emboli continue distally into small arteries or arterioles. The lower lobes are more often involved than the upper lobes and multiple emboli are usually present at the time of diagnosis. Only 10% to 20% of emboli cause infarction, usually in patients with preexisting cardiopulmonary disease.

III. **Risk factors for DVT and PE**

A. Prior venous thromboembolism.

B. Factors promoting stasis such as bed rest, congestive heart failure, or inactivity.

C. Endothelial damage such as lower extremity surgery or trauma.

D. Hypercoagulable states such as factor Leiden, prothrombin mutation, antithrombin III deficiency, lupus anticoagulant, and antiphospholipid antibody.

E. Malignancy. Approximately 15% of patients with venous thromboembolic disease who have no known risk factors for DVT or PE will have an occult malignancy diagnosed within 2 years.

IV. **Clinical manifestations**

A. **Symptoms and signs**

1. **DVT.** Many lower extremity venous thrombi are asymptomatic, probably because they remain non-

occlusive or because of the development of collaterals. Symptomatic thrombi classically produce calf pain, edema, venous distention, and pain on passive dorsiflexion of the foot (Homan's sign). These symptoms and signs are nonspecific. Prospective studies of outpatients with symptoms suggestive of DVT actually find DVT by objective testing in only a third of patients. In patients with leg symptoms suggesting DVT but in whom venography is normal, musculoskeletal injuries, Baker's cysts, and chronic lymphatic or venous insufficiency are the usual explanations.

2. **PE.** Autopsy series suggest that many pulmonary emboli are silent. When clinically apparent, symptoms and signs depend on the size of embolized material. Symptoms of small to medium emboli include dyspnea, chest pain, and cough. Tachypnea and tachycardia are present in most patients. Mild fever below 39°C is common. Wheezing occurs in less than 5% of patients. If infarction occurs, hemoptysis, pleuritic pain, and pleural rub are present. Massive emboli often produce cardiovascular findings. Symptoms include syncope, chest pain, and dyspnea along with signs of right ventricular dysfunction (e.g., a right ventricular heave, a right ventricular S_3, jugular venous distention, or a murmur of tricuspid regurgitation).

B. **Hemodynamic findings.** After pulmonary embolism, cardiac output is usually normal, but in hypotensive patients with massive pulmonary embolism the cardiac output is low. In this setting, right ventricular diastolic and right atrial mean pressures are always elevated. Pulmonary artery pressure tends to be increased but correlates poorly with the size of the embolus and may be normal even in cases of massive pulmonary embolism.

C. **Differential diagnosis.** Smaller pulmonary emboli can mimic pneumothorax, hyperventilation, asthma, myocardial infarction, congestive heart failure, pleurodynia, or serositis. If infarction is present, clinical findings can resemble pneumonia, bronchial obstruction by mucus or tumor, or pleural effusion. The differential diagnosis for massive pulmonary emboli includes right ventricular infarction, pericardial tamponade, and venous air embolism.

V. **Laboratory evaluation**

A. **The electrocardiogram (ECG)** is often abnormal in small to medium pulmonary emboli, but findings are nonspecific. The ECG is normal in 23% of patients with submassive embolism, and in 6% of patients with massive pulmonary embolism.

B. **Chest radiography.** Even without infarction, radiographic abnormalities occur in most patients with pulmonary emboli, including elevation of a hemidiaphragm, atelectasis, and effusion. An infarct classically appears as a pleural-based infiltrate with a convex margin directed toward the hilum.

C. **Noninvasive studies for DVT. Color-flow Doppler** with compression ultrasound (referred to as venous ultrasound) has high sensitivity (89% to 100%) and specificity (89% to 100%) in comparison with venography for the detection of proximal DVT, and slightly less sensitivity and specificity for calf vein thrombi. Venous ultrasound is also useful for the detection of a Baker's cyst. Sensitivity falls dramatically when venous ultrasonography is used for asymptomatic, high risk patients (33%). **Impedance plethysmography (IPG)** also offers high sensitivity, slightly less specificity, and lower cost in comparison with venous ultrasound. IPG is not accurate for the detection of calf vein thrombi.

D. D-dimers are usually present in the serum of patients with pulmonary emboli, but are nondiagnostic. However, a level below 500 U/ml has a high negative predictive value of 91% (95% confidence: interval 77% to 98%). Because the rapidly available and inexpensive red cell agglutination assay is negative below a level of 500 D-dimer units/ml, a negative test makes DVT or PE unlikely, particularly in patients with low pretest probabilities for PE.

E. **Lung scintigraphy.** Perfusion lung scans are performed by injection of radiolabeled albumin macroaggregates or microspheres. Scans are sensitive; a negative perfusion scan virtually excludes pulmonary embolism (Table 22-1). Results are also nonspecific. Because pulmonary arterioles constrict in response to hypoxia, perfusion defects, especially if nonsegmental, may be secondary to a ventilatory abnormality and not to obstruction of flow by an embolism. Perfusion scans may be abnormal in atelectasis, asthma, chronic airways obstruction, or other causes of regional hypoventilation. A large multicenter study (PIOPED) of the accuracy of ventilation perfusion scans compared with pulmonary angiography suggested that multiple segmental or larger perfusion defects, not matched by ventilation defects, are fairly consistent with the presence of pulmonary emboli and have a false–positive finding rate of about 14%. Most patients with a high probability lung scan and a negative angiogram have either chronic pulmonary emboli or cancer with vascular involvement. Multiple subsegmental perfusion defects that are matched by ventilation defects are uncommonly associated with pulmonary emboli with a false–negative finding rate of 15%. The combination of clinical probability assessments and lung scan probability assessments are complementary (Table 22-1).

F. **Noninvasive diagnostic approach.** Unfortunately, many of the clinical and scan probabilities fall in the nondiagnostic zone (low or intermediate). In such patients, noninvasive assessment for DVT may be helpful. If venous ultrasound is positive for DVT, then the

Table 22-1. PIOPED: percent with pulmonary emboli

Scan category	Clinical science probability (%)		
	High	Intermediate	Low
High	95	86	56
Intermediate	66	28	15
Low	40	15	4
Near normal through normal	0	6	2

From the PIOPED Investigators. Value of the ventilation/perfusion scan in acute pulmonary embolism. Results of the prospective investigation of pulmonary embolism diagnosis (PIOPED). *JAMA* 1990;263:2753–2759.

indication and rationale for anticoagulation therapy are the same as for confirmed pulmonary embolism. More than a third of patients with angiographic evidence of PE have negative leg studies for DVT. Such patients either have false–negative findings for leg studies, thrombi that originated from calf vein thrombi that were missed by noninvasive leg studies, a source of emboli other than the legs, or the entire lower extremity clot burden embolized in one clinical event.

G. **Outcome studies.** The safety of withholding anticoagulation in patients with suspected pulmonary embolism (low or moderate suspicion), nondiagnostic lung scans, and negative serial leg studies (over 2 weeks) has recently been shown in a large, five-hospital outcome study. Substituting a single negative D-dimer for serial leg studies in this approach was supported in a parallel study of the same cohort.

H. **Pulmonary angiography.** Despite the advantages of noninvasive techniques, a significant proportion of patients require angiography to confirm or exclude pulmonary embolism with certainty. Angiography is the definitive diagnostic technique in this disease. It is performed by injecting radiocontrast dye into a pulmonary artery branch after percutaneous catheterization, usually transfemorally. The injection catheter should be advanced at least into the right or left pulmonary arteries to achieve good dye concentration in the pulmonary vessels. A positive result consists of a filling defect or sharp cutoff of small vessels. The procedure carries a mortality rate of less than 0.5%. Morbidity occurs in about 5%, usually related to catheter insertion and contrast reactions.

I. **Contrast spiral computed tomography (CT)** appears to have 60% to 80% sensitivity for pulmonary emboli lodged in segmental or larger vessels and 80% to 95% specificity. High specificity requires reader expertise, and emboli in smaller vessels are not reliably detected with this technique.

    J. **Magnetic resonance angiography (MRA)** has high sensitivity and specificity. Limited emergency availability of MRA and the appropriate monitoring for unstable patients in the scanner are potential limitations.

VI. **Prophylaxis for DVT and PE**

    A. **High risk** patients include those immobilized or at bed rest and who have:

        1. **Severe head injury** (Glasgow Coma scale ≤ 8).

        2. **Severe blunt chest** or **abdominal injury.**

        3. **Pelvic fractures.**

        4. **Severe lower extremity injuries.**

        5. **Selected burns,** especially electrical burns.

    B. **Relatively immobile patients** should receive prophylaxis, if possible, if they have additional risk factors such as:

        1. **Previous history of DVT or PE.**

        2. **Obesity.**

        3. **Aged more than 60 years.**

        4. **Presence of femoral venous catheter.**

        5. **Pregnancy.**

        6. **Cancer.**

        7. **Marginal cardiopulmonary reserve.**

    C. **Prophylaxis includes nonpharmacologic and pharmacologic measures.**

        1. **Elastic stockings and sequential compression boots** are routine, but their efficacy appears marginal. Increasing patient mobility reduces venous stasis and the formation of DVT. Usually, these measures should be supplemented by pharmacologic prophylaxis.

        2. **If no contraindication to anticoagulation exists,** consider administration of continuous intravenous heparin, followed by oral coumadin in high risk patients (section **VII**).

        3. **If a mild to moderate risk of bleeding exists, subcutaneous heparin** (in the adult, 5,000 U every 12 hours, or every 8 hours for patients > 100 kg) or **dalteparin** (Fragmin; 5,000 U subcutaneously, once daily) can be administered.

        4. **If anticoagulation is contraindicated,** periodic systematic screening for DVT with venous ultrasound (section **V.C.**) should be conducted. This is usually performed twice a week in high risk patients.

        5. **If surveillance cannot be adequately performed,** consider prophylactic placement of an **inferior vena caval filter** in high risk patients (section **VII.E.**).

VII. **Treatment**

    A. **Unfractionated heparin**

        1. **Dose.** The constant intravenous infusion of unfractionated heparin is the current standard of care for most patients with DVT or PE. A bolus of 75 U/kg

should be followed by approximately 18 U/kg/h in most patients. An activated partial thromboplastin time (aPTT) of 1.5 to 2.5 times the mean laboratory control should be achieved within 24 hours, and this should correspond to a heparin level of 0.2 to 0.4 U/ml in plasma. Fatal recurrences on anticoagulant therapy usually happen within the first week after diagnosis; failure to reach a therapeutic aPTT increases the risk for recurrence or extension of DVT tenfold.

2. **The duration** of heparin therapy should be 5 to 7 days, with 5 days of overlap with warfarin. For massive PE and ileofemoral thrombosis, a longer period of heparin therapy may be considered.

3. **Complications.** Hemorrhage is the major complication of heparin therapy, occurring in approximately 1% of patients per day after the first day. Heparin can also cause thrombocytopenia (3% to 4%) with or without thrombosis (see Chapter 12).

4. **Contraindications.** Absolute contraindications to heparin are intracranial bleeding or tumors, active gastrointestinal bleeding, retroperitoneal hemorrhage, proliferative retinopathy with hemorrhage, heparin-associated thrombocytopenia, and malignant pericarditis. A known bleeding diathesis and recent surgery are relative contraindications.

B. **Fractionated or low molecular weight (LMW) heparins** (such as dalteparin) are derived from unfractionated heparin and have smaller molecular weights. They are typically administered by subcutaneous injection, have more predictable dose–response characteristics than unfractionated heparin, and can be given without the need for monitoring of an anticoagulant effect. They are equally effective and possibly safer than unfractionated heparins. LMW heparins currently are approved in the United States only for prophylaxis, but will probably also soon receive approval for treatment. Importantly, **spinal or epidural hematomas** have been associated with spinal or epidural anesthesia and lumbar punctures in patients receiving fractionated heparins or heparinoids. The risk of epidural hematoma formation is increased in patients who have indwelling epidural catheters or are also receiving other drugs that may adversely affect hemostasis.

C. **Oral anticoagulants**

1. **Onset of action.** Because the antithrombotic effect of warfarin is caused by prothrombin (factor II) depletion, and because it takes roughly 5 days for prothrombin to fall to an effective antithrombotic level (roughly 20% of normal), warfarin should not be used alone in the acute setting.

2. **Monitoring.** An international normalized ratio of 2.5 should be targeted for most patients.

3. **Treatment duration.** A 6-week course of warfarin is sufficient for calf vein thrombosis; a course of 3 to 6 months is recommended for patients with proximal DVT and for patients with PE. Idiopathic venous thrombosis is likely to recur even after 6 months of warfarin (2-year incidence up to 27%) and 6 to 12 months of anticoagulation are reasonable in this setting. Life-long anticoagulation is considered for recurrent episodes or a first event with a nonreversible risk factor such as cancer, homozygous factor V Leiden carriers, or antiphospholipid antibody syndrome.

D. **Thrombolytic therapy**

1. **Indications.** Thrombolytic therapy is approved for proximal DVT and massive pulmonary emboli (filling defects in 2 or more lobar vessels or emboli causing hemodynamic instability). Some authors recommend lytic therapy for those with echocardiographic evidence of right ventricular dysfunction during acute embolization. Because mortality is similar and complications are less with heparin, we favor the use of thrombolytic therapy only for acute massive PE with hemodynamic compromise.

2. **The objective** of thrombolysis for DVT is complete and rapid removal of thrombus and preservation of venous valvular function, leading to a reduction in postphlebitic complications. Severe postphlebitic complications (e.g., edema, pain, and ulceration) are probably reduced with streptokinase compared with heparin, but the effect is small. The objective of use of thrombolytic agents for pulmonary embolism is to accelerate clot lysis, reduce pulmonary artery pressure, improve right ventricular function, and improve survival. Although no reduction in mortality has been shown in comparison with heparin in large prospective series, a recent smaller study of tissue-type plasminogen activator (tPA) suggested a survival advantage with lysis, although the heparin dosing schedule was suboptimal. Thrombolytic therapy may allow improved pulmonary function after recovery, and a recent long-term follow-up study has suggested improved exercise tolerance 7 years after thrombolysis.

3. **Contraindications.** Absolute contraindications include intracranial bleeding, or a strong possibility thereof, or other major bleeding. Relative contraindications are recent (10 days) surgery or trauma.

4. **Choice of thrombolytic agent.** The three thrombolytic agents currently approved for the treatment of pulmonary embolism and their recommended doses and costs are shown in Table 22-2. Conclusive data do not currently suggest that any one of these agents is either more effective or safer than another.

Table 22-2.   Choice of thrombolytic agents for pulmonary embolism

Drug	FDA approved dose	Alternative dose	Cost
Streptokinase	250,000 U × 20 min, 100,000 U/h × 24–72 h	1,500,000 U × 1 h	$350
Urokinase	4,400 U/kg bolus, 4,400 U/kg/h × 12 h	3,000,000 U × 2 h	$2,000– 2,700
tPA	100 mg × 2 h	0.6 mg/kg × 3–15 min	$2,000– 4,200

tPA, tissue plasminogen activator.

Urokinase and tPA are expensive. Streptokinase is antigenic in humans and reacts with antistreptococcal antibodies. tPA appears to be as effective as other thrombolytic agents in the treatment of pulmonary embolism, but it is not necessarily safer at the currently recommended doses. Three recent studies of weight-adjusted bolus dosing of tPA (0.6 mg/kg over 3–15 minutes) show similar efficacy but no reduction in bleeding complications.

   5.   Complications. Bleeding complications correlate poorly with coagulation parameters but are increased by performing invasive procedures. Patients in whom thrombolytic therapy is considered should have procedures performed in distal vessels, if possible. As many as one third of patients treated with streptokinase develop mild fever, and a smaller percentage have allergic reactions, usually manifested by urticaria, itching, or flushing. Hypotension can occur in approximately 10% of patients, which limits the use of this agent in unstable patients.

E.   Inferior vena caval filters. If anticoagulation is strongly contraindicated, or if emboli recur despite adequate anticoagulation, an inferior vena cava interruption procedure should be performed to prevent further embolization from leg or pelvic veins.

F.   Pulmonary embolectomy. The utility of emergency pulmonary embolectomy for massive pulmonary embolus is uncertain. Of those who die from emboli, 80% do so in the first hour. Only rarely can an embolectomy be accomplished in this time frame. Mortality during thromboembolectomy is extremely high (57% in emergency procedures and 25% in semiurgent procedures). Randomized comparison with thrombolytic therapy has not been performed. Transvenous catheter embolectomy or catheter fragmentation can be considered as an alternative to operative embolectomy in nonsurgical candidates.

SELECTED REFERENCES

Anand SS, Wells PS, Hunt D, et al. Does this patient have deep vein thrombosis? *JAMA* 1998;279:1094–1099.

Becker DM, Philbrick JT, Selby JB. Inferior vena cava filters. *Arch Intern Med* 1992;152:1985–1994.

Goldhaber SZ, Haire WD, Feldstein ML, et al. Alteplase versus heparin in acute pulmonary embolism: randomized trial assessing right-ventricular function and pulmonary perfusion. *Lancet* 1993; 341:507–511.

Goldhaber SZ. Contemporary pulmonary embolism thrombolysis. *Chest* 1995;107:45S–51S.

Gulba DC, Schmid C, Borst HG, et al. Medical compared with surgical treatment for massive pulmonary embolism. *Lancet* 1994;343: 576–577.

Hirsh J. Heparin. *N Engl J Med* 1991;324:1565–1574.

Hyers TM. Venous thromboembolism. *Am J Respir Crit Care Med* 1999;159:1–14.

Kearon C, Ginsberg JS, Hirsh J. The role of venous ultrasonography in the diagnosis of suspected deep venous thrombosis and pulmonary embolism. *Ann Intern Med* 1998;129:1044–1049.

Kearon C, Julian JA, Math M, et al. Noninvasive diagnosis of deep venous thrombosis. *Ann Intern Med* 1998;128:663–677.

Koning R, Cribier A, Gerber L, et al. A new treatment for severe pulmonary embolism: percutaneous rheolytic thrombectomy. *Circulation* 1997;96:2498–2500.

Meyer G, Tamisier D, Sors H, et al. Pulmonary embolectomy: a 20-year experience at one center. *Ann Thorac Surg* 1991;51:232–236.

Price DT, Ridker PM. Factor V Leiden mutation and the risks for thromboembolic disease: a clinical perspective. *Ann Intern Med* 1997;127:895–903.

Stein PD, Terrin ML, Hales CA, et al. Clinical, laboratory, roentgenographic and electro-cardiographic findings in patients with acute pulmonary embolism and no pre-existing cardiac or pulmonary disease. *Chest* 1991;100:598–603.

The PIOPED Investigators. Value of the ventilation/perfusion scan in acute pulmonary embolism. Results of the prospective investigation of pulmonary embolism diagnosis (PIOPED). *JAMA* 1990;263: 2753–2759.

Wells PS, Ginsberg JS, Anderson DR, et al. Use of a clinical model for safe management of patients with suspected pulmonary embolism. *Ann Intern Med* 1998;129:997–1005.

Renal Disease

Adam Sapirstein

I. **Introduction**
   A. **Overview of renal disease in the intensive care unit (ICU).** In health, the kidneys excrete metabolic wastes and maintain homeostasis of the body's fluid volume and composition. **Acute renal failure (ARF)** remains a relatively common complication in critically ill patients. Patients who have **chronic renal failure (CRF)** are at increased risk for further loss of renal function during critical illness. Patients with **end-stage renal disease (ESRD)** can become functionally anephric and require hemodialysis. This chapter focuses on the diagnostic and management strategies for patients with ARF and discusses principles that are generally applicable to the care of all patients with renal disease who are critically ill.
   B. **Acute renal failure** is characterized by a rapid deterioration in renal function that results in the accumulation of nitrogenous wastes and an imbalance of fluids and electrolytes. Up to 5% of hospitalized patients and approximately 20% of patients in the ICU will develop ARF. The magnitude of the problem is best indicated by the fact that the associated mortality of renal failure in the ICU is between 30% and 50%.

II. **Pathogenesis and natural history**
   A. **ARF** is a multifactorial disease that is often reversible. The infectious and inflammatory conditions that often affect patients in the ICU play a role in the pathogenesis of acute renal injury, but we have only a rudimentary understanding of this process.
   B. **Ischemic ARF** frequently is used as a model for the pathogenesis of renal failure. Injury occurs first at the proximal tubules where disrupted cellular metabolism and enzyme activation result in membrane alterations, a loss of epithelial cell polarity, and eventually cell death. The loss of epithelial integrity results in back diffusion of solute and water. Debris from dead and infiltrating inflammatory cells causes obstruction of the tubular lumen that leads to the formation of tubular casts. Tubular obstruction decreases glomerular filtration rate (GFR) and increases back pressure, which leads to a further decline in renal blood flow.
   C. **Natural history.** The initiation phase of ARF is followed by the maintenance phase of renal failure in which a marked decrease in GFR and a steady increase in the serum concentrations of urea nitrogen and creatinine occurs. Patients can be oliguric or have normal urinary outflow during this time. Assuming recovery

of renal function, the duration of this phase varies from days to weeks depending on the degree of injury. The maintenance phase of ARF is followed by the recovery phase in which both renal functional parameters and urine flow return to normal.

III. **Causes of ARF.** The causes of ARF are classified as **prerenal, intrarenal** (intrinsic), and **postrenal.** This is an important classification because different causes require different therapies.

A. **Prerenal causes.** Hypovolemia, or decreases in the functional circulating blood volume as occurs in sepsis, is a frequent occurrence in the critically ill patient. Advanced age, atherosclerotic disease, diuretics, and nonsteroidal antiinflammatory drug use all predispose to prerenal failure. Prompt recognition and treatment of the underlying cause usually restores renal function; ongoing renal hypoperfusion, however, will result in intrinsic renal injury.

B. **Intrinsic causes**

1. **Tubular necrosis** is the most common cause of ARF in the critically ill patient (~ 85%). Advanced age, trauma, hypotension, sepsis, and preexisting renal disease are predisposing conditions.

   a. **Ischemia and reperfusion injury** (50% of cases) is the most common cause of perioperative renal failure. Operations involving the abdominal aorta or those using extracorporeal circulation have increased risk for the development of this complication.

   b. **Toxins** are responsible for about 35% of the cases of acute tubular necrosis. Critically ill patients are frequently exposed to nephrotoxins such as aminoglycoside antibiotics, amphotericin B, myoglobin (after crush or burn injuries), hemoglobin (from hemolysis), intravascular radio-contrast agents, and cisplatin.

   c. **Interstitial nephritis** (10% of cases) may be a hypersensitivity reaction seen in response to sulfonamides, nonsteroidal antiinflammatory drugs, or penicillins. Autoimmune diseases and infections can also present as interstitial nephritis. Fever, rash, eosinophilia, and eosinophiluria are suggestive of this diagnosis. Discontinuation of the inciting drug usually resolves the renal failure.

   d. **Acute glomerulonephritis** (5% of cases) is a rare cause of ARF, but needs to be considered because prompt immunosupressive therapy may be indicated.

C. **Postrenal causes.** Urinary tract obstruction can be caused by bilateral ureteral obstruction, unilateral obstruction of a single functioning kidney, or bladder outlet obstruction. Although not a common cause of ARF, it should be considered because it is readily treated by decompression. The degree of renal injury is proportional to the duration of obstruction. Common causes of obstruction include bladder, prostatic, or cervical cancers; prostatic hypertrophy; intraureteral crystal or myeloma light chain deposition; and neurogenic bladder obstruction.

D. **Specific causes** of ARF that frequently occur in the ICU include:

1. **Sepsis.** A major precipitating cause of renal failure, the pathogenesis is likely to be multifactorial and includes cytokine toxicity and disruption of systemic and regional hemodynamics.

2. **Amphotericin B.** The traditional formulation of amphotericin B and sodium deoxycholate at therapeutic doses will cause a reproducible increase in serum creatinine concentration (Chapter 27). Pretreatment with intravenous (IV) saline is recommended when possible because it ameliorates the fall in GFR caused by amphotericin B treatment. For patients with established CRF or those at high risk for developing ARF, newer formulations of amphotericin B within a lipid vehicle are available (ABELCET, The Lipsome Co., Princeton, NJ; Amphotec ALZA Corp., Mountain View, CA; AmBisome, Gilead Sciences, Foster City, CA). These lipid-based formulations appear to have an equivalent efficacy to amphotericin B with sodium deoxycholate, but they greatly reduce nephrotoxicity. Their primary disadvantage at this time is their high cost and unproved benefit in defined clinical situations.

3. **Liver failure.** Most cases of renal failure associated with hepatic failure likely are secondary to alterations in renal and systemic hemodynamics. The **hepatorenal syndrome** produces a unique form of renal failure that can progress to acute tubular necrosis (ATN) (Chapter 24). Blood flow to the kidney is not compromised and structural injury is not observed.

4. **Hemolytic uremic syndrome.** This can be caused by toxins produced by *Escherichia coli* in diarrheal illnesses or it can be associated with other diseases such as transplanted graft rejection or malignant hypertension. The diarrheal form is most common in pediatric patients and patients with the human immunodeficiency virus (HIV) infection. The treatment is largely supportive, but infusion of fresh frozen plasma (FFP) and plasmapheresis has been suggested to limit renal failure in the nondiarrheal form of the disease.

5. **Renal vascular emboli.** Large emboli usually produce flank pain and hematuria. Microvascular emboli are often silent.

6. **HIV-associated nephropathy.** The acquired immune deficiency syndrome (AIDS)-associated nephropathy is characterized by proteinuria, glomerulosclerosis, and rapidly deteriorating renal function that leads to ESRD in several weeks.

Acute tubular necrosis can develop because of co-morbid conditions or from direct nephrotoxicity. The hemolytic uremic syndrome is also more frequent in HIV-infected patients.

7. **Disseminated intravascular coagulation (DIC)** and **vasculitis** are common in critically ill patients, but infrequently cause renal failure.

IV. **Evaluation of patients with ARF.** The first sign of renal failure is often oliguria; the diagnosis, however, needs to be considered whenever serum creatinine increases significantly.

A. **History and physical examination** should attempt to determine current fluid status and identify possible initiating events.

1. **Recent fluid losses and administration** should be estimated and the fluid balance calculated.

2. **Daily weights** give an indication of the total body water balance, but are poorly reproducible in the ICU setting. Measurement of patient weight is often imprecise and total body water correlates poorly to intravascular volume of the critically ill patient.

3. **Intravascular volume is assessed** to determine the presence of signs of hypervolemia (e.g., jugular venous distention) or hypovolemia (e.g., tachycardia, hypotension). Invasive measurements of central vascular pressures (e.g., central venous pressure, pulmonary capillary occlusion pressure) and cardiac output are often necessary (Chapter 1).

4. **Response** to an IV fluid challenge frequently differentiates early ARF from prerenal azotemia. In most patients, this can be done safely by infusing 250 to 500 ml of normal saline or lactated Ringer's solution over 15 minutes. Increases in blood pressure, cardiac output, or urine output suggest a temporary repletion of intravascular volume and point to a prerenal cause.

B. **Evaluation of the urine.** Urinalysis and determination of the urine indexes are simple and rapid tests that provide useful diagnostic information. A summary is found in Table 23-1.

1. **Urine dipstick.**

a. **Proteinuria** is usually associated with glomerular lesions, but may also be seen with tubular injury. Glomerular injury permits large proteins to pass into the urine as indicated by a reading of 3+ to 4+ on dipstick testing. Tubular injury of ATN can prevent the normal reabsorption of small, filtered proteins as indicated by mild proteinuria of 1+ to 2+.

b. **Blood positive dipstick** tests, without red blood cells in the urinary sediment, suggest **hemoglobinuria** or **myoglobinuria.** The former is associated with pink plasma, whereas the supernatant of a centrifuged blood sample will be clear in the case of myoglobinemia.

Table 23-1. Diagnostic studies and indexes of urine

	Prerenal	Renal	Postrenal
Dipstick	0 or trace protein	Mild—moderate protein, hemoglobin, leukocytes	0 or trace protein, red and white cells
Sediment	Few hyaline casts	Granular and cellular casts[a]	Crystals and cellular casts possible
Urine osmolality	>500	<350	<350
Urine/serum plasma creatinine	>40	<20	<20
Urine/serum plasma urea	>8	<3	<3
FE_{Na}	<1%	>1%	>1%

FE_{Na}, fractional excretion of sodium; $FE_{Na} = (U_{Na}/P_{Na}) \div (U_{cr}/P_{cr})$.
[a] Composition of casts depends on cause of renal failure (see text).

2. **Microscopic examination** of the urine sediment provides insight into the pathogenesis of ARF. Tubular casts are an indirect indication of ongoing processes in the kidney.

   a. **Hyaline casts** are acellular and are consistent with prerenal azotemia.

   b. **Granular casts** contain degenerating renal tubular epithelial cells and may indicate a process of ARF caused by ischemic or nephrotoxic injuries. The casts typically are pigmented in hemoglobin- and myoglobin-induced renal failure.

   c. **White blood cell casts** indicate an inflammatory process and may be seen in pyelonephritis and acute interstitial nephritis.

   d. **Red blood cell casts** indicate glomerular pathology (e.g., glomerulonephritis).

3. **Diagnostic indexes**

   a. **Oliguria from prerenal causes** has urine that reflects intact renal mechanisms of salt and water balance. The urine is highly concentrated and the urine-to-plasma ratios of creatinine and urea are increased.

   b. **Disruption of tubular function** in ARF usually produces a defect in urinary concentrating ability and the production of isotonic urine. The fractional excretion of sodium (FE_{Na}) will be increased (Table 23-1).

   c. **Specific limitations of urinary indexes**

      (1) **Preexisting renal disease** can affect salt and water homeostasis, which makes interpretation of urine electrolytes difficult.

      (2) **Diuretic administration** blocks tubular reabsorption of solute and can complicate data interpretation for up to 24 hours.

      (3) **Nonoliguric ATN** can present with a normal FE_{Na}, particularly in the early phase of the disease.

      (4) **Early urinary tract obstruction, acute glomerulonephritis, or renal emboli** can present with decreased GFR with normal tubular function. Highly concentrated urine is expected in this setting.

C. **Imaging techniques** generally are used to exclude reversible urinary tract obstruction or traumatic injury.

   1. **Ultrasonography** is the most valuable tool in the initial evaluation of obstruction. It can be performed at the bedside in unstable patients.

   2. **Radiographs** of the abdomen assess kidney size and shape and may demonstrate renal urinary calculi, if present.

3. **Intravenous pyelography** is indicated only for the evaluation of renal trauma and has no role in the diagnosis of ARF.

4. **Antegrade and retrograde pyelography** can be used to pinpoint the urinary tract obstruction and to accomplish drainage.

5. **Computed tomography (CT)** and magnetic resonance imaging are frequently obtained as part of an evaluation of intraabdominal pathology. They can provide detailed anatomic information on the kidneys, bladder, and urinary collecting system.

6. **Radionuclide studies** may be useful to assess renal perfusion.

D. **Renal biopsy** is not indicated in most cases because history, physical examination, and noninvasive testing will indicate the cause of the renal failure. Biopsy may be indicated in cases of intrinsic ARF not caused by ischemia or toxins and to determine the cause of graft dysfunction after renal transplantation. The morbidity of renal biopsy is relatively low.

V. **Management of ARF**

A. **Prophylaxis.** Extensive and conflicting literature is found regarding the use of prophylactic measures to reduce the occurrence of ARF in populations at risk. Experimental evidence has suggested benefit from the use of diuretics such as mannitol and furosemide. Other potential strategies include the use of dopamine, calcium channel blockers, and volume loading prior to an ischemic or nephrotoxic insult. Unfortunately, none have been proved to be of benefit in prospective human studies. Despite limited supporting evidence, the use of prophylactic measures in certain clinical settings seems justified by experimental data and clinical experience.

B. **Therapy for established ARF.** Therapy begun after acute renal failure occurs is aimed at decreasing the maintenance phase of renal failure and improving the chance of functional recovery.

1. **Diuretic therapy** has received considerable attention in the literature and is of benefit in some models.

a. Diuretics are proposed to limit injury by maintaining urine flow, thus preventing tubular obstruction and its sequelae. Human studies have not supported this theory.

b. Although spontaneous nonoliguric renal failure has a lower mortality rate than oliguric renal failure, it is not clear that diuretic induction of urine flow improves outcome. Many nephrologists believe that diuretic responsiveness is simply a marker of less severe renal injury.

c. Diuretics, and in particular **the combination of furosemide and mannitol,** can convert some cases of oliguric renal failure to nonoliguric failure. Clinically, furosemide (in doses of up to 3 g/d) has been used for this purpose. At the Massachusetts General Hospital, a continuous IV infusion of 2 mg/ml furosemide in 20% mannitol often is started at a dose of 10 mg/h for this purpose.

2. **Vasoactive drugs** have long been postulated to be beneficial because of a belief that altering renal blood flow and GFR might improve outcome.

   a. Vasoactive drugs have both systemic and renal effects. It is not possible to attribute clinical effects to one system or the other.

      (1) Dopamine, calcium channel blockers, and atrial naturietic peptide have been used to improve renal hemodynamics.

      (2) Vasopressors such as norepinephrine have been used to increase renal blood flow in settings of systemic hypoperfusion.

   b. Whereas animal models have shown the expected effects of these therapies on renal perfusion, patient-based studies have not convincingly demonstrated any improvement. Some studies have shown increased morbidity related to these therapies.

3. **Recommendations.** It is reasonable to attempt to improve both urine flow and renal hemodynamics. The failure of many studies to demonstrate clinical benefits from the use of any pharmacologic adjuvants in intrinsic renal failure, however, and the potential of these agents to exacerbate injury, suggest the following recommendations.

   a. Systemic hemodynamics and central blood volume should be optimized prior to initiating any specific renal therapy.

   b. Because the morbidity of ARF is high and volume management of the oliguric patient is difficult, measurement of central vascular pressures and cardiac output should be used to guide fluid therapy. After assessment and treatment of systemic hemodynamics, diuretics can be used in an attempt to treat oliguria.

C. **Specific agents**

1. **Mannitol** is an inert sugar that is freely filtered at the glomerulus and is not reabsorbed; thus, it causes an osmotic diuresis even in the presence of hypovolemia. Mannitol also dilates the renal vasculature and increases renal blood flow, an effect mediated in part by renal prostaglandins. Mannitol is a free radical scavenger at high doses, but this effect is unlikely to be important at clinically relevant dosing. Mannitol may be beneficial in several specific situations.

   a. **Prevention of ARF in transplanted kidneys.** The incidence of ATN following cadaveric renal transplant is between 20% and 40%.

Hydration and infusion of mannitol prior to removal of a donor kidney may reduce graft injury.

b. **Hemoglobinuria and myoglobinuria** usually are treated by inducing a brisk diuresis and alkalinizing the urine. This is usually accomplished by infusing a solution of 5% dextrose in half-normal saline (D5-1/2NS) to which 40 mEq/L of sodium bicarbonate and 10 g/L of 20% mannitol is added.

c. **Interruption of renal blood flow,** as occurs during aortic cross-clamping or circulatory arrest, often is treated prophylactically with mannitol (12.5–25 g IV).

2. **Loop diuretics,** of which **furosemide** is the most widely used, differ from other classes of diuretics because they increase renal blood flow. Furosemide often is used in combination with mannitol in attempts to convert oliguric to nonoliguric renal failure.

3. **Dopamine** is a naturally occurring catecholamine with actions mediated through dopamine, alpha, and beta-adrenergic receptors.

a. **Dopamine receptor-mediated effects** are believed to predominate at low dose infusions (1–4 µg/kg/min), whereas escalating doses additionally lead to β-adrenergic receptor and then α-adrenergic receptor mediated effects. At low doses, dopamine produces renal and splanchnic vasodilation with a resultant increase in renal blood flow and GFR.

b. **Diuresis and naturesis** produced by dopamine is believed to be mediated both through direct renal effects and its hemodynamic actions.

c. **Warnings** against the use of dopamine as either a prophylactic or a therapeutic option have been voiced.

(1) **β-adrenergic effects** can cause dangerous tachycardias.

(2) **Effects on the splanchnic circulation** can cause "splanchnic steal" and bowel ischemia in susceptible patients.

d. Currently, dopamine often is used as an adjuvant therapy for refractory oliguria.

VI. **Management of the complications of ARF.** In health, the kidneys maintain normal intravascular volume, osmolality and pH; eliminate excess potassium, phosphorous, magnesium, many pharmacologic agents and endogenous wastes; and produce hormones that are important in the maintenance of normal levels of serum calcium and the production of erythrocytes. A variety of problems arises when the kidneys do not function normally.

A. **Volume overload**

1. An average human requires approximately 500 ml fluid each day to carry nonvolatile solute. Fluid in-

take is offset by urinary, gastrointestinal, wound, and insensible losses. In patients with renal failure, the inability to balance fluid intake by urinary elimination can lead to volume overload.

2. Most patients in the ICU require the administration of fluid volumes in the form of drugs and nutrition that are far in excess of the volume required to carry solute.

3. Treatment options to minimize the risk of or treat fluid overload include:

    a. Induce diuresis. Fluid management often can be facilitated in renal failure when an oliguric condition responds to diuretic therapy. Forced diuresis should never be attempted until prerenal oliguria has been excluded.

    b. Minimize excess fluid administration.

        (1) Use low flow, constant flush systems on pressure-monitoring catheters and infusion pumps for IV administration.

        (2) Concentrate drugs to their solubility or safety limits.

        (3) Avoid any unnecessary fluid administration (e.g., convert medications to enteral formulations whenever practical).

    c. Dialysis or hemofiltration inevitably will be required in the anuric patient or when conservative therapy fails.

B. Hyponatremia is most often the result of excessive antidiuretic hormone (ADH) secretion, but can also develop as a result of defective concentrating mechanisms in renal failure. The first line of treatment in either of these cases is fluid restriction (< 800 ml/d) but this may be impractical. Treatment with normal saline and a loop diuretic may be necessary (Chapter 26).

C. Metabolic acidosis results from the body's production of organic acids.

1. Organic acids are normally produced at a rate of 1 mEq/kg/d, but production can be greatly increased in catabolic, critically ill patients. Serum bicarbonate can decrease at a daily rate of 2 mEq/L or more.

2. Treatment is usually not necessary until the bicarbonate concentration falls below 15 mEq/L.

3. Overaggressive correction of acidosis can precipitate acute hypocalcemia and tetany because of the rapid lowering of ionized calcium levels by bicarbonate.

4. Management

    a. Sodium bicarbonate (40–80 mEq/d) can usually maintain pH within the normal range.

    b. Dialysis may be necessary when the acid load is very high or when volume overload or hypernatremia limits the amount of sodium bicarbonate that can be safely administered.

      c. **Hyperventilation** can be used as a temporizing measure in patients receiving mechanical ventilation.

      d. **Sedation and neuromuscular blockade** can decrease the contribution of muscular activity to acid production.

D. **Hyperkalemia** is a potentially life-threatening complication of ARF.

    1. **Electrocardiographic (ECG) changes** may be diagnostic. Peaking of the T waves and shortening of the QT interval usually are the earliest changes, followed by prolongation of the PR interval and a decrease in the amplitude of the P wave. As hyperkalemia progresses, depression of the ST segment and widening of the QRS complex follow, eventually producing a sinusoidal waveform.

    2. **Treatment** depends on the degree of hyperkalemia and the severity of ECG changes. A widened QRS complex is an indication for prompt treatment with IV calcium, bicarbonate, glucose, and insulin. Less pronounced changes such as T-wave peaking can be managed with the more slowly acting cation exchange resins.

    3. **Specific treatment guidelines**

      a. **Calcium gluconate** (15–30 mg/kg IV) or calcium chloride (5–10 mg/kg IV), administered over 2 to 5 minutes, directly antagonizes the effect of potassium on the myocardium.

      b. **Sodium bicarbonate** (50–100 mEq IV) partly reverses the acidosis and will cause a redistribution of potassium into cells. In mechanically ventilated patients, hyperventilation can be used to create a respiratory alkalosis, which will have the same effect.

      c. **Glucose and insulin** [1—2 ampules of 50% glucose (dextrose) in water and 10 U of regular insulin IV] should be given over a 5-minute period. Redistribution of potassium into cells occurs within minutes.

      d. **Sodium polystyrene sulfonate (Kayexalate)** is a sodium-potassium ion exchange resin given via the gastrointestinal tract that directly removes potassium from the body. Approximately 1 mEq of potassium is exchanged for each 1 mEq of sodium per gram of sodium polystyrene sulfonate; Kayexalate (25–50 g in 100 ml of a 20% sorbitol solution) can be given orally or as a retention enema. Because of its slow rate of potassium removal, it should not be used as sole therapy for life-threatening hyperkalemia.

      e. **Dialysis** is indicated for the urgent treatment of life-threatening hyperkalemia.

E. **Hypermagnesemia** is rarely seen in renal failure, except when supplemental magnesium, such as in some antacids, is administered.

F. **Hyperphosphatemia** is common in ARF. Although phosphorous has no toxic effects, in excess it decreases serum calcium concentration. Phosphorous binding antacids (Amphojel, AlternaGEL) usually are given to decrease plasma phosphorous levels and maintain calcium levels within a normal range. Overuse of antacids can produce hypophosphatemia.

G. **Anemia** in patients with ARF has many causes. **Erythropoietin,** produced by the kidney, stimulates erythrocyte production within the bone marrow. Absence of this hormone likely contributes to anemia in ARF. Erythropoietin therapy is used routinely for patients with chronic renal failure, but is not used for treatment of anemia in ARF.

H. **Altered mental status** with renal failure results from retention of endogenous wastes.
   1. **Manifestations** range from tremor, myoclonus, asterixis, and frank seizures to lethargy, disorientation, and coma.
   2. **Dialysis** usually results in improvement of mental status when obtundation is caused by uremia.
   3. Many other metabolic derangements and drug effects can contribute to encephalopathy in critically ill patients (Chapter 29).

I. **Decreased drug elimination.** Many drugs are eliminated by the kidneys, including several neuromuscular blocking agents and potentially toxic drugs such as aminoglycoside antibiotics and digoxin. The dosages of renally excreted drugs must be adjusted when renal function is impaired. It should be remembered that in early ARF, the serum creatinine concentration does not fully reflect the reduction in GFR.

J. **Uremic pericarditis** occurs for unknown reasons. Cardiac tamponade and infective pericarditis are potential complications. Patients should be examined daily for the presence of a pericardial friction rub, and cardiac tamponade should be considered if unexplained cardiovascular decompensation occurs. Pericarditis may be an indication for emergency dialysis.

K. **Bleeding abnormalities** are common in patients with renal failure and are generally attributed to abnormal platelet function. **Management** of bleeding problems (Chapter 12) can include:
   1. **Dialysis** often temporarily corrects platelet abnormalities, but also can activate complement and platelets and exacerbate a coagulopathy.
   2. **Desmopressin acetate (DDAVP)** (0.3–0.4 µg/kg) IV, subcutaneously, or intranasally may improve platelet function in uremic patients.
   3. **Conjugated estrogen** therapy produces a long-lasting improvement in the bleeding tendency of uremic patients.

L. **Infectious complications** are responsible for most of the deaths in patients with ARF. The ability to fight infection is impaired with uremia and the usual manifestations of infection can be blunted.

M. Nutritional support is an important ancillary measure in critically ill patients with ARF (Chapter 8).

  1. Providing adequate nutritional support for these patients is complicated by the need for volume restriction and the concern that supplemental protein can result in the production of additional nitrogenous wastes.

  2. Carbohydrates have a protein-sparing effect. Nutritional supplements, when administered with essential amino acid preparations, can be provided that do not significantly increase serum urea nitrogen concentration.

  3. Enteral nutrition is preferred to parenteral nutrition, when possible.

  4. Continuous renal replacement therapies permit an increased volume of feedings with less concern of volume overload. Renal replacement therapies also eliminate nutrients as they do wastes. Glucose is usually infused with the replacement fluid and amino acid solutions can be increased to account for the loss.

VII. Management of patients with CRF

  A. These patients often have problems related to cardiovascular disease, advanced age, and diabetes mellitus.

  B. Vascular access complications are common in patients with ESRD and the need for nephrectomy, transplantation, and urologic reconstructive surgeries increases the need for perioperative care. Studies have suggested that up to one third of patients on chronic dialysis require major operations during a 3-year period.

  C. Specific concerns related to CRF.

   1. Volume status. Maintenance of adequate intravascular volume forms the cornerstone of hemodynamic management in patients with CRF. Careful monitoring of intake and output and frequent measurement of central vascular pressures and cardiac function are used to ensure adequate circulatory stability.

   2. Hyperkalemia can result from tissue trauma, metabolic acidosis, ischemic injuries, and infections. Early intervention is indicated if hyperkalemia develops (see section **VI.D.**)

   3. Infections are more common because of immunosupression. Problems with wound healing and infections are frequent.

VIII. Renal replacement therapy (RRT) refers to techniques that utilize a semipermeable membrane to remove waste from the blood of a patient. The most familiar example of RRT is **intermittent hemodialysis (HD).**

  A. Indications for RRT

   1. Traditional indications include treatment of uremic syndrome (e.g., encephalopathy, pericarditis), acidosis, hyperkalemia, and fluid overload.

2. **In critically ill patients,** RRT, especially continuous venovenous hemofiltration, sometimes is used **expectantly** to treat progressively worsening azotemia and fluid overload.

B. **Extracorporeal techniques**

1. **Intermittent RRT** uses a high flow arteriovenous or venovenous extracorporeal circuit with a high efficiency dialysis cartridge to remove blood-borne wastes and fluid. **Hemodialysis** (see below) is the usual mode of intermittent RRT. In HD, blood flow rates are typically 200 to 300 ml/min, whereas typical dialysate flow is 500 ml/min. Dialysis run times are on the order of several hours, but may need to be lengthened in some patients to avoid hemodynamic instability.

    a. **Advantages** of intermittent HD include:
        (1) High efficiency.
        (2) Rapid removal of toxins and wastes.
        (3) Dedicated machines and specialized staffing.

    b. **Disadvantages** of intermittent HD include:
        (1) **Hemodynamic instability** with hypotension.
        (2) **Limited ability to remove volume** because of hypotension and the relatively brief duration of treatment.
        (3) **Disequilibrium syndrome,** characterized by confusion, restlessness, gastrointestinal symptoms, and sometimes seizures, can occur. Disequilibrium syndrome is thought to be caused by rapid changes in the osmolarity of nerve cells. Slowing the rate of dialysis is usually helpful.

2. **Continuous RRT**

    a. As with traditional hemodialysis, continuous RRT requires an extracorporeal blood circuit created by vascular access to the patient (Fig. 23-1). Initial **arteriovenous circuits** used arterial pressure as the driving pressure for flow across a filter or dialysis membrane and returned the blood through a venous catheter. These have largely been replaced by pump-driven **venovenous** extracorporeal systems. Venovenous systems have more stability and control, because the driving pressure does not depend on the arterial blood pressure of the patient. They also eliminate the need for high flow arterial catheterization. Instead, access usually is accomplished through a single large-bore, double-lumen catheter that is placed percutaneously in the femoral or subclavian vein.

    b. **Continuous RRT** is recommended for patients who are hemodynamically unstable,

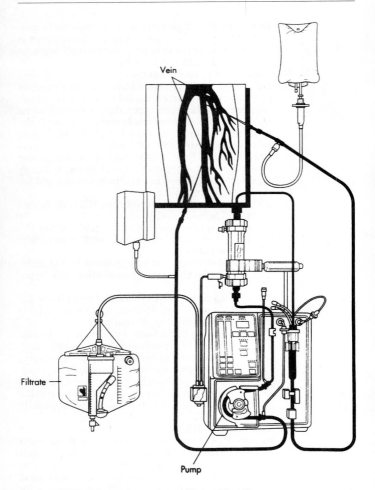

Fig. 23-1.   Continuous venovenous hemofiltration.

        have cerebral edema and multiple organ system dysfunction, or require ongoing fluid removal.

  c. Continuous RRT has been advocated for the removal of inflammatory cytokines in septic patients. Although studies have demonstrated that continuous RRT can increase clearance of cytokines from the circulation, no proof exists that such therapy is helpful.

  d. **Advantages** of continuous RRT over intermittent HD include improved hemodynamic stability and the ability to remove large volumes of fluid. Whether the use of continuous RRT improves resolution of renal failure or survival of patients when compared with intermittent hemodialysis remains unproved.

e. **Complications of RRT**

(1) **Pump errors.** Pumps can have varied responses and accuracy, particularly when variable negative and positive pressures are applied to their inlets and outlets. Even when using dedicated, specially designed pumps, it should never be assumed that the pump settings accurately reflect the true flow rate. Fluid inputs and outputs must be meticulously and directly measured. Because the pumped volumes are so large, small deviations from the prescribed flow rates can result in life-threatening volume alterations.

(2) **Clotting** of the membrane is the most common technical limitation in providing continuous RRT, decreasing both the life expectancy and efficiency of the dialysis membrane.

(3) **Systemic anticoagulation** by heparin administration via the inflow limb prevents clotting, but increases the risk of bleeding complications. Local, prefilter administration of heparin with reversal by a protamine infusion postfilter can be used in patients who cannot tolerate heparin. Alternatively, **citrate anticoagulation** by infusion of sodium citrate solution can be used. This anticoagulation technique requires supplemental administration of Ca^{2+} and a modified (no base) dialysis solution. Heparinized priming of the circuit can lead to heparin binding and a local anticoagulation effect. In patients who are most at risk for bleeding complications, it may be necessary to use a system without any anticoagulation. In most cases, the life expectancy of the filters will be greatly diminished.

(4) **Vascular access complications** include infection, bleeding, and the potential for air embolism. Systems should be equipped with air traps and air and disconnect detectors.

3. **Modes of RRT.** Several different modes of renal replacement are available. Each has unique advantages and disadvantages. The two major modes are hemofiltration and hemodialysis.

a. **Hemofiltration (HF)**

(1) **Hemofiltration** is performed by directing blood flow over a semipermeable membrane (Fig. 23-1). The pressure gradient across the membrane produces an ultrafiltrate of plasma consisting of plasma water and non–protein-bound solutes. Molecules of small and medium size are carried across the membrane by convection with the ultrafiltrate. This technique has the ability to remove 10 to 15 L/d of ultrafiltrate and requires such volumes for effective solute clearance. The volume of ultrafiltrate produced is controlled by placing a pump on the ultrafiltrate side of the filter. The ultrafiltrate is replaced with a suitable electrolyte solution such as lactated Ringer's solution supplemented with Mg^{2+} and Ca^{2+}. The volume of replacement solution will determine the patient's fluid balance. Replacement solution can be infused into the extracorporeal circuit either before (predilution) or immediately after (postdilution) the filter. Hemofiltration will remove non–protein-bound drugs from the plasma. Drug doses should be adjusted as if the creatinine clearance was 7 ml/min for every 10 L of ultrafiltrate produced per day.

(2) **Advantages** of HF include ease of implementation, removal of high volumes, and high efficiency of solute removal.

(3) **Disadvantages** of HF arise from the need to filter large volumes for effective solute removal. Practical and technical limitations often decrease the theoretical efficiency of HF.

b. **Hemodialysis** has the highest clearance rate for urea and is now the continuous RRT of choice in many institutions.

(1) **The principle** is the same as in intermittent HD. Blood is pumped forward through a dialysis cartridge while dialysis solution is pumped over the other side of the dialysis membrane in a countercurrent direction. Small waste molecules are efficiently removed from the blood by diffusion. During continuous HD, the blood flow rate typically is 100 to 150 ml/min and the dialysis flow rates are approximately 15 ml/min. These flows are greatly reduced from those used during intermittent dialysis, but permit the efficient removal of waste in a volume of be-

tween 3 and 6 L/d. The rate of dialysate flow is determined by calculating the required urea clearance. Commercially prepared dialysis solutions are available for continuous therapy. Alternatively, peritoneal dialysis solutions with the appropriate sodium (140 mEq/L) and glucose (~ 100 mg/dl) concentrations can be used. The volume of ultrafiltrate is set as the difference between blood flow and dialysis flow. Antibiotics and other therapeutic drugs also are removed from the circulation through diffusion, and dosages should be adjusted by determining serum drug levels when available.

(2) **Advantages** of continuous HD include high efficiency of urea clearance, control of ultrafiltrate composition, and decreased volume of ultrafiltrate for waste clearance (when compared with HF).

C. **Peritoneal dialysis (PD)** uses the capillaries of the peritoneum as a semipermeable exchange membrane. The dialysate is infused into the peritoneum through an indwelling catheter. Peritoneal dialysis is less efficient than the other forms of dialysis. It is rarely used in the adult ICU patient because of the risk of infection and the high incidence of other intraabdominal pathology in critically ill adult patients.

SELECTED REFERENCES

Better OS, Stein JH. Early management of shock and prophylaxis of acute renal failure in traumatic rhabdomyolysis. *N Engl J Med* 1990;322:825–829.

Daugirdas JT, Ing TS. *Handbook of dialysis.* Philadelphia, Lippincott-Raven; 1994.

McCarthy JT. Prognosis of patients with acute renal failure in the intensive-care unit: a tale of two eras. *Mayo Clin Proc* 1996;71:117–126.

Nissenson AR. Acute renal failure: definition and pathogenesis. *Kidney Int Suppl* 1998;66:S7–S10.

Patel R. Antifungal agents. Part I. Amphotericin B preparations and flucytosine. *Mayo Clin Proc* 1998;73:1205–1225.

Rao TK. Acute renal failure syndromes in human immunodeficiency virus infection. *Semin Nephrol* 1998;18:378–395.

Ronco C, Bellomo R. Continuous renal replacement therapy: evolution in technology and current nomenclature. *Kidney Int Suppl* 1998;66: S160–S164.

Solomon R, Werner C, Mann D, et al. Effects of saline, mannitol, and furosemide to prevent acute decreases in renal function induced by radiocontrast agents. *N Engl J Med* 1994;331:1416–1420.

Thadhani R, Pascual M, Bonventre JV. Acute renal failure. *N Engl J Med* 1996;334:1448–1460.

Thompson BT, Cockrill BA. Renal-dose dopamine: a siren song? *Lancet* 1994;344:7–8.

Liver Disease

Fritz Daudel and Kenneth L. Haspel

I. **Postoperative complications after liver surgery**
   A. **Hemorrhage**
      1. **Insufficient surgical hemostasis.** Some bleeding must be anticipated after surgery. Surgical techniques resecting the segmental structure of the liver (i.e., anatomic resection) and the use of argon beam coagulators have decreased both intraoperative and postoperative blood loss. Wedge resections tend to bleed more postoperatively than whole lobectomies, because more raw surface remains.
      2. **Postoperative coagulopathy** (Chapter 12)
      3. **Management**
         a. Restoration of **normovolemia** with crystalloids, colloids, and packed red blood cells.
         b. Restoration of **normothermia.**
         c. If the hematocrit does not stabilize or hemodynamic instability occurs despite the above-mentioned measures, ongoing bleeding must be suspected that requires **surgical reintervention.** Hepatic angiography and embolization may be valuable options.
   B. **Coagulopathy** can occur secondary to massive operative blood losses, hypothermia, hyperfibrinolysis, or to decreased production of clotting factors in the remaining liver. Coagulopathy is corrected with transfusion of fresh frozen plasma, platelets, cryoprecipitate, and so on. (Diagnosis and management are discussed in Chapter 12.)
   C. **Fever.** Postoperative pyrexia may reflect resorption of hematoma or necrotic tissue, or it may be a sign of peritonitis or abscess formation.
   D. **Biliary fistulas.** Leaking bile ducts can form bile collections. Suction drains should be left in place or new drains should be inserted by interventional radiology. Usually, biliary fistulas close on their own within 3 weeks.
   E. **Hepatic aneurysm.** Anemia, leukocytosis, and abdominal pain can indicate a late complication after hepatic trauma, namely the development of a false aneurysm after an injury of the hepatic vasculature. Therapeutic embolization is considered the treatment of choice.
   F. **Intra- or perihepatic abscess.** The risk of abscess formation is increased with concomitant colonic or pancreatic injury, large collections of hematoma or bile, and open drains. Prolonged postoperative pyrexia in combination with leukocytosis and increasing right upper quadrant pain should raise the suspicion of a peri- or intrahepatic abscess. Treatment includes drainage by

interventional radiology or surgical revision, in combination with intravenous antibiotics.

G. **Postoperative liver failure.** In normal livers (i.e., liver surgery for removal of a metastatic lesion or adenoma), resections of up to 80% of the liver mass are generally well tolerated. Complications can arise when:
   1. The remaining liver is too small to maintain full hepatic function.
   2. Alterations in hepatic blood flow lead to ischemia.

II. **Postoperative liver dysfunction after nonhepatic surgery**
   A. **Causes include:**
      1. Infections (e.g., viral hepatitis, exacerbation of chronic hepatitis, sepsis).
      2. Ischemia secondary to hypotension, congestive heart failure, and hepatic artery ligation or injury.
      3. Hypoxia.
      4. Drug- and toxin-induced (e.g., alcohol, halothane, acetaminophen) injury.
      5. Bile duct obstruction or injury.
      6. Pancreatitis.
      7. Bilirubin overload secondary to hematomas, blood transfusions, hemolysis, and so forth.
   B. **Preexisting hepatic disease** makes the liver much more vulnerable to the above-mentioned stress factors.
   C. **Symptoms** are often nonspecific; they include right upper quadrant pain, nausea, vomiting, indigestion, pruritus, fatigue, fever, mental confusion, and encephalopathy.
   D. **Signs** include jaundice, right upper quadrant tenderness, palmar erythema, spider nevi, splenomegaly, ascites, portosystemic collaterals (e. g., caput medusae, hemorrhoids, gastroesophageal varices), coagulopathy, anemia, and gynecomastia.
   E. **Management** (see section **III.C.**)

III. **Fulminant hepatic failure**
   A. **Fulminant hepatic failure** is characterized as a fast onset of severe impairment of liver function. Patients with chronic liver disease are excluded. Fulminant hepatic failure can be subdivided further in **hyperacute** (0–7 days), **acute** (8–28 days), and **subacute** (29 days to 12 weeks) failure, depending on the time interval between first symptoms and signs of liver failure.
   B. **Causes**
      1. **Infections**
         a. **Viral** (e.g., hepatitis A, B, C, D, E; yellow fever, cytomegalovirus, Epstein-Barr virus).
         b. **Bacterial** (e.g., liver abscess, Legionella pneumophila, sepsis, Q fever).
      2. **Toxins, drugs, and chemicals,** including acetaminophen, carbon tetrachloride, designer drugs (e.g., "Ecstasy"), mushroom toxins (*Amantia phalloides*), halothane, isoniazid, valproic acid.
      3. **Ischemia, hypoxia,** or both of any cause, but also specifically caused by venous congestion of the liver

(e.g., right ventricular failure, Budd-Chiari syndrome), tumors that impair blood flow to the liver, and trauma to the liver and its supplying vessels.

4. **Metabolic causes** (e.g., Reye's syndrome, acute fatty liver of pregnancy, Wilson's disease, and heat stroke).

C. **Complications and management**

1. **Cerebral edema** is the leading cause of death in fulminant hepatic failure. Cerebral edema is present in up to 80% of cases of hepatic failure that proceed to stage IV encephalopathy (Table 24-1). Theories for the development of cerebral edema include impaired cerebral autoregulation and decline of cerebral blood flow, disruption of the blood–brain barrier, and intracellular accumulation of osmotically active molecules. Focal neurologic signs do not usually occur and can indicate intracranial bleeding or early cerebral herniation. (**Management** of cerebral edema is discussed in Chapter 11 and Chapter 29, section **IV**).

2. **Cardiovascular.** Arteriovenous shunting and vasodilation from decreased clearance of vasoactive metabolites by the liver produce a high output state characterized by tachycardia, increased cardiac output, and decreased systemic vascular resistance. An important differential diagnosis in these immunocompromised patients is sepsis. (Diagnosis and management are discussed in Chapters 1, 9, and 10.) If increased intracranial pressure (ICP) is present, special attention is required to maintain a cerebral perfusion pressure greater than 60 mm Hg.

3. **Respiratory**

   a. **Endotracheal intubation** may be required if protective airway reflexes are lost.

   b. **Hypoxemia** which may require intubation and ventilation can occur in patients with hypoventilation, atelectasis, pleural effusions, pulmonary shunting, and pulmonary edema.

   c. **Hyperventilation** may be necessary as a temporary treatment for increased intracranial pressure (Chapter 11).

Table 24-1.   Clinical stages of hepatic encephalopathy

Stage 1. Altered behavior, impairment of sleep, change of handwriting, slurred speech.

Stage 2. Drowsiness, disorientation, restlessness, brisk tendon reflexes, increased muscle tone, clonus.

Stage 3. Somnolent, but arousable; marked confusion, disturbance of speech, hyperreflexia, miosis.

Stage 4. Coma, mydriasis, hypo- or areflexia, unresponsiveness to painful stimuli.

4. **Coagulopathies** may be secondary to decreased production of clotting factors and to increased thrombolysis. Thrombocytopenia and impaired platelet function are common (Chapter 12). Transfusion of coagulation factors in the absence of active bleeding is controversial, but may be indicated prior to invasive procedures or when invasive ICP monitoring devices are in place.

5. **Renal failure,** which complicates about half of the cases of fulminant hepatic failure, commonly is caused by **hepatorenal syndrome.** (Renal failure and hepatic disease are discussed in detail in section **IV.H.**)

6. **Electrolyte and acid-base disorders,** which are varied, include:
   a. Respiratory alkalosis.
   b. Metabolic alkalosis.
   c. Hypokalemia.
   d. Hyponatremia, secondary to reduced free water clearance.
   e. Hypernatremia, secondary to dehydration after mannitol therapy.
   f. Hypoglycemia, because of impaired glycogen mobilization, gluconeogenesis, and insulin metabolism.

D. **Liver transplantation in fulminant hepatic failure**
   1. **Indications.** Orthotopic liver transplantation may be an option for patients with fulminant hepatic failure. Accurate predictions of whether a patient's liver will be able to recover with medical treatment alone may avoid unnecessary liver transplantation or suggest early transplantation, which may improve outcome. The **King's college criteria for liver transplantation** provide a comparatively fast and inexpensive assessment of liver function that can be frequently repeated (Table 24-2). **Factor V levels** also have been used to determine indications for liver transplantation in patients with viral hepatitis. Encephalopathy associated with a factor V level of less than 20% of normal (in patients aged < 30 years) or less than 30% of normal (in patients aged > 30 years) are considered indications for transplantation. Because these assessment protocols are not perfect, it has been advocated to list all patients with fulminant hepatic failure for transplantation as soon as the diagnosis is made. The patient is reevaluated when a donor liver becomes available, and the decision made to transplant or continue to follow is made at that time.
   2. **Contraindications** to transplantation include sepsis, acute respiratory distress syndrome, and cerebral edema that is unresponsive to treatment. **Relative contraindications** include rapidly de-

Table 24-2. King's College criteria for liver transplantation in fulminant hepatic failure

Acetaminophen intoxication

Arterial pH <7.3 (irrespective of grade of encephalopathy) or a combination of:
  –Encephalopathy grade III or IV
  –Prothrombin time >35 s (USA) or INR >7.7
  –Serum creatinine >3.4 mg/dl

Nonacetaminophen patients

INR >7.7 (irrespective of grade of encephalopathy), or any three of the following variables (irrespective of the grade of encephalopathy):
  –Cause is non-A non-B hepatitis, halothane hepatitis, or idiosyncratic drug reaction
  –Duration of jaundice before onset of encephalopathy >7 d
  –Prothrombin time >25 s (INR >3.85)
  –Serum bilirubin >18 mg/dl

INR, International normalized ratio.

veloping hemodynamic instability requiring increasing vasopressor support, psychiatric disturbances (e.g., noncompliance with medications, multiple suicide attempts), and advanced age.

IV. **Cirrhosis** can be seen as an irreversible final pathway of chronic liver diseases. Hepatocyte necrosis and destruction of the connective tissue network lead to irregular nodular regeneration of hepatic parenchyma, extensive fibrosis, and distortion of the hepatic vasculature.

  A. **Causes include:**
    1. **Alcoholic cirrhosis,** which accounts for most cases in the Western world.
    2. **Viral hepatitis** following chronic hepatitis B, C, and D infection. Of chronic hepatitis C cases, 20% progress to cirrhosis.
    3. **Primary biliary cirrhosis,** which is idiopathic.
    4. **Secondary biliary cirrhosis** as a result of prolonged obstruction of the biliary tract.
    5. **Prolonged congestive heart failure.**
    6. **Metabolic diseases** (e.g., hemochromatosis, Wilson's disease, glycogen storage diseases, and α_1-antitrypsin deficiency).
    7. **Drug-related toxicities** (e.g., methotrexate, isoniazid, methyldopa).
    8. **Parasitic infections** (e.g., *Echinococcus, Schistosomiasis*).

  B. **Portal hypertension and bleeding from gastroesophageal varices.** Although other causes (e.g., Budd-Chiari syndrome, portal vein thrombosis) are seen, cirrhosis is the most common underlying disease leading to portal hypertension. Cirrhosis creates portosystemic collaterals that can form varices with a risk of bleeding.

1. **Patients with esophageal bleeding** present with hematemesis, melena, and hematochezia. The diagnosis must be confirmed by **esophagogastroscopy,** because bleeding frequently occurs from duodenal or gastric ulcers or the Mallory-Weiss syndrome.

2. **Endoscopic sclerotherapy and variceal ligation** are commonly used to manage esophageal varices and esophageal bleeding. The procedures are highly successful and can immediately follow diagnostic esophagogastroscopy.

3. **Portal vein pressures** can be measured by catheterization of the portal vein (percutaneous transhepatic) or indirectly by transjugular or transfemoral catheterization of the hepatic veins.

4. **Nonselective β-adrenergic blockers** (e.g., **propranolol**) administered prophylactically reduce the risk of bleeding, although mortality is unaffected. Propranolol reduces portal pressure by constricting the splanchnic vasculature and, to a smaller degree, by reducing cardiac output.

5. **Vasopressin** reduces blood flow and pressure in the portal system, including its collaterals. Vasopressin should be administered through a central line because infiltration can cause tissue necrosis. The infusion dose is 0.1 to 0.4 U/min. Side effects include myocardial ischemia, gastrointestinal ischemia, acute renal failure, and hyponatremia. Concomitant infusion of nitroglycerin may reduce the side effects of vasopressin.

6. **Somatostatin** is a naturally produced peptide hormone that acts as a vasoconstrictor in supraphysiologic doses. Fewer side effects are reported with somatostatin than with vasopressin.

7. **Octreotide** is a synthetic analog of somatostatin that has a much longer half-life. The dose is 25 to 50 μg/h.

8. **Balloon tamponade** is only recommended if medical therapy, sclerotherapy, or variceal ligation is unsuccessful. Different tubes are available. The **Sengstaken-Blakemore** tube is a triple lumen tube with a gastric balloon, an esophageal balloon, and a gastric tube. The **Minnesota tube** has an additional port for esophageal aspiration and a larger gastric balloon. The **Linton-Nachlas** tube has only a gastric balloon. When tubes with a double balloon are used, the gastric balloon is inflated first and placed on gentle traction. If the bleeding does not stop, the esophageal balloon is also inflated. Major complications include esophageal rupture and pulmonary aspiration of gastric contents. Aspiration risks can be reduced by endotracheal intubation prior to insertion of the esophageal tube.

9. **Emergency surgical shunt operations** and **surgical ligations** are only used as last resorts. **Transjugular intrahepatic portosystemic shunt** (TIPS) procedures use a percutaneously placed expandable metal stent to form a direct portocaval channel within the liver. All these procedures are associated with high complication rates, and are usually reserved for patients who have recurrent bleeding despite repeated sclerotherapies.

C. **Hepatic encephalopathy** appears to be caused by multiple factors. Hepatic clearance of cerebrotoxic substances such as ammonia, mercaptans, and short-chain fatty acids is reduced. In addition, experimental evidence suggests that the damaged liver is no longer able to produce certain substances that are crucial for normal brain function. The isolation of benzodiazepinelike compounds from brains of patients with hepatic encephalopathy, and partial antagonism of hepatic encephalopathy by flumazenil, suggest that the γ-aminobutyric acid (GABA)-ergic system may be altered.

1. **Diagnosis of hepatic encephalopathy** is made clinically. Ammonia levels do not correlate with the severity of the encephalopathy. In contrast to fulminant hepatic failure, increased intracranial pressure is associated with chronic hepatic encephalopathy only rarely.

2. **Management** includes the elimination of any precipitating factors (e.g., gastrointestinal bleeding) if possible. A nasogastric tube should be inserted to document and evacuate any upper gastrointestinal bleeding (if present) and permit administration of lactulose.

3. **Lactulose** acidifies the bowel contents and increases diffusion of ammonia into bowel lumen where it can be eliminated. The initial dose is 20 ml/h orally or by nasogastric tube until diarrhea occurs. The dose is then adjusted to produce three to four soft stools per day. Lactulose also can be administered as an enema (300 ml of 50% lactulose in 700 ml of water three times daily). Side effects include hypokalemia, dehydration, and hypernatremia. Alternatively, **neomycin** (1 g) orally or by nasogastric tube, four times daily, may be helpful. **Corticosteroids** have no beneficial effect in hepatic encephalopathy.

D. **Ascites** is produced in cirrhosis by the combination of portal hypertension, hypoalbuminemia, and fluid retention. Greater than 500 ml ascites usually is evident clinically by a distended abdomen, bulging flanks, everted umbilicus, shifting abdominal dullness, and an abdominal fluid wave. The diagnosis can be confirmed by ultrasonography. Other causes of ascites should be excluded by a diagnostic paracentesis. Ascites can be classified as transudative or exudative.

1. **Transudative ascites** is caused by movement of fluid across the hepatic sinusoids and the intestinal capillaries, which results from increased hydrostatic pressure from portal hypertension. In transudative ascites from portal hypertension, the total protein content tends to be less than 2.5 g/dl and the difference between the albumin concentrations of the serum and ascites is frequently greater than 1 g/dl. **Other causes** of transudative ascites include congestive heart failure, inferior vena cava occlusion, Budd-Chiari syndrome, and Meigs' syndrome.

2. **Exudative ascites** develops secondary to exudation of the fluid from the peritoneum. Portal hypertension is absent. In exudative ascites (with normal portal pressure), the protein content usually exceeds 2.5 to 3 g/dl and the difference between the albumin concentrations of the serum and ascites is often less than 1 g/dl. **Other causes** of exudative ascites include neoplasms (e.g., peritoneal carcinomatosis), peritoneal infections (e.g., tuberculosis, pyogenic peritonitis), chylous ascites, pancreatitis, and nephrogenic ascites.

3. **On diagnostic paracentesis,** the ascites should be sent for laboratory studies: cell count, Gram's stain, bacterial culture, amylase level, lactate dehydrogenase, carcinoembryonic antigen, and triglycerides.

4. **Mainstays of therapy for ascites in cirrhosis** are a salt-restricted diet, containing a level of sodium as low as 11 mmol/d to induce a negative sodium balance and stop ascitic fluid accumulation. Diuretics are added if necessary. As one cause for the fluid retention in cirrhosis is secondary hyperaldosteronism, **spironolactone** is the diuretic of first choice. Other diuretics can be added cautiously if needed. Overly aggressive diuresis can result in azotemia and hypotension secondary to hypovolemia. The effectiveness of the treatment is monitored by daily weighing. Daily weight loss should not exceed 0.5 to 1 kg. Patients refractory to medical therapy may require additional paracenteses. Plasma and urinary electrolytes should be monitored regularly, especially during diuretic treatment.

E. **Splenomegaly** can produce thrombocytopenia or pancytopenia, but rarely requires treatment.

F. **Spontaneous bacterial peritonitis (SBP)** is an infection of ascitic fluid without a primary intraabdominal focus.

1. **Signs and symptoms** can range from subtle to severe abdominal pain with rebound tenderness, fever, chills, nausea, and vomiting. Because symptoms may be absent, **diagnostic paracentesis** for culture and cell count is recommended in the assessment of patients with ascites. Gastrointestinal hemorrhage, which is often associated with bac-

teremia, puts the cirrhotic patient at risk of developing SBP. The most important sources of contamination of the ascites are the gastrointestinal tract, urinary tract, pneumonias, and endoscopic procedures. Greater than 90% of the cases of SBP are caused by a single bacterial species. Enteric gram-negative bacteria are most frequently isolated (70%), followed by gram-positive cocci (*Streptococcus pneumoniae, Enterococcus, Staphylococcus*) in approximately 20% of the cases, and anaerobes in approximately 5%. **Polymicrobial infections in SBP are rare and should trigger a search for bowel perforation.**

2. **Treatment.** Because the mortality of untreated SBP is high, antibiotic therapy should be initiated immediately after samples of the ascites are taken. Empiric antibiotics that are active against gram-negative, gram-positive, and anaerobic bacteria should be administered initially and then modified based on cultures. Potential regimens include:

   a. A β-lactam such as ampicillin plus aminoglycoside.

   b. A third generation nonpseudomonal cephalosporin (e.g., **ceftriaxone** or **cefotaxime**).

   c. A β-lactam/β-lactamase inhibitor (e.g., **timentin**).

   d. **Vancomycin** should be added to each of the above regimens if methicillin-resistant *Staphylococcus aureus* (MRSA) is suspected.

3. **Prophylaxis.** Patients with cirrhosis who are admitted with gastrointestinal bleeding can be prophylactically treated with cefotaxime. To prevent recurrence of SBP, consider prophylactic treatment with a fluoroquinolone or trimethoprim-sulfamethoxazole, especially for liver transplant candidates.

G. **Hepatopulmonary syndrome.** Pathologic **dilation of intrapulmonary vessels** in cirrhosis increases right-to-left shunting of blood flow through the lungs. The diagnosis can be made with contrast-enhanced echocardiography or radio-labeled macroaggregated albumin. The degree of hypoxemia is variable, and is inconsistently improved by administration of supplemental oxygen. Partial or complete improvement of hypoxemia after liver transplantation has been reported.

H. **Hepatorenal syndrome (HRS)** is characterized by worsening renal function, sodium retention, and oliguria without an identifiable cause in a patient with cirrhosis and ascites. Renal failure is thought to be caused by inappropriate renal vasoconstriction, which reduces renal blood flow and glomerular filtration rate. Significant morphologic abnormalities are absent. Clinical signs usually include oliguria, azotemia, hyperkalemia, and hyponatremia. Other causes of renal failure, such as prerenal azotemia, acute tubular necrosis, and glomerulonephritis must be excluded (Chapter 23). In hepatorenal syndrome, the urinary sediment is unremarkable and marked sodium retention is present. The urinary sodium is often less than 5 mmol/l, which is less than that observed in prerenal azotemia, and is unresponsive to volume expansion. Treatment of hepatorenal syndrome usually is unsuccessful and the mortality rate is high. Because the kidney is extremely susceptible to further injury and hypotension, nephrotoxic drugs and nonsteroidal antiinflammatory drugs should be avoided.

  I. **Grading of liver disease.** Originally designed to assess the surgical risk in patients undergoing surgery, Pugh's modification of Child's classification (Table 24-3) is also used to assess the course of patients with cirrhosis.

V. **Drug-induced liver disease**

  A. The liver is the central organ for the metabolism of most drugs. Drug excretion through the kidneys and the bile is made possible by transformation to more hydrophilic compounds (biotransformation). In most cases, hepatotoxicity is not caused by the originally administered drug, but rather by its metabolites.

  B. **Hepatotoxicity** has been classified into **direct hepatotoxic reactions** and **idiosyncratic reactions.**

   1. **Direct hepatotoxins** damage the liver in a dose-dependent fashion and characteristically produce hepatocyte necrosis in a particular region of the liver lobule.

   2. **Idiosyncratic hepatotoxins** account for most of the cases; they are unpredictable and occur even when the drugs are administered in the normal therapeutic range. The histology shows diffuse liver injury consisting of necrosis, cholestasis, or both, and usually is associated with a significant inflammatory reaction. Rash, febrile reaction, eosinophilia, or a serum sickness syndrome can be present. In some instances, autoantibodies to cytochrome P_{450}

Table 24-3. Child-Pugh's classification

	Classification points		
	1	2	3
Encephalopathy	None	Grades I and II	Grades III and IV
Ascites	Absent	Slight–moderate	Tense
Bilirubin (mg/dl) *or*	<2.0	2–3	>3.0
If primary biliary cirrhosis	<4	4–10	>10
Albumin (g/dl)	>3.5	2.8–3.5	<2.8
Prothrombin (sec above control)	1–4	4–6	>6

Points from each of the five categories are summed to yield a total score: grade A: 5–6 points, grade B: 7–9 points, grade C: 10–15 points. The mortality of cirrhotic patients rises dramatically with increasing Child scores. The 1-year mortality rate for ≤10% for Child A, 20% to 30% for Child B, and 50% to 60% for Child C.

Table 24-4. Classification of drug-induced hepatic disease

Type of lesion	Examples	Comments
Acute viral hepatitis-like reaction	Diclofenac, halothane, isoflurane, isoniazid, methyldopa, phenytoin	Mortality rate much higher than that for viral hepatitis; pattern of bridging necrosis in severe cases
Zonal necrosis	Acetaminophen, carbon tetrachloride	Dose-dependent, negligible inflammatory response, lesions predominantly restricted to one lobular zone
Steatohepatitis Alcoholic hepatitis-like reaction	Amiodarone, perhexiline, nifedipine, valproic acid	
Steatohepatitis Microvesicular	Aspirin, tetracycline, zidovudine (AZT)	
Cholestasis	ACE-inhibitors, carbamazepine, chlorpromazine, cimetidine, cotrimoxazole, dextropropoxyphene, erythromycin, estrogens, flucloxacillin, haloperidol, sulphonamides, tricyclic antidepressants	Histologically, inflammatory, noninflammatory forms with bile duct destruction can be recognized
Granulomatous hepatitis	Allopurinol, diltiazem, quinidine, phenytoin, procainamide, sulfonamides	Histiocytes and eosinophiles in the granulomas reflect a hypersensitivity reaction
Veno-occlusive disease	Chemotherapeutic drugs	Lesions are dose-dependent
Chronic hepatitis	Amiodarone, aspirin, diclofenac, isoniazid, methyldopa, phenytoin, nitrofurantoin, trazodone	Occurs with continued exposure to a drug; in most cases, hepatitis resolves after discontinuation of the drug
Adenomas, hepatocellular carcinomas	Estrogens, anabolic hormones	

ACE, angiotensin-converting enzyme.

and other microsomal enzyme groups can be demonstrated.
3. This classification is blurred, however, because of considerable interindividual variation in susceptibility to direct hepatotoxins. Some idiosyncratic reactions seem to occur when a combination of host, environmental, or both, factors is present. Variables such as enzyme polymorphism, interactions among drugs, age, and obesity influence the extent of both direct and idiosyncratic hepatotoxic reactions.

C. **Diagnosis** is based on a history of exposure to a certain drug (reactions usually occur within 90 days after first administration), but is especially difficult in the ICU setting wherein patients are exposed to multiple drugs. Clinical and laboratory data are used to support the diagnosis. Other causes of liver dysfunction must be excluded.

D. **The differential diagnosis** of drug-induced liver disease includes viral hepatitis, worsening of chronic liver disease, biliary obstruction (e.g., tumor, gallstones, injury), postoperative liver dysfunction, sepsis, congestive heart failure, and pancreatitis.

E. Some drugs are associated with characteristic histologic lesions, whereas others can vary or show considerable overlap in their histologic presentation. Results of liver biopsies often are inconclusive. Table 24-4 lists some examples of drugs associated with liver disease. Virtually any drug, however, can affect the liver.

VI. **Total parenteral nutrition (TPN) and liver disease**
A. **Fatty liver.** Parenteral feeding may be associated with complications that affect the liver. Serum hepatic aminotransferases and bilirubin concentrations can increase progressively with increasing duration of TPN. The histopathologic correlate in adults usually is a fatty liver (i.e., macro- and microvesicular steatosis). It is usually asymptomatic and benign in character. Overfeeding (Chapter 8) appears to be the most important factor contributing to the steatosis.

B. **Cholestasis.** Cholecystokinin (CCK), a hormone derived from the intestine, is released after stimulation by food. Total parenteral nutrition creates a fasting-like state for the gut and decreases CCK release, which diminishes gallbladder emptying and promotes biliary sludge formation. Acalculous and calculous forms of cholecystitis can be distinguished by ultrasonography.

SELECTED REFERENCES

Caraceni P, Van Thiel DH. Acute liver failure. *Lancet* 1995;345: 163–169.

Christenson E, Schlichting P, Fauerholdt L, et al. Prognostic value of Child-Turcotte criteria in medically treated cirrhosis. *Hepatology* 1984;4:430–435.

Infante-Rivard C, Esnaola S, Villeneuve J-P. Clinical and statistical validity of conventional prognostic factors in predicting short-term survival among cirrhotics. *Hepatology* 1987;7:660–664.

Lee WM. Acute liver failure. *N Engl J Med* 1993;16:1862–1872.

O'Grady JG, Alexander GJ, Hayllar KM, et al. Early indicators of prognosis in fulminant hepatic failure. *Gastroenterology* 1989;97:439–445.

Shellman R, Fulkerson W, DeLong E, et al. Prognosis of patients with cirrhosis and chronic liver disease admitted to the medical intensive care unit. *Crit Care Med* 1988;16:671–678.

Sherlock S, Dooley J. *Diseases of the liver and biliary system,* 10th ed. Oxford: Blackwell Science Inc.; 1997.

Zakim D, Boyer T. *Hepatology: a textbook of liver disease,* 3rd ed. Philadelphia: WB Saunders; 1996.

Gastrointestinal Disease

Luat T. Nguyen, Horacio Hojman, and Jean Kwo

I. **Gastrointestinal (GI) diseases** in critically ill patients pose a diagnostic and therapeutic challenge. Critically ill patients are less likely to present with the classic symptoms seen in otherwise healthy patients. Because of concomitant illnesses, treatment options often are limited and must be tailored to the individual case.

II. **Stress ulceration**

  A. **Pathogenesis**

    1. **Stress ulcers** have also been termed "stress erosions" and "stress erosive gastritis." These are gastric mucosal lesions that occur in the setting of trauma, shock, sepsis, and other severe medical illnesses. Typically found in the fundus of the stomach and the first part of the duodenum, these lesions usually heal with the clinical improvement of the patients. The incidence of patients bleeding from stress ulcers in the intensive care unit (ICU) is approximately 5%.

    2. **Contributing factors** include:

      a. **High intragastric acidity.**

      b. **Mucosal ischemia** associated with hypotension secondary to shock or sepsis.

      c. **Inhibition of prostaglandin production** by aspirin and other nonsteroidal antiinflammatory drugs. Prostaglandins enhance the mucosal barrier by increasing mucosal blood flow and mucus secretions, and decreasing acid secretion at high doses.

      d. **Glucocorticoids,** which decrease the rate of epithelial cell turnover, can affect mucus secretion.

      e. **Reflux of bile salts** enhances ulcerations by increasing the permeability to hydrogen ions.

  B. **Diagnosis** is made by endoscopy. Endoscopy offers a means for therapy and is useful to exclude other lesions.

  C. **Prophylactic therapy**

    1. Because of cost and the potential side effects, stress ulcer prophylaxis is not indicated in all patients in the ICU (Table 25-1). Improvement of the patient's underlying condition is likely to promote healing and decrease bleeding.

    2. Those patients who may benefit from stress ulcer prophylaxis because of an increased risk of bleeding include those with severe burns, sepsis, multiple organ failure, trauma, prolonged mechanical ventilation (> 3 days), or a history of upper GI bleeding.

    3. **Reduction of intragastric acidity**

      a. **Antacids** neutralize gastric acidity. By increasing gastric pH, antacids inhibit the pro-

**Table 25-1.   Common drugs
used for stress ulcer prophylaxis**

H₂ blockers	Cimetidine	300 mg IV every 6 to 8 h or 150–300 mg IV bolus followed by infusion of 37.5–50 mg/h
	Ranitidine	50 mg IV every 8 h or 50 mg IV bolus followed by infusion of 6.25 mg/h
	Famotidine	20 mg IV every 12 h
Proton pump inhibitors	Omeprazole	20 to 40 mg/d orally
Cytoprotection	Sucralfate	1 g orally every 6 h
	Misoprotol	200 µg orally every 6 h

IV, intravenous.

teolytic activity of pepsin. Antacids are titrated to maintain gastric pH greater than 3.5.

   b. **H₂ antagonists** are similar in their ability to suppress acid production. **Cimetidine** has the greatest degree of antiandrogenic and central nervous system (CNS) effects. Cimetidine also inhibits the cytochrome P_{450} oxidase system, affecting the metabolism of other drugs.

   c. **Proton pump inhibitors** are potent acid suppressants. Compared with H₂ antagonists, proton pump inhibitors have fewer side effects. Oral **omeprazole** appears as safe and effective against stress ulceration as H₂ blockers.

4. **Cytoprotection**

   a. **Sucralfate** is the basic aluminum salt of sulfated sucrose, a polysaccharide with antipeptic activity. In acidic gastric juice, the complex dissociates into the aluminum ion and the nonabsorbable polar form of the drug. Sucralfate forms an ulcer-adherent complex with the mucus layer and offers local cytoprotection. It is the most cost-effective drug, but it appears less effective than ranitidine.

   b. **Prostaglandins** at low dosages stimulate mucus and bicarbonate secretion and improve mucosal blood flow. At high dosages, they can suppress acid production.

D. **Surgical therapy** is usually not necessary to treat hemorrhagic gastritis. Modalities advocated to treat this condition when medical treatment fails include vagotomy and drainage procedures, vagotomy and antrectomy, and total gastrectomy. A particularly challenging group of patients are those with **portal hyper-**

tension, who require procedures to decompress the portal system (Chapter 24).

III. **Acute and chronic GI bleeding**
   A. **Initial assessment and stabilization**
      1. **Clinical signs and symptoms** include hematemesis, melena, hematochezia, occult blood loss, or symptoms of hypovolemia.
      2. **Stabilization** of the patient must begin while assessment is underway. Blood should be analyzed for type and cross-matching, hematocrit, and coagulation. Assessment of the degree of hypovolemia may require measurement of central vascular pressures and cardiac output in patients with significant cardiac disease. Crystalloids and blood products should be administered as appropriate. Dilutional thrombocytopenia and coagulopathy may need to be corrected with blood products. Serial assessments of hematocrit, coagulation parameters, and hemodynamics should be done to follow the patient's course.
   B. **Diagnosis**
      1. **Hematemesis** and **melena** are common manifestations of acute GI bleeding. **Hematemesis** indicates bleeding above the ligament of Treitz. **Melena** indicates that blood has remained in the GI tract long enough for bacterial degradation to occur. **Hematochezia** is usually caused by lower GI bleeding, except in cases of massive upper GI hemorrhage. Colonic bleeding rarely produces melena but presents as occult blood or hematochezia. A nasogastric (NG) tube should be placed and gastric lavage performed to diagnose upper GI bleeding. The NG aspirate may be clear in up to 10% of duodenal ulcers because of pyloric edema or spasm.
      2. **Localization of upper GI bleeding**
         a. **Endoscopy** allows for diagnosis as well as therapy and is the technique of choice for most cases.
         b. **Angiography** also can identify the sources of bleeding. Therapeutic embolization can be performed.
      3. **Localization of lower GI bleeding**
         a. **Colonoscopy** is the procedure of choice to evaluate lower GI bleeding. Anoscopy and sigmoidoscopy may be used if distal lesions are suspected.
         b. **Angiography** is useful in massive hemorrhage; it allows for therapeutic treatment in the form of vasopressin infusion or embolization.
         c. **Radionuclide scanning** in the form of Technetium-99^m sulfur colloid or labeled red blood cells (RBC) can be used to detect occult bleeding. ^{99m}Tc sulfur colloid is cleared by the liver, spleen, and the other parts of the reticu-

loendothelial system. Activity visualized apart from this system represents extravasation of blood.

C. Specific lesions and therapy
  1. Upper GI bleeding
    a. Mallory Weiss lesions are mucosal tears at the gastroesophageal (GE) junction that often are caused by severe vomiting. Most tears are located on the gastric side of the GE junction. Most of these lesions spontaneously stop bleeding and have a slight chance of rebleeding. Medical treatment with **vasopressin** infusion controls bleeding in more than 90% of cases. If medical treatment is unsuccessful, endoscopic electrocoagulation or angiographic therapy may be necessary. Surgery is rarely required.

    b. Gastroesophageal varices secondary to portal hypertension can cause bleeding (Chapter 24). Risk factors include the severity of the liver disease and the size of the varices. Medical prevention involves treatment with a nonselective beta-blocker or nitrates to lower the portal pressure (Table 25-2).

      (1) Initial management of an acute bleed should involve establishment of adequate intravenous (IV) access and aggressive fluid resuscitation.

      (2) The need for **airway protection** with an endotracheal tube should be constantly evaluated.

      (3) Endoscopic variceal ligation and **sclerotherapy** are highly effective treatments. Variceal ligation is performed by applying an elastic band around the mucosa surrounding the varix. It is more effective than sclerotherapy in controlling variceal bleeding. The success rate in controlling bleeding is between 80% and 100%, with a rebleeding rate between 25% and 36%.

      (4) In the event that endoscopy is not readily available, drug treatment with vasopressin, somatostatin, octreotide, or

Table 25-2. Common regimens for prophylaxis of variceal bleeding

Medication	Dose (oral)
Propranolol	20–40 mg twice a day
Nadolol	40 mg/d
Isosorbide mononitrate	20–40 mg twice a day

balloon tamponade can be attempted (Chapter 24).

(5) Transjugular intrahepatic portocaval shunt (TIPS) is an expandable stent that is placed, from a transjugular approach, within the liver to connect the portal and systemic circulations (Chapter 24). It is effective in controlling acute bleeding when other methods have failed, and in preventing rebleeding while awaiting transplantation. Its use is complicated by occlusion and the development of hepatic encephalopathy in some patients.

c. **Peptic ulcer disease** is the most common cause of upper GI bleeding.

(1) Important pathogenic factors include acid production, *Helicobacter pylori* infection, and the use of nonsteroidal anti-inflammatory drugs.

(2) The characteristic appearance of an ulcer on endoscopy can be of prognostic significance. Large ulcers and actively bleeding lesions have a high risk of rebleeding. An ulcer with an adherent clot or a visible vessel has a moderate risk of recurrent bleeding, whereas an ulcer with a clean base is at low risk for rebleeding.

(3) Treatment starts with prompt resuscitation. **Endoscopy** is the diagnostic procedure of choice because it allows for hemostatic therapy. Selective **arterial embolization** and **vasopressin** infusion are other therapeutic options. Approximately 10% of patients require **surgery** to control the hemorrhage. Immediate operation is recommended for patients with rapidly exsanguinating hemorrhage and for patients with active bleeding and failure of endoscopic management to control bleeding.

(4) Patients with comorbid disease and hemodynamic instability associated with bleeding, and those who develop recurrent bleeding may benefit from an early **elective operation** after initial endoscopic therapy.

(5) Medical therapy with H$_2$ antagonists and proton pump inhibitors has not been successful in stopping active bleeding or in preventing rebleeding. Nevertheless, it is reasonable to institute this therapy to increase gastric pH and enhance healing.

(6) Eradication of H. pylori infection decreases the rate of future rebleeding more than antisecretory therapy alone, although little role is seen for *H. pylori* eradication in the acute setting. Various regimens have been reported (Table 25-3). Therapy with a single antimicrobial agent is not recommended because of the potential for the development of antimicrobial resistance.

d. **Aortoenteric fistulas** can be primary, arising without a prior history of aortic repair, or secondary, which occurs after a vascular grafting procedure. In primary abdominal aortic fistulas, the erosions occur between the abdominal aorta and the overlying third and fourth portion of the duodenum. Secondary fistulas, which are more common, develop between the proximal aortic graft anastomosis and the adjacent duodenum. Mechanical erosion, suture line leak, and aortic graft infection are contributing factors. Diagnostic evaluation depends on the patient's status on presentation. If the patient is hemodynamically unstable, immediate fluid resuscitation and emergent exploratory laparotomy are required. In stable patients, endoscopy, computed tomography (CT), and angiography can be used to localize the fistula.

e. **Dieulafoy's lesion** is an abnormally large submucosal artery that ruptures into the gastric lumen, causing acute bleeding. Bleeding can be massive and recurrent. These lesions can be difficult to identify unless actively bleeding. Surgical resection and endoscopic thermal therapy have been reported to be successful in treating them.

2. **Small intestinal hemorrhage,** which accounts for approximately 3% to 5% of lower GI hemor-

Table 25-3.   Regimens for eradication of *Helicobacter pylori* infection

Omeprazole: 40 mg once followed by a 2-week course of 20 mg orally once daily and

Clarithromycin: 500 mg orally three times daily for 2 weeks

Ranitidine bismuth citrate: 400 mg orally twice daily for 4 weeks and

Clarithromycin: 500 mg orally three times daily for 2 weeks

Metronidazole: 250 mg orally every 6 h and

Tetracycline: 500 mg orally every 6 h and

Bismuth subsalicylate: 525 mg orally every 6 h for 2 weeks

rhage, can be difficult to diagnose. The most common cause of bleeding is **angiodysplasia.** Other causes include tumors, regional enteritis, ileal diverticula, small bowel varices, and focal ulcers caused by medications. Treatment of small intestinal sources of bleeding is directed at the underlying disease.

3. **Colonic bleeding**

   a. **Hemorrhoids** are a common cause of bright red blood from the rectum. Conservative treatment includes sitz baths and fiber supplementation. Surgery is reserved for refractory cases.

   b. **Diverticular disease** is the most common cause of lower GI bleeding, although significant hemorrhage only occurs in a small percentage of patients. Most episodes are self-limited. Urgent therapy is needed in 20% of the cases, and rebleeding occurs in 25% of the patients. **Colonoscopy** and **angiography** can locate the site of bleeding and offer means for therapy. **Vasopressin** infusion may decrease the rate of bleeding. Recurrent hemodynamically significant bleeding is an indication for operative resection.

   c. **Inflammatory bowel disease** often presents with a history of frequent bouts of bloody diarrhea and abdominal pain. Medical therapy involves hydration, bowel rest, and steroids. Colonoscopy with biopsies will assist in the diagnosis. The risk of life-threatening hemorrhage is low. Rarely, a colectomy or small bowel resection is needed for uncontrollable bleeding.

   d. **Arteriovenous malformations** (angiodysplasia), which occur with increasing frequency with advancing age, are present in up to 30% of the elderly population. They are commonly found in the ascending colon. Bleeding is characteristically chronic, slow, and recurrent. Colonoscopic coagulation is the initial treatment of choice. Surgery is reserved for recalcitrant cases.

   e. **Colorectal neoplasms** account for approximately 25% of cases of severe lower GI bleeding. Occult bleeding or iron deficiency anemia in an elderly patient warrants a search for neoplasm. Treatment involves surgical resection, chemotherapy, or radiation.

IV. **Acute pancreatitis**

   A. **Etiology.** The exact inciting agent of acute pancreatitis often is unknown. Gallstones are the most common cause of acute pancreatitis, (~ 45% of cases), followed by alcohol (35% of cases), miscellaneous causes (~ 10% of cases), and idiopathic (10% of cases).

   B. **Pathogenesis.** The central event in the pathogenesis of acute pancreatitis is the release of activated pancreatic enzymes within the gland and the surrounding pancreatic tissue, which produces a variable inflammatory response. Factors such as the acute obstruction of the pancreatic duct, exposure to toxins, and ischemia can initiate the process, although the exact mechanism is unknown. The intraacinar activation of **trypsin** is one of the initiating events. Trypsin activates other enzymes and the release of pancreatic digestive enzymes in the pancreatic bed, leading to pancreatic necrosis. Pathologic findings in the pancreas range from interstitial edema and fat necrosis to areas of pancreatic and peripancreatic necrosis and hemorrhage. Systemic complications arise from the release of pancreatic enzymes, inflammatory mediators, vasoactive substances, and hormones, sometimes leading to shock, respiratory insufficiency, and renal failure.

C. **Diagnosis**
   1. Patients usually present with epigastric pain, back pain, or both and often have diffuse abdominal tenderness, ileus, and rebound tenderness on palpation.
   2. **The differential diagnosis** is extensive and includes gastritis, perforated duodenal ulcer, small bowel obstruction, ruptured ectopic pregnancy, leaking abdominal aortic aneurysm (AAA), and sickle cell crisis. Supine and upright plain abdominal radiographs should help to exclude perforated viscus or small bowel obstruction.
   3. **Elevated serum amylase levels** usually pinpoint the diagnosis, except for patients with a history of chronic pancreatitis in whom a rise in serum amylase may not occur. Patients with renal failure may have elevated amylase levels because of decreased renal clearance of amylase. An **elevated serum lipase level** is a more specific test because lipase, for the most part, originates from the pancreas. The simultaneous determination of amylase and lipase gives a 90% to 95% sensitivity and specificity for the diagnosis of acute pancreatitis.
   4. **Contrast-enhanced CT** is the imaging method of choice for delineating the pancreas and determining the severity of many of the complications of pancreatitis.

D. **Prognostic indicators**
   1. **The clinical course** is mild and easily treated with fluid replacement, analgesia, and bowel rest in 75% to 80% of patients with acute pancreatitis.
   2. **Approximately 25% of attacks of pancreatitis are severe** and lead to complications. These patients should be admitted to a facility with (a) resources to care for critically ill patients, (b) expertise with dynamic CT and percutaneous needle aspiration and drainage procedures, and (c) ability to perform endoscopic procedures. Prognostic assessment allows for the early identification of patients at risk for major complications and death.

3. **Ranson** et al. have developed commonly used combinations of clinical and laboratory data that can indicate the severity of acute pancreatitis (Table 25-4). Their first five criteria assess the severity of the acute inflammatory process, whereas the criteria measured at 48 hours determine the systemic effects of circulating enzymes and toxins. Very low mortality rates are found in patients with fewer than three of these risk factors. Morbidity and mortality rates increase, however, as the number of risk factors increases.

4. **The appearance of the pancreas on CT scan** has been used to estimate the severity of pancreatitis. Patients with early evidence (within 3–10 days of admission) of extensive pancreatic necrosis (> 30% of gland) and extrapancreatic fluid collections are more likely to develop infected necrosis and require surgical intervention.

5. **The Acute Physiology and Chronic Health Evaluation (APACHE) II** scoring system also has been used to assess the initial severity of acute pancreatitis. This system also provides a means for ongoing monitoring of illness severity.

6. **The mortality rate of acute pancreatitis** is about 10%. Mortality rates increase to greater than 50% with the development of complications. Mortality within the first week usually is attributed to the systemic complications of acute pancreatitis, such as renal failure or acute respiratory distress syndrome (ARDS), whereas mortality after the first week usually is caused by pancreatic necrosis complicated by infection.

E. **Treatment**
1. **Initial treatment** of acute pancreatitis is largely supportive. Patients with mild disease are treated

Table 25-4.   Ranson's criteria for determining the severity of pancreatitis

At admission or diagnosis:
Age >55 y
White blood cell count >16,000/μl
Blood glucose >200 mg/dl
Serum lactic dehydrogenase (LDH) >350 IU/L
Serum glutamic oxaloacetic transaminase (SGOT) >250 U/dl

During initial 48 hours:
Hematocrit decrease of >10%
Blood urea nitrogen (BUN) increase of >5 mg/dl
Serum calcium <8 mg/dl
Arterial P_{O_2} <60 mm Hg
Base deficit >4 mEq/L
Estimated fluid sequestration >6L

with stopping oral intake, starting IV hydration, and providing parenteral analgesia. Immediate endoscopic removal of gallstones and endoscopic sphincterotomy may reduce mortality. In severe acute pancreatitis, the activation of inflammatory mediators leads to cardiovascular, respiratory, and renal dysfunction. **Aggressive fluid resuscitation** should be instituted early. Severe third-space fluid losses into the peritoneum, retroperitoneum, and gut lumen occur. Because pancreatitis leads to the release of inflammatory mediators and vasoactive substances, hypotension may be secondary to volume depletion, reduced systemic vascular tone, or cardiac depression. Measurement of central venous pressure, pulmonary artery occlusion pressure, and cardiac output may be necessary to properly guide the resuscitation. **Respiratory insufficiency** secondary to compressive atelectasis or ARDS often accompanies severe pancreatitis. Endotracheal intubation and mechanical ventilation are often necessary.

2. **Therapeutic maneuvers** to moderate the inflammatory response, "rest" the pancreas, and inhibit or remove toxic substances released by the inflamed pancreas have been tried. **Nasogastric tubes** are used to decompress the stomach and decrease the stimulation of the pancreas. Agents that decrease pancreatic secretion (e.g., somatostatin, fluorouracil, and glucagon) and agents that inhibit pancreatic proteases (e.g., aprotinin and gabexate) can interfere with the autodigestive process and reduce the severity of acute pancreatitis. Their efficacy remains unproved. **Total parenteral nutrition (TPN)** is used for nutritional support in patients who are unable to tolerate enteral feedings for extended periods.

3. **Prophylactic antibiotics.** Secondary infection of necrotic pancreatic and peripancreatic tissue is the major determinant of morbidity and mortality. Infection occurs from contamination of devitalized tissues by common GI organisms. **Fluoroquinolones** and **imipenem** readily penetrate the pancreas and achieve effective tissue concentrations. Controlled clinical studies demonstrate that antibiotic prophylaxis reduces the rate of pancreatic infection in severe acute pancreatitis. Mortality rate, however, is not reduced consistently by prophylactic antibiotics.

4. **Infected necrosis** develops in 40% to 70% of patients with necrotizing pancreatitis. The main determinant of infection is the presence and extent of intra- and extrapancreatic necrosis. The timing of presentation is variable. Using fine needle aspiration, bacteria can be demonstrated in areas of necrosis at a median of 6 days after the onset of

acute pancreatitis. Approximately 70% of specimens are contaminated after 2 weeks of necrotizing pancreatitis. The mortality rate of patients with infected necrosis ranges from 15% to 80%, whereas that of patients with sterile necrosis is about 10%.

  a. Contrast-enhanced computed tomography is the standard for detecting pancreatic necrosis. Serial examinations allow for the assessment of the extent of pancreatic and peripancreatic necrosis and the detection of peripancreatic fluid collections and pseudocysts.

  b. Guided percutaneous fine needle aspiration with Gram's stain and culture of the aspirate is necessary to detect infected pancreatic necrosis. Interventional radiologic drainage techniques can be used to treat infected pancreatic fluid collections and pseudocysts.

5. **Surgical treatment.** Traditional indications for surgery include exploration in patients with an acute abdomen, removal of impacted gallstones, drainage of pancreatic fluid collections, and debridement of necrotic tissue. Patients with infected necrotic tissue should undergo surgical debridement.

F. **Complications**
  1. **Vascular complications**
      a. Hemorrhage usually occurs from the retroperitoneal vessels, but also can occur from the splenic, middle colic, and pancreaticoduodenal vessels. Initial treatment consists of resuscitation with blood products. Coagulopathies are common in this setting and should be aggressively treated. Operative intervention is reserved for patients who continue to bleed.

      b. Thrombosis of the splenic vein can occur as it courses along the posterior surface of the pancreas and becomes involved in peripancreatic inflammation. Esophageal, gastric, and duodenal varices can occur secondary to splenic vein thrombosis and can lead to hemorrhage. Splenectomy is usually curative in this situation. Thrombosis of the mesenteric vessels, leading to visceral ischemia, also can occur.

      c. Pseudoaneurysms affecting the splenic, hepatic, gastroduodenal, and pancreaticoduodenal arteries occur rarely. Patients usually present with pain caused by expansion and pressure on adjacent structures, or hemorrhage. The diagnosis is made by Doppler ultrasonography and mesenteric angiography. Treatment involves angiography and embolization.

  2. **Pancreatic pseudocyst** is defined as a fluid collection enclosed by a fibrous capsule; it occurs in 10% to 15% of patients. Operative intervention is delayed for 6 to 8 weeks after the radiologic diagnosis of pancreatic pseudocyst is made, because

approximately 20% of pseudocysts can resolve spontaneously. Asymptomatic pseudocysts less than 6 cm in diameter can be followed for even longer periods, because they can resolve over many months. Major complications that can occur while waiting include abscess formation, rupture of the pseudocyst, and erosion into a major artery (e.g., splenic artery).

3. **Pancreatic fistulas** usually result from interventions such as open or closed drainage of a pseudocyst or pancreatic debridement. The diagnosis usually is made by the finding of an increased amylase concentration in the drainage. **Endoscopic retrograde cholangiopancreatography (ERCP)** can define the presence of proximal ductal obstruction or connection between the fistula and the pancreatic duct. If proximal ductal obstruction is present, endoscopic placement of a stent or distal surgical decompression may be needed. Conservative treatment includes controlling the fistula drainage, protecting the skin, and providing nutritional support. **Octreotide** is helpful in the management of high output fistulas. Low output fistulas usually will close without operative intervention.

V. **Gastrointestinal motility problems**
    A. **Diarrhea**
        1. **Pathophysiology.** Under normal conditions, 9 L of fluid enter the bowel each day from oral intake and intestinal secretions. The majority is absorbed in the small bowel, leaving 1 to 1.5 L to enter the colon. The remaining fluid is absorbed in the proximal half of the colon. Changes in GI motility and epithelial mucosal integrity can drastically affect fluid absorption. Water is absorbed secondary to active and passive transport of sodium and osmotic flow of the products of digestion.
        2. **Etiology.** Common causes of diarrhea in the critically ill patient include infections, enteral nutrition, and medications. Ischemic colitis is a particular concern in patients after vascular surgery. Less common causes include fecal impaction, intestinal fistula, neoplasm, pancreatic insufficiency, sepsis, and hypoalbuminemia.
            a. **Infectious diarrhea** in the ICU setting is caused most commonly by *Clostridium difficile* (Chapter 28). Clinical presentation varies from asymptomatic carriage to fulminant colitis. **Pseudomembraneous colitis,** which is the classical presentation of this disease, is found most commonly in the left colon. Most of the patients will respond to medical therapy once a diagnosis is made. Complications include dehydration, secondary infection, and toxic dilation and perforation of the colon. Surgery is

rarely required. Other bacterial and viral infections causing diarrhea in critically ill patients are rare. Stool cultures and ova and parasite examinations are of low yield after the initial 2 days of hospitalization.

b. **Enteral nutrition** as a cause of diarrhea is a diagnosis of exclusion. Osmotic diarrhea is secondary to malabsorption of nutrients and usually stops with fasting. Intestinal atrophy can reflect overall nutritional status or luminal nutritional deprivation; it plays a significant role in causing malabsorption.

c. **Medications** implicated as a cause of diarrhea include antibiotics, sorbitol additives, theophylline, magnesium antacids, H_2 blockers, antineoplastic agents, antidysrhythmic agents, antihypertensive agents, cholesterol medications, and thyroid hormone.

   (1) **Sorbitol** is a poorly absorbed polyalcohol sugar that is present as an inactive ingredient in many medications. It can cause an osmotic diarrhea if given in sufficient quantity.

   (2) **Antibiotics** can be associated with diarrhea independent of an infectious cause. This may result from altered muscularis motor activity or a change in the bacterial milieu, decreasing the fermentation of carbohydrate to absorbable short chain fatty acids.

   (3) **Chemotherapeutic agents** cause diarrhea by causing intestinal epithelial damage.

d. **Ischemic colitis** can be secondary to atherosclerosis, vasculitis, hypercoagulable states, or hypoperfusion. It is a complication after abdominal aortic surgery because of iatrogenic inferior mesenteric artery ligation or intraoperative hypotension. The left colon is most commonly affected. In low flow states, the right colon, splenic flexure, and recto-sigmoid colon are most likely to be injured. Common signs and symptoms include abdominal pain and distention, nausea and vomiting, and GI bleeding. In severe ischemia with necrosis, laboratory evaluation may show hyperkalemia, lactic metabolic acidosis, hyperphosphatemia, and elevated alkaline phosphate levels. The diagnosis is made by colonoscopy. Most cases can be managed medically with supportive care and treatment of the underlying illness. Indications for surgery include peritonitis, colonic perforation, and clinical deterioration despite adequate medical therapy.

e. **Miscellaneous causes of diarrhea**
   (1) **Hypoalbuminemia** has been associated with enteral feeding diarrhea. Mucosal atrophy or edema appears to play a contributory role.
   (2) **Fecal impaction** can paradoxically lead to diarrhea as a result of decreased rectal tone, mucus secretion, and impaired anorectal sensation.
   (3) **Inflammatory bowel disease** commonly presents as bloody diarrhea and abdominal cramps, usually with a prior history of similar episodes.
   (4) **An altered enterohepatic circulation,** leading to increased bile acid in the colon, can induce net fluid secretion. This is seen in diseases of the ileum, fatty acid malabsorption, and altered bowel flora.

3. **Diagnosis and management**
   a. **Initial supportive care** includes replacement of lost fluids and electrolytes.
   b. **A careful review** of current and recent medications is warranted. **Physical examination** may reveal fecal impaction in which case manual disimpaction and enemas are the treatment of choice. Blood in the stool suggests an infectious or ischemic cause.
   c. **An infectious cause** must be considered. Leukocytes in the stool are a nonspecific marker for inflammation. Because the sensitivity of the toxin assay for *C. difficile* is greater than 90%, testing one to two stool samples should be adequate for diagnosis. Visualization of pseudomembranes on flexible sigmoidoscopy may confirm the diagnosis. Along with supportive measures and discontinuation of the implicated antimicrobial agent, *C. difficile* co-litis must be treated with metronidazole or vancomycin (Chapter 28).

   If an osmotic diarrhea is suspected, stool electrolyte concentrations and osmolality can be determined $\{2 \times ([Na^+] + [K^+])\}$ and the osmolar gap calculated. The **osmolar gap** is the difference between the measured stool osmolality and the calculated stool osmolality. An osmolar gap of greater than 100 mOsm/kg is suggestive of an osmotic diarrhea.
   d. **Switching to a peptide-based enteral formula** may alleviate diarrhea associated with tube feedings. Little data support adjusting formula osmolality, temperature, or fat content. Similarly, elemental formulas and fiber supplements have not provided any consistent advantage.

      e. Once an infectious cause is excluded, diarrhea can be treated symptomatically with several agents (Table 25-5).

B. **Ileus** is the failure of the GI contents to pass in the absence of mechanical obstruction. Patients present with nausea and vomiting, abdominal distention, and poorly localized abdominal discomfort. Significant fluid can be sequestered in the bowel, leading to electrolyte disturbances and hypovolemia. The chance for perforation is increased with bowel distention.

    1. **Pathophysiology.** After an uncomplicated abdominal operation, small bowel motility generally returns within 24 hours. Gastric motility follows within 48 hours and colonic motility returns in 3 to 5 days. Ileus is thought to result from the loss of organized contraction by the intrinsic activity of the bowel (Table 25-6).

    2. **Diagnosis.** Abdominal radiographs typically show distention of the small and large intestine with intraluminal air present throughout. Bowel sounds are reduced or absent. Rarely, radiographic contrast studies are needed to exclude mechanical obstruction.

    3. **Treatment**

        a. **Supportive care** begins with fluid and electrolyte repletion. Patients with abdominal distention and significant nausea or vomiting should have nasogastric tubes placed to decompress their GI tracts. Potential causes of ileus should be reviewed. In postsurgical patients, ileus can be an early sign of intraabdominal infection.

        b. **Pharmacologic agents** have been used in the treatment of postoperative ileus. The prokinetic effect of **metoclopramide** is achieved through peripheral dopaminergic blockade and cholinergic enhancement. **Cisapride** is an indirect cholinergic agonist. It exerts its prokinetic effect throughout the GI tract. Because cisapride can cause serious ventricular dysrhythmias, including ventricular tachycardia

Table 25-5. Agents used to treat diarrhea

Diphenoxylate with atropine (Lomotil)	A constipating meperidine congener, diphenoxylate is extensively metabolized to the active metabolite difenoxine.
Loperamide (Imodium)	Inhibits peristalsis and slows intestinal activity.
Bismuth subsalicylate (Pepto-Bismol)	Has antisecretory, antimicrobial, and antiinflammatory effects.

Table 25-6.   Causes of ileus

Electrolyte derangements
  –Hypokalemia
  –Hyponatremia
  –Hypomagnesemia
  –Hypermagnesemia
Postoperative
  (Especially following operations in the peritoneal cavity)
Drugs
  –Calcium channel blockers
  –Narcotics
  –Anticholinergics
Retroperitoneal hemorrhage and inflammation
Sepsis
Sympathetic hyperactivity

and fibrillation, its use is not recommended for seriously ill patients. **Erythromycin** is a motilin receptor agonist. None of these agents, however, effectively alters the course of postoperative ileus.

    c. **Colonoscopic or operative decompression** can be performed for impending perforation.

C. **Constipation.** Many disease states and medications can produce constipation. A careful review of the history and medications should be undertaken (Table 25-7). Treatment is aimed at correcting the underlying disease (Table 25-8). Fiber supplementation and various laxatives can be administered once the cause is identified.

VI. **The acute abdomen in the critically ill patient**

    A. **Initial assessment.** The abdomen is a potential source of occult, and sometimes serious, infection in critically ill patients. These patients are difficult to assess because the classical signs of an acute abdomen, tenderness and guarding, may not be present. Nonspecific findings (e.g., fever, positive blood cultures, or shock) may suggest intraabdominal sepsis, but these are not diagnostic. Consequently, one must maintain a high index of suspicion that intraabdominal pathology may be present.

    B. **Diagnostic evaluation**

        1. **Ultrasonography** can be used to evaluate the gallbladder and biliary tract. It is less helpful for distinguishing between small abscesses and fluid-filled loops of bowel. Large amounts of intestinal gas can severely hinder ultrasonographic evaluation.

        2. **Computed tomography** can localize abdominal abscesses and delimit organs that may have marginal or no blood flow. Free intraperitoneal air or

Table 25-7. Causes of constipation

Medications
> Narcotics
> Anticholinergics
> Aluminum hydroxide antacids
> Calcium channel blockers
> Iron
> Barium

Endocrine
> Hypothyroidism
> Hypercalcemia
> Diabetes

Intestinal obstruction
> Tumor
> Volvulus
> Diverticulitis
> Endometriosis

Neurologic
> Cerebral vascular accident
> Parkinson's disease
> Alzheimer's disease
> Spinal cord disease
> Chagas disease
> Hirshsprung's disease

Systemic
> Scleroderma
> Amyloidosis
> Hypokalemia
> Uremia

Functional
> Immobilization
> Low fiber diet
> Irritable bowel syndrome

fluid from a recent laparotomy can confuse interpretation of the radiographic study. Occasionally, the patient's condition precludes transportation to the CT scanning suite.

3. **Laparoscopy** has been suggested as a possible tool for evaluating the abdomen in the critically ill patient. This can be performed at the bedside in some institutions; however, its efficacy for evaluation has not been fully determined.

4. **Laparotomy** may be indicated in critically ill patients with occult sources of sepsis or organ failure. The laparotomy is more likely to be therapeutic in patients who have received a prior abdominal operation or if the laparotomy is directed by evidence supporting an acute intraabdominal process.

Table 25-8.   Agents to treat constipation

Bulk producing	Methylcellulose Psyllium Polycarbophyl	Holds water in stool; most physiologic.
Irritant/ stimulant	Bisacodyl Senna Cascara Phenolphthalein Casanthranol Castor oil	Direct action on the intestinal mucosa; stimulates myenteric plexus.
Lubricant	Mineral oil	Retards colonic absorption of fecal water; softens stool.
Surfactants	Docusate	Detergent activity; softens stools.
Saline-based	Magnesium sulfate Magnesium hydroxide Magnesium citrate Sodium phosphate Sodium phosphate and biphosphate enema	Attracts and retains water in intestinal lumen.
Miscellaneous	Lactulose Glycerin suppository	Osmotically active molecules.

C.   **Acute acalculous cholecystitis** is associated with trauma, surgery, burns, prolonged parenteral nutrition, and prolonged use of narcotics. Functional obstruction of the bile duct can occur secondary to viscous bile, decreased cystic artery perfusion, bacterial colonization, and reflux of pancreatic juice. Of patients with acalculous cholecystitis, 50% develop gangrenous changes in the gallbladder, and 8% to 15% develop perforation of the gallbladder.

1.   **Pathology.** The gallbladder is markedly edematous. Present may be focal necrosis of the gallbladder wall, arteries, and veins and thrombosis. This arterial and venous involvement is not seen in the gallbladder with gallstone disease, suggesting that vascular occlusion is central to the pathogenesis of acute acalculous cholecystitis.

2.   **Diagnosis.** Acalculous cholecystitis should be considered in every critically ill patient who has sepsis without an obvious source. Because of associated critical illness, the diagnosis may not be readily apparent. Fever, leukocytosis, and hyperbilirubinemia are common but nonspecific findings. Examination of the abdomen generally is unreliable.

a.   **Ultrasonography** of the gallbladder is the primary diagnostic modality. It can be performed rapidly and accurately at the bedside. Thickening of the gallbladder wall (> 3.5 mm) is a reliable diagnostic criterion. Other helpful ultrasonographic findings include sludge in the gallbladder, pericholecystic fluid, intramural gas, and a lucent intramural layer representing intramural edema.

    b. **Computed tomography** is also highly accurate in the diagnosis of acute acalculous cholecystitis.

  3. **Treatment. Percutaneous drainage** is the first choice for treatment in critically ill patients. Drainage can be performed safely under ultrasonographic guidance at the bedside. **Traditional surgical management** consists of either surgical cholecystostomy or cholecystectomy. **Antibiotic therapy** should be directed toward organisms identified by Gram's stain and culture. Prior antibiotic therapy can alter the host flora and select resistant strains of common pathogens. Anaerobes are relatively common in the bile of patients with diabetes mellitus, those aged more than 70 years, or those whose biliary tracts have previously been instrumented.

D. **Mesenteric ischemia and intestinal necrosis**

  1. **Acute mesenteric ischemia** occurs predominantly in the geriatric population, especially those with significant cardiovascular and systemic disorders. **Superior mesenteric artery emboli** are responsible for 40% to 50% of episodes. The embolus usually originates from a left atrial or ventricular mural thrombus that is dislodged during a dysrhythmia or following cardiac catheterization. Emboli lodge at points of normal anatomic narrowing, usually distal to the origin of a major branch. Ischemic injury occurs when vasoconstriction develops in arteries both proximal and distal to the embolus.

  2. **Nonocclusive mesenteric ischemia** accounts for 20% to 30% of episodes of acute mesenteric ischemia. It is caused by splanchnic vasoconstriction secondary to vasoactive medications or by hypoperfusion from hypotension, dysrhythmias, myocardial depression, or hypovolemia. Vasoconstriction can persist even after the precipitating cause has been eliminated or corrected.

  3. **Intestinal ischemia** can produce a range of injury—from changes in capillary permeability leading to interstitial edema and fluid movement into the lumen of the bowel to transmural bowel necrosis. Ischemia causes marked increases in gut mucosal permeability. Increased permeability allows bacterial endotoxins to enter the systemic circulation, which can produce septic shock, myocardial depression, acute renal failure, and even death.

4. **Diagnosis.** Early identification of acute mesenteric ischemia requires a high index of suspicion in patients who have significant risk factors associated with the disease. Most patients experience acute abdominal pain, often out of proportion to physical findings. In nonocclusive disease, up to 25% of patients do not experience pain. Unexplained GI distention or bleeding may be the only indication of mesenteric ischemia. Rebound tenderness and muscle guarding occurs if transmural necrosis develops. The stool may contain occult blood. Hyperkalemia and metabolic lactate acidosis may be present. Angiography is diagnostic.

5. **Treatment.** Initial treatment of acute mesenteric ischemia is aimed toward resuscitation, supportive care, and correcting the precipitating cause of ischemia.

   a. **Intra-arterial infusion of papaverine** through a catheter placed at the origin of the superior mesenteric artery during angiography can relieve mesenteric vasoconstriction.

   b. **Laparotomy** is necessary to restore intestinal arterial flow after an embolus or thrombosis and to resect irreparably damaged bowel. Reexploration (second look) is required within 12 to 24 hours to assess the need for further bowel resection.

   c. **Broad-spectrum antibiotics** should be started as soon as the diagnosis of acute mesenteric ischemia is made and continued into the postoperative period. The ischemic bowel allows translocation of intraluminal bacteria into the systemic circulation. Blood cultures often are positive and can help guide further antibiotic therapy.

VII. Abdominal compartment syndrome (ACS)

A. **ACS** is a condition of increased intraabdominal pressure that is associated with hemodynamic, respiratory, and renal dysfunction.

B. **Causes** include intraabdominal bleeding after blunt and penetrating abdominal trauma, particularly after abdominal packing for uncontrollable bleeding, aggressive fluid resuscitation with the resultant bowel edema, ascites, pancreatitis, and liver transplantation.

C. **Treatment for intraabdominal hypertension** should be directed toward prevention: avoiding closure of the abdominal wall under tension and gradual closure of the wound when increased intraabdominal pressure is suspected. Once significant intraabdominal hypertension develops, treatment is by decompressive laparotomy. See Chapter 33 for additional details concerning diagnosis and management.

SELECTED REFERENCES

Avgerinos A, Nevens F, Raptis S, et al. Early administration of somatostatin and efficacy of sclerotherapy in acute oesophageal variceal bleeds: the European Acute Bleeding Oesophageal Variceal Episodes (ABOVE) randomised trial. *Lancet* 1997;350:1495–1499.

Beger HG, Rau B, Mayer J, et al. Natural course of acute pancreatitis. *World J Surg* 1997;21:130–135.

Cook D, Guyatt G, Marshall J, et al. A comparison of sucralfate and ranitidine for the prevention of upper gastrointestinal bleeding in patients requiring mechanical ventilation. Canadian Critical Care Trials Group. *N Engl J Med* 1998;338:791–797.

Cullen DJ, Coyle JP, Teplick R, et al. Cardiovascular, pulmonary, and renal effects of massively increased intra-abdominal pressure in critically ill patients. *Crit Care Med* 1989;17:118–121.

Fernandez-del Castillo C, Rattner DW, Makary MA, et al. Debridement and closed packing for the treatment of necrotizing pancreatitis. *Ann Surg* 1998;228:676–684.

Ivatury RR, Diebel L, Porter JM, et al. Intra-abdominal hypertension and the abdominal compartment syndrome. *Surg Clin North Am* 1997;77:783–800.

Laine L. Acute and chronic gastrointestinal bleeding. In: Sleisenger MH, Fordtran JS, eds. *Gastrointestinal disease: pathophysiology/diagnosis/management,* 6th ed. Philadelphia: WB Saunders, 1998: 198–219.

Martin RF, Flynn P. The acute abdomen in the critically ill patient. *Surg Clin North Am* 1997;77:1455–1464.

Mithofer K, Fernandez-del Castillo C, Ferraro MJ, et al. Antibiotic treatment improves survival in experimental acute necrotizing pancreatitis. *Gastroenterology* 1996;110:232–240.

Powell JJ, Miles R, Siriwardena AK. Antibiotic prophylaxis in the initial management of severe acute pancreatitis. *Br J Surg* 1998;85: 582–587.

Ringel AF, Jameson GL, Foster ES. Diarrhea in the intensive care patient. *Crit Care Clin* 1995;11:465–477.

Tryba M, Cook D. Current guidelines on stress ulcer prophylaxis. *Drugs* 1997;54:581–596.

Turnage R, Bergen P. Intestinal obstruction and ileus. In: Sleisenger MH, Fordtran JS, eds. *Gastrointestinal disease: pathophysiology/diagnosis/management,* 6th ed. Philadelphia: WB Saunders, 1998: 1807–1808.

Endocrine Disorders

Robert A. Peterfreund and Stephanie L. Lee

Endocrine disorders are common comorbid conditions that can complicate management of critically ill patients in the postoperative period. Diabetes mellitus is the endocrine condition most likely to be encountered, but other conditions significantly contribute to comprehensive care of the severely compromised patient.

I. **Diabetes mellitus**
   A. **Physiology overview.** Diabetes mellitus (DM) is a chronic systemic disease caused by the absolute (**type 1 DM**) or relative (**type 2 DM**) lack of insulin, which results in hyperglycemia. Elevated glucose levels, normally stimulate insulin secretion from pancreatic beta cells. Catecholamines inhibit insulin secretion. Insulin facilitates glucose and potassium transport across cell membranes, enhances glycogen synthesis, and inhibits lipolysis. Insulin production continues at a low basal level even during periods of fasting, which prevents catabolism and ketoacidosis. States of physiologic stress, including surgery, infection, and cardiopulmonary bypass, are associated with peripheral resistance to the effects of insulin. The liver and kidney metabolize insulin. Prolonged insulin action commonly is encountered with renal insufficiency.
      1. **Type 1 DM.** Autoimmune destruction of pancreatic beta cells results in the absolute insulin deficiency of type 1 DM. The condition was formerly known as juvenile or insulin-dependent (IDDM) diabetes; this terminology is no longer recognized. Patients generally present at a younger age and are sensitive to small amounts of insulin. They are susceptible to ketosis, but not obesity. Therapy is with human insulin. Insulin is absolutely required even during fasting to prevent ketoacidosis.
      2. **Type 2 DM.** Peripheral resistance to insulin necessitates high circulating insulin levels to maintain euglycemia in patients with type 2 DM, who represent 90% of all diabetics. Patients are generally older, obese, and ketosis-resistant. They are susceptible to hyperosmolar complications. Management is with diet alone, exercise, oral hypoglycemic agents, or insulin. Terms no longer recognized for this condition include "noninsulin-dependent," and "adult-onset" diabetes (AODM).
      3. **Other causes of insulin insufficiency.** Cystic fibrosis, chronic pancreatitis, hemochromatosis, toxic effects of pentamidine, and pancreatic surgery or

resection can result in hyposecretion of insulin from the pancreas. Glucagonoma, pheochromocytoma, acromegaly, and glucocorticoid excess often increase insulin resistance, resulting in glucose intolerance.

B. Acute complications of diabetes

   1. Diabetic ketoacidosis (DKA). DKA occurs almost exclusively in type 1 diabetics. Ketoacidosis results from the absolute insulin deficiency or resistance to insulin seen during stress (e.g., infection, surgery, and trauma).

   a. Circulatory depression. Acidosis and metabolic derangements depress myocardial contractility and peripheral vascular tone. Preexisting coronary artery disease (CAD), cardiomyopathy, or peripheral vascular disease (PVD) can contribute to hemodynamic instability. Hyperglycemia (and concurrent hyperosmolarity) produces an osmotic diuresis leading to profound hypovolemia.

   b. Electrolyte abnormalities include hyperglycemia (although glucose is usually < 500 mg/dl), intracellular dehydration, hyperkalemia, and hyponatremia. Serum K^+ levels are elevated because acidosis drives K^+ out of cells. Insulin concentrations are insufficient to maintain intracellular K^+ levels so that total body K^+ is actually depressed (3–10 mEq/kg body weight). Measured Na^+ concentrations are artifactually lowered ~1.6 mEq/L for every 100 mg/dl that the glucose is elevated. Hypophosphatemia and hypomagnesemia commonly result from urinary losses.

   2. Hyperglycemic, hyperosmolar, nonketotic state (HONK)

   a. Presentation. HONK is often triggered by infection, dehydration, an acute cardiovascular event [including silent myocardial infarction (MI) or stroke], trauma, or surgery in elderly type 2 diabetic patients. HONK may be the initial presentation of type 2 DM.

   b. Characteristics. Serum glucose levels often exceed 500 mg/dl. Osmotic diuresis initially results in hypovolemia with profound fluid deficits (5–10 L), electrolyte abnormalities (prerenal azotemia, hypernatremia, hypokalemia, hypophosphatemia and hypomagnesemia, but usually no anion gap), hemoconcentration, and central nervous system (CNS) dysfunction (depressed sensorium, seizures, or coma). Insulin levels are usually sufficient to block lipolysis and ketogenesis so that ketoacidosis is not typically encountered. Sustained, profound hypovolemia can result in lactic acidosis with an anion gap and renal failure.

C. **Chronic complications of diabetes**
1. **Atherosclerosis.** Diabetes is a strong risk factor for vascular disease, which tends to occur more extensively and at an earlier age than in the general population. Microvascular disease (retinopathy and nephropathy) and macrovascular disease (coronary artery, cerebrovascular, and peripheral vascular) are prevalent among diabetics. Diabetes is the most common cause for blindness, renal failure leading to dialysis, and vascular insufficiency necessitating amputation.
2. **Neuropathy.** Peripheral sensory neuropathies can cause pain and numbness. Central ventilatory responses to hypoxia can be diminished, and sensitivity to CNS depressants can increase. Autonomic neuropathy is common with postural hypotension, gastroparesis, and bladder atony. A feature of diabetic autonomic neuropathy is symptomatically "silent" cardiac ischemia. Diabetics have an increased risk of sudden cardiac death caused by autonomic cardiac dysfunction.
3. **Other manifestations.** Infection and poor wound healing are major complications.

D. **Diabetes therapy**
1. **Oral hypoglycemic agents** (Table 26-1) are commonly used for first line, chronic therapy of type 2 DM. It is important to recognize that the various agents have different mechanisms, onset times, and durations of action. Side effects also differ. **Sulfonylureas** act by increasing pancreatic insulin release. Certain preparations can induce hypoglycemia up to 50 hours after administration in the fasting patient. Some sulfonylureas increase the effectiveness of thiazide diuretics, barbiturates, and anticoagulants by altering protein binding. A nonsulfonylurea agent, **repaglinide,** also increases insulin secretion in the presence of hyperglycemia. The biguanide **metformin** and the thiazolidinediones **troglitazone** and **rosiglitazone** inhibit hepatic glucose production and increase sensitivity to insulin, but no increase in insulin secretion occurs. **Acarbose,** an α-glucosidase inhibitor, delays digestion and absorption of complex carbohydrates from the intestine. Single agent therapy with metformin, acarbose, or troglitazone is not associated with hypoglycemia in the fed or fasting state. Troglitazone therapy is associated with a risk of elevation in liver enzymes and possible hepatic dysfunction. Fulminant hepatic failure is a rare complication of troglitazone therapy. In prerelease testing, rosiglitazone was associated with a reduced incidence of hepatic enzyme elevation compared with troglitazone. The profile of rosiglitazone's toxic effects will not be fully defined until the drug is used by a large number of patients. Metformin can cause life-threatening lactic acido-

Table 26-1. **Oral agents used to treat diabetes mellitus**

Agent	Time to onset (h)	Duration of action (h)
Sulfonylurea[a]		
—Tolbutamide (Orinase, Oramide)	1	6–12
—Glipizide (Glucotrol)	1	6–12
—Glipizide XL	1–4	10–24
—Acetoheximide (Dymelor)	1	8–12
—Tolazamide (Tolinase)	4–6	10–15
—Glyburide (Micronase, Diabeta)	1–4	10–24
—Glimepiride (Amaryl)	1	18–24
—Chlorpropamide (Diabinase)	1	24–72
Alpha glucosidase inhibitor[b,c]		
—Acarbose (Precose)	Immediate	<0.3
Biguanide[c,d]		
—Metformin (Glucophage)	1	8–12
Thiazolidinedione[c,d]		
—Troglitazone (Rezulin)	1	24
—Rosiglitazone (Avandia)	1	24
—Piaglitazone (Actos)	1	24
Meglitinide[a,e]		
—Repaglinide (Prandin)	≤0.25	3–4

[a] Increases insulin secretion.
[b] Nonsystemic. Delays digestion and absorption of complex carbohydrates from the intestine.
[c] When used as the *sole agent* for treatment, hypoglycemia (insulin reaction) is unlikely; may be taken on the morning of surgery.
[d] Inhibits hepatic glucose production. Increases sensitivity to insulin. No increase in insulin secretion.
[e] Closes ATP-dependent potassium channels, depolarizing pancreatic β cells leading to calcium channel opening and enhanced insulin release. Nonsulfonylurea. Peak effect at 1 h. Usually administered before meals.

sis in patients with renal failure. Metformin should be stopped immediately if renal dysfunction is suspected. In situations where renal failure is likely, such as after intravenous contrast radiographic studies in diabetic patients, metformin should be held until normal renal function has been verified 2 days later.

2. **Insulin** (Table 26-2) is available in several preparations for parenteral administration in the management of type 1 or type 2 DM. Currently, most insulin-treated patients take human insulin (**humulin**); it is associated with decreased antigenicity compared with the animal insulins used in the past. Occasionally, patients still using animal insulin preparations will be encountered. Outpatient therapy is typically with subcutaneous administration.

3. **Routine glucose management in the ICU.** Therapy is designed to maintain serum glucose be-

Table 26-2. Insulin preparations for diabetes mellitus therapy

Agent	Time to onset (h)	Peak	Duration of action (h)
Insulin (SC administration)			
–Lispro (Humalog)	≤0.25	1	3.5–4.5
–Regular	0.5–1	1–5	5–8
–Semilente	0.5–3	2–10	12–16
–NPH	1–4	4–12	24–28
–Lente	1–3	6–15	22–28
–Protamine zinc	1–6	14–24	≥36
–Ultralente	2–8	10–30	≥36

Note: When regular insulin is administered IV, the onset of action is immediate and the duration of action is ~1h..
SC, subcutaneously.

tween 120 and 200 mg/dl. Management is usually with insulin administered intravenously (IV), subcutaneously (SC), or intramuscularly (IM).

a. **Monitoring.** Frequent monitoring of blood sugar is recommended. Patients on stable IV insulin infusions should have blood glucose checked every 2 hours. Blood glucose should be checked approximately 1 hour after an adjustment in the rate of IV insulin infusion. Patients receiving regular insulin SC should have blood glucose checked every 4 hours after administration. Patients treated with NPH insulin SC should have blood glucose checked every 8 hours after administration. Patients receiving total parenteral nutrition containing insulin should have blood glucose monitored twice a day.

b. **Insulin therapy.** Unreliable absorption of SC or IM insulin is encountered in the critically ill patient with hypothermia, edema, hemodynamic instability, or vasopressor support. **Intravenous regular insulin** is the preferred therapy in such patients. Routine maintenance dosing guidelines for hyperglycemic patients are listed in Table 26-3. The insulin regimen must be individually titrated. All patients receiving exogenous insulin should have an exogenous source of carbohydrate available, which can be given via enteral feeding, total parenteral nutrition, or IV glucose. The typical adult glucose infusion is 5 g/h of glucose, supplied as 5% dextrose (D5) in one half normal saline (NS) infused at 100 ml/h.

c. **Signs and symptoms of hypoglycemia** include evidence of elevated sympathetic out-

Table 26-3. Guidelines for
routine regular insulin infusions

Starting infusion rate (regular insulin, 25 U/250 ml saline), units/h

Type I DM (female)	0.5
Type I DM (male)	1.0
Type II DM (male or female)	1.0

Adjustment of regular insulin infusion rate, units/h

Blood glucose	Infusion change	Other treatment
<70 mg/dl	Hold 30 min	Administer D50, 15–20 ml Recheck glucose after 30 min Repeat glucose administration until serum glucose >70 mg/dl
70–120	–0.3 U/h	
121–180	No change	
181–240	+0.3 U/h	
241–300	+0.6 U/h	
>300	+1.0 U/h	

Note: Guidelines assume the patient is fasting, and not in diabetic ketoacidosis. Patients should have a source of exogenous carbohydrate available or infusing, such as glucose at 5 g/h. **Dosing must be individualized titrated based on frequent serum glucose monitoring.**

flow (e.g., tachycardia, tremulousness, palpitations, diaphoresis) along with headache, seizures, or a depressed level of consciousness ranging from confusion to coma. These may all be masked by other features of the critically ill patient's condition. Patients with chronically tight blood sugar control often lose the sympathetic response to hypoglycemia, a condition known as "hypoglycemic unawareness." Ketoacidosis or hyperosmolar coma must be prevented without inducing hypoglycemia. Fasting (NPO) patients who are not receiving adequate exogenous carbohydrate are at risk for hypoglycemia.

(1) **Oral hypoglycemic agents.** Some sulfonylurea agents have extended durations of action. Prolonged hypoglycemic effects should be anticipated if chloropropramide or another long-acting agent had recently been ingested.

(2) **Insulin therapy.** Some insulin preparations have extended durations of action. Hypoglycemic effects can persist in patients who have recently received any of the long-acting preparations, particularly in the setting of renal insufficiency.

d. **Type 1 diabetics.** These patients must always receive some insulin to prevent ketoacidosis. Glucose infusions may be required to prevent hypoglycemia when insulin is administered.

4. **Management of DKA in type 1 DM:**
   a. **Regular** insulin, bolus (0.1 U/kg, IV or 10 U IV push); then continuous insulin infusion (starting at 0.1 U/kg/h).
   b. **Hourly** glucose and electrolyte determinations to guide adjustment of insulin dose.
   c. **Adjustments** to insulin infusion:
      (1) If serum glucose falls less than 10% or if anion gap and pH are unchanged, double the insulin infusion rate.
      (2) Maintain the insulin infusion rate until glucose level is less than 250 mg/dl or serum bicarbonate corrects to more than 18 mEq/L.
      (3) Reduce insulin infusion rate to 2 to 3 U/h. Add dextrose 5% when serum glucose falls below 250 mg/dl in order to continue insulin infusion until anion gap and serum bicarbonate are normal.
   d. **Volume** replacement, initially with NS then one half NS.
   e. **Electrolyte** replacement (K^+, Mg^{2+}, PO_4^-). Potassium and phosphate are essential for insulin action and should be replaced carefully. Verify normal kidney function first.

   Serum K^+ <3 mEq/L, give K^+ 40 mEq/h
   Serum K^+ <4 mEq/L, give K^+, 30 mEq/h
   Serum K^+ <5 mEq/L, give K^+, 20 mEq/h
   Serum K^+ > 5 mEq/L, no replacement

   f. **Consider** bicarbonate therapy only for severe acidosis (pH < 7), hemodynamic instability or cardiac rhythm disturbances.
5. **Management of hyperglycemic, hyperosmolar, nonketotic state in type 2 DM:**
   a. **Vigorous** volume replacement with NS can reduce plasma glucose load up to 50% over several hours. Typical adult replacement is with one-half NS. Lower rates of volume replacement are recommended for patients with cardiovascular disease.

   First hour, 1.5 L
   Second and third hours, 1 L
   After 3 hours, 0.5–1 L/h

   b. **Careful** monitoring of volume status is necessary, especially in elderly patients with cardiovascular or renal disease. Consider invasive monitoring.
   c. **Hourly** glucose and electrolyte determinations to guide adjustment of insulin dose.
   d. **Regular** insulin bolus (10 U IV push), then continuous insulin infusion starting at 0.1 U/kg/h. Double insulin infusion rate if the glucose concentration is unchanged after 2 to 4 hours. Titrate insulin infusion to maintain glucose less

than 250 mg/dl and until cardiovascular, electrolyte and metabolic parameters are normal.

    e. **Electrolyte** replacement. Note that the absence of acidosis in type 2 DM decreases the likelihood of severe potassium depletion.

II. Thyroid disease

A. **Physiology overview.** Thyroid hormones alter the speed of cellular biochemical reactions, total body oxygen consumption, and heat production. Thyrotropin-releasing hormone (TRH) from the hypothalamus stimulates the secretion of thyroid-stimulating hormone (TSH) from the anterior pituitary. TSH controls iodine uptake by the thyroid gland and iodine incorporation into tyrosine residues of thyroglobulin (organification). The hormones L-thyroxine (T_4) and triiodothyronine (T_3) are formed and stored in the thyroid gland. A low basal level of thyroid hormone secretion is enhanced by TSH and inhibited by thyroid hormone. Circulating thyroid hormone also exerts negative feedback on the hypothalamus and pituitary to control TRH and TSH release. Both forms of thyroid hormone are extensively (> 99%) bound to plasma proteins. Only the free (unbound) thyroid hormone is biologically active. Peripheral tissues convert T_4 to T_3, which is 100 times more potent than T_4 but has a shorter half-life.

B. **Evaluation and laboratory studies.** Thyroid function tests must be used in close conjunction with observation of the patient's clinical status because no single test is completely diagnostic for all types of thyroid disease. A careful history and physical examination are essential (Table 26-4). The most useful initial laboratory test for assessing thyroid function is measurement of serum TSH. Starvation, glucocorticoids, stress, dopamine, and fever depress TSH levels. The level of free T_4 may aid diagnosis under these conditions. The profile of test results in different thyroid conditions is outlined in Table 26-5. Note that normal values for thyroid function tests vary among institutions. Local normal values must be used for reference and diagnosis.

C. **Hyperthyroidism**

    1. **Causes.** The most common cause of hyperthyroidism is Graves' disease. Toxic multinodular goiter, subacute thyroiditis (acute phase), toxic adenoma, and a variety of tumors also can lead to hyperthyroidism. Iatrogenic overdosing or surreptitious ingestion of excessive amounts of thyroid hormone should not be overlooked.

    2. **Clinical features of hyperthyroidism**

        a. **Hyperthyroidism** is a hypermetabolic state. Nervousness, tachycardia, heat intolerance, muscle weakness, tremors, and weight loss are presenting complaints. The elderly may not manifest all of these features. Cardiovascular signs, often the only indication of hyperthyroidism in the elderly, include dysrhythmias (e.g., sinus tachycardia, atrial fibrillation), sys-

Table 26-4.   Clinical features of thyroid disease

Hyperthyroidism/Thyrotoxicosis

Symptoms	Signs
Nervousness	Motor hyperkinesis
Fatigue	Tachycardia or atrial
Weakness	fibrillation
Increased perspiration	Systolic hypertension
Irregular menses	Warm, moist skin
Palpitations	Tremor
Increased appetite	Proximal muscle weakness
Weight loss despite	Eyelid retraction
increased appetite	Lid lag
Frequent bowel movements	Stare
or diarrhea	Elevated liver function tests
	Decreased cholesterol

Hypothyroidism

Symptoms	Signs
Fatigue	Slow movement
Sleepiness	Slow speech
Depression	Hoarseness
Cold intolerance	Bradycardia
Weight gain	Dry, sallow skin
Constipation	Periorbital edema
Irregular menses with	Nonpitting edema (myxedema)
menorrhagia	Delayed relaxation of deep
Paresthesias	tendon reflexes
Carpal tunnel syndrome	Enlarged tongue
	Hypertension (especially
	diastolic)
	Low voltage ECG
	Elevated cholesterol
	Elevated CPK
	Enlarged cardiac silhouette on
	radiography

ECG, electrocardiogram; CPK, creatine phosphokinase.

tolic murmurs, and high output or ischemic congestive heart failure (Table 26-4). Associated findings include mild leukopenia, thrombocytopenia, and hypothrombinemia.

b. **Thyroid storm** is a state of extreme thyrotoxicosis with physiologic decompensation. The presentation includes fever out of proportion to any evidence of infection, dehydration (from fever, vomiting, diaphoresis, or diarrhea), tachydysrhythmias and hypotension often resistant to pharmacologic therapy, and alterations in mental status that range from confusion and agitation to psychosis, stupor, and coma. Progression to cardiovascular collapse and death is likely without prompt recognition and treatment. Thyroid storm can mimic malignant hyperthermia, neuroleptic malig-

Table 26-5. Laboratory tests of thyroid function

Condition	Total T₄	Free T₄	T₃	FTI[a]	THBR[b]	TSH
Hyperthyroidism	↑	↑	↑[c]	↑	↑	↓
Hypothyroidism-1°	↓	↓	↓[d]	↓	↓	↑
Hypothyroidism-2°	↓	↓	↓[d]	↓	↓	↓ or inappropriately Nl
Euthyroid sick						
Mild	Nl to low	Nl	↓	Nl to low	Nl	Nl to low
Severe	↓	Nl to low	↓	↓	Nl[e]	↓
Pregnancy	↑	Nl	↑	Nl to high	↓	Nl[f]

T₄, thyroxine; THBR, thyroid hormone-binding ratio (similar to T₃ uptake [T₃RU/T₃U]); TSH, thyroid-stimulating hormone; ↑, increased; ↓, decreased; Nl, normal.

[a] Free Thyroxine Index, T₄ × THBR.
[b] Also T₃RU, T₃U.
[c] 5% of patients have only elevated T₃, not T₄.
[d] T₃ may be maintained in near normal range until severe hypothyroidism.
[e] If plasma protein normal.
[f] 13% have transiently low TSH and normal free T₄ at the end of the first trimester.

nant syndrome, sepsis, hemorrhage, or reactions to transfusions or drugs. Thyroid storm can be precipitated by surgical stress but is usually seen 6 to 18 hours postoperatively. Other precipitants include myocardial infarction, stroke, infection, or trauma. Patients with untreated thyrotoxicosis or a history of thyrotoxicosis should be evaluated for abnormal thyroid hormone levels.

3. **Treatment of hyperthyroidism**
    a. **Chronic thyroid hormone excess** is treated with specific antithyroid drugs [e.g., **propylthiouracil** (PTU) and **methimazole**]. Thyroid hormone levels may not begin to normalize for 2 to 6 weeks. The most serious side effects of antithyroid agents are hepatitis and agranulocytosis. Ablation of the gland can be accomplished with surgery or radioactive iodine therapy.
    b. **Thyroid storm.** The first line of treatment for thyroid storm is cardiovascular resuscitation with volume repletion (NS, 5% dextrose). After rehydration, β-adrenergic blockers are used to control tachycardia. Specific treatment includes antithyroid medication in large doses. **Propylthiouracil** (300–400 mg, orally every 4 hours) is preferred over methimazole because it prevents conversion of T_4 to the more bioactive T_3. Graves' disease patients (but not patients with toxic multinodular goiter or toxic adenoma) are also treated with **iodine** (SSKI, five drops orally every 6 hours) with the dose given at least 1 hour *after* the first administration of PTU. Fever is treated with acetaminophen and external cooling. **Meperidine** may be useful to attenuate shivering, thereby reducing heat production. **High dose glucocorticoids** (dexamethasone, 2 mg, every 6 hours) will partially inhibit the release of thyroid hormone and prevent relative adrenal insufficiency resulting from the physiologic stress and increased glucocorticoid metabolism caused by thyrotoxicosis. Management of thyroid storm should be carried out in consultation with an endocrinologist. Even with prompt institution of appropriate therapy, mortality in thyroid storm can be as high as 20% to 30%, usually from cardiovascular collapse.

4. **Special considerations in hyperthyroid states**
    a. **Sympathetic stimulation** (pain, ketamine, pancuronium) can complicate the management of the thyrotoxic patient. If anesthesia is required, thyrotoxic patients may benefit from the sympathectomy produced by regional techniques, particularly epidural blockade.

b. **Hypotension.** Thyroid hormone excess results in systemic vasodilation that can produce hypotension. Treatment is with direct-acting vasoconstrictors. Fluid resuscitation is important in the patient rendered volume-depleted by excessive perspiration and increased insensible fluid losses.

c. **Heart failure.** Thyrotoxicosis may precipitate heart failure in patients (particularly the elderly) with underlying heart disease, (e.g., ischemia or valvular lesions) who are unable to tolerate tachycardia and the hormone-induced increases in contractility. Such patients may benefit from β-adrenergic blockade. In patients without heart disease, alterations in ventricular contractility are attributed to sustained elevations in heart rate, as are commonly seen in long-standing thyrotoxicosis. Cardiac function will not return to normal until after the treatment of thyrotoxicosis and rate control is achieved. Patients also can suffer from volume overload with "high output" failure in the setting of high filling pressures and decreased diastolic filling time. Ventricular performance may be normal. These patients may benefit from diuretics.

d. **Enhanced drug metabolism** is a feature of thyrotoxicosis; anticipate high sedative and analgesic requirements. Dose requirements for anticoagulants are decreased because of a reduction in coagulation factor levels.

e. **Myasthenia gravis** may be seen in some Graves' disease patients (30 times increased incidence), so neuromuscular blocking agents should be titrated carefully.

D. **Hypothyroidism**
1. **Causes.** In adults, **Hashimoto's thyroiditis** is the most common cause of hypothyroidism; it can be associated with other autoimmune processes, including systemic lupus, rheumatoid arthritis, primary adrenal insufficiency, pernicious anemia, diabetes mellitus, or Sjögren's syndrome. Thyroid ablation (surgery, radioiodine) or radiation therapy can decrease the synthesis of thyroid hormone. Iodine deficiency, drug therapy (lithium or phenylbutazone), and late phase subacute thyroiditis may be causative. Reduced thyroid hormone synthesis can also be congenital. Clinically significant hypothyroidism is unlikely immediately after thyroid surgery because the half-life of T_4 is 7 to 10 days. A significant reduction in measured T_4 levels is not evident until 3 to 7 days postoperatively.

2. **Clinical features of hypothyroidism**
a. **Hypothyroidism is a hypometabolic state.** Features include lethargy, CO_2 insensitivity, constipation, cold intolerance, facial edema

with an enlarged tongue, reversible cardiomyopathy, pericardial effusion, ascites, anemia, dilutional hyponatremia from decreased water
excretion, and an adynamic ileus with delayed
gastric emptying. Adrenalitis with decreased
cortisol production may be present. Hemodynamic derangements include elevated systemic vascular resistance (SVR), bradycardia,
diminished baroreceptor reflexes, and reduced
cardiac output (Table 26-4).

b. Sick euthyroid state, a condition characterized by central suppression of the thyroid axis,
is also known as "nonthyroidal illness syndrome." In mild states, only a low T_3 and an increase in reverse T_3 (rT_3) is observed. In severe
states, T_4 levels fall with an inappropriately
normal or (more commonly) suppressed TSH
level. In the critically ill patient, a T_4 level less
than 4 µg/dl is associated with a probability of
death approaching 50%; a T_4 level less than
2 µg/dl correlates with mortality of approximately 80%. The mechanism of the sick euthyroid state is controversial. No clear consensus
is found as to whether this is a hypothyroid
state that should be treated with thyroid hormone to reproduce normal physiologic levels,
or whether the condition is an adaptation
to critical illness. In the setting of clinically
significant depression of cardiac function,
however, short-term thyroid hormone supplementation may be beneficial.

In the sick euthyroid state, T_4 is not converted to T_3. Therapy is with T_3, (usually 15 µg
IV, every 8 hours). In replacement doses, T_3 is
generally well tolerated, but elderly patients
or patients with significant CAD should be
treated cautiously to reduce the chance of precipitating ischemia or dysrhythmias. The T_3
level should be monitored every 2 days and adjusted to the low normal range, usually 70 to
100 ng/ml.

c. Myxedema coma (profound hypothyroidism)
is a clinical diagnosis defined by decreased
mental status. It is associated with hyporre-
sponsiveness to CO_2, congestive heart failure
(CHF), hypothermia, and exaggerated signs
and symptoms of severe hypothyroidism. In the
severely hypothyroid patient, surgery, drugs,
trauma, and infection can precipitate this de-
compensated state.

**3. Laboratory diagnosis and evaluation of hypo-
thyroidism** is usually based on the measurement
of TSH. High-dose glucocorticoid therapy or high-
dose dopamine infusions will blunt the elevation of

TSH in the critically ill hypothyroid patient. Thus, the degree of elevation of TSH may not directly reflect the magnitude of thyroid hormone deficiency. Additional thyroid function tests [free T_4, total T_4, or free thyroxine index (FTI)] will help characterize the condition. The diagnosis of Hashimoto's autoimmune thyroiditis, the most common cause of hypothyroidism, is confirmed with antithyroid antibody titers and measurement of antithyroperoxidase (TPO) antibodies.

4. **Treatment.** Chronic treatment involves exogenous oral supplementation with thyroid hormone. Thyroxine requires 7 to 10 days to have an effect. Oral T_3 begins to have an effect in 6 hours. *Cautious IV* thyroid hormone loading will hasten recovery and is indicated for myxedema coma. The agent of choice is T_3. The adult loading dose is 25 to 50 µg; this should be reduced to 10 to 20 µg in cases of known or suspected cardiac disease. The typical T_3 requirement is approximately 65 µg/d, administered in divided doses every 4 to 6 hours based on clinical responses. For patients on chronic oral T_4 replacement requiring long-term IV thyroid hormone, the convention is to administer T_4 daily, starting with 50% of the usual oral dose. TSH levels should be checked after 7 days and the T_4 dose adjusted to keep TSH levels in the normal range.

5. **Critical care considerations in hypothyroidism**
   a. **Increased CNS and respiratory sensitivity** to all depressant medications is a feature of hypothyroidism.
   b. **Cortisol supplementation** may be required because of adrenalitis that decreases corticosteroid production.
   c. **Intravascular volume repletion** and invasive monitoring may be required to assess volume status.
   d. **Correct anemia.**
   e. **Potential airway problems** include an enlarged tongue, relaxed oropharyngeal tissues, and poor gastric emptying.

III. **Calcium metabolism and parathyroid disease**
   A. **Physiology overview.** Calcium is essential for neuromuscular excitability, coagulation, muscle contraction, neurotransmission, hormone secretion, and hormone action. Plasma calcium is partly ionized (60%) and partly complexed (40%) with protein (mainly albumin) or organic ions. Ionized calcium is the biologically active entity. Acidosis increases and alkalosis decreases ionized calcium because of alterations in albumin binding. Abnormal total calcium levels can be "corrected" if the albumin level is known. Hypoalbuminemia decreases the total serum calcium concentration by ap-

proximately 0.8 mg/dl for each gram per deciliter of albumin below normal (4.0 g/dl). Although ionized calcium levels are technically easy to measure, improper sample handling can lead to nonreproducible measurements.

B. **Extracellular calcium.** Calcium concentrations are maintained within a narrow physiologic range by **parathyroid hormone (PTH)** and **vitamin D**. PTH increases intestinal calcium absorption, decreases renal clearance of calcium, and enhances formation of 1,25 dihydroxy-vitamin D by the kidney. **Calcitonin** from thyroid "C" cells antagonizes PTH by lowering both calcium and phosphorous concentrations.

1. **Hypercalcemia**
   a. **Clinical features** of hypercalcemia include anorexia, nausea, vomiting, dehydration, constipation, peptic ulcer disease, impaired memory, somnolence, depression, lethargy, nephrolithiasis, polyuria, electrocardiographic (ECG) abnormalities and changes (e.g.,prolonged PR interval with a short QT interval) and hypertension (Table 26-6). Hypercalcemia is considered an emergency when the total calcium level is greater than 15 mg/dl.
   b. **Causes.** Multiple medical conditions predispose to hypercalcemia, including hyperparathyroidism, malignancy, immobilization, granulomatous diseases, vitamin D intoxication, familial hypocalciuric hypercalcemia, thyrotoxicosis, and adrenal insufficiency (Table 26-7). **Malignant hypercalcemia** is caused by the release of a PTH-like molecule (PTH-

Table 26-6.   Hypercalcemia: signs and symptoms

Gastrointestinal	Central nervous system
—Nausea/vomiting	—Seizures
—Anorexia	—Disorientation/psychosis
—Constipation	—Memory loss
—Pancreatitis	—Sedation/lethargy/coma
—Peptic ulcers	Renal
Hemodynamic	—Polyuria
—Dehydration	—Nephrolithiasis
—Hypertension	—Oliguric failure (late)
—ECG/conduction changes	
—Digitalis sensitivity	
—Dysrhythmias	
—Catechol resistance	
Osteopenia/Osteoporosis	
Weakness/Atrophy/Fatiguability	

ECG, electrocardiogram.

Table 26-7. Causes of hypercalcemia

Endocrine
  —Hyperparathyroidism (1°, 3°)
  —Hyperthyroidism
  —MEN syndromes
  —Acromegaly
  —Pheochromocytoma
  —Adrenal insufficiency
Malignancy
  —Squamous cell cancers
    (i.e., lung)
  —Pancreatic cancer
  —Hypernephroma
  —Myeloma
  —Breast cancer
  —Lymphoma/leukemia (rare)
AIDS
Renal diseases (various)
Familial/genetic causes (various)
Immobilization

Granulomatous disease
  —Sarcoidosis
  —Histoplasmosis
  —Coccidiomycosis
  —Tuberculosis
  —Berylliosis
Drugs
  —Iatrogenic administration
  —Theophylline
  —Lithium
  —Thiazides
  —Vitamin D
  —Antacids (calcium con-
    taining)
  —Vitamin A

MEN, multiple endocrine neoplasia; AIDS, acquired immune deficiency syndrome.

related protein, PTH-RP) from tumors (primarily lung, breast, gut, urinary tract) and cytokine-mediated or direct bone destruction resulting in resorption of calcium from the skeleton. **Hyperparathyroidism** usually is caused by a parathyroid adenoma. It is characterized by hypercalcemia, hypophosphatemia, and an elevated PTH level. Four-gland **parathyroid hyperplasia** is found in only 10% of hyperparathyroidism cases. Parathyroid hyperplasia can be associated with medullary thyroid carcinoma and pheochromocytoma in multiple endocrine neoplasia type I. **Parathyroid carcinoma** is a rare cause of hyperparathyroidism and hypercalcemia.

  c. **Surgical management.** Treatment of a parathyroid adenoma or carcinoma is removal of the abnormal gland, with intraoperative sampling of the remaining glands to rule out hyperplasia. Intraoperative rapid measurement of immunoreactive PTH also can be used to evaluate the resection. Successful resection is indicated by a 50% reduction in circulating PTH levels 10 minutes following removal of the adenoma. Removal of three and one half to four glands with optional frozen storage or forearm reimplantation is the treatment for hyperplasia.

  d. **Medical management.** Management includes limiting oral intake of calcium to 0.5 to 1.0 mg/d, hydration with normal saline (6–10 L/d, IV), and diuresis with furosemide or ethacrynic acid. The patient must be closely observed for fluid overload, hypokalemia, and hypomagnesemia. Administration of oral phosphate (1–2 mg/d) will limit intestinal absorption and increase skeletal reuptake of calcium. Phosphate is effective but poorly tolerated because of diarrhea. Elevations in serum phosphorus levels (> 5 mg/dl) must be avoided. When the calcium-phosphate product (total calcium concentration × phosphate level) rises above 60, an increased risk is seen for soft tissue calcification.

e. **Severe hypercalcemia.** Palmidronate, mithramycin, and calcitonin, which decrease bone resorption, are used in life-threatening cases of hypercalcemia.

   (1) **Mithramycin** (25 μg/kg body weight, IV, over 30 minutes) will correct hypercalcemia in 48 hours. A lower dose of mithramycin (5–15 μg/kg body weight) can be given in less critical cases. Rarely used because of toxicity, mithramycin can produce nausea, thrombocytopenia, and hepatic and renal toxicity.

   (2) **Palmidronate** is the preferred treatment for severe hypercalcemia. Serum calcium levels greater than 13.5 mg/dl in patients with normal renal function are treated with palmidronate (90 mg, IV, administered in saline over 4 hours). Calcium levels less than 13.5 mg/dl can be treated with 60 mg IV over 4 to 24 hours. Maximal decrease in the calcium concentration occurs between 4 and 7 days and lasts about 2 weeks. A side effect of therapy is fever. Lower doses are used in renal dysfunction.

   (3) **Calcitonin.** Hypercalcemia may also respond to salmon calcitonin (4–8 IU/kg IV every 12 hours). Tachyphylaxis reduces the utility of calcitonin for long-term therapy.

f. **Critical care considerations in hypercalcemia**

   (1) **Neuromuscular blockade.** Hypercalcemia has an unpredictable effect on neuromuscular blockade. Neuromuscular blocking agents should be carefully titrated.

   (2) **Careful positioning** is required, because hypercalcemic patients can have significant osteoporosis.

   (3) **Parathyroidectomy.** After parathyroid surgery, patients may have transient or

permanent hypocalcemia requiring calcium and vitamin D supplementation. The onset of hypocalcemia usually is within a few hours of surgery, but may not occur until a few days postoperatively.

2. **Hypocalcemia**
   a. **Clinical features** (Table 26-8). Hypocalcemia is defined as a low ionized calcium concentration in the absence of abnormalities in pH, or a corrected total calcium concentration less than 8.5 mg/dl. Symptomatic hypocalcemia is unusual until the serum calcium level falls below 7.5 mg/dl, especially if calcium concentrations decline slowly. Acute hypocalcemia (e.g., after neck surgery and removal of or damage to the parathyroid glands) produces neuromuscular irritability with carpal-pedal spasm and circumoral and acral paresthesias. Severe hypocalcemia results in stridor, laryngospasm, tetany, apnea, and focal or grand mal seizures unresponsive to conventional therapy. Bedside demonstration of facial nerve irritability to percussion (Chvostek's sign) or carpal spasm with tourniquet ischemia for 3 minutes (Trousseau's sign) indicates the need for expeditious calcium supplementation. However, 10% to 15% of normocalcemic patients will have a positive Chvostek's sign. Calcium is a cofactor in the coagulation cascade and clotting function can be

Table 26-8. Hypocalcemia: Signs and symptoms

Muscle spasms
  –Stridor
  –Laryngospasm
  –Carpal/pedal spasm
  –Chvostek's Sign
  –Trousseau's Sign
  –Tetany
Dysrhythmia
Coagulopathy
Weakness
Hypotension
Congestive heart failure
Altered mental status
Paresthesias (acral, perioral)
Apnea
Seizures
Catechol resistance

Particularly when symptomatic, hypocalcemia should be treated if total calcium is <7.5 mg/dl. Of note, alkalosis decreases *ionized* calcium 0.1 mg/dl (0.25 mEq/l) for every increase of 0.1 pH unit. Total calcium is not affected by pH changes.

compromised. Patients may have hypotension with relative insensitivity to β-adrenergic agonists and a prolonged QT interval on ECG, which can lead to 2:1 heart block.

b. Causes (Table 26-9).The most common causes of hypocalcemia are planned removal or inadvertent disruption of the parathyroid glands with neck surgery. "Hungry bone syndrome" is an unusual postoperative complication of thyroidectomy for Graves' disease with severe thyrotoxicosis; calcium is extensively sequestered in bone after surgery. Extensive burns and pancreatitis cause sequestration of calcium. Hypocalcemia can be worsened by respiratory or metabolic alkalosis, rapid infusions of multiple units of cit-rated blood products, hypothermia, and renal dysfunction. Hypoparathyroidism is usually caused by underproduction of PTH. Other causes of hypoparathryoidism leading to hypocalcemia include autoimmune destruction, radiation therapy, hemosiderosis, infiltrative processes (e.g., malignancy or amyloidosis), severe hypomagnesemia, and severe vitamin D deficiency or malabsorption. Rarely, end-organ tissues resist the effects of PTH.

c. Treatment. Symptomatic, severe hypocalcemia should be treated with IV calcium. A 10 ml ampule of **calcium gluconate** contains only 93 mg (4.6 mEq) of elemental calcium,

Table 26-9. Causes of hypocalcemia

Hypoparathyroidism	Critical illness
–Primary	–Alkalosis
–Surgical	–Burns
–Idiopathic	–Toxic shock
–Autoimmune	–Pancreatitis
–Hypomagnesemia	–Fat embolism
–Peripheral resistance	Anticonvulsant therapy
(pseudohypoparathyroidism)	Hypoalbuminemia
–Hemosiderosis	Osteoblastic metastases
–Amyloidosis	Loop diuretics
Hyperphosphatemia	Contrast media containing EDTA
–Rhabdomyolysis	Intestinal malabsorption
–Phosphate therapy	Massive transfusion (citrate
–Renal failure	intoxication with chelation of
–Chemotherapy/tumor lysis	calcium)
Vitamin D deficiency	
–Liver failure	
–Renal failure	
–Lack of sun exposure	
–Dietary deficiency	

whereas a 10 ml ampule of **calcium chloride** contains 273 mg (13.6 mEq) of elemental calcium. For urgent therapy, two ampules of calcium gluconate IV or one ampule of calcium chloride IV may be administered slowly (10–20 minutes). Therapy can be continued by infusing calcium at a rate of 15 mg/kg over 6 to 8 hours. Parenteral therapy must be monitored by serum calcium measurements every 4 to 8 hours. **Oral supplementation with calcium and vitamin D** is the usual therapy for mild to moderate hypocalcemia. Patients require 1.5 to 3 g/d of elemental calcium (3,750–7,500 mg of calcium carbonate) in divided doses with food. In acute symptomatic hypocalcemia treated with oral calcium, **1,25 dihydroxyvitamin D** (calcitriol; Rocaltrol, 0.25–3.0 μg/d in divided doses) is given to allow GI absorption. For chronic replacement, oral **vitamin D** (ergocalciferol, 50,000 IU, 1 to 3 times weekly) is given. Therapeutic goals are a serum calcium concentration near 8 mg/dl and a low urinary calcium level. Phosphorus and magnesium levels should also be evaluated. Elevated phosphorus levels are treated with oral phosphate binders, whereas low magnesium levels (< 1 mg/dl) that suppress PTH secretion are treated with parenteral magnesium sulfate.

IV. Adrenal cortical disease

   A. Physiology overview. The adrenal gland consists of an outer cortex that secretes steroid hormones and an inner medulla that secretes catecholamines. Together, these hormones maintain homeostasis during states of physiologic stress including surgery, fasting, trauma, or shock. The adrenal cortex produces three classes of steroid hormones: glucocorticoids, mineralocorticoids, and androgens.

   1. Glucocorticoids. Cortisol is the principal hormone of this class. **Adrenocorticotropic hormone (ACTH)** from the anterior pituitary stimulates the release of cortisol in a diurnal pattern and in response to stress. Approximately 30 mg of cortisol is produced daily under basal conditions. Cortisol has multiple effects on carbohydrate, protein, and fatty acid metabolism. It decreases cellular uptake of glucose and promotes gluconeogenesis and hepatic glycogen synthesis. It is crucial for the conversion of norepinephrine to epinephrine in the adrenal medulla; it is required for the production of angiotensin II and adequate vascular tone. Cortisol acts as an antiinflammatory agent by stabilizing microsomes and promoting capillary stability. It is metabolized by the liver and also filtered and excreted unchanged by the kidney.

2. **Mineralocorticoids. Aldosterone** is an important regulator of extracellular fluid volume and potassium homeostasis. The renin–angiotensin system and, to a lesser extent, potassium concentration regulate aldosterone secretion. Aldosterone's principal effect is on the renal tubule to stimulate absorption of Na^+ and transport it to the extracellular fluid. The resulting excess of anions in the tubule causes a passive transfer of K^+ and H^+ into the tubule with excretion in the urine.

3. **Androgens.** Abnormal secretion of these sex hormones may indicate abnormalities in biosynthesis of multiple steroids, including cortisol. The most common cause of increased adrenal androgen secretion is **congenital adrenal hyperplasia,** resulting in hirsuitism and menstrual irregularities in women. **Adrenal cortical carcinoma** is a rare cause of excess adrenal androgen production.

B. **Adrenal cortical hyperfunction**

1. **Clinical features.** Patients can present with truncal obesity, hypertension, hypernatremia, excess intravascular volume, hyperglycemia, hypokalemia, cutaneous striae, poor wound healing, muscle wasting and weakness, osteoporosis, aseptic osteonecrosis, hypercoagulability with thromboembolism, mental status changes, emotional lability, benign intracranial hypertension, pancreatitis, peptic ulceration, glaucoma, and infection.

2. **Adrenal hyperfunction** is usually (80% of cases) the result of ACTH-induced adrenal hyperplasia. By definition, patients have **Cushing's disease** when excess secretion of ACTH from a pituitary tumor drives overproduction of adrenal cortical steroids. Hyperadrenalism from any other cause (e.g., ectopic production of ACTH by carcinoids or tumors, adrenal adenoma or bilateral adrenal micronodular hyperplasia, steroid therapy) is defined as **Cushing's syndrome.** Cushing's syndrome is most commonly iatrogenic, resulting from therapeutic administration of glucocorticoids.

3. **Management**

    a. **Hypertension** can be difficult to treat. Combinations of antihypertensive agents in high doses may be required.

    b. **Excess intravascular volume** can be reduced with diuretics, but potassium must be replaced.

    c. **Serum glucose** must be monitored frequently.

    d. **Osteoporosis** makes careful positioning of the patient necessary.

C. **Adrenal cortical hypofunction**

1. **Clinical features.** Primary adrenal insufficiency (**Addison's disease**) is associated with low levels of cortisol and aldosterone. Findings include weight loss, weakness, fatigue, anorexia, nausea, vomiting,

abdominal pain, postural hypotension, diarrhea or constipation, and hyperpigmentation. Glucocorticoid deficiency can present with abdominal pain associated with episodic fever and hypotension that is difficult to distinguish from an acute surgical abdomen. Mineralocorticoid deficiency will lead to decreasing urinary sodium conservation and to decreased response to circulating catecholamines, and hyperkalemia. In secondary adrenal insufficiency caused by abnormalities in ACTH excretion, cortisol levels are low, and aldosterone function is preserved.

2. **Causes.** Idiopathic autoimmune atrophy, surgical removal, radiation therapy, metastatic destruction, infection [e.g., fungus, tuberculosis, human immunodeficiency virus (HIV), cytomegalovirus], hemorrhage [e.g., septicemia, Waterhouse-Friedrichsen syndrome (in meningococcemia), anticoagulant therapy], drugs (e.g., ketoconazole, rifampin, metyrapone), or loss of ACTH stimulation can produce adrenal cortical hypofunction. Exogenous steroid administration can suppress the pituitary–adrenal axis for 12 months or more after cessation of therapy. Additional steroid supplementation may be indicated in states of physiologic stress such as critical illness or major surgery. A small number of critically ill patients (1%) exhibit relative central suppression of the hypothalamic-pituitary-adrenal (HPA) axis and relative adrenal insufficiency. These patients are often hypotensive and unresponsive to fluid or vasopressor support. Hemodynamics may improve rapidly with glucocorticoid therapy.

3. **Laboratory evaluation of HPA function.** Cortisol secretion is episodic. Although random cortisol determinations are not predictive of adrenal function, a random cortisol level higher than 20 μg/ dl suggests adequate adrenal function. Provocative testing to assess HPA function includes the insulin tolerance test with induction of hypoglycemia, ACTH (cosyntropin) stimulation tests, and responses to lysine vasopressin or metyrapone. The **insulin tolerance test** is physiologically the most reliable evaluation; however, this test is not routinely administered to the unstable patient. The standard **cosyntropin test** measures serum cortisol following the administration of cosyntropin (250 μg IV or IM). An abnormal response is an increase in cortisol levels at 30 or 60 minutes after stimulation of less than 8 μg/dl over the baseline value. A second criterion is a maximal stimulated cortisol level less than 18 to 20 μg/dl.

The standard cosyntropin test uses supraphysiologic doses of cosyntropin and may not be sufficiently sensitive to identify patients with subtle central adrenal insufficiency. An alternative test is the low-dose cosyntropin test that uses 1 µg of ACTH as the stimulus, with measurements of serum cortisol levels 30 minutes later. A normal response is a serum cortisol level higher than 18 to 20 µg/dl. Experience with the low-dose cosyntropin test is limited and the results must be carefully assessed. Borderline results can be confirmed with additional tests. A "stress dose" of steroids for 2 to 3 days will stabilize a patient with adrenal insufficiency without causing significant harm to patients with normal HPA function.

4. **Treatment**
   a. **Acute adrenal insufficiency (Addisonian crisis)** is a medical emergency presenting with hypotension and tachycardia that are unresponsive to fluids. Treatment includes fluids (D5NS), steroid replacement (hydrocortisone 75 mg IV or dexamethasone 2 mg IV, then hydrocortisone 200 mg over 24 hours by continuous IV infusion), inotropes as necessary, and correction of electrolyte imbalances. **In a suspected acute adrenal crisis,** immediately treat the patient with dexamethasone, 2 mg IV and then perform cosyntropin testing to confirm the diagnosis. A single dose of dexamethasone will not interfere with stimulation testing carried out within 12 hours.
   b. Causes precipitating adrenal crises must be detected and treated. Hydrocortisone dosage can decrease by 50% every 1 to 3 days, depending on the clinical status. Primary adrenal insufficiency requires replacement of both glucocorticoids and mineralocorticoids. Once the hydrocortisone dose is below 75 mg daily, mineralocorticoid must be added as **fludrocortisone** [(Florinef) 0. 05–0.2 mg daily].
   c. A variety of synthetic steroids is available. They differ in their relative potencies, half-lives, and ratios of glucocorticoid to mineralocorticoid effects (Table 26-10). Of note, the synthetic glucocorticoid dexamethasone lacks mineralocorticoid activity.

5. **Perioperative and ICU considerations**
   a. Under basal conditions, the usual **hydrocortisone replacement** is 20 to 30 mg daily (20 mg on awakening and 10 mg at 4 p.m.) or prednisone (5–7.5 mg once daily). Recommendations for IV "stress" glucocorticoid supplementation have recently changed and are based on a reassessment of endogenous cortisol production during stress. For settings of extreme stress (e.g., major surgery, trauma), the current recommendations for glucocorticoid supplementation are to administer hydrocortisone 100–150 mg/d for 2–3 days. For

Table 26-10. Glucocorticoid and mineralocorticoid hormones

Steroid	Relative potency		Equivalent dose (mg)	Duration (h)
	Glucocorticoid	Mineralocorticoid		
Short-acting				
–Cortisol	1.0	1.0	20	8–12
–Cortisone	0.8	0.8	25	8–12
–Aldosterone	0.3	3,000	—	8–12
Intermediate-acting				
–Prednisone	4.0	0.8	5	12–36
–Prednisolone	4.0	0.8	5	12–36
–Methylprednisolone	5.0	0.5	4	12–36
–Fludrocortisone	10.0	125	—	12–36
Long-acting				
–Dexamethasone	25–40	0	0.75	>24
				>24

moderately stressful situations, the recommendation is hydrocortisone 50–75 mg/d for
1–2 days. The supplemental dosage of hydrocortisone for situations of minor stress is
25 mg/d for 1 to 2 days (Table 26-11). These
guidelines may not meet the requirements of
all patients and perioperative or stress steroid
replacement should be individually tailored.

b. Any patient who has received more than a
14-day treatment with superphysiologic steroids in the past year should receive glucocorticoid supplementation (i.e., "stress steroid
coverage") perioperatively.

c. **Etomidate** should be avoided because of its
propensity for adrenal suppression.

d. Sedative, anesthetic, and vasoactive drugs
must be titrated carefully, as patients with
adrenal hypofunction are exquisitely sensitive
to drug-induced myocardial depression.

e. After unilateral or bilateral adrenalectomy,
steroid replacement should begin immediately
postoperatively. Following unilateral adrenalectomy, glucocorticoid supplementation is necessary until the remaining adrenal cortex
resumes normal glucocorticoid output, typically after several months. Endogenous mineralocorticoid secretion from the remaining
gland is usually adequate. Both glucocorticoid
and mineralocorticoid replacement are permanently required with bilateral adrenalectomy.

V. Adrenal medullary disease

A. Physiology overview. Preganglionic fibers of the
sympathetic nervous system end in the adrenal medulla and stimulate catecholamine release [norepi-
nephrine (20%), epinephrine (80%)]. Catecholamines
cause chronotropic and inotropic stimulation of the
heart; vasomotor changes; enhanced hepatic glycogenolysis; and inhibition of insulin release. Metaneph-
rine and vanillylmandelic acid (VMA) generated by the
liver and kidney are the primary biotransformation
products of catecholamines.

B. Pheochromocytoma

1. Physiology. Pheochromocytoma is usually a tumor
of the adrenal medulla. It can occur in a variety
of other locations, most often within sympathetic
ganglia (paraganglioma). Tumors are typically solitary, but 10% are bilateral and 10% are metastatic
in the adult. Ten percent of pheochromocytomas are
familial and occur as part of multiple endocrine neoplasia syndromes types II and III; they can also be
associated with von Recklinghausen's disease. Most
tumors secrete both epinephrine and norepinephrine, and their release is independent of neurogenic
control.

Table 26-11. Perioperative hydrocortisone supplementation guidelines

Anticipated surgical stress	Preoperative	Intraoperative	Postoperative
Minor[a]	25 mg or usual dose	None, unless complications	Resume usual replacement POD 1
Moderate[b]	50–75 mg or usual steroid dose, whichever is higher	50 mg IV	20 mg IV every 8 h on POD 1; then resume preoperative replacement dose on POD 2
Major[c]	100–150 mg or usual steroid dose, whichever is higher, within 2 h of start of procedure	50 mg IV every 8 h after initial dose	50 mg IV every 8 h, or 150 mg continuously over 24 h for 2–3 days; then reduce dose by 50% per day until preoperative regimen is reached

Note that these guidelines may not meet the requirements of all patients and perioperative or stress steroid replacement should be individually tailored.

[a] Inguinal herniorrhaphy, minor urologic or gynecologic procedures, oral surgery, plastic surgery.

[b] Total joint replacement, open cholecystectomy, lower extremity revascularization.

[c] Thoracotomy, cardiac surgery, major abdominal surgery.

POD, postoperative day.

2. **Signs and symptoms** result from excess catecholamine release. The **classic triad** includes palpitations, headache, and diaphoresis in an episodically hypertensive patient, but 10% of patients are not hypertensive. Pheochromocytoma is a rare cause of chronic hypertension. Other signs and symptoms include flushing, anxiety, tremor, hyperglycemia, hypovolemia-induced orthostatic hypotension, polycythemia, and weight loss. Patients with pheochromocytoma are usually dehydrated and hemoconcentrated because of increased insensible losses and vasoconstriction. Chronic exposure to high catecholamine concentrations can ultimately produce a cardiomyopathy. Of note, physical examination (especially of the abdomen) with manipulation of a tumor can cause the release of catecholamines and precipitate a crisis. Extirpative surgery is the definitive treatment, but only after pharmacologic and volume stabilization of the patient. Endogenous catecholamine levels should return to normal within a few days after successful removal of the tumor.

3. **Perioperative considerations**
   a. **Hypertensive crisis.** Treatment alternatives include **nitroprusside** infusion or **phentolamine** [bolus 1–5 mg IV or as an infusion (10 mg/L in saline)] titrated to blood pressure along with aggressive hydration (normal saline) for volume expansion. After controlling blood pressure, tachycardia can be treated with cautious **β-adrenergic blockade.** A risk is seen for vasoconstriction and exacerbation of hypertension if β-adrenergic blockers are administered before complete α-adrenergic blockade is established.
   b. **Preoperative preparation**
      (1) **α-adrenergic receptor blockade** is often initiated with oral **phenoxybenzamine,** a long-acting α_1 and α_2-adrenergic blocker (starting with 20–30 mg/d and increasing to 60–250 mg/d until blood pressure is controlled). Achieving adequate α-receptor blockade may require 10 to 14 days. Features include postural hypotension, nasal stuffiness, and decreased sweating. **Prazosin,** a shorter-acting α_1 blocker, may be preferred. The shorter duration of action allows reversal of α blockade soon after resection of the pheochromocytoma. Prazosin lacks α_2-adrenergic blocking activity. Treatment with prazosin thus preserves physiologic presynaptic α_2-adrenergic receptor activity that suppresses sympathetic outflow. Adequate volume repletion is reflected

by a fall in the hematocrit along with hemodynamic data.

(2) **β-adrenergic blockade** is instituted only after the onset of adequate alpha blockade, and only if tachycardia persists.

(3) **Preoperative depletion of catecholamine stores** can be accomplished with **α-methyl-L-tyrosine** (Demser) therapy. This drug inhibits tyrosine hydroxylase, which is the rate-limiting enzyme in catecholamine synthesis, thereby inhibiting catecholamine biosynthesis. The starting dose is 250 mg orally, four times a day, which can be increased in increments, up to a maximum of 4 g/d. The maximal effect is achieved by 2 to 3 days of adequate therapy, but preoperative administration of the maximum tolerated dose for at least 7 to 14 days is recommended.

VI. Pituitary disease

A. Anterior pituitary

1. **Physiology.** The anterior pituitary gland secretes a variety of hormones that regulate the thyroid and adrenal glands, the ovaries and testes, growth, and lactation. **Growth hormone** (GH) and **prolactin** (PRL) act directly on target tissues, whereas **ACTH, TSH, follicle-stimulating hormone** (FSH), and **luteinizing hormone** (LH) act by stimulating other endocrine glands. Control over anterior pituitary hormone production is achieved with stimulation or inhibition by specific hypothalamic factors and feedback inhibition by peripheral hormones. Pituitary tumors are usually benign adenomas characterized by the hormone secretion profile (i.e., nonsecreting, prolactinoma, or GH-, ACTH-, TSH-, and gonadotropin-secreting adenomas). Adenomas can lead to excess secretion of hormones. A variety of conditions leads to pituitary insufficiency (discussed below).

2. **Hyperfunction**

   a. **Hyperfunctioning adenomas** are usually benign pituitary tumors that cause no special perioperative problems. The hyperthyroidism of a TSH-secreting adenoma and the hyperadrenalism (Cushing's disease or syndrome) of the ACTH-secreting adenoma are treated as described in previous sections.

   b. **Acromegaly**

      (1) **Airway concerns.** Excess GH secretion in the adult will lead to **prognathism,** soft-tissue overgrowth of the lips, tongue, epiglottis, and vocal cords, with subglottic narrowing of the trachea. Difficulties with airway management and endotracheal intubation should be anticipated.

(2) **Special considerations.** The cardiovascular status should be thoroughly evaluated because acromegaly predisposes to congestive heart failure, dysrhythmias, and an increased incidence of morbidity and mortality from coronary artery disease. Glucose intolerance is commonly encountered; thus, serum glucose levels should be carefully monitored. Carpal tunnel syndrome, peripheral neuropathies, and colon carcinoma are associated with acromegaly. Some patients suffer from skeletal muscle weakness that can contribute to respiratory insufficiency.

3. **Hyposecretion (panhypopituitarism)**
   a. **Causes of pituitary failure.** Postpartum hemorrhagic shock can cause vasospasm and subsequent pituitary necrosis and hypofunction, which is known as **Sheehan's syndrome.** Other causes include trauma, radiation therapy, pituitary apoplexy, lymphocytic hypophysitis, infiltrative diseases (e.g., sarcoidosis or histiocytosis), and tumors (e.g., metastatic carcinoma or craniopharyngiomas). Surgical removal of the pituitary is performed for tumor resection. Pituitary carcinoma is a rare cause of isolated or complete pituitary insufficiency.
   b. **Special considerations**
      (1) **Glucocorticoid therapy** is essential for patients with a history of adrenal insufficiency.
      (2) **Hypothyroidism.** No special treatment or supplementation is necessary for mild to moderate hypothyroidism. Management of severe hypothyroidism is discussed above.
      (3) **The onset of pituitary insufficiency** after pituitary surgery or apoplexy is delayed. Adrenal insufficiency develops over 4 to 14 days after destruction or removal of the pituitary gland. Glucocorticoid, but not mineralocorticoid, replacement is required. Because of the long half-life of thyroid hormone (7–10 days), symptomatic hypothyroidism does not occur until 2 to 3 weeks following pituitary surgery or apoplexy.

B. **Posterior pituitary**
   1. **Physiology.** The main functions of **oxytocin** are to regulate uterine contractions in labor and lactation. **Antidiuretic hormone** (ADH, vasopressin) regulates plasma osmolarity and extracellular fluid volume by facilitating renal tubular resorption of water and increasing urinary osmolarity.

Antidiuretic hormone secretion is enhanced by several commonly encountered stimuli, including decreases in intravascular volume; pain from trauma or surgery; nausea; and positive airway pressure.

2. **Diabetes insipidus (DI)**

   a. **Causes.** Insufficient ADH secretion by the posterior pituitary gland is known as **central diabetes insipidus.** Central DI can be caused by intracranial trauma, hypophysectomy, metastatic disease to the pituitary gland or hypothalamus, and infiltrative diseases such as histiocytosis and sarcoidosis. **Nephrogenic DI** describes the failure of the renal tubules to respond to ADH. Causes of nephrogenic DI include hypokalemia, hypercalcemia, sickle cell anemia, chronic myeloma, obstructive uropathy, chronic renal insufficiency, lithium therapy, and a rare X-linked hereditary disorder. Nephrogenic DI can also be seen in the third trimester of pregnancy.

   b. **Diagnosis.** Clinical evidence for DI is a urine production of greater than 1 L/h in the setting of pituitary surgery or head trauma. Suspected DI is diagnosed by examining simultaneous serum and urine osmolality values. Serum osmolality is high (310–320 mOsm/kg). The urine is inappropriately dilute with a specific gravity less than 1.001 and urine osmolality less than 200 mOsm/kg. Serum Na^+ levels will be elevated.

   c. **Central DI.** Clinical features include polydipsia and polyuria. Central DI can be treated with the synthetic vasopressin analog **desmopressin** (DDAVP) 1–2 µg (0.25–0.5 ml) subcutaneously or IV every 6 to 24 hours, as needed. Nasal inhalers or oral preparations can be used in appropriate patients. Side effects of DDAVP include hyponatremia and coronary artery vasospasm.

   d. **Nephrogenic DI.** The polyuria of nephrogenic DI is associated with hypotonic urine, normal or high levels of plasma vasopressin, and failure of exogenous vasopressin to reduced urinary volume. No specific therapy exists for nephrogenic DI. Adequate oral or parenteral hydration must be assured. Inhibition of prostaglandin synthesis (with ibuprofen, indomethacin, or aspirin) or mild salt depletion with a thiazide diuretic may reduce urine volume.

   e. **Management of DI** includes careful monitoring of urine output and specific gravity, serum sodium levels, plasma volume, and plasma osmolality. The total body water deficit can be estimated as:

$$\text{Water deficit (liters)} = \left[0.6 \times \text{body weight (kg)}\right]$$
$$\times \left\{([Na^+] - 140)/140\right\}$$

where body weight is the initial weight in kilograms before dehydration.

Initial therapy is volume expansion with IV isotonic fluids (normal saline). Once plasma osmolality falls below 290 mOsm/kg, hypotonic fluids (half normal saline) are usually used. Mild DI (daily urinary volumes of 2–6 L) does not require treatment in patients with an adequate thirst mechanism who are able to drink fluids freely.

3. **Syndrome of inappropriate ADH secretion (SIADH)**
   a. **Causes. SIADH** is persistent secretion of ADH with hyponatremia in the absence of an osmotic stimulus. SIADH can be caused by carcinoma (bronchogenic, duodenal, pancreatic, ureteral, prostatic or bladder); other malignancies (lymphoma, leukemia, thymoma, mesothelioma); CNS disorders (trauma, infections, tumors); pulmonary disorders (tuberculosis, pneumonia, positive-pressure ventilation); drugs (nicotine, narcotics, chlorpropramide, clofibrate, vincristine, vinblastine, cyclophosphamide); hypothyroidism; Addison's disease; and porphyria.
   b. **Diagnosis.** Suspected SIADH is diagnosed by examining simultaneous serum and urine Na^+ and osmolality values. SIADH is associated with a high urine osmolality (higher than serum value), a urinary Na^+ concentration greater than 20 mEq/L, and a serum Na^+ concentration less than 130 mEq/L. If serum Na^+ levels fall below 110 mEq/L, cerebral edema and seizures may result.
   c. **Management of SIADH. Fluid restriction** (800–1,000 ml daily) is the primary treatment for the mild hyponatremia of SIADH. Chronic hyponatremia without symptoms has virtually no mortality. Resuscitation using hypertonic Na^+-containing solutions is reserved for symptomatic, severe hyponatremia (serum $Na^+ <$ 120 mEq/L). Hyponatremia should be corrected slowly, no faster than an increase of 0.5 mEq/L/h, because overly aggressive replacement can result in central pontine myelinolysis. In volume-contracted states, serum Na^+ is partially corrected to 125 mEq/L or a serum osmolality of 250 m Eq/L over a period of 6 to 8 hours with 3% to 5% hypertonic saline. To calculate the Na^+ requirement:

$$\text{Required mEq of } Na^+ = (125\, mEq/L$$
$$- \text{serum } [Na^+]) \times 0.6$$
$$\times \text{body weight} (kg)$$

Hypertonic saline is potentially dangerous in volume-expanded, salt-retaining states such as congestive heart failure. In SIADH associated with volume expansion, administration of hypertonic saline alone is ineffective because the excess Na^+ is excreted. Treatment is with parenteral hypertonic saline plus a furosemide-induced diuresis to produce a hypotonic urine.

VII. Carcinoid

  A. Carcinoid tumors. Most carcinoid tumors arise from the embryonic foregut (bronchus, stomach, pancreas), midgut (midduodenum to midtransverse colon), or hindgut (descending colon and rectum). The most common location of carcinoid tumors is the appendix, followed by the ileum and rectum. Carcinoid tumors frequently metastasize to the liver; less commonly, they spread to the breast, head or neck, lung, gonads, genitourinary system, and thymus.

    The biochemical hallmark of carcinoid tumors is the overproduction of serotonin, the serotonin precursor 5-hydroxytryptophan, or both, along with an increased excretion of the degradation product 5-hydroxyindoleacetic acid (5HIAA) in the urine. Carcinoid tumors arising from the foregut secrete primarily 5-hydroxytryptophan. Carcinoid tumors arising from the embryonic midgut secrete serotonin (5-hydroxytryptamine). Tumors of the hindgut do not secrete large amounts of either 5-hydroxytryptophan or serotonin. In addition to serotonin, mediators secreted by carcinoid tumors include bradykinin, histamine, prostaglandins, and kallikrein. Stimuli for the release of mediators include catecholamines, histamine, and tumor manipulation.

  B. Carcinoid syndrome. Clinical features of the carcinoid syndrome depend on the tumor's location and extent of liver metastasis. The syndrome includes **episodic flushing, bronchoconstriction, gastrointestinal hypermotility, and mild hyperglycemia.** Cardiac manifestations include supraventricular tachycardias and valve cusp distortions. The possibility of left-sided cardiac lesions should not be overlooked. Peripheral vasodilation can produce profound hypotension. Of patients with carcinoids located in the small bowel and the proximal colon, 40% to 50% will have the symptom complex. Symptoms are less frequent with bronchial carcinoids, rare in appendicial carcinoids, and not seen with rectal carcinoid tumors. Compounds released by the tumor are typically metabolized during their first pass through the liver, and symptoms usually are seen only in cases of extensive hepatic metastases or with a tumor located outside the portal system.

C. **Management considerations**

1. **Critical care management** of the symptomatic carcinoid patient can be difficult. A carcinoid crisis may be refractory to conventional therapeutic measures such as fluid resuscitation and direct-acting vasopressors (e.g., phenylephrine). Treatment should then be initiated with the somatostatin analog **octreotide** (Sandostatin, 50–100 μg IV). This prevents the release of serotonin and its precursors and may block the peripheral actions of serotonin, kinins, and other mediators. Infusions of dilute octreotide (10 μg/ml, rate titrated to blood pressure) can be used for maintenance therapy. Depending on the secretion profile of the particular tumor, other agents that can potentially be useful in the management of a carcinoid crisis include H_1 and H_2 histamine antagonists, the kallikrein inhibitor, aprotinin, and serotonin antagonists.

2. **Paroxysmal bronchoconstriction** always occurs concurrently with a flushing episode and is associated with release of mediators from the tumor. In addition to the usual treatment of bronchoconstriction, **octreotide** can be given to decrease release of mediators. Note that **catecholamines can enhance tumor mediator release,** worsening a carcinoid crisis.

3. **Endocardial disease.** Plaquelike thickening on the endocardium of the cardiac valve leaflets, atria, and ventricles occurs in 20% of patients with carcinoid, and usually is associated with high levels of serotonin. Thickening of the endocardium commonly results in **pulmonic stenosis** and **tricuspid insufficiency,** which can produce right ventricular failure.

SELECTED REFERENCES

Diabetes

Baker JR. Autoimmune endocrine disease. *JAMA* 1997; 278:1931–1937.

Foster DW, McGarry JD. The metabolic derangements and treatment of diabetic ketoacidosis. *N Engl J Med* 1983;309:159–169.

Gavin LA. Perioperative management of the diabetic patient. *Endocrinol Metab Clin North Am* 1992;21:457–475.

Genuth SM. Diabetic ketoacidosis and hyperglycemic hyperosmolar coma. *Curr Ther Endocrinol Metab* 1997;6:438–447.

Mahler RJ, Adler ML. Clinical review 102: type 2 diabetes mellitus: update on diagnosis, pathophysiology and treatment. *J Clin Endocrinol Metab* 1999;84:1165–1171.

Milaszkiewicz RM. Diabetes mellitus and anesthesia: what is the problem? *Int Anesthesiol Clin* 1997;35:35–62.

Thyroid

Brent GA, Hershman JM. Thyroxine therapy in patients with severe nonthyroidal illnesses and lower serum thyroxine concentration. *J Clin Endocrinol Metab* 1986;63:1–8.

Broderick TJ, Wechsler AS. Triiodothyronine in cardiac surgery. *Thyroid* 1997;7:133–137.

Dabon-Almirante CLM, Surks MI. Clinical and laboratory diagnosis of thyrotoxicosis. *Endocrinol Metab Clin North Am* 1998;27:25–36.

De Groot LJ. Dangerous dogmas in medicine: the nonthyroidal illness syndrome. *J Clin Endocrinol Metab* 1999;84:151–164.

Dillmann WH. Thyroid storm. In: Bardin CW, ed. *Current therapy in endocrinology and metabolism,* 6th ed. New York: Mosby, 1997: 81–85.

Gomberg-Maitland M, Frishman WH. Thyroid hormone and cardiovascular disease. *Am Heart J* 1998;135:187–196.

Hofbauer LC, Heufelder AE. Coagulation disorders in thyroid diseases. *Eur J Endocrinol* 1997;136:1–7.

Klein I, Ojamaa K. Thyrotoxicosis and the heart. *Endocrinol Metab Clin North Am* 1998;27:51–62.

Klemperer JD, Klein I, Gomez M, et al. Thyroid hormone treatment after coronary artery bypass surgery. *N Engl J Med* 1995;333: 1522–1527.

McIver B, Gorman CA. Euthyroid sick syndrome: an overview. *Thyroid* 1997;7:125–132.

Pittman CS, Zayed AA. Myxedema coma. In: Bardin CW, ed. *Current therapy in endocrinology and metabolism,* 6th ed. New York: Mosby, 1997:98–101.

Saad, H. Clinical implications of the interaction between hypothyroidism and the cardiovascular system. *Clev Clin J Med* 1997; 64:93–98.

Calcium

Adams J, Andersen P, Everts E, et al. Early postoperative calcium levels as predictors of hypocalcemia. *Laryngoscope* 1998;108:1829–1831.

Bushinsky DA, Monk RD. Calcium. *Lancet* 1998;352:306–311.

Adrenals

Barquist E, Kirton O. Adrenal insufficiency in the surgical intensive care unit. *J Trauma* 1997;42:27–31.

Dickstein G, Shechner C, Nicholson WE, et al. Adrenocorticotropin stimulation test: effects of basal cortisol level, time of day and suggested new sensitive low dose test. *J Clin Endocrinol Metab* 1991;72:773–778.

Horton R, Nadler JL. Hypoaldosteronism. In: Bardin CW, ed. *Current therapy in endocrinology and metabolism,* 6th ed. New York: Mosby, 1997:164–167.

Lamberts SWJ, Bruining HA, de Jong FH. Corticosteroid therapy in severe illness. *N Engl J Med* 1997;337:1285–1292.

Malchoff CD, Carey RM. Adrenal insufficiency. In: Bardin CW, ed. *Current therapy in endocrinology and metabolism,* 6th ed. New York: Mosby, 1997:142–147.

Napolitano LM, Chernow B. Guidelines for corticosteroid use in anesthetic and surgical stress. *Int Anesthesiol Clin* 1988;26:226–232.

Oelkers W. Adrenal insufficiency. *N Engl J Med* 1996;335:1206–1212.

Salem M, Tainsh RE, Bromberg J, et al. Perioperative glucocorticoid coverage. *Ann Surg* 1994;219:416–425.

Thaler LM, Blevins LS. The low dose (1-μg) adrenocorticotropin stimulation test in the evaluation of patients with suspected central adrenal insufficiency. *J Clin Endocrinol Metab* 1998;83:2726–2729.

Pheochromocytoma

Kenady DE, McGrath PC, Sloan DA, et al. Diagnosis and management of pheochromocytoma. *Curr Opin Oncol* 1997;9:61–67.

O'Riordan JA. Pheochromocytomas and anesthesia. *Int Anesthesiol Clin* 1997;35:99–127.

Pituitary

Kumar S, Berl T. Sodium. *Lancet* 1998;353:220–228.

Lombardi G, Colao A, Ferone D, et al. Effect of growth hormone on cardiac function. *Horm Res* 1997;48(Suppl 4):38–42.

Singer I, Oster JR, Fishman LM. The management of diabetes insipidus in adults. *Arch Int Med* 1997;157:1293–1301.

Van den Berghe G, de Zegher F, Bouillon R. Acute and prolonged critical illness as different neuroendocrine paradigms. *J Clin Endocrinol Metab* 1998;83:1827–1834.

Carcinoid

Kulke MH, Mayer RJ. Carcinoid tumors. *N Engl J Med* 1999;340:858–868.

Vaughan DJA, Brunner MD. Anesthesia for patients with carcinoid syndrome. *Int Anesthesiol Clin* 1997;35:129–142.

General Considerations in Infectious Disease

Judith Hellman

I. **Introduction**
   A. **Diagnosis of infection** in patients in the intensive care unit (ICU) can be difficult because they often develop clinical signs of infection (e.g., fever, hemodynamic instability, and so forth) from noninfectious causes, and often have multiple potential sites of infection (Table 27-1). The incidence of multiple system organ failure and death is increased in patients with infection in the ICU. A systematic, thorough evaluation of the patient with symptoms and signs of infection is essential to localize the site(s) of infection and exclude noninfectious causes, so that medical or surgical intervention can be initiated in a logical manner.
   B. Multiple risk factors exist for the development of serious infections in the ICU (Table 27-2). Many infections that occur in patients in the ICU are nosocomial. **Nosocomial infections** are hospital-acquired infections occurring after 48 hours of hospitalization. Such infections tend to be caused by organisms with increased virulence, antimicrobial resistance, or both. Infections are caused by a variety of microorganisms, including gram-negative and gram-positive aerobic and anaerobic bacteria, fungi, viruses, and parasites. Common organisms and abbreviations are shown in Table 27-3. **Aerobic bacteria** require oxygen for growth, whereas **facultative anaerobes** grow in the presence or absence of oxygen, and **anaerobes** will not grow in the presence of oxygen.

II. **Antibacterial agents**
   A. **β-lactam** antimicrobial agents, including **penicillins, cephalosporins, monobactams,** and **carbapenems,** interfere with bacterial cell wall synthesis. The spectrum of activity of various β-lactam agents varies widely. β-Lactam agents have bactericidal activity against susceptible organisms. They have only bacteriostatic activity against *Enterococcus* spp. A synergistic combination of a β-lactam (or vancomycin) plus an aminoglycoside is necessary for bactericidal activity against *Enterococcus* spp. **Resistance** to β-lactams results from production of β-lactamase, altered binding to penicillin-binding proteins (PBPs), or decreased antibiotic penetration into the bacteria. Treatment of *Enterobacter* spp, *Citrobacter* spp, and *Acinetobacter* spp with β-lactams can be complicated by rapid development of resistance because they harbor an inducible chromosomal β-lactamase.

Table 27-1.   Potential sites of infection in ICU patients

Site	Infection
Surgical	Superficial and deep wound infection, anastomotic breakdown, abscess
Chest	Pneumonia, tracheobronchitis, mediastinitis, lung abscess, empyema, endocarditis
Abdomen	Peritonitis, abscess, cholecystitis, cholangitis, urinary tract infection, *Clostridium difficile* colitis
Head and neck	Sinusitis, parotitis, central nervous system infection, periotonsillar abscess
Indwelling catheters	Urinary, intravascular

B.   **Penicillins (penicillin, nafcillin, ampicillin, ticarcillin, piperacillin)**
   1.   **Spectrum of activity**
      a.   **Penicillin** and **nafcillin** are active against aerobic and anaerobic gram-positive bacteria. **Penicillin** is active against gram-positive cocci such as *Streptococcus* spp (*Strep.* spp), gram-positive rods such as *Listeria monocytogenes,* and many anaerobes. *Staphylococcus aureus* or *S. epidermidis* are often resistant. **Nafcillin** is effective against *S. aureus,* excluding methicillin-resistant *S. aureus* (MRSA). Nafcillin is less active than penicillin against *Strep.* spp.
      b.   **Ampicillin** is active against many gram-positive cocci and enteric gram-negative bacilli, including *Escherichia coli, Proteus* spp, and *Serratia* spp. The addition of the β-lactamase inhibitor, sulbactam, to ampicillin (**Unasyn**), increases the activity against *S. aureus* (not MRSA), β-lactamase producing gram-negatives, and anaerobes.

Table 27-2.   Risk factors for infections in the ICU

   1. Age >70 y
   2. Shock
   3. Major trauma
   4. Coma
   5. Prior antibiotics
   6. Mechanical ventilation
   7. Drugs that affect the immune system (steroids, chemotherapy)
   8. Indwelling catheters
   9. Prolonged ICU stay (>3 d)
   10. Acute renal failure

Table 27-3.   Classification of microorganisms causing infections in the ICU

General groups	Specific microorganisms
Bacteria: gram-positive aerobes	*Staphylococcus aureus (S. aureus), Staphylococcus epidermidis* (coagulase-negative staphylococcus), *Streptococcus* spp (*Strep.* spp), *Enterococcus* spp
Bacteria: enteric gram-negative aerobes and facultative anaerobes	*Escherichia coli (E. coli), Klebsiella pneumonia (K. pneumoniae), Proteus mirabilis (P. mirabilis), Enterobacter cloacae (E. cloacae)* and other *Enterobacter* spp, *Acinetobacter* spp, *Citrobacter* spp, *Serratia marcescens (S. marcescens), Salmonella* spp
Bacteria: non-enteric gram-negative aerobes and facultative anaerobes	*Pseudomonas aeruginosa (P. aeruginosa), Pseudomonas cepacia (P. cepacia), Neisseria* spp, *Haemophilus influenzae (H. influenzae), Haemophilus parainfluenzae (H. parainfluenzae)*
Bacteria: anaerobes (gram-positive and gram-negative)	*Bacteroides fragilis (B. fragilis)* and other *Bacteroides* spp, *Clostridium difficile (C. diff.)* and other *Clostridium* spp, *Peptostreptococcus* spp
Fungi	*Candida* spp, *Torulopsis glabrata (T. glabrata), Aspergillus* spp, *Histoplasma capsulatum*
Viruses	Herpes zoster virus (HZV), herpes simplex virus (HSV) I and II, cytomegalovirus (CMV), Epstein-Barr virus (EBV)
Parasites	*Pneumocystis carinii*

spp, species.

    c. **Ticarcillin** and **piperacillin** are active against gram-positive, gram-negative, and anaerobic bacteria. Their resistance to β-lactamase confers broader gram-negative coverage than ampicillin that can include *Pseudomonas* spp and *Enterobacter* spp. **Piperacillin** is also active against some species of *Klebsiella*. Although these antipseudomonal penicillins are active against many gram-positive bacteria, *S. aureus* is often resistant. The addition of the β-lactamase inhibitor clavulanate to ticarcillin (**Timentin**), and tazobactam to piperacillin (**Zosyn**), broadens the spectrum of activity to include

S. aureus (except MRSA), *Bacteroides fragilis,* and some aerobic β-lactamase producing gram-negative bacteria.

2. **Adverse reactions** to penicillins include hypersensitivity reactions ranging from rash to anaphylaxis; bleeding caused by impaired platelet function (ticarcillin); volume overload or hypernatremia because of a large salt load (ticarcillin, piperacillin); interstitial nephritis (especially nafcillin); neutropenia (nafcillin at high doses); fever; and central nervous system (CNS) toxicity. A history of "**allergy**" to penicillin is often elicited in patients without clear documentation that an actual allergic reaction has occurred. **Skin testing** may be useful in diagnosing true allergy to β-lactams. In situations where a β-lactam is essential for optimal treatment of a life-threatening bacterial infection in a patient with a documented severe allergy to β-lactams, desensitization may be an option. Rapid desensitization can be achieved by intravenous (IV) administration of escalating doses of the desired antibiotic in a carefully monitored setting. Because of the potential for serious complications, a physician who is trained in this procedure should perform the desensitization.

C. **Cephalosporins**
   1. **Spectrum of activity.** Cephalosporins are classified into four generations based on their spectrum of activity.
      a. **First generation cephalosporins** such as **cefazolin** are active against many gram-positive and some gram-negative bacteria. Enteric gram-negative rods such as *E. coli,* some *Klebsiella* spp, and gram-positive oral anaerobes are often susceptible. *Enterococcus* spp, methicillin-resistant *S. epidermidis* (MRSE), and gram-negative anaerobes such as *Bacteroides* spp are resistant to cefazolin.
      b. **Second generation cephalosporins** are more active against gram-negative bacteria and less active against gram-positive bacteria than first generation agents. Two major subgroups of second generation cephalosporins exist. One group, which includes **cefuroxime,** is active against *Haemophilus influenzae.* The other group, which includes **cefoxitin** and **cefotetan,** is active against anaerobes such as *Bacteroides* spp.
      c. **Third generation cephalosporins** have greater activity against gram-negative bacilli than second generation agents. They are active against most enteric and some nonenteric (*H. influenzae* and *Neisseria* spp) gram-negative

bacilli. *Enterobacter* spp, *Citrobacter* spp, and *Acinetobacter* spp often become resistant to third generation cephalosporins because of inducible production of β-lactamase. **Ceftazidime** has strong activity against *Pseudomonas* spp, but is poorly active against gram-positive bacteria. **Ceftriaxone** and **cefotaxime** have activity against some gram-positive bacteria (not *Enterococcus* spp, *Listeria monocytogenes,* MRSA, or MRSE), but are often ineffective against *Pseudomonas* spp. Third generation cephalosporins have good CNS penetration and are often used to treat bacterial meningitis.

- **d. Fourth generation cephalosporins** such as **cefepime** have a similar spectrum of activity as ceftriaxone against gram-positive cocci, but broader gram-negative coverage that includes bacteria with inducible β-lactamase, such as *Enterobacter* spp, and *Citrobacter* spp. They can also be active against some ceftazidime-resistant *P. aeruginosa.*

- **2. Adverse reactions** to cephalosporins include hypersensitivity reactions (5% to 10% incidence of cross-reactivity with penicillin allergy), and bleeding because of inhibition of vitamin K-dependent coagulation factor synthesis (cefotetan).

D. Carbapenems have broad antimicrobial activity and can be used to treat infection originating at multiple sites. They offer the advantage of very broad coverage of gram-positive and gram-negative bacteria, and anaerobes. It is prudent to reserve carbapenem agents for treating documented nosocomial infections caused by antibiotic-resistant bacteria.

- **1. The spectrum of activity of imipenem–cilastatin** and **meropenem** are similar. They are active against most gram-negative bacteria, many gram-positive cocci, and anaerobes. Although they have the broadest spectrum of activity of the β-lactams, some pathogenic strains remain resistant. Resistant strains have included *Stenotrophomonas* (previously *Xanthomonas) maltophilia, P. cepacia,* and occasionally *P. aeruginosa, E. cloacae,* and *S. marcescens.* Resistant gram-positive bacteria have included some *Enterococcus* spp, MRSA, *Corynebacterium* spp, and *Bacteroides* spp.

- **2. Adverse reactions** include seizures and hypersensitivity reactions. The increased incidence of seizures in patients receiving imipenem–cilastatin who have renal failure or a seizure disorder may limit the use of this drug in some patients. Meropenem does not seem to induce seizures as frequently as imipenem–cilastatin.

E. Monobactams have a narrow spectrum of activity.

- **1. Spectrum of activity. Aztreonam** is active against many gram-negative aerobes and facultative anaerobes. It is not active against anaerobes or gram-positive aerobes. Some nonenteric gram-negative bacteria are resistant, including *S. maltophilia* and *Acinetobacter* spp, and *P. aeruginosa*.

2. **Adverse reactions** include hypersensitivity reactions. Despite the β-lactam structure, aztreonam seems to have very little cross-reactivity with other β-lactams and is often used in patients who have had minor allergic responses to β-lactams. The safety of aztreonam in patients with a history of anaphylaxis has not been clearly established.

F. **Glycopeptides,** including **vancomycin** and **teicoplanin,** interfere with bacterial cell wall synthesis.

1. **Spectrum of activity.** Glycopeptides are bactericidal for most gram-positive bacteria. They are active against the highly resistant staphylococcal strains, MRSA and MRSE, as well as *Enterococcus* spp and *Streptococcus* spp. As with the β-lactams, vancomycin is not bactericidal for *Enterococcus* spp, and should be combined with an aminoglycoside for synergistic coverage if bactericidal activity against enterococci is required. Teicoplanin, which is not currently available for use in the United States, may be more active against vancomycin-resistant *Enterococcus* (VRE) than vancomycin.

2. **Adverse reactions** to vancomycin include "red man" syndrome, rash, ototoxicity, nephrotoxicity, and neutropenia. "Red man" syndrome is a histamine-release syndrome characterized by flushing of the face, neck, and trunk, and variable degrees of hypotension. This reaction is not allergic in nature, occurs frequently, and is generally mild and transient (20 minutes); it can be minimized by delivering the drug in a large volume, reducing the dosage, slowing the rate of infusion, and premedicating with an antihistamine. The other adverse effects listed above are rare. Ototoxicity often is not reversible and can be associated with a persistent gait disturbance.

3. **Vancomycin-resistant gram-positive bacteria.** Vancomycin-resistant isolates of *Enterococcus* (VRE) are a problematic consequence of vancomycin therapy. Although *Enterococcus* spp generally are not pathogenic, they have emerged as nosocomial pathogens that cause significant infection in debilitated critically ill patients. Of great concern is the possibility that vancomycin resistance will emerge in more virulent gram-positive bacteria, such as MRSA or *Strep. pneumoniae*. Thus, vancomycin should be used cautiously and for very clear indications. Alternatives for treatment of serious infections caused by vancomycin-resistant gram-positives (such as chloramphenicol, tetracycline, and teicoplanin) are limited

and unreliable. Drugs under investigation include linezolid and quinapristin-dalfopristin (Synercid).

G. **Aminoglycosides** are bactericidal agents that interfere with bacterial protein synthesis. The most commonly used aminoglycosides in the ICU are **gentamicin, tobramycin,** and **amikacin.**

1. **Spectrum of activity.** Aminoglycosides are active primarily against gram-negative bacteria. Most enteric gram-negative bacteria are sensitive. *P. aeruginosa* is often sensitive, but *P. cepacia* and *S. maltophilia* are often resistant. Aminoglycosides are synergistic with the cell wall active agents (β-lactams, vancomycin) against *Enterococcus* spp, *Staphylococcus* spp, and *S. viridans*.

2. **Adverse reactions** include nephrotoxicity, ototoxicity, weakness, and potentiation of neuromuscular blockade. Nephrotoxicity, the most common adverse effect, is generally mild, nonoliguric, and reversible. Risk factors for nephrotoxicity include advanced age, overall debilitation, baseline renal insufficiency, hypotension, hypovolemia, and concomitant administration of other nephrotoxins such as amphotericin B or IV contrast agents. These risk factors are not absolute contraindications to aminoglycoside administration. Aminoglycosides can be extremely useful in some life-threatening infections (for instance, endocarditis caused by *Enterococcus* spp or *Pseudomonas* spp), and in some situations may have to be administered despite the potential for renal toxicity.

3. **Low pH and low oxygen tension** significantly diminish aminoglycoside antibacterial activity. Thus, they are not considered to be effective in acidic fluids (e.g., ascites) or under anaerobic conditions (e.g., within abscesses and poorly perfused tissues).

4. **Tissue concentrations** of aminoglycosides are variable. Low concentrations are achieved in tracheobronchopulmonary secretions, and penetration into the CNS is poor.

5. **Monitoring aminoglycoside levels** is controversial. Peak serum concentrations often are measured to verify that bactericidal levels are achieved, and trough levels are measured to assure adequate clearance of the drug in the hopes of preventing nephrotoxicity and ototoxicity.

6. **Once-a-day administration** with a large loading dose has gained popularity recently. Potential advantages include maximization of concentration-dependent bactericidal activity, a "postantibiotic effect," whereby bacterial growth is suppressed even after the serum level drops below the minimal inhibitory concentration, and less renal toxicity. Although studies have not conclusively shown improved eradication of serious infections in adults,

multiple laboratory and clinical studies have demonstrated decreased nephrotoxicity with a single daily dose. Studies are incomplete in patients with abnormal or changing renal function.

H. Fluoroquinolones are bactericidal agents that act by inhibiting DNA synthesis. Enteral absorption of **ofloxacin** and **levofloxacin** is excellent (approaching 95%), but is decreased by concomitant administration of iron, zinc, antacids (particularly those containing aluminum and magnesium), and sucralfate. Fluoroquinolones are concentrated in the urine, prostate, kidney, bowel, and lung, but penetrate the CNS poorly. They are potentially useful for many conditions including bone and joint infections, complicated urinary tract infections, bacterial gastroenteritis, and intra-abdominal infection.

1. **Spectrum of activity. Ciprofloxacin, ofloxacin,** and **levofloxacin** are primarily active against aerobic gram-negative bacilli, including *P. aeruginosa*. They are not consistently active against anaerobes, and have some activity against aerobic gram-positive bacteria. **Levofloxacin** often is used in combination with agents that cover gram-positive bacteria and anaerobes, such as clindamycin. The newer agents, **grepafloxacin, sparfloxacin**, and others, have extended the spectrum of activity to include some aerobic gram-positive cocci (not MRSA), and show promise for the treatment of a variety of different anaerobic and polymicrobial infections. Fluoroquinolones are also active against atypical bacteria such as *Legionella* spp, *Chlamydia* spp, and some *Mycobacteria* spp. Later generation agents have activity against penicillin-resistant *Strep. pneumoniae*.

2. **Adverse reactions** include gastrointestinal (GI) upset, CNS toxicity (headache, dizziness, confusion, hallucinations, seizures), and hypersensitivity reactions. Administration of ciprofloxacin to patients taking theophylline can result in theophylline toxicity. Metabolism via the hepatic P_{450} enzyme system predicts extensive drug interactions that merit consideration.

I. Metronidazole is bactericidal and acts by cleaving bacterial DNA. It is well absorbed from the GI tract and is metabolized in the liver.

1. **The spectrum of activity** of metronidazole is limited to gram-positive and gram-negative anaerobes. It is often used alone for the treatment of pseudomembranous (*C. difficile*) colitis, and in combination with other agents for treatment of peritoneal infections arising from the GI tract.

2. **Adverse reactions** are uncommon and include GI symptoms (metallic taste, anorexia, nausea) and neurologic dysfunction (peripheral neuropathy, seizures, ataxia, vertigo).

J. Clindamycin is a bacteriostatic agent and inhibits bacterial protein synthesis. It is well absorbed from the GI tract. It penetrates poorly into the CSF. Clindamycin is metabolized in the liver.

1. **Spectrum of activity.** Clindamycin is active against most anaerobes and gram-positive aerobes. Resistant organisms include gram-negative aerobes and facultative anaerobes, *Enterococcus* spp, and some isolates of *B. fragilis*. It can be used alone or with other agents to treat aspiration pneumonia.

2. **Adverse reactions** include GI upset, rash, and elevated liver enzymes. Clindamycin is notorious for promoting *C. difficile* colitis.

K. Macrolides are bacteriostatic and inhibit bacterial protein synthesis. **Erythromycin** is well absorbed from the GI tract and undergoes hepatic metabolism and biliary excretion. Penetration into the CNS is poor. The main indication for erythromycin in critically ill patients is atypical pneumonia. Newer agents of this class (e.g., azithromycin, clarithromycin) have a broader spectrum of activity with activity against mycobacteria and *H. influenzae* (azithromycin).

1. **Spectrum of activity.** Erythromycin is active against many gram-positive cocci, (especially *Streptococcus* spp), *Legionella* spp, *L. monocytogenes*, *Chlamydia pneumoniae* (TWAR), and *M. pneumoniae*.

2. **Adverse reactions** include GI upset with enteral administration, thrombophlebitis with IV administration, tinnitus, and transient deafness (rare).

L. Chloramphenicol inhibits protein synthesis.

1. **Spectrum of activity.** Chloramphenicol is active against a wide range of gram-positive and gram-negative aerobic and anaerobic organisms.

2. **Adverse reactions.** Because of the rare but serious side effect of aplastic anemia, chloramphenicol is rarely used. Current indications include serious infections that cannot be treated with alternative regimens, such as meningitis or endocarditis caused by VRE. Chloramphenicol can cause adverse hematologic effects, ranging from dose-dependent, but reversible bone marrow depression to fatal aplastic anemia ($\sim$ 1/25,000–50,000). Other adverse effects include GI upset, hypersensitivity reactions, and optic neuritis.

III. Antifungal agents

A. Amphotericin B exerts its antifungal effect by creating pores in the cell membrane. It is administered IV or via intrathecal routes, and by local instillation into the bladder. The pharmacokinetics of amphotericin B are uncertain. Amphotericin B is still considered the treatment of choice for life-threatening systemic fungal infections.

1. **Spectrum of activity.** Amphotericin B is broadly active against most *Candida* spp, *Torulopsis glabrata,* and many isolates of *Aspergillus.*
2. **Adverse reactions**
   a. **Fever and rigors** are common with administration of amphotericin B. Hypotension and hypoxemia also occur. **Pretreatment** with acetaminophen, antihistamines, low dose corticosteroids, or meperidine decreases the incidence and severity of these side effects. In some cases, reduction of the daily dose is necessary to allow continued treatment.
   b. Some degree of **renal dysfunction** occurs in most patients treated with amphotericin B. Adverse renal effects include azotemia, renal tubular acidosis, impaired ability to concentrate urine, electrolyte imbalances (hypokalemia, hypomagnesemia), and decreased production of erythropoietin. Severe renal failure occurs primarily in patients receiving other nephrotoxic drugs, patients with preexisting renal disease or renal transplantation, and severely ill patients who are hypotensive, hypovolemic, or both. Alternate day dosing and administration of saline (1 L/d in excess of baseline fluid requirements) may be of benefit in preventing or blunting renal toxicity.
   c. **Other** adverse effects include anemia and GI upset.
   d. **Test dose.** Therapy should be initiated carefully. Although some physicians favor administration of a 1 mg IV test dose, given over 15 minutes followed by close observation for 1 hour, no clear data support this practice. An unfavorable reaction to the test dose should not prompt a dosage reduction in a critically ill patient, but rather a prolongation of infusion time, increases in the volume of fluid used to administer the drug, and treatment of symptoms.
3. **Lipid formulations** of amphotericin B include **amphotericin B lipid complex, amphotericin B colloidal suspension,** and **liposomal amphotericin B.** These agents are extremely costly. Their role in the management of invasive fungal infections is still being defined, and controlled comparative studies are limited. The available data suggest that lipid formulations are generally as effective as standard formulations and cause less renal toxicity. Lipid formulations of amphotericin B have been used in some immunocompromised patients with *Fusarium* species infection, unexplained fever in neutropenia, and in those intolerant of standard amphotericin B therapy.
B. **Triazoles,** including **ketoconazole, fluconazole,** and **itraconazole,** act by inhibiting fungal membrane

sterol synthesis. Itraconazole use in the ICU is limited by the lack of parenteral formulations (other than voriconazole, a newer agent). Enteral absorption of fluconazole is excellent (≥90%) in patients who are tolerating enteral feedings, and CNS penetration is reasonably good. Potential uses of fluconazole include prophylaxis against invasive fungal infections in immunocompromised hosts (e.g., leukemia, HIV, organ transplant recipients), treatment of candidemia, and treatment in stable patients of invasive mycosis caused by *Candida* spp, excluding *C. krusei* and most *C. glabrata*. Preliminary noncontrolled studies in patients with candiduria suggest that fluconazole may be more effective in preventing dissemination and sepsis than amphotericin B bladder irrigation.

1. **Spectrum of activity.** Triazoles are active against many *Candida* spp (*C. albicans, C. parapsilosis,* and *C. tropicalis*) and *Cryptococcus neoformans. C. krusei* and *T. glabrata* are frequently resistant. The newer agent, voriconazole, has a broader spectrum of activity.

2. **Adverse reactions** include GI upset, rash, headaches, increased hepatocellular enzyme levels, exfoliative dermatitis (rare), and severe hepatotoxicity (rare).

3. **Drug interactions.**
   a. **Coumadin.** Further prolongation of the prothrombin time.
   b. **Phenytoin** and **cyclosporine** levels are increased by fluconazole.
   c. **Rifampin** increases fluconazole levels.
   d. **Cisapride** administration with fluconazole can cause QT-prolongation on the electrocardiogram and, rarely, polymorphic ventricular tachycardia.

C. **5-Fluorocytosine** (flucytosine) is an antimetabolite that inhibits fungal protein and DNA synthesis. It is sometimes used with amphotericin B for synergistic treatment of severe systemic candidiasis or cryptococcal meningitis. Toxicity (primarily hematologic) correlates with high serum levels.

IV. **Antiviral agents**

A. **Acyclovir** is available in enteral and parenteral formulations. Parenteral administration is recommended for treatment of serious infection such as varicella pneumonia or herpes encephalitis.

1. **Spectrum of activity.** Acyclovir is active against herpes simplex virus (HSV) I and II, varicella zoster virus (VZV), and Epstein-Barr virus (EBV). Cytomegalovirus (CMV) is resistant.

2. **Adverse reactions** include renal dysfunction, particularly in hypovolemic patients or in those with preexisting renal disease. Neurotoxicity also occurs, resulting in confusion, tremulousness, and seizures. Intravenous acyclovir is the treatment of choice for

serious HSV and VZV infections. Oral acyclovir can
be used for treatment of mucocutaneous HSV.

B. **Famciclovir** and **valacyclovir** are newer antiviral
agents with a similar spectrum of activity as acyclovir.
Only enteral formulations are currently available.

C. **Ganciclovir** is used to treat CMV infections, including
retinitis, colitis, and pneumonitis in immunocompromised patients. It is also used as prophylaxis against
CMV infections in transplant recipients.

1. **Spectrum of activity.** Ganciclovir is active against
HSV, VZV, and CMV.

2. **Adverse reactions.** Myelosuppression and nephrotoxicity are the major adverse effects of ganciclovir.

3. **Alternatives. Foscarnet** and **cidofovir** also
have activity against CMV, but nephrotoxicity is
common.

V. **Sepsis and septic shock.** Sepsis is an important cause of
morbidity and mortality in the ICU. Sepsis is caused by a
variety of microorganisms, including bacteria, fungi, and,
rarely, viruses, which originate from virtually any site of
infection. The mortality rate for septic shock is extremely
high (≥30%) despite the multitude of available antibiotics
and improved supportive care in the ICU (Chapter 9).

A. **Definitions**

1. **The systemic inflammatory response syndrome (SIRS)** has infectious and noninfectious
causes (e.g., pancreatitis, major trauma, transfusion reaction). Criteria for SIRS include fever
(> 38°C) or hypothermia (< 36°C), tachypnea (> 20
breaths/min) or hypocarbia ($Paco_2$ < 32 mm Hg),
tachycardia (heart rate > 90 bpm), and leukocytosis
(> 12,000/μl), leukopenia (< 4,000/μL), or more than
10% immature (band) forms.

2. **Sepsis** is the systemic inflammatory response to
invasion by microorganisms.

3. **Severe sepsis** is sepsis with hypotension or hypoperfusion and dysfunction of at least a single
organ (acute respiratory failure, acute renal failure, metabolic acidosis, mental status changes).

4. **Septic shock** is defined as severe sepsis with hypotension that does not promptly respond to fluid
administration. Septic shock can progress to **refractory septic shock** when hypotension persists for more than 1 hour despite appropriate fluid
resuscitation.

5. **Multiple organ dysfunction syndrome
(MODS)** is failure of more than one organ that requires external support to maintain stability (i.e.,
dialysis for renal failure, mechanical ventilation
for acute respiratory failure).

B. **Pathophysiology**

1. **Microbial toxins** such as endotoxin, peptidogly-
can, lipoteichoic acid, and secreted exotoxins trigger a complex inflammatory cascade in the host.

2. **Host responses** against infection are crucial. They can have deleterious effects on the host, and can ultimately cause cardiovascular collapse, MODS, and death. A variety of mediators are involved in the host response:

   a. **Cytokines** such as tumor necrosis factor-alpha (TNF_α) and the interleukins mediate a variety of signs and symptoms, including fever, tachycardia, increased vascular endothelial permeability, disseminated intravascular coagulation (DIC), and shock.

   b. **Vasodilator substances** such as nitric oxide, prostaglandin E_2, and prostacyclin.

C. **Manifestations and complications of sepsis** vary widely. Early signs include hyperventilation, tachycardia, fever, and progressive disorientation. Fever is variably present, and its absence can be misleading. Later signs include shock with hypotension, obtundation, respiratory failure, acute renal failure, and DIC. **Vascular endothelial injury** occurs, leading to extravasation of intravascular fluid into the extravascular space, microthrombosis, and activation of the coagulation–fibrinolytic system.

   1. **Shock** results from vasodilation, variable degrees of myocardial dysfunction, and intravascular hypovolemia from extravasation of intravascular fluid. Hemodynamic assessment usually reveals a high cardiac output with decreased peripheral vascular tone.

   2. **Respiratory failure.** Arterial oxygenation can decline because of extravasation of fluid across leaky alveolar capillaries. The **acute respiratory distress syndrome (ARDS)** frequently occurs with severe sepsis and septic shock that results from pulmonary and extrapulmonary infections.

   3. **Renal dysfunction** ranges from mild oliguria to acute tubular necrosis, which requires dialysis. It can result from hypotension with impaired renal perfusion or direct damage to the kidneys.

   4. **Metabolic acidosis** is common in sepsis, although initially patients may be alkalemic from hyperventilation.

   5. **Hematologic complications** include thrombocytopenia and DIC. Thrombosis most commonly occurs in the microcirculation and can produce ischemic necrosis of the digits.

   6. **MODS** often complicates sepsis. The mortality of MODS is high.

D. **Management** of patients with sepsis includes, at minimum, antibiotics and supportive care of vital functions. A thorough evaluation for the source of infection and prompt removal of identified sources of infection is crucial for successful management.

   1. **Antibiotic choices** depend on the microorganisms involved. Empiric, broad-spectrum coverage

is generally initiated before culture data become available. Specific choices will depend on the suspected origin of the infection. Once the patient is stabilized, antibiotics should be adjusted based on culture and sensitivity data.

2. **Supportive care**

   a. **Hemodynamic management** should focus on restoration of intravascular volume and tissue perfusion. Usually this requires administration of a combination of IV fluids and vasopressors. Patients initially may require massive volumes of IV fluid to offset "third-space" losses. Pressors are added when fluid administration fails to restore adequate perfusion pressure (Chapters 9 and 10).

   b. **Mechanical ventilation** (Chapters 4 and 20) is frequently necessary and may need to be continued well beyond resolution of the episode of sepsis and ARDS.

   c. **Hemodialysis** or **hemofiltration** may be required if severe acidemia, hyperkalemia, uremia, or hypervolemia complicate acute renal failure (Chapter 23).

   d. **Severe DIC** is treated with transfusions of platelets and fresh frozen plasma as indicated by coagulation profile and platelet count (Chapter 12).

3. **Removal of the source of sepsis.** Choice of surgery, catheter drainage, or other invasive procedures depends on the source of sepsis. Abscesses can often be drained using percutaneous catheters, whereas open peritoneal contamination requires surgical correction.

4. **Experimental therapies** developed for adjunctive treatment of sepsis target microbial toxins [i.e., anti-lipopolysaccharide syndrome (LPS) antibodies, bactericidal/permeability-increasing protein], or intervene in the inflammatory cascade triggered by the infection (i.e., antibodies against TNF_α, soluble TNF receptors). Many of these therapies appeared protective in experimental models, but none have been convincingly effective in clinical trials. New agents continue to be developed and evaluated, including bactericidal/permeability-increasing protein, reconstituted forms of high-density lipoprotein, and lipid A antagonists.

VI. **Infections in immunocompromised hosts** Immunocompromised hosts are at increased risk of community-acquired, nosocomial, and opportunistic infections. Prompt intervention is required to successfully treat these infections, but their diagnosis often is difficult because of the lack of clear localizing signs. A thorough search for the source of infection must be undertaken. At minimum, this includes cultures of blood, urine, and sputum, and a chest radiograph. Immunocompromise results from many causes, including immunosupressive therapy, burns, malignancy, HIV infection, chemotherapy, corticosteroids, and severe malnutrition. Because different aspects of the immune response can be altered in these conditions, the infectious disease complications are variable. The lung is the most common site of infection in the immunocompromised patient.

A. Infections in neutropenic patients

   1. **Neutropenia** most often is a result of leukemia, chemotherapy, or bone marrow transplantation; less frequently, it is caused by drug reactions or aplastic anemia. Bacteria, particularly enteric and nonenteric gram-negatives and gram-positives, and fungi (*Candida* spp, *Aspergillus* spp, *T. glabrata*) characteristically cause infection in neutropenic patients, although severe viral infections (HSV, CMV, EBV) can also occur.

   2. **Fever** in patients with severe neutropenia [absolute neutrophil count (ANC) < 100/μL] should be assumed to result from infection.

   3. **Treatment of neutropenic fever**

      a. **Initial treatment. Broad-spectrum antibacterial agents** directed against gram-positive and gram-negative bacteria, including *Pseudomonas* spp, should be administered initially. Antibiotics should be continued for a minimum of 10 days or until the ANC rises above 500/μL (whichever is later).

         (1) **Monotherapy** using a broad-spectrum agent such as imipenem–cilastatin or a third generation antipseudomonal cephalosporin may be sufficient in patients who are not critically ill.

         (2) **Combination therapy** should be administered to critically ill patients, using agents that are likely to treat nosocomial antibiotic-resistant organisms, and organisms such as *Enterobacter* spp and *Citrobacter* spp that rapidly become resistant to β-lactams. Potential combinations include a third generation antipseudomonal β-lactam (e.g., ceftazidime or piperacillin) and either an aminoglycoside or a fluoroquinolone. Aminoglycosides can be problematic, particularly in patients with renal dysfunction or those receiving cyclosporine. Vancomycin should be added if suspicion exists of gram-positive infection from MRSA.

      b. **Subsequent treatment. Ongoing fever for 4 to 7 days** despite broad antibacterial therapy warrants antifungal treatment with amphotericin B.

B. Infections in transplant recipients. Transplant recipients are most susceptible to life-threatening infections during the first 6 months after organ transplantation. During this time, they are maximally immuno-suppressed; they are exposed to many nosocomial organisms and may be experiencing allograft rejection or graft-versus-host disease (GVHD). Infections are caused by bacteria, fungi, viruses, protozoa, parasites, and mycobacteria. Bacterial infections are caused by aerobic gram-positive and gram-negative bacteria. Fungal infections are most commonly caused by *Candida* spp and *Aspergillus* spp. Some infections such as CMV are transmitted from the organ to the recipient or via transfused blood products. Fever in the absence of localized findings is often the first manifestation of infection.

Short courses of parenteral antibiotics are generally given before and after solid organ transplantation. Patient and environmental factors dictate antibiotic choice. Some antibiotics have significant interactions with immunosuppressive agents. Metabolism of cyclosporine by the cytochrome P_{450} system can be increased or decreased by administration of fluoroquinolones, macrolides, fluconazole, rifampin, and isoniazid. Aminoglycosides, amphotericin B, vancomycin, pentamidine, and high-dose trimethoprim–sulfamethoxazole enhance the nephrotoxicity of cyclosporine. Cyclosporine levels should be monitored in patients receiving these agents.

1. Solid organ transplantation

   a. In the first month after transplantation, infections are usually caused by the same bacteria and fungi that cause infections in immunocompetent postsurgical patients. **Early posttransplant** infections are usually nosocomial, occurring at the surgical site, or are a result of the prolonged presence of indwelling catheters or endotracheal intubation.

   b. Between 1 and 6 months, viral and opportunistic infections, (e.g., *Pneumocystis carinii* pneumonia and aspergillosis) predominate.

   c. After 6 months, infections depend on the level of immunosuppression and environmental exposures. Patients on minimal immunosuppressive therapy develop similar infections as normal hosts. High doses of immunosuppressive agents predispose patients to infections with opportunistic microbes such as *P. carinii, L. monocytogenes, Aspergillus fumigatus,* and *Cryptococcus neoformans.* Preexisting viral infections can progress and cause severe damage to infected organs. Cytomegalovirus infection often causes isolated fever, hepatitis, pneumonitis, hypotension, enterocolitis, and glomerulnephritis. Manifestations of CNS infections (generally caused by *L. monocytogenes* or opportunistic pathogens) can be atypical. Computed tomography (CT) of the head and lumbar puncture are necessary for transplant patients with unexplained fever or headache. Chest CT is often useful in the evaluation of transplant patients with pulmonary symptoms given that the typical radiographic signs of inflammation are often attenuated.

2. **Bone marrow transplantation.** Allogeneic and autologous bone marrow transplants are done to treat acute and chronic leukemias, lymphoma, solid tumors, multiple myeloma, and severe aplastic anemia. As for other types of organ transplantation, three phases of infectious disease complications occur after bone marrow transplantation:

   a. **The first month** is characterized by ongoing neutropenia from prior chemotherapy. Bacterial, fungal, and viral infections occur. Bacterial infections are caused by gram-positive aerobes, including coagulase-negative staphylococcus, *Strep. viridans*, *S. aureus*, and *Corynebacterium* spp, and enteric and nonenteric gram-negative aerobes and facultative anaerobes. Reactivation of HSV can also occur during this period.

      Empiric antibiotic therapy for febrile neutropenic bone marrow transplant patients should include agents that cover gram-negative aerobes and facultative anaerobes and gram-positives. Antipseudomonal coverage should be included. Empiric coverage is often undertaken using a combination of β-lactams [one antipseudomonal cephalosporin and one antipseudomonal penicillin (e.g., piperacillin or mezlocillin)] or vancomycin plus an antipseudomonal β-lactam (or imipenem–cilastatin). Fevers persisting despite broad antibacterial coverage raise the possibility of invasive fungal infections and often are treated with amphotericin B.

   b. **From 1 to 3 months,** patients are susceptible to viral infections (CMV), opportunistic infections, and bacterial infections (gram-positive and gram-negative).

   c. **After 3 months,** patients with GVHD are predisposed to late infections. Late infections often involve the respiratory tract; they are caused by respiratory viruses and encapsulated organisms such as *Strep. pneumoniae* or *H. influenzae*. Mucocutaneous damage caused by GVHD also predisposes these patients to infections with skin flora such as staphylococci.

C. **HIV.** Infection with HIV predisposes patients to opportunistic infections and immunosuppression-related malignancies. Progresses in treatment with antiretroviral therapy and prophylaxis against opportunistic infections have resulted in longer survival. Similarly, survival in HIV-infected patients admitted to the ICU has improved considerably over the last decade. The **T4 helper (CD4)** count is an accurate predictor of sites and organisms involved in infection in HIV patients as indicated in Table 27-4. HIV infection also increases susceptibility to infection with encapsulated bacteria, including *Strep. pneumoniae* and *H. influenzae.*

1. **Pulmonary infections** in the HIV-infected patient are caused by a variety of microorganisms, depending on the CD4 count (Table 27-4) and the geographical location. In patients with normal CD4 counts, pneumonia may be caused by community-acquired organisms. As the CD4 count drops, the likelihood that pulmonary infection is caused by opportunistic infections, particularly *P. carinii* and CMV, increases. Evaluation for the cause of pneumonitis should be prompt, and should include induced sputum examination, deep aspiration, or bronchoscopy with bronchoalveolar lavage. Empiric antibiotic therapy should cover the most likely pathogens based on the CD4 count and geographic location. Above a CD4 count of approximately 200 to 300/μL antibiotics should cover community-acquired organisms. Below a CD4 count of 200, treatment also should cover *P. carinii.*

2. **CNS infections,** such as brain abscess, meningitis, and encephalitis, can be caused by a variety of organisms, including bacteria, fungi, viruses, and parasites, in patients infected with HIV. Evaluation for CNS infections, including CT scans or magnetic resonance imaging of the brain and lumbar puncture should be done if CNS infection is suspected, and empiric antibiotics should be administered while awaiting the results.

VII. **Infection control in the ICU**

A. **Nosocomial (hospital-acquired) infections** are frequent in ICU patients. Patient and environmental factors are important in the development of nosocomial infections. Impaired host defenses, use of drugs that shift the endogenous colonizing flora (such as

Table 27-4.   Relationship of CD4 count to infection in HIV patients

CD4 count (per μl)	Microbiologic predisposition
>800	Community-acquired organisms
<800	*Mycobacterium tuberculosis* (pulmonary)
<500	*Candida* spp, *Cryptococcus neoformans, Histoplasma capsulatum, Coccidioides* spp
<300	*Pneumocystis carinii*
<100	*Mycobacterium avium intracellulare, M. tuberculosis* (disseminated), *Cryptosporidium,* CMV

spp, species; CMV, cytomegalovirus.

antibiotics), invasive monitors, and transmission of microorganisms to patients by personnel, equipment, solutions, and ventilation systems contribute to the development of nosocomial infections. The hospital environment facilitates colonization with antibiotic-resistant microorganisms.

B. Infection control measures are necessary to decrease the risk of nosocomial infection and to prevent transmission of blood-borne pathogens such as HIV, HBV, and hepatitis C virus (HCV) between patients and ICU staff. General control measures are designed to prevent transmission of infection between hospital personnel and patients, to decrease colonization of surfaces and equipment with microorganisms, and to minimize the development of antibiotic-resistant pathogens. Each hospital maintains specific guidelines and policies for infection control. Such guidelines emphasize:

1. **Routine hand washing** with antiseptic-containing solutions before and after contact with patients or after contact with contaminated materials.

2. **Wearing gloves** when hands are likely to be exposed to blood or other bodily fluids. Gloves must be changed (and hands washed) before and after contact with each patient.

3. **Sterilization of reusable equipment** such as bronchoscopes, laryngoscopes, and surgical instruments.

4. **Isolation precautions.**

   a. **Universal precautions** apply to all patients, regardless of underlying diseases. Barrier precautions are required when potential exists for contact with blood and other bodily secretions and fluids, as these can harbor infectious agents. Barriers include gloves, protective eyewear or face shields, and gowns.

   b. **Special precautions** including **contact, airborne,** and **droplet precautions** are used to limit the transmission of antibiotic-resistant bacteria among patients and healthcare workers, to limit the spread of viruses and bacteria present in respiratory secretions, and to protect immunocompromised hosts from infection.

      (1) **Contact precautions** are used for patients colonized or infected with antibiotic-resistant bacteria, such as VRE, and require that gloves be worn when entering the room, and gowns be worn when in direct contact with the patient, or equipment or surfaces in the patient's room.

      (2) **Airborne** and **droplet precautions** limit the spread of pathogens in respiratory secretions.

         (a) **Droplet precautions** are used to limit spread of infectious agents such as *Neisseria meningitidis, H. in-*

fluenzae, Mycoplasma pneumoniae, adenovirus, and rubella virus. Personnel and visitors who come in close proximity to patients on droplet precautions must wear a surgical mask. A private room is preferred, but a negative-pressure isolation room is not required.

(b) **Airborne precautions** are used to limit spread of *Mycobacterium tuberculosis,* VZV, rubeolla, and multiple other viruses. A private negative-pressure isolation room is required for patients on airborne precautions.

5. **To decrease transmission of blood-borne pathogens** (HIV, HBV, HCV), used needles should not be recapped, but should be immediately discarded into special puncture-proof receptacles. The risk of transmission of disease from a needle stick contaminated with blood from an infected patient is estimated to be between 6% and 30% for hepatitis B; approximately 3% for hepatitis C; and 0.3% per occurrence for HIV. Hollow needles are thought to be riskier than solid (suture) needles. A needle that passes through a glove before piercing the skin may have a lower infection rate. The use of specially designed needles and blunt-tipped or needle-free systems for drug administration and phlebotomy effectively reduces the incidence of needle stick injuries.

6. **Limiting the use of antibiotics.** The frequent use of broad-spectrum antibiotics in the ICU has resulted in the emergence of microorganisms that are resistant to multiple antibiotics. The recent emergence of vancomycin-resistant *Enterococcus* is concerning, particularly because it suggests that other more virulent gram-positives, such as MRSA, may also become resistant to vancomycin. To decrease the likelihood of selecting for antibiotic-resistant organisms, the narrowest spectrum of antibiotics should be chosen. When broad empiric antibiotic therapy is required, the regimen should be rapidly narrowed, based on results of cultures. Prophylactic perioperative antibiotics should be administered only when necessary, and should be limited to the immediate perioperative period (24 hours). Many institutions have policies that limit the use of various antibiotics, require justification for use of certain agents, and have guidelines for routine perioperative antibiotic prophylaxis.

SELECTED REFERENCES

Ambrose PG, Owens RC, Quintilian R, et al. Antbiotic use in the critical care unit. *Crit Care Clin* 1998;14:283–308.

Bone RC, Balk RA, Cerra FB, et al. Definitions for sepsis and organ failure and guidelines for the use of innovative therapies in sepsis. *Chest* 1992;101:1644–1655.

Boyce JM. Vancomycin-resistant Enterococcus: detection, epidemiology, and control measures. *Infect Dis Clin N Am* 1997;11:367–384.

Diekhaus KD, Cooper BW. Infection control concepts in critical care. *Crit Care Clin* 1998;14:55–70.

Fishman JA, Rubin RH. Infection in organ-transplant recipients. *N Engl J Med* 1998;338:1741–1751.

Nichols RL. Surgical infections: prevention and treatment—1965 to 1995. *Am J Surg* 1996;172:68–74.

The Sanford guide to antimicrobial therapy. Vienna, Virginia: Antimicrobial Therapy, Inc., 1998

Wheeler AP, Benard GR. Treating patients with severe sepsis. *N Engl J Med* 1999;340:207–214.

Wong-Beringer A, Jacobs RA, Guglielmo BJ. Lipid formulations of amphotericin B: clinical efficacy and toxicities. *Clin Infect Dis* 1998;27:603–618

Specific Infections

Judith Hellman

This chapter provides a brief overview of specific infections encountered in critically ill patients and emphasizes their clinical presentation, microbiology (see Table 27-3), and diagnostic and therapeutic approaches. A detailed review of each entity is beyond the scope of this chapter, and the reader is referred to textbooks of infectious diseases for more complete discussions. Because of the complexity of infectious complications in critically ill patients, management often requires the contribution of physicians specifically trained in infectious diseases.

I. **Thoracic infections**
   A. **Community-acquired pneumonia (CAP)** is an infection of the lower respiratory tract that is acquired outside of the hospital. Although the overall mortality of CAP is low, the mortality of patients in the intensive care unit (ICU) with CAP is high. Risk factors for poor outcome include advanced age, coexisting chronic diseases (e.g., heart disease, pulmonary disease, diabetes), immunosuppression, and neoplastic disease. Clinical findings on admission also predict outcome. Increased respiratory rate, hypotension, fever, altered mental status, high or low white blood cell count (WBC), hypoxemia, and multilobar involvement are associated with higher mortality.
      1. **Microbiology.** The most frequent pathogen is *Streptococcus pneumoniae.* CAP is also caused by *Haemophilus influenzae* and other gram-negative bacteria such as *Klebsiella pneumoniae* and *Pseudomonas aeruginosa* (particularly in patients with underlying lung disease), gram-positive bacteria such as *Staphylococcus aureus,* atypical pathogens such as *Legionella pneumophila*, *Mycoplasma pneumoniae,* and *Chlamydia pneumoniae,* and viruses. *Moraxella catarrhalis* can cause CAP in patients with chronic obstructive pulmonary disease (COPD) and chronic bronchitis. Immunocompromised patients can develop pneumonia from standard pathogens as well as opportunistic organisms.
      2. **Diagnosis.** Findings on chest radiography can be variable, depending on the underlying condition of the host and the pathogen. Infiltrates can be unilobar or multilobar, and may not be apparent on initial chest radiographs of severely hypovolemic patients. Whenever possible, the causative microorganism should be identified. Analysis of the sputum by Gram's stain should reveal more than

25 neutrophils and less than 10 epithelial cells per low-power field. The causative organism may be suggested by the abundance and morphology of the bacteria on a well-collected sample. In some cases, it may be necessary to perform bronchoscopy to obtain adequate sputum samples. Sputum cultures can be helpful in identifying the organism and defining the antimicrobial sensitivity, although often a specific pathogen is not identified. Blood cultures can also be helpful in defining the organism. If pneumonia is accompanied by a significant pleural effusion, the pleural fluid should be analyzed for Gram's stain and culture, pH, lactate dehydrogenase, glucose, and protein concentration. Serologic tests can be useful for identifying infection from atypical pathogens. *L. pneumophila* antigen may be detected in the sputum or urine.

3. **Treatment.** Initial management of CAP is usually empiric, and is guided by the condition of the patient and the results of the Gram's stained sputum specimen. Outcome is improved with early administration of antibiotics. Clinical presentation does not reliably predict the pathogens involved, and frequently the causative microorganism is not identified. The potential for antibiotic resistance should influence the choice of antibiotics (for instance, *Strep. pneumoniae* can be penicillin-resistant). Antibiotics for early broad empiric therapy should cover typical as well as atypical microorganisms. Therapy should be adjusted based on results of cultures and serologic tests. Potential regimens for severely ill patients in the ICU include:

   a. A fluoroquinolone such as levofloxacin plus a β-lactam (second generation cephalosporin such as cefuroxime or β-lactam/β-lactamase inhibitor such as ampicillin–sulbactam).

   b. A macrolide such as erythromycin for coverage of atypical microorganisms plus a third or fourth generation cephalosporin with gram-positive coverage such as ceftriaxone, cefotaxime, or cefipime.

   c. A macrolide plus a β-lactam/β-lactamase inhibitor combination such as ampicillin–sulbactam.

   d. A macrolide plus a carbapenem such as imipenem or meropenem.

B. **Nosocomial pneumonia,** which is common in surgical and trauma patients, is associated with the highest mortality of all nosocomial infections. It occurs most frequently in patients requiring prolonged mechanical ventilation. Bacteria enter the lungs through various routes, including aspiration of oropharyngeal secretions or esophageal or gastric contents; inhalation of airborne droplets; hematogenous spread from other sites; and direct inoculation from colonized hospital personnel or contaminated equipment or devices.

1. **Microbiology.** The microorganisms causing nosocomial pneumonia differ substantially from those causing CAP. Infections are often polymicrobial. Enteric gram-negative bacteria (such as *Escherichia coli, Klebsiella* spp, *Proteus* spp, *Enterobacter* spp and *S. aureus)* most frequently cause nosocomial pneumonia. Other bacteria include nonenteric gram-negatives such as *Pseudomonas aeruginosa* and *H. influenzae,* anaerobes, and gram-positives such as *Enterococcus* spp and *Strep. pneumoniae.* Antibiotic-resistant bacteria are very common.

2. **Diagnosis** of nosocomial pneumonia in patients in the ICU can be difficult. Signs such as fever, leukocytosis, purulent secretions, and even the presence of infiltrates on chest radiographs are nonspecific and may not indicate actual pulmonary infection. Considerable variability is seen in the approach to diagnostic evaluation. Controversy exists over whether sputum samples should be collected using invasive methods, and whether quantitative bacterial cultures (which must be obtained via invasive means) are necessary.

   a. **Nonquantitative cultures** are often performed on sputum samples (obtained by noninvasive and invasive means). Most agree that cultures of expectorated sputum and samples from blind endotracheal suctioning are unreliable for definitive diagnosis of pneumonia or for defining with certainty the causative microorganism. It is likely, however, that the pathogen will be among the bacteria cultured, and sensitivity data may help to define the antimicrobial resistance patterns. Thus, with limitations, this relatively noninvasive means of obtaining sputum can be useful in guiding antibiotic choices.

   b. **Invasive collection** using protected-brush bronchoscopy or bronchoalveolar lavage (BAL) provides lower respiratory tract samples for **quantitative cultures.** Quantitative cultures may be more reliable for diagnosis of infection and identification of the specific pathogen(s). Pneumonia is diagnosed for protected-brush bronchoscopy concentrations of more than 10^3 colony forming units/ml and BAL concentrations of more than 10^4 or 10^5 colony forming units/ml. These samples can also be more useful in defining the specific pathogen. Unfortunately, these techniques can be limited by the invasiveness of the procedures, the lack of standardization for obtaining such samples, and the potential failure to definitively diagnose pneumonia in the early stages when bacterial counts are likely to be lower. With all sampling techniques, the sensitivity of sputum cultures decreases with even short courses of antibiotics prior to sample collection.

3. **Treatment.** Often antibiotics must be initiated empirically until culture data are available. The clinical setting, including severity of illness, underlying and coexisting diseases, duration of hospitalization, and the local flora of the hospital influence the choice of antibiotics.

   a. **Uncomplicated mild to moderate disease** (i.e., without respiratory failure, hemodynamic instability, or signs of injury to other organs) occurring early during the hospitalization (< 5 days) is often treated with a single antibiotic such as a second or third generation nonpseudomonal cephalosporin, or a fluoroquinolone in patients who are allergic to penicillins. A number of studies suggest that **monotherapy** is safe and effective when used properly, and may decrease the likelihood of infection from antibiotic-resistant microorganisms. If anaerobes are a possibility, a β-lactam/β-lactamase inhibitor combination such as ampicillin–sulbactam or ticarcillin–clavulanate can be used as monotherapy. Alternatively, clindamycin or metronidazole can be used in combination with a β-lactam or fluoroquinolone for adequate anaerobic coverage.

   b. **Severe hospital-acquired pneumonia** (i.e., respiratory failure, hemodynamic instability, extrapulmonary organ damage) is treated with combination therapy. Combination therapy should also be considered when **mild to moderate pneumonia** occurs later in the hospitalization, in patients with significant underlying diseases, or in patients who have recently received antibiotics. These situations increase the likelihood that pneumonia is caused by *P. aeruginosa,* other multiresistant enteric gram-negatives such as *Enterobacter* spp, *Klebsiella* spp, and methicillin-resistant *S. aureus* (MRSA). Generally, combination therapy includes a β-lactam (such as ceftazidime, ticarcillin, piperacillin, ceftazidime, imipenem–cilastatin, or aztreonam) plus a fluoroquinolone or an aminoglycoside. Vancomycin should be added when a possibility of MRSA pneumonia exists. Antibiotics should be modified as soon as possible based on culture and sensitivity data.

C. **Lung abscess** results from destruction of the pulmonary parenchyma leading to large fluid-filled cavities. The most frequent predisposing factor for lung abscess is **aspiration pneumonia,** followed by periodontal disease and gingivitis. Bronchiectasis, pulmonary infarction, septic embolization, and bacteremia also predispose to lung abscess.

1. **Microbiology.** Bacteria causing aspiration pneumonia and subsequent abscess formation differ depending on whether aspiration occurs on an outpatient or an inpatient basis. Hospital-acquired aspiration pneumonia is caused by anaerobes, gram-positive bacteria such as *S. aureus,* and gram-negative bacteria such as *P. aeruginosa* and *K. pneumoniae.* Abscesses resulting from hematogenous spread of infection are usually peripheral and multifocal, and are most commonly caused by *S. aureus.* Anaerobes and gram-negative bacilli also cause abscesses in this setting. *Mycobacterium tuberculosis, Nocardia* infections, amoebae, and fungi are rarer causes of lung abscess.

2. **Diagnosis** of lung abscess is based on chest radiograph or chest computed tomography (CT). Cultures of expectorated sputum are unreliable. Samples should be collected using protected-brush bronchoscopy or BAL.

3. **Treatment.** Prolonged (2–4 months) antibiotic therapy is the primary treatment for lung abscess. Antibiotic choices will depend on culture isolates. Postural drainage is an important aspect of the management, and bronchoscopy can be helpful in facilitating drainage or removing foreign bodies. Occasionally, a lung abscess is treated with surgical resection; however, this is not a first line of therapy. Complications of lung abscess include empyema, bronchopleural fistula formation, and bronchiectasis.

D. **Empyema** usually originates from intrapulmonary infection such as lung abscess or pneumonia, but also can be introduced from the outside as in trauma or thoracic surgery.

1. **Microbiology.** The most common bacterial cause of empyema is *S. aureus.* Enteric and nonenteric gram-negative bacteria, gram-positive bacteria, anaerobic bacteria, fungi, and *M. tuberculosis* also can cause empyema.

2. **Diagnosis** requires direct analysis of pleural fluid for pH, total protein, red blood cell (RBC) and leukocyte (WBC) count and differential, Gram's stain and bacterial cultures (anaerobic and aerobic), and possibly fungal smear and culture. Smears and cultures for acid-fast bacilli should be performed if *M. tuberculosis* is suspected.

3. **Treatment.** Empyema is treated with a combination of antibiotics and drainage via a thoracoscopy

tube. Occasionally, open drainage or decortication of the empyema sac is required.

E. **Mediastinitis** can result from spontaneous perforation of the esophagus, leakage from an esophageal anastomosis, trauma, cardiothoracic surgery, head and neck infections, and dental procedures.

1. **Microbiology.** Mediastinitis following cardiothoracic surgery that does not involve the esophagus is generally monomicrobial—most often caused by gram-positive aerobic bacteria, although gram-negative aerobic bacteria, facultative anaerobic bacteria, and fungi also cause mediastinitis. Mediastinitis arising from infections in the head and neck or disruption of the esophagus is usually polymicrobial and is caused by mixed anaerobic bacteria (*Peptococcus* spp, *Peptostreptococcus* spp, *Fusobacterium* spp, and *Bacteroides* spp), aerobic gram-positive bacteria, enteric and nonenteric gram-negative bacteria, and fungi (*Candida albicans, Torulopsis glabrata*).

2. **Diagnosis.** Chest pain may be a presenting symptom. Other manifestations include fever and other systemic signs, crepitus and edema of the head and neck, and sepsis. Widening of the mediastinum, pleural effusion, and subcutaneous or mediastinal emphysema may be evident on chest radiograph and chest CT.

3. **Treatment** must be initiated rapidly, in most cases with a combination of antibiotics and surgical intervention, including drainage, debridement, and removal or repair of the source of infection. In some situations, contained rupture or small perforations of the esophagus can be treated medically. Broad empiric antibiotic coverage should be used initially. Antibiotics should then be adjusted based on results of intraoperative cultures. Coverage for head and neck sources (including esophageal disruption) should include anaerobes, gram-positive aerobes, and gram-negative aerobes and facultative anaerobes. Combination therapy with penicillin G or clindamycin plus agents against gram-negative bacteria (e.g., a third generation cephalosporin or a fluoroquinolone) is effective. Metronidazole also provides adequate anaerobic coverage. Broadly active β-lactams (e.g., ticarcillin–clavulanate and imipenem–cilastatin) also are reasonable early coverage. Empiric coverage for postsurgical mediastinitis should include an antistaphylococcal agent such as nafcillin or vancomycin (for MRSA or for patients who are allergic to penicillin).

II. **Intraabdominal infections** usually arise from sources within the gastrointestinal (GI) tract. Infection can also result from contiguous spread from the urogenital or reproductive tract, from hematogenous or lymphatic spread; it can be introduced from the outside (as occurs with trauma). Infections are often polymicrobial and include enteric gram-negative rods (*E. coli, Klebsiella* spp, *Enterobacter* spp, and *Proteus* spp), *P. aeruginosa,* aerobic gram-positive cocci (*Enterococcus* spp and *Streptococcus* spp), and gram-positive and gram-negative anaerobes (*Clostridium* spp, *Bacteroides* spp, *Fusobacterium* spp, and *Peptostreptococcus* spp). Management of intraabdominal infection depends on the cause and the site(s).

A.   Microflora of abdomen and pelvis

   1.   Gastrointestinal tract. Normally, concentrations of bacteria increase progressively from the stomach through the small bowl and colon. Bacteria in the stomach and proximal small bowel include *Streptococcus* spp, *Lactobacillus* spp, and anaerobes such as *Peptostreptococcus* spp, but generally not *Bacteroides* spp. The concentration of enteric gram-negative bacilli (e.g., *E.coli*) and anaerobic gram-negatives (e.g., *Bacteroides* spp) increases progressively in the distal small bowel and colon. Colonic bacteria include enteric gram-negative rods, gram-positive aerobes (e.g., *Enterococcus* and *Lactobacillus*) and anaerobes (e.g., *Bacteroides* spp, *Clostridium* spp, and *Peptostreptococcus* spp). Many factors alter either the quantity or quality of the GI microflora, resulting in increases in the concentration as well as a shift in the spectrum of bacteria to include antibiotic-resistant bacteria, including nonenteric strains such as *P. aeruginosa*. Such factors include:

   a. pH (antacids, H_2 blockers).
   b. Antibiotics.
   c. GI dysmotility.
   d. Small bowel obstruction, ileus, regional enteritis.
   e. Bowel resection or intestinal bypass procedures.
   f. Hospitalization or residence in a chronic nursing facility prior to developing infection.

   2.   Genital tract microflora include gram-positive aerobic bacteria such as *Streptococcus, Lactobacillus,* and *Staphylococcus* spp, and anaerobic bacteria such as *Peptostreptococcus, Clostridium,* and *Bacteroides* spp.

B.   Specific intraabdominal infections

   1.   Peritonitis. Peritoneal infections can occur spontaneously; they can result from perforation of an abdominal viscus or can be introduced from the outside (as with trauma or the presence of foreign bodies such as peritoneal dialysis catheters).

   a.   Spontaneous bacterial peritonitis (SBP) occurs in susceptible individuals, such as those with ascites from chronic liver disease or congestive heart failure. It is believed to result from hematogenous or lymphatic spread or translocation of bacteria across the bowel wall. Generally, SBP is caused by a single organism (Chapter 24, section **IV.F.**). The presence of anaerobic bacteria or more than one organism should prompt an evaluation for secondary peritonitis.

b.   **Secondary peritonitis** usually results from perforation or necrosis of a solid viscus, or suppurative infections of the biliary and female reproductive tracts.

   (1)   **Diagnosis** can often be made with assistance of plain abdominal radiograph films and scans [e.g., CT, magnetic resonance (MR) imaging, ultrasonography]. Exploratory laparotomy may be necessary to diagnose and treat the source of peritonitis.

   (2)   **Treatment** requires identification and removal of the source of infection. Treatment usually involves a combination of surgery and broad-spectrum antibiotics that are active against gram-positive bacteria, gram-negative bacteria, and anaerobic bacteria.

   (a)   Peritonitis that occurs very early in the hospitalization and without recent antibiotic therapy is unlikely to result from antibiotic-resistant bacteria. Potential treatment regimens include:

   (i)   A second generation cephalosporin with antianaerobic properties such as cefoxitin or cefotetan (for milder infection).

   (ii)   A β-lactam/β-lactamase inhibitor such as ampicillin–sulbactam.

   (iii)   An antianaerobe (clindamycin or metronidazole) plus a third generation cephalosporin (ceftriaxone, cefotaxime, ceftizoxime).

   (iv)   An antianaerobe that provides coverage of aerobic gram-positive organisms (clindamycin) and fluoroquinolone.

   (v)   Aztreonam and clindamycin.

   (vi)   The traditional "triple antibiotic" regimen of ampicillin, gentamicin, and metronidazole.

   (b)   Peritonitis that develops during hospitalization or residence in a chronic nursing facility, or in the context of recent therapy with antibacterial agents may be caused by antibiotic-resistant microorganisms and should be treated with antibiotics that cover resistant bacteria.

(i) An antianaerobe plus third generation cephalosporin (ceftazidime if *Pseudomonas* spp are suspected). Consider adding a fluoroquinolone if infection with *Pseudomonas* spp or *Enterobacter* spp is suspected.

(ii) An antianaerobe with coverage of aerobic gram-positives (clindamycin) and a fluoroquinolone may be useful in patients allergic to β-lactams or if infection with *Pseudomonas* spp is suspected.

(iii) Carbapenem (imipenem–cilastatin or meropenem).

(iv) Vancomycin should be added to each of the above regimens if infection with MRSA is a possibility.

2. **Intraabdominal abscess** can result from persistence of bacteria after secondary peritonitis, or hematogenous spread of extraabdominal infection. Abscesses can cause fever, peritonitis, sepsis, and multiple-organ dysfunction syndrome.

a. **Microorganisms** commonly cultured from abscesses include *Bacteroides* spp (especially *B. fragilis*), gram-negative aerobic bacteria, facultative anaerobic bacteria, and gram-positive aerobic bacteria such as *Enterococcus* spp and *S. aureus.*

b. **Diagnosis.** CT is useful for diagnosing and localizing abscesses. Ultrasonography can be done at the bedside, and can be particularly useful in diagnosis of right upper quadrant, renal, and pelvic abscesses. Indium-labeled WBC and gallium scans are occasionally useful in localizing abscesses, but have low specificity and must be followed up with more definitive tests. Rarely, exploratory laparotomy must be performed for diagnosis.

c. **Treatment** of intraabdominal abscess includes drainage and antibiotics. The method of drainage (percutaneous under CT or ultrasound guidance versus operative) depends on a variety of factors, including the location of the abscess, whether the abscess is associated with perforation or gangrene, and the presence of loculations that make drainage with a single catheter unlikely. Often culture data are available to guide antibiotic selection. Empiric coverage should include agents active against gram-positive (including *Enterococcus* spp), gram-negative, and anaerobic bacteria. It is reasonable to use one of the combinations suggested above for treating secondary peritonitis in hospitalized patients. Ceftazidime may be favored over ceftriaxone because it has better activity against *P. aeruginosa*.

3. **Infections of the hepatobiliary system**
   a. **Acute cholecystitis** results from biliary tract obstruction or instrumentation of the biliary tract and involves the gall bladder and cystic duct. **Complications** include perforation of the gall bladder with subsequent peritonitis, empyema of the gall bladder caused by persistent cystic duct obstruction, and emphysematous cholecystitis. **Empyema of the gallbladder** can cause gram-negative sepsis; it increases the likelihood of perforation. **Emphysematous cholecystitis** occurs when acute calculous or acalculous cholecystitis is complicated by ischemia or gangrene and has high mortality.
      (1) **Microbiology.** Bacteria include enteric gram-negative bacteria such as *E. coli, Klebsiella* spp, *Proteus* spp, and *Enterobacter* spp, gram-positive bacteria such as *Enterococcus* spp, and anaerobic bacteria such as *Clostridium* spp and *Bacteroides* spp. Emphysematous cholecystitis is caused by *Clostridium* spp, gram-negative aerobic bacteria, and facultative anaerobic bacteria.
      (2) **Diagnosis.** Abdominal ultrasonography may reveal gallstones, thickening of the gallbladder wall, a dilated gall bladder, or a pericholecystic fluid collection.
      (3) **Treatment** includes antibiotics and surgery. The timing of surgery depends on a number of factors. Surgery is often performed on an urgent basis when the more severe complications of acute cholecystitis described above occur. Surgery can be delayed until the patient is stabilized or the patient with serious medical conditions is prepared. Cholecystitis can be treated with the antibiotic regimens described for secondary peritonitis.
   b. **Cholangitis** is usually caused by partial or complete common bile duct (CBD) obstruction.
      (1) **Diagnosis.** The classic presentation is jaundice, fevers, chills, and biliary colic. Blood cultures are often positive.
      (2) **Treatment** differs depending on whether the CBD obstruction is partial or com-

plete. **Nonsuppurative cholangitis,** which results from partial CBD obstruction, often responds to antibiotic therapy. **Suppurative cholangitis,** which results from complete CBD obstruction causing pus under pressure, bacteremia, and septic shock, must be treated as early as possible with a combination of antibiotics and surgical or endoscopic decompression. Cholangitis can be treated with the antibiotic regimens described for secondary peritonitis.

  c. **Liver abscess** results from local or hematogenous spread of infection. The most common local source is the biliary system. Abscesses can be solitary or multiple. Manifestations range from fever with leukocytosis and right upper quadrant pain, to sepsis.

  (1) **Microbiology.** The organisms involved vary, depending on the source of infection. Abscesses arising from the biliary tract often contain gram-negative bacteria and *Enterococcus* spp. Those arising from peritoneal infections often contain anaerobic bacteria, gram-positive bacteria, and gram-negative bacteria. Abscesses derived from hematogenous spread generally contain a single organism such as *S. aureus* or *Streptococcus* spp. Candidal abscesses also occur.

  (2) **Diagnosis** is generally made by CT scan or ultrasonography.

  (3) **Treatment** includes drainage and antibiotics. The choice of initial empiric antibiotics depends on the origin of the infection. Abscess arising from the biliary tract or peritoneum should be treated with antibiotics directed against the organisms involved in the initial infection. Abscess resulting from hematogenous spread should be treated with agents active against gram-positive aerobes.

4. **Splenic abscess** is rare, but has high mortality if left untreated. It usually results from hematogenous spread, but can result from splenic trauma or contiguous spread. The diagnosis of splenic abscess should prompt a search for **bacterial endocarditis** as the source.

  a. **Microbiology.** The most common organism isolated on culture is *Streptococcus* spp, followed by *S. aureus*. *Salmonella* spp and, rarely, anaerobic bacteria also cause splenic abscess.

  b. **Diagnosis** is suggested by left upper quadrant pain, fever, leukocytosis, and a left-sided pleural effusion.

    c. **Treatment.** Splenic abscess is usually treated with splenectomy and antibiotics.

5. **Pseudomembranous** or *Clostridium difficile* (*C. difficile*) colitis occurs as a complication of antibiotic therapy and is caused by overgrowth of *C. difficile,* which produces toxins that damage the bowel wall (Chapter 25). *C. difficile* is an anaerobic, gram-positive, spore-forming bacillus. The spores are heat resistant and can persist in the environment for months. The carrier rate is 3% in the general population and 20% in patients treated with antibiotics. Although clindamycin, cephalosporins, and ampicillin are the most frequent offenders, almost all antibiotics have been implicated, including vancomycin and metronidazole. Antibiotics alter the normal flora, providing an environment for the conversion of *C. difficile* spores to vegetative forms, which in turn results in rapid replication and toxin production. Epidemic outbreaks can occur because of environmental contamination, transmission by healthcare workers, and oral–fecal spread. Manifestations include watery or bloody diarrhea, abdominal cramps, toxic megacolon, bowel perforation, and peritonitis. Leukocytosis can be marked, sometimes in excess of 50,000 cells/μL.

    a. **Diagnosis.** Stool examination may reveal leukocytes, red blood cells, and *C. difficile* toxin. Stool cultures for *C. difficile* are not helpful, because *C. difficile* is usually present at low concentrations in the stool. Sigmoidoscopy with visualization of "pseudomembranes" can be helpful in making the diagnosis.

    b. **Treatment.** *C. difficile* colitis is treated with oral metronidazole or vancomycin and, if possible, with discontinuation of causative antibiotic(s). Unless contraindicated, therapy should begin with metronidazole to decrease the selection pressure for vancomycin-resistant gram-positive bacteria such as vancomycin-resistant *Enterococcus* (VRE). The efficacy of intravenous (IV) metronidazole for managing *C. difficile* colitis is controversial. Generally, treatment is continued for 10 days, although some practitioners favor continuing treatment until antibacterial agents are discontinued, or until three stool assays for *C. difficile* toxin are negative. However, repetitive testing for *C. difficile* toxin is costly. Suggested enteral doses are:

      (1) Metronidazole 250 mg orally every 6 hours, or 500 mg every 8 hours.

      (2) Vancomycin 125–500 mg orally every 6 hours.

III. Wound infections. Multiple factors influence the development and severity of wound infections. The incidence of postoperative wound infection from antibiotic-resistant bacteria increases with the length of hospitalization prior to surgery. Prophylactic measures are effective in preventing wound infections.

A. Classification of surgical wounds
1. **Clean.** No entry into internal organs that harbor bacteria.
2. **Clean-contaminated.** Organs are entered in elective surgery without spillage of contents.
3. **Contaminated.** Spillage of organ contents occurs without formation of pus.
4. **Dirty.** Spillage of contents occurs with pus formation.

B. Microbiology. Bacteria causing wound infections reflect the site of origin of the infection, and are altered by recent treatment with antibiotics, prolonged preoperative hospitalization, and coexisting diseases. **Clean surgical wound infections** are most often caused by *S. aureus,* coagulase-negative *Staphylococcus,* and *Streptococcus* spp. Severe wound infections that occur in the first 48 hours after surgery may be caused by *Clostridium* or group A streptococcus (*Strep.* pyogenes). Infections of **contaminated wounds** will reflect the origin of contamination [respiratory, GI, or genitourinary (GU) tract].

C. Clinical presentation and diagnosis. Wound infections vary in severity from superficial infections of the skin and subcutaneous tissues, to deep and severe infections involving the underlying fascia or muscles. Superficial wound infections are most frequently manifested by erythema, warmth, and edema. Fever is variably present.

D. Prevention. Detection and treatment of active infection at other sites, limiting the duration of hospitalization prior to surgery, proper surgical technique, and proper preoperative scrubbing of the patient and surgical team members are important measures. Whereas recommendations vary for clean procedures that do not involve placement of foreign material, **prophylactic antibiotics** are routinely administered for clean procedures involving placement of foreign material and for all procedures that enter or are complicated by spillage from internal organs. Prophylactic antibiotics should be given within the 30 minutes prior to incision, and for clean or clean-contaminated operations should be discontinued within 24 hours of surgery to minimize the risk of colonization with antibiotic-resistant organisms. Longer courses of antibiotics are generally given for contaminated or dirty wounds. Choices of prophylactic antibiotics are guided by site and type of surgery, duration of hospitalization prior to surgery, and recent use of antibiotics. Many institutions have established specific guidelines for prophylactic antibiotics.

E. **Treatment**
   1. **Mild superficial wound infections** can be treated with removal of sutures or staples and opening of the wound to drain fluid collections.
   2. **Severe wound infections,** particularly those causing systemic signs of infection, are treated with a combination of parenteral antibiotics and surgical debridement. Cultures of fluid or tissue collected in a sterile fashion should be used to guide antimicrobial therapy. Initial empiric antibiotic coverage is dictated by the setting. First generation cephalosporins are reasonable coverage for uncomplicated postoperative wound infections. Clindamycin is an alternative in patients allergic to β-lactams. Vancomycin should be reserved for cases wherein a reasonable likelihood is seen that the infection is caused by MRSA. Gram-negative coverage should be considered for infections originating in the GI, GU, and respiratory tracts.

F. **Necrotizing soft tissue infections. Necrotizing fasciitis** and **myonecrosis** (clostridial and nonclostridial) are life-threatening deep infections that involve the fascia and subcutaneous tissue (necrotizing fasciitis) and muscle (myonecrosis). These infections have the propensity to spread rapidly and cause severe systemic toxicity even early in the course of infection. The mortality from necrotizing soft tissue infections is high, particularly if delays occur in surgical or medical intervention.
   1. **Microbiology**
      a. **Necrotizing fasciitis.** *Streptococcus* spp are most commonly isolated from wound cultures. Polymicrobial infections with anaerobes, enteric gram-negative bacteria, and *Streptococcus* spp also occur.
      b. **Myonecrosis.** Clostridial myonecrosis (gas gangrene) is a severe, fulminant skeletal muscle infection caused by *Clostridium* spp. Exotoxins released by bacteria are important in the pathogenesis of clostridial myonecrosis. Nonclostridial myonecrosis is generally polymicrobial, caused by streptococci, enteric gram-negative rods (*E. coli, K. pneumoniae, Enterobacter* spp), and anaerobic bacteria.
   2. **Diagnosis.** Early features of necrotizing soft tissue infections are pain out of proportion to the local findings, and systemic toxicity. Gas gangrene is characterized by the presence of gas in soft tissues leading to crepitus.
   3. **Treatment**
      a. **Debridement.** Immediate recognition and prompt surgical exploration and debridement are crucial for all deep necrotizing infections. Frequent surveillance of the wound is essen-

tial; often, repeated surgical debridement is necessary.

b. **Antibiotics** are chosen based on the presentation and the likely source of infection. Gram's stain of intraoperative wound samples can guide initial therapy. Empiric therapy should be broad, and include coverage of *Streptococcus* and *Staphylococcus* spp, enteric gram-negative bacteria, and anaerobes.

c. The role of **hyperbaric oxygen** for necrotizing soft tissue infections caused by anaerobic bacteria is not yet clear; some experts advocate hyperbaric oxygen therapy, especially for *Clostridium* infections, if available.

IV. **Urinary tract infections.** The range of severity of urinary tract infections (UTIs) varies from urethritis and cystitis, which are often treated in the outpatient setting, to pyelonephritis, renal or perinephric abscess, which can produce septic shock. Predisposing factors include indwelling urinary catheters, neurologic or structural abnormalities of the urinary tract, and nephrolithiasis. Urinary tract infections are the most common nosocomial infection, causing up to 30% of gram-negative bacteremias in hospitalized patients.

A. **Microbiology.** Because bacteria usually enter the urinary tract via the urethra, and then spread to more proximal segments, the same microorganisms tend to cause both upper and lower UTIs. Occasionally, hematogenous seeding (especially with *S. aureus*) or spread from contiguous peritoneal infection can result in upper UTIs (especially perinephric and renal abscesses). The most common organisms cultured from the urine are gram-negative rods, including *E. coli, Klebsiella* spp, *Proteus* spp, and sometimes *Enterobacter* spp. *Serratia* spp and *Pseudomonas* spp are additional causes of catheter-related infections. Gram-positive organisms, including *S. saprophyticus, Enterococcus* spp, and *S. aureus,* sometimes are involved. Urethritis can also be caused by *Chlamydia trachomatis, Neisseria gonorrhoeae, Trichomonas, Candida* spp, and herpes simplex virus (HSV). Fungal infections of the urinary tract are discussed in section **VIII.**

B. **Diagnosis.** Distinguishing colonization from infection can be difficult. Asymptomatic bacteriuria is present in up to 50% of elderly men and women. Analysis of the urinary sediment for leukocytes in conjunction with urine cultures can be useful in determining whether a true infection is present, and whether the infection is in the upper or lower urinary tract. White blood cell casts in the urinary sediment suggest that infection involves the kidneys or tubules. Urine cultures are essential to guide antimicrobial therapy.

C. **Specific UTIs**

1. **Cystitis** is infection of the urinary bladder characterized by dysuria and frequency, cloudy or bloody urine, and localized tenderness of the urethra and suprapubic regions. More severe symptoms such as high fever, nausea, and vomiting suggest renal involvement.

2. **Acute pyelonephritis** is a pyogenic infection of the renal parenchyma and pelvis. It is characterized by costophrenic angle tenderness, high fevers, shaking chills, nausea, vomiting, and diarrhea. Laboratory analysis reveals leukocytosis, pyuria with leukocyte casts, occasional hematuria, and bacteria that are often visible on Gram's stain of unspun urine. Evaluation of the urinary tract should be considered, because a significant proportion of pyelonephritis is associated with structural abnormalities resulting in stasis or obstruction to urinary flow. Treatment includes antibiotics and removal or correction of the source of infection. Complications of pyelonephritis include papillary necrosis, impaired urine concentrating ability, urinary obstruction, and sepsis.

3. **Renal and perinephric abscesses** are uncommon; they usually are caused by ascending infection from the bladder and ureters. Major risk factors include nephrolithiasis, structural urinary tract abnormalities, urologic trauma or surgery, and diabetes mellitus. Most common bacteria are *E. coli, Klebsiella* spp, and *Proteus* spp. *Candida* spp rarely may cause renal and perinephric abscesses. Renal and perinephric abscesses may present nonspecifically with fever, leukocytosis, and pain (flank, groin, abdomen). Urine cultures may be negative, particularly if the patient has already received antibiotics for a UTI. Diagnosis can be made by abdominal ultrasound or CT scan. Treatment is drainage and antibiotics.

4. **Prostatitis** is an infrequent infection that can occur as a result of bladder catheterization of patients in the ICU. Symptoms and signs include fevers, chills, dysuria, and an enlarged, tender, and boggy prostate. Treatment includes antibiotics and, if possible, removal of the urinary catheter.

D. **Treatment of UTIs.** Antibiotic choices depend on the source and severity of infection, and the microbiology. Prior to receiving culture results, empiric broad therapy should be initiated to cover likely organisms. Fluoroquinolones or third generation cephalosporins are often used. Ceftazidime may be selected if infection with *Pseudomonas* spp is likely. If *Enterococcus* spp is suspected, broader coverage can be obtained with ampicillin plus an aminoglycoside. Rarely, imipenem–cilastatin may be used for infections caused by antibiotic-resistant bacteria.

V. **Intravascular catheter-related infections** can be localized to the site of insertion (site infections) or can be disseminated (catheter-related bacteremia). Catheters in the central circulation (central venous and pulmonary artery) are responsible for most catheter-related infections. Peripheral venous and arterial catheters rarely cause significant catheter-related infections. The most common pathogen is coagulase-negative *Staphylococcus,* followed by *S. aureus,* although a variety of gram-negative and gram-positive organisms and fungi can cause catheter-related infections. Fever is the most common presenting feature and localized signs of infection at the insertion site often are absent. Site infections or unexplained fever should prompt assessment for line infection.

A. **Risk factors and prevention.** The likelihood of infection is increased by prolonged catheterization. Although no demonstrable benefit is seen for routine replacement of catheters, some practitioners still empirically change central lines after approximately 1 week. Important preventive measures include strict sterile technique during placement and care of catheters, and routine dressing changes. Catheter-related infections, particularly fungal infections, are more frequent in patients receiving total parenteral nutrition. Catheter-related infections can be more frequent with multiple-lumen as opposed to single-lumen catheters. Antibiotic-bonded catheters are associated with fewer infections.

B. **Management**

   1. **Catheter removal.** Institutional guidelines for the management of suspected catheter-related infections vary. At some institutions, catheters suspected of being infected are changed over a guidewire and quantitatively cultured. If the blood or quantitative tip cultures are positive, then the catheter is changed to a new site. A strong suspicion that the catheter is the source of fever or septic complications, however, should prompt a change in site and, at minimum, blood cultures.

   2. **Antibiotics.** Use of antibiotics (agent and duration) is dictated by the clinical situation and culture data. Empiric therapy often is started with vancomycin if systemic signs of infection are present or if preliminary blood culture results indicate gram-positive bacteremia. Often an additional agent is added to cover gram-negative bacteria or for synergistic coverage of *Enterococcus* spp. Further therapy should be tailored to the specific organism identified. For uncomplicated catheter-related bacteremia, antibiotics are generally continued for 7 to 14 days (14 days if *S.aureus* is isolated from the blood). Fungal infections are treated longer, particularly in immunocompromised hosts.

VI. **Infective endocarditis (IE)**

A. **Infective endocarditis** is caused by microbial invasion of the endocardium. IE most commonly involves the cardiac valves, but can also occur in the septal or mural myocardium. IE can involve native valves [**native valve endocarditis (NVE)**] and prosthetic valves [**prosthetic valve endocarditis (PVE)**]. PVE occurring within 2 months of valve replacement (early PVE) results from colonization of the valve by microbes at the time of surgery, and most commonly is caused by *Staphylococcus* spp. Late PVE is similar to NVE.

B. **Microorganisms gain entry** into the bloodstream via direct inoculation during procedures (GI, GU, and dental procedures, bronchoscopy, endotracheal intubation), or from a focus of existing infection such as pneumonia or dental abscess. **Acute IE** is characterized by abrupt onset and rapid progression. **Subacute IE** is characterized by insidious onset and slower progression. Predisposing factors for IE include abnormalities of the heart (such as those caused by rheumatic heart disease and degenerative valvular lesions) and IV drug abuse. Endocarditis also occurs in previously normal hearts. Intravascular devices such as central venous catheters, pacemaker wires, hemodialysis shunts, and prosthetic valves increase the chance of developing infective endocarditis.

C. **Physical examination** may reveal a heart murmur, petechiae, nail-bed splinter hemorrhages, retinal hemorrhages (Roth's spots), red or purple nodules on digital pads (Osler's nodes), and flat red lesions on the palms or soles (Janeway lesions).

D. **Microbiology.** IE is most commonly caused by bacteria but can also be caused by fungi, viruses, and Rickettsiae.

1. **Gram-positive bacteria** cause acute and subacute IE. *Streptococcus* spp are the most common pathogens, particularly the viridans group (such as *Strep. sanguis, Strep. mutants,* and *Strep. intermedius*). *Enterococcus* spp also cause endocarditis, particularly in elderly patients who have undergone GU procedures, and in IV drug abusers. *Staphylococcus* spp, particularly *S. aureus,* often cause infective endocarditis. *S. aureus* endocarditis often is severe and more commonly is complicated by myocardial and valve ring abscesses, emboli, and metastatic lesions [e.g., lung, central nervous system (CNS), and splenic abscess]. Endocarditis caused by *Strep. bovis* is often the result of a GI lesion such as colon cancer; identification of this bacteria should prompt a workup for a GI source.

2. **Gram-negative bacteria** infrequently cause infective endocarditis, but IV drug abusers and patients with prosthetic valves are more susceptible. Manifestations generally are severe with abrupt onset and high mortality. A characteristic NVE of abnormal valves is caused by a group of gram-negative bacteria, collectively called HACEK

group bacteria (**H**aemophilus spp, **A**ctinobaccillus actinomycetemcomitans, **C**ardiobacterium hominis, **E**ikenella corrodens, and **K**ingella spp), and is characterized by a subacute course, large vegetations, and frequent embolic events.

E. **Diagnosis**

1. **Blood cultures** are moderately sensitive for IE. Several (three or more) sets of blood cultures should be obtained within the first 24 hours in patients suspected of having IE. Rarely, blood cultures can be negative, particularly when IE is caused by intracellular organisms such as Rickettsiae, anaerobic bacteria, the HACEK group of bacteria, and fungi. Special media may be necessary to isolate the responsible microorganism.

2. **Echocardiography** is an important tool for diagnosing and managing IE. Transthoracic echocardiography (TTE) is far less sensitive than transesophageal echocardiography (TEE) for detecting vegetations, particularly in patients receiving mechanical ventilation. In addition to detection of vegetations, echocardiography can be used to follow both the progression of known vegetations and the complications such as valvular insufficiency, valve ring or myocardial abscesses, pericardial effusions, and heart failure.

F. **Treatment** of IE involves prolonged administration of antibiotics and sometimes surgery.

1. **Antibiotics.** Prolonged courses of bactericidal antibiotics are used for the treatment of IE because host defenses are inadequate at assisting with sterilization. For acute bacterial endocarditis, it may be necessary to begin antibiotics prior to definitive diagnosis. Blood cultures, however, should be obtained prior to the first dose of antibiotics. Empiric therapy should be started in (a) critically ill patients in whom is seen a strong suggestion of endocarditis, (b) patients likely to have endocarditis who are to undergo cardiac surgery, (c) patients with positive blood cultures, (d) when the diagnosis seems certain (such as vegetations documented by echocardiography in the setting of fever and other clinical parameters consistent with IE), and (e) patients suspected of having PVE. Sometimes treatment of subacute NVE is delayed until results of blood cultures are available. **Prolonged antibiotic therapy** should be based on results of blood cultures and sensitivity data. Determinations of minimal inhibitory and bactericidal concentrations are extremely important in deciding the optimal regimen. Blood cultures should be obtained during therapy to assess clearance. Failure to clear bacteremia may indicate abscess.

a. **Empiric initial therapy for acute NVE** should include agents that are active against *Streptococcus* spp, *Enterococcus* spp, and *Staphylococcus* spp. Potential regimens:

   (1) Ampicillin or penicillin plus nafcillin plus aminoglycoside (gentamicin).

   (2) Vancomycin plus aminoglycoside (gentamicin). Enterococcal infection should be treated with a combination of ampicillin or vancomycin plus an aminoglycoside, because ampicillin and vancomycin are only bacteriostatic for *Enterococcus* spp.

b. **Empiric initial therapy for early or late PVE:**

   (1) Vancomycin plus aminoglycoside (gentamicin) plus rifampin.

2. **Surgery.** Valve replacement or valvulectomy (tricuspid) can be an essential aspect in the management of IE. Indications for surgery, which vary depending on the valve infected, include severe and refractory heart failure, valve obstruction, fungal endocarditis, prosthetic valve instability, and failure to clear bacteremia with appropriate antibiotic therapy. Surgery also may be indicated for recurrent IE, extension to the myocardium or paravalvular region, two or more embolic events, or periprosthetic leaks.

G. **Complications**

   1. **Cardiac**

      a. **Valvular insufficiency** and **heart failure** result from inflammatory damage to the valve. The most common cause of death in patients with IE is heart failure.

      b. **Myocardial and paravalvular abscess.**

      c. **Heart block** can result from extension of a paravalvular abscess.

      d. **Obstruction.** Rarely, large vegetations can cause obstruction, particularly when IE is caused by fungi.

      e. **Purulent pericarditis** occurs most commonly with endocarditis caused by *Staphylococcus* spp.

   2. **Extracardiac**

      a. **Immune complex disease** can damage distant organs such as the kidneys.

      b. **Embolic events** can lead to ischemia and infarction. Abscesses can occur at sites of embolization. Left-sided endocarditis predisposes to emboli to the kidneys, brain, spleen, and heart, whereas right-sided endocarditis predisposes to pulmonary emboli. The site of embolization will determine manifestations.

      c. **Mycotic aneurysms,** which result from local infection of the blood vessel with dilation of the vessel, generally are diagnosed following subarachnoid or intracerebral hemorrhage.

d. **Neurologic complications** include toxic encephalopathy, meningitis, cerebritis, brain abscess, and stroke (infarction or hemorrhage).

e. **Renal failure.**

f. **Sepsis.**

VII. **Miscellaneous infections**

A. **Sinusitis.** Facial trauma and the presence of nasotracheal or nasogastric tubes predispose patients in the ICU to sinusitis.

1. **Microbiology.** Sinusitis is usually caused by gram-negative bacteria, *S. aureus,* and anaerobes.

2. **Diagnosis** can be difficult. Many experts recommend CT scans of the face and sinuses. Needle aspiration of the sinuses may provide helpful bacteriologic data, particularly in patients who have been hospitalized for prolonged periods and may be infected with antibiotic-resistant organisms.

3. **Treatment** is often initiated based on the clinical constellation of fever of unclear cause, presence of nasal tubes or history of head and neck trauma, and purulent nasal discharge. Treatment includes removal of nasal tubes to allow drainage of the obstructed sinus outflow tract, nasal humidification and decongestants, and antibiotics that target likely pathogens. Surgical drainage is rarely indicated.

B. **Central nervous system infections**

1. **Meningitis.** Generally, infection is limited to the subarachnoid space and cerebral ventricles and does not involve the brain parenchyma, but occasionally meningitis is complicated by brain abscess. Bacterial meningitis can result from hematogenous seeding, direct invasion from trauma or surgery, or extension of infection from a contiguous structure such as rupture of a brain or epidural abscess into the subarachnoid space.

a. **Microbiology.** Many organisms cause meningitis. Community-acquired pathogens include *Strep. pneumoniae, H. influenzae, N. meningitidis,* and *L. monocytogenes.* Meningitis caused by enteric and nonenteric gram-negative bacteria and *S. aureus* can result from trauma, neurosurgery, or bacteremia. *Staphylococcus aureus* meningitis can originate from infections (e.g., pneumonia, sinusitis, and endocarditis) at other sites. Meningitis associated with cerebrospinal fluid (CSF) shunts are most often caused by *S. epidermidis.*

b. **Diagnosis.** Collection of CSF for analysis of glucose, protein, cell count and differential, Gram's stain, and bacterial culture is essential. Other specialized tests of CSF, including cryptococcal antigen, VDRL, bacterial antigen tests, and fungal smear and culture may be indicated depending on other patient factors such as immunocompromise. In patients suspected of having cerebral edema, a CT scan of the brain should be done prior to the lumbar puncture. Blood cultures should be obtained before starting antibiotics.

c. **Treatment.** The choice of antibiotics will be determined by the clinical situation and the ability of various antibiotics to penetrate the CNS. Because host defenses are impaired in the CNS, bacterial meningitis must be treated with bactericidal antibiotics. Emergence of penicillin-resistant community-acquired pathogens has resulted in a shift in treatment to third generation non-antipseudomonal cephalosporins (e.g., ceftriaxone), which penetrate the CNS well. Vancomycin is often added if concern exists about resistance to β-lactam antibiotics. *Listeria monocytogenes* meningitis should be treated with penicillin G or ampicillin, or with trimethoprim–sulfamethoxazole in penicillin-allergic patients, possibly in conjunction with an aminoglycoside. Meningitis caused by gram-negative bacteria is frequently treated with a third generation cephalosporin. If *P. aeruginosa* is suspected, ceftazidime should be used. *S. aureus* meningitis is usually treated with nafcillin or vancomycin in penicillin-allergic patients or if MRSA is the pathogen.

2. **Paradural abscesses include epidural and subdural abscesses.** Epidural abscesses most frequently occur in the vertebral column, whereas subdural abscesses usually occur in the cranium. Paradural abscesses result from trauma, neurosurgery, invasion of the paradural space (such as with epidural catheter placement), local spread from contiguous structures (e.g., the paranasal sinuses or paravertebral region), and hematogenous spread from distant sites. Paradural abscess can rapidly progress and can cause considerable irreversible damage to underlying neural structures. Thus, rapid diagnosis and institution of therapy is essential. Drainage of the abscess is crucial for microbiologic diagnosis as well as for treatment.

   a. **Microbiology.** Bacteria causing subdural abscesses reflect the source of infection. Infections can be caused by *Strep. pneumoniae,* *Staphylococcus* spp, *H. influenzae,* enteric gram-negative bacteria, and anaerobes. *S. aureus* is the most common cause of epidural abscess. Enteric gram-negative bacteria also cause epidural abscesses, particularly in patients with UTIs, or following vertebral surgery.

   b. Diagnosis. Severe localized spinal pain is the most common presenting symptom of epidural abscess. CT scans are helpful in diagnosing and localizing subdural abscesses. Magnetic resonance imaging is the diagnostic test of choice for epidural abscesses. CT and myelography also can be helpful.

   c. Treatment includes antibiotics and drainage. Initial antibiotic therapy should be based on likely pathogens for the situation and then modified based on results of cultures. *S. aureus* should be treated with nafcillin. Vancomycin can be substituted in penicillin-allergic patients or if MRSA is the pathogen. Third generation cephalosporins (antipseudomonal if *P. aeruginosa* is the pathogen) are often used for gram-negative infections.

VIII. Fungal infections. Fungi act as opportunistic or, less commonly, as virulent pathogens, causing a variety of different syndromes ranging from superficial mucocutaneous infection to systemic infection with visceral organ involvement.

   A. *Candida*

   1. ***Candida*** spp are the most common cause of opportunistic fungal infections occurring in surgical and medical ICUs. The incidence of nosocomial candidal infections has increased dramatically in the last 10 years, and *Candida* species are now the fourth most common organisms isolated from blood cultures.

   2. **Risk factors** include treatment with broad-spectrum antibiotics, presence of indwelling devices (urinary, peritoneal, and intravascular), immunocompromise [human immunodeficiency virus (HIV), transplantation, hematologic malignancy, chemotherapy, neutropenia, and burns], and total parenteral nutrition.

   3. **Clinical manifestations**

      a. Candiduria can be caused by infection or it can reflect colonization of an indwelling urinary catheter. Candiduria should raise concerns about possible fungal balls, pyelonephritis, or candidemia.

      b. Mucocutaneous infections include oropharyngeal candidiasis, esophagitis, GI candidiasis, vulvovaginitis, and intertrigo.

      c. Candidemia is characterized by positive blood cultures, and can be associated with dissemination to visceral organs. The mortality is very high, especially with *T. glabrata*. Patients with positive blood cultures should be evaluated closely for indwelling vascular line and/or deep organ infections. Quantitative cultures of catheter tips can be performed. Growth of $\geq$ 15 colony-forming units from the catheter tip of the same isolate as cultured from the blood is indicative of a catheter-related candidal infection.

d. **Disseminated or invasive candidiasis.** Deep organ infections can result from hematogenous spread, by direct extension from contiguous sites, or by local inoculation. Diagnosis can be difficult, since blood cultures are frequently negative. Positive superficial cultures (e.g., urine, sputum, and wounds) may represent colonization or contamination, and diagnostic serologic tests are not available. A high level of suspicion must be maintained in patients with the risk factors described above. Definitive criteria for disseminated infection include positive cultures from the infected tissue or peritoneal fluid, actual invasion (histologically) of burn wounds, and endophthalmitis. Suggestive criteria include two positive blood cultures at least 24 hours apart, with one positive culture drawn at least 24 hours after the removal of vascular cannulae, and (in the right population) three or more colonized sites.

(1) **Hepatosplenic candidiasis** is most common in patients with hematologic malignancy. The diagnosis is suggested by right upper quadrant pain, persistent fevers, elevated alkaline phosphatase, and multiple "bull's eye" lesions on abdominal ultrasonography or CT scan, although the liver may also appear homogeneous in these studies. Diagnosis can be confirmed by histologic analysis of a liver biopsy.

(2) **Candidal peritonitis** results from perforation of the intestines or stomach, or infection of a peritoneal dialysis catheter.

(3) **Cardiac candidiasis** includes myocarditis, pericarditis, and endocarditis. Valvular vegetations can be large, and major embolic events are common and devastating.

(4) **Renal candidiasis** results from ascending infection from the bladder, resulting in fungus balls and papillary necrosis, or from hematogenous spread resulting in pyelonephritis and abscess formation.

(5) **Ocular candidiasis** can cause blindness.

(6) **Other sites of disseminated candidiasis** include the CNS and musculoskeletal system.

4. **Treatment of candidal infections.** Few controlled trials have been done to define the best therapeutic modalities. Antifungal therapy should be tailored to available culture data, with particular attention to the presence of fluconazole-resistant organisms.

   a. **Candiduria** can be treated with amphotericin or nystatin bladder irrigation, or oral fluconazole. The choice should be guided by the organism identified (*Torulopsis* is often resistant to fluconazole), as well as the likelihood of renal involvement. Because urinary catheters often have a thick fungal sediment attached, replacement of indwelling urinary catheters is also recommended.

   b. **Mucocutaneous candidiasis** is initially treated with topical agents such as nystatin, mycostatin, chlotrimazole, or ketoconazole. Systemic therapy with oral fluconazole may be indicated when patients do not respond to topical therapy.

   c. **Candidemia** is treated with systemic antifungal therapy. Venous and arterial catheters should be replaced at new sites, and catheter tips should be cultured. Tunneled central venous lines are often left in place unless there is failure to clear the fungemia with antibiotics. The decision to treat with amphotericin B or fluconazole is based on the patient's overall clinical status. Amphotericin B is the treatment of choice in unstable patients.

   d. **Disseminated candidiasis** requires a combination of systemic antifungal therapy, drainage or debridement of infected areas, removal of intravascular catheters, and sometimes removal of infected valves and other foreign bodies. Although a general consensus exists that *Candida* spp grown from the peritoneal cavity (i.e., not just peritoneal drains) should be treated, opinions differ with respect to whether amphotericin B or fluconazole should be used and whether the toxic agent 5-fluorocytosine should be added for synergy. The same is true for hepatosplenic candidiasis. Lack of response to fluconazole is an indication to change to amphotericin B. Severe endophthalmitis is treated with amphotericin B.

B. **Aspergillus** is a cause of invasive opportunistic infection in immunocompromised patients in the ICU. Distinguishing colonization from infection can be difficult. Diagnosis of infection is based on serologic data, tissue histology, and culture results. Positive sputum cultures do not necessarily indicate disease and negative cultures do not rule out disease. Thus, it is helpful, although not always clinically feasible, to get pulmonary tissue for analysis.

1. **Clinical manifestations** range from localized pulmonary disease to disseminated disease.
   a. **Invasive pulmonary disease** occurs in immunocompromised patients, and presents with fever and pulmonary infiltrates. Pathologic analysis reveals infarction and hemorrhage. Pulmonary thrombosis can occur when the organisms invade vessel walls. Diagnosis is made by direct analysis of pulmonary tissue. Many patients with locally invasive disease also have disseminated disease.
   b. **Dissemination** to a variety of organs occurs because of vascular invasion. Abscesses occur in the CNS, lung, liver, and myocardium. Budd-Chiari syndrome and myocardial infarctions can occur.
   c. **Other pulmonary manifestations**
      (1) **Aspergillomas** are fungus balls that occur in cavities in the upper lobes of the lungs, especially in bullae and occasionally in old tuberculous cavities. Patients present with cough, hemoptysis (which can be life threatening), fever, and dyspnea.
      (2) **Allergic bronchopulmonary aspergillosis** causes episodic asthmatic symptoms, and usually occurs in patients with chronic asthma or cystic fibrosis. Radiographic findings range from segmental infiltrates to transient nonsegmental infiltrates. Eosinophilia is present in the sputum and blood.
2. **Treatment of aspergillosis**
   a. **Disseminated disease** and **invasive pulmonary disease** are treated with IV amphotericin B. Surgical resection may be indicated when systemic antifungal therapy has failed. Itraconazole can be used as a second-line agent for disseminated disease when the patient has failed or is intolerant to amphotericin B.
   b. **Localized pulmonary manifestations**
      (1) **Aspergilloma.** Surgery is indicated in patients with recurrent hemoptysis. A role may also be seen for corticosteroid treatment. Systemic amphotericin B does not improve outcome compared with supportive measures.
      (2) **Allergic bronchopulmonary aspergillosis** is treated with systemic corticosteroids (aerosolized steroids are not of benefit), and sometimes aerosolized antifungals. The benefits of long-term corticosteroid therapy have not been proved.

IX.   Viral infections
- **A.   Cytomegalovirus (CMV)** is an important cause of infection in immunocompromised patients. It is the most common cause of infection in solid organ and bone marrow transplant recipients. Primary infection occurs in seronegative individuals, whereas secondary infection occurs in cases of activation of latent infection or reinfection of a seropositive host. Primary infection in immunocompetent hosts is often asymptomatic, although rarely severe disease occurs. Diagnosis of CMV infection requires detection of viral components or an increase in antibodies directed to CMV.
  - **1.   Manifestations of CMV in immunocompromised patients.**
    - **a.   Self-limited febrile illness** is common.
    - **b.   Interstitial pneumonitis.** CMV pneumonitis resulting in respiratory failure requiring mechanical ventilation has a high mortality rate.
    - **c.   CMV hepatitis** is usually mild, but can be severe, particularly in liver transplant patients.
    - **d.   GI.** Diarrhea, GI bleeding.
    - **e.   Retinitis.**
  - **2.   Treatment.** CMV infection is very difficult to treat and infection recurs rapidly after cessation of antiviral agents. **Ganciclovir** and **foscarnet** are both used to treat CMV retinitis in patients with acquired immune deficiency syndrome (AIDS). Ganciclovir is also given for CMV infection in organ transplant recipients. Foscarnet is used in patients with CMV who are intolerant of ganciclovir. Severe CMV disease is sometimes treated with a combination of CMV immunoglobulin and ganciclovir. Administration of hyperimmune globulin to bone marrow transplant recipients with pneumonitis has resulted in improved outcome.
- **B.   Herpes simplex virus (HSV) I and II**
  - **1.   Manifestations** of HSV infection include:
    - **a.   Mucocutaneous** and **genital** disease.
    - **b.   Respiratory tract infection.**
      - **(1)**   Tracheobronchitis.
      - **(2)**   HSV pneumonia generally occurs in debilitated or immunocompromised patients.
    - **c.   Ocular infection** such as blepharitis, conjunctivitis, keratitis, corneal ulceration, and blindness.
    - **d.   Esophagitis.**
    - **e.   Encephalitis, meningitis.**
  - **2.   Disseminated HSV** usually occurs in patients who are extremely debilitated or immunocompromised, but occasionally occurs during pregnancy. Manifestations include necrotizing hepatitis, pneumonitis, cutaneous lesions from hematoge-

nous spread, fever, hypotension, disseminated intravascular coagulation, and CNS involvement.
3. **Diagnosis.** Wright's, Giemsa's stain (Tzanck smear), or Papanicolaou's stain of material scraped from lesions can be helpful, but are insensitive and do not distinguish between HSV and varicella zoster virus (VZV) infection. Viral culture, histologic examination of tissue or skin biopsy, and DNA or protein staining of viral antigens are other diagnostic tests. Brain biopsy may be necessary for diagnosis of HSV encephalitis.
4. **Treatment**
    a. **Severe HSV infections,** including CNS infections, pneumonitis, and disseminated HSV are treated with IV **acyclovir. Vidarabine,** an alternative therapy, is more toxic, and may be less effective than acyclovir.
    b. **Mucosal, cutaneous,** and **genital infections** can be treated with **acyclovir, famciclovir,** or **valacyclovir.** Although normal hosts do not always require treatment, consideration should be given to treating critically ill or debilitated patients even if they do not fit classic criteria for immunocompromise.
    c. **Ocular infection** can be treated with topical agents such as acyclovir, and should be managed in consultation with an ophthalmologist.
C. **Varicella Zoster virus** infection may be encountered in the ICU as a primary infection (chicken pox) or reactivation infection (herpes zoster or shingles); it can cause mild to life-threatening disease.
    1. **Primary VZV** infection in adults can have severe systemic effects and pulmonary involvement that results in respiratory failure. Immunocompromised patients are susceptible to severe systemic disease with involvement of lungs, kidneys, CNS, and liver.
    2. **Herpes zoster** usually manifests as a dermatomal cutaneous infection from reactivation of VZV that has been dormant in the sensory ganglia. Rarely, reactivated herpes zoster causes CNS disease such as encephalitis and cerebral vasculitis.
    3. **Treatment. Intravenous acyclovir** is used for serious VZV infection (i.e.: pneumonia, encephalitis) in immunocompromised or immunocompetent hosts.

SELECTED REFERENCES

American Thoracic Society (consensus statement). Hospital-acquired pneumonia in adults: diagnosis, assessment of severity, initial antimicrobial therapy, and preventative strategies. *Am J Respir Crit Care Med* 1995;153:1711–1725.

Chapnick EK, Abter EI. Necrotizing soft-tissue infections. *Infect Dis Clin North Am* 1996;10:835–855.

Cunha BA. Intravenous line infections. *Crit Care Clin* 1998;14:339–346.

Cunha BA. Severe community-acquired pneumonia. *Crit Care Clin* 1998;14:105–118.

Edwards Jr JE, Bodey GP, Bowden RA, et al. International conference for the development of a consensus on the management and prevention of severe Candidal infections. *Clin Infect Dis* 1997; 25:43–59.

Keys TF. Diagnosis and management of infective endocarditis. *Cleve Clin J Med* 1990;57:558–562.

McClean KL, Sheehan GJ, Harding GKM. Intraabdominal infection: a review. *Clin Infect Dis* 1994;19:100–116.

Nichols RL. Surgical infections: prevention and treatment—1965 to 1995. *Am J Surg* 1996;172:68–74.

Paradisi F, Corti G, Mangani V. Urosepsis in the critical care unit. *Crit Care Clin* 1998;14:165–180.

Richardson JD, Carrillo E. Thoracic infection after trauma. *Chest Surg Clin of N Am* 1997;7:401–427.

The Sanford guide to antimicrobial therapy. Vienna, Virginia: Antimicrobial Therapy, Inc., 1998.

Shands Jr JW. Empiric antibiotic therapy of abdominal sepsis and serious perioperative infections. *Surg Clin North Am* 1993;73:291–306.

Acute Cerebral Injuries

Alan Z. Segal, Jonathan Rosand, and
Lee H. Schwamm

I. **Stroke** is the acute onset of a focal neurologic deficit or disturbance in the level of arousal. It can be caused by ischemia, hemorrhage, or cerebral venous occlusion. Therapy is aimed at restoring cerebral blood flow and preventing secondary brain injury.

    A. **Acute ischemic stroke** is caused by acute vascular occlusion. In a **transient ischemic attack (TIA),** the reduction in cerebral blood flow is temporary and full function is restored within minutes to hours. The transition from reversible to irreversible injury is a function of duration and depth of ischemia. Symptoms often include sudden onset of visual loss, weakness or numbness on one side of the body, ataxia or unexplained falling, or aphasia. **Thrombosis-in-situ** can occur in diseased segments of small penetrating vessels (i.e., lacunar stroke) or larger arteries (e.g., atherosclerotic stenosis, arterial dissection), and **emboli** may be liberated from proximal sites (e.g., heart, aorta, carotid) to lodge in normal major cerebral arteries or their distal branches.

        1. **Lacunar strokes** tend to occur in patients with diabetes and chronic hypertension. They can be clinically silent or present as pure motor hemiparesis, pure sensory loss, or a variety of well-defined syndromes (e.g., dysarthria-clumsy hand, ataxic-hemiparesis). Descending, compact white matter tracts or brainstem gray matter nuclei are injured, often producing widespread and striking initial deficits. The prognosis for recovery with lacunar stroke is better than with a large artery territory stroke. For this reason, many centers favor using antiplatelet therapy (e.g., aspirin, clopidogrel) or conservative management rather than thrombolytic therapy for uncomplicated lacunar stroke. The risk of hemorrhagic transformation or edema in these patients is extremely low. Because the initial clinical presentation can be deceiving, particularly when involving the posterior circulation, all patients presenting with acute ischemic symptoms should undergo some form of neurovascular imaging to establish large vessel patency [e.g., computed tomographic (CT) angiography, magnetic resonance (MR) angiography, ultrasound, or conventional contrast angiography].

        2. **Large artery occlusion** is divided into disorders of the anterior (internal carotid artery and

branches) and posterior (vertebrobasilar arteries and branches) circulation. These strokes carry the risk of edema and hemorrhagic conversion.

a.   **Middle cerebral artery (MCA) occlusion** is characterized by weakness of the contralateral face, arm, and leg with hemianopia and a preference of the eyes and head toward the side of the involved hemisphere. Additional findings include aphasia in dominant hemisphere injury, and hemineglect (patient "ignores" the left side of the body, the surroundings, or the presence of the deficit itself) in nondominant hemisphere injury. Involvement restricted to branches of the MCA can produce fragments of this syndrome, often with sparing of leg strength.

b.   **Anterior cerebral artery (ACA) occlusion,** which is much rarer, causes isolated weakness of the lower limb. If both ACAs are affected, a generalized decrease in initiative (abulia) can occur. **Border zone** or watershed infarction is the result of insufficient blood flow to distal territories of the major cerebral vessels. This develops most commonly in the setting of severe, sustained hypotension (e.g., cardiac arrest) or in the presence of severe atherosclerotic narrowing of the carotid arteries. Because the cerebral circulation is formed by end arteries, hypotension produces ischemia and infarction in the tissues supplied by the most distal branches of these arteries. The classic presentation is proximal arm or leg weakness with preservation of distal strength, the so-called "man in a barrel."

c.   **Posterior circulation infarction** involves the brainstem, cerebellum, thalamus, and occipital lobes. Consequently, patients can present with bilateral limb weakness or sensory disturbance, cranial nerve deficits, ataxia, nausea and vomiting, or coma. The full-blown syndrome results from occlusion of the basilar artery trunk, with fragments of the syndrome produced by branch occlusions. Edema and mass effect from cerebellar stroke can be life threatening because of the confined space of the posterior fossa, with resulting upward or downward transtentorial herniation (See section on cerebellar hemorrhage).

3.   **Conditions mimicking stroke** include seizure, migraine, toxic-metabolic derangement, and amyloid spells. Diffusion-weighted MR imaging helps distinguish cerebral infarction from stroke mimics by identifying areas of intracellular swelling (i.e., cytotoxic edema) associated with ischemia.

a. Whereas partial complex **seizures** can mimic stroke, especially if speech is impaired, post-ictal neurologic deficits ("Todd's" phenomena) can masquerade as any focal neurologic deficit, including weakness, sensory loss, or aphasia lasting hours to days after a seizure.

b. The aura associated with a **migraine** headache can include focal neurologic deficits such as weakness, numbness, or aphasia; it can occur in the absence of headache (acephalgic migraine).

c. **Toxic-metabolic states** such as hypoglycemia, hyponatremia, or intoxication can produce focal or global neurologic deficits. Laboratory evaluation including electrolytes should be performed in all cases.

d. Patients with **amyloid angiopathy** can have transient neurologic dysfunction associated with microscopic hemorrhages that are suggestive of TIAs. Diagnosis may be made on MR imaging gradient-echo sequences with blooming in areas of hemosiderin deposition.

4. Important **causes** of stroke include cardiac and arterial thromboemboli, intracranial and extracranial atherosclerosis, endocarditis, paradoxical emboli, arterial dissection, vasculitis, and inherited and acquired hypercoagulable disorders. **Carotid or vertebral artery dissection** can occur spontaneously, after trauma, or in connective tissue disease (fibromuscular dysplasia). It can be seen by angiography or axial T1 MR imaging. **Vasculitis** can occur in primary central nervous system (CNS) disease or as part of a systemic syndrome such as systemic lupus erythematosis (SLE). **Hypercoagulability** can result from clotting factor imbalance (protein C, S, antithrombin III deficiency) or autoimmunity (antiphospholipid antibodies).

5. **Acute evaluation for intravenous (IV) thrombolysis** should be performed in all patients presenting to an appropriate facility within 3 hours of symptom onset. Evaluation includes neurologic assessment, CT or MR imaging to exclude hemorrhage and early ischemic changes, laboratory exclusion of stroke mimics, hemostatic profile [platelet count, prothrombin (PT) and activated partial thromboplastin times (aPTT)] and historical and imaging findings consistent with acute ischemia. If available, echo-planar MR with diffusion- and perfusion-weighted imaging or functional CT may provide further insight into vascular anatomy and tissue injury. Alternatively, **ultrasound** can permit rapid and repeatable neurovascular assessment of the carotid bifurcation, cervical vertebrals, and intracranial arterial branches. Medical centers with endovascular specialists may offer intraarterial **(IA)** thrombolytics that have a longer

therapeutic window of 6 hours in the anterior circulation and perhaps up to 24 hours in the posterior circulation. The only drug approved for use in acute ischemic stroke is IV **recombinant tissue plasminogen activator (rt-PA).** See http://www.acutestroke.com for acute stroke protocols.

6. **Subacute evaluation** should identify the cause and help define the risk for recurrent stroke. **Electrocardiography (ECG)** is indicated in all patients to exclude acute myocardial infarction and dysrhythmias. **Echocardiography** with agitated saline contrast injection excludes intracardiac thrombus; and it assesses left ventricular size and function, left atrial size, mitral and aortic valvular disease, and right-to-left shunt. **Transesophageal** studies are more sensitive to left atrial thrombus and atheromatous disease of the aortic arch. A 24-hour **Holter monitor** may identify paroxysmal atrial fibrillation.

7. **Acute treatment**

   a. If the time of onset is clearly established to be less than 3 hours and intracranial hemorrhage and early signs of stroke have been excluded with a cranial CT, those patients with significant nonresolving deficits and the clinical diagnosis of ischemic stroke are candidates for **IV rt-PA.** A 0.9 mg/kg (maximum of 90 mg) dose is infused over 60 minutes with 10% of total dose administered as an initial IV bolus over 1 minute. Contraindications to IV rt-PA include suspected subarachnoid hemorrhage, active internal bleeding, platelet count less than 100,000/mm^3, aPTT more than the upper limit of normal, PT longer than 15 seconds, recent intracranial surgery, serious head trauma, previous stroke or intracerebral hemorrhage (ICH), and systemic hypertension defined as a systolic blood pressure greater than 185 mm Hg or diastolic blood pressure less than 110 mm Hg despite therapy with nitroglycerin, IV labetalol, or nitroprusside. Patients aged more than 75 years or with severe strokes have a higher rate of hemorrhage after rt-PA.

   b. **Intraarterial thrombolytic** administration should be considered in patients with confirmed large artery occlusion and those past the 3-hour IV rt-PA window according to locally developed protocols. Doses of up to 1.25 million units of urokinase or 20 mg rt-PA have been used in conjunction with mechanical clot disruption to recanalize proximal arteries and restore function. Proximal artery occlusions are less likely to recanalize with IV rt-PA and are more likely to produce severe clinical deficits.

    c. Continuous full-dose IV **unfractionated heparin** is often used in presumed embolic infarction in patients ineligible for thrombolysis, although its efficacy is unproved. Heparin also should be considered in patients with basilar insufficiency, cervical artery dissection, critical carotid stenosis in the setting of a less than maximal MCA infarct, fluctuating deficits, or suspected cardiac embolism. The aPTT should be monitored every 6 hours, with the rate adjusted to maintain the aPTT in the range of 60 to 80 seconds. An initial heparin bolus can increase the risk of hemorrhage and is deferred except in fluctuating deficits or acute basilar thrombosis. Any patient with a clinical deterioration while on heparin must be imaged immediately to exclude acute hemorrhage.

    d. **Aspirin** in doses ranging from 160 to 1,000 mg daily can benefit patients with acute stroke for whom thrombolytics or anticoagulants are not indicated. Other antiplatelet agents such as **ticlopidine, clopidogrel,** or IV **abciximab** are promising agents in acute ischemic stroke, although their efficacy has not yet been proved.

    e. Urgent **carotid endarterectomy** or **carotid stenting** may be indicated in cases of stroke in which are seen a critical degree of carotid stenosis, a small distal infarction, and a large territory of vulnerable brain. Revascularization of larger strokes can be associated with **acute reperfusion injury** (Chapter 37) and should be delayed by weeks to months.

    f. In some patients with stenosis of major vessels, **pharmacologically induced hypertension** with **phenylephrine** may ameliorate symptoms and rescue viable brain tissue.

8. Subacute treatment

    a. Hypovolemia and hyponatremia should be avoided.

    b. **Fever** should be aggressively controlled, because even mild hyperthermia worsens outcome.

    c. **Cerebral edema** is maximal at 2 to 5 days after stroke onset, and standard management of intracranial pressure (ICP) should be initiated. In massive hemispheric or cerebellar infarction, **decompressive surgery** can be life saving and may improve outcome in survivors.

    d. **When intracerebral hemorrhage is suspected** in patients receiving thrombolysis, obtain immediate cranial CT, emergent neurosurgical and hematologic consultation, and laboratory evaluation of coagulation (PT, aPTT, complete blood count, D-dimer and fibrinogen levels). Treatment includes **fresh frozen plasma** to replete factors V and VII, large volumes of **cryoprecipitate** to replete fibrinogen, and **platelet transfusions,** as necessary. Patients having anticoagulant therapy with heparin should have its effects reversed with **protamine** 1 mg IV (slowly) for every 100 U of unfractionated heparin given in the preceding 4 hours. Follow coagulation profiles hourly until bleeding is brought under control. If these measures fail to control bleeding, then consider **aminocaproic acid** (5 g IV over 1 hour).

B. **Primary ICH.** The most common locations for ICH are basal ganglia, thalamus, cerebral white matter, pons, and cortical lobar surface; 8% to 10% occur in the cerebellum. Long-standing hypertension is the most common cause (75%), although other causes include aneurysm, trauma, vascular malformations, amyloid angiopathy, coagulopathies, neoplasms, sympathomimetic drugs, and vasculitis. Metastases, especially adenocarcinoma, can present with cerebellar hemorrhage or swelling. ICH as a primary process should be differentiated from hemorrhagic transformation of ischemic infarction, in which a bland ischemic stroke develops petechial bleeding or turns into a space-occupying hematoma.

1. **Clinical presentation.** ICH often presents with headache, nausea, vomiting, and focal neurologic signs similar to those seen in ischemic strokes. The evolution of symptoms can occur more slowly than in ischemic stroke, or ICH can cause an acute devastating picture. As a rule, patients with ICH present with systolic hypertension. In patients who were normotensive at baseline, this usually resolves over the first week; in chronically hypertensive patients, aggressive therapy is often required to control blood pressure. In contrast with most cortical hemorrhages, the progression to death from cerebellar hemorrhage can be rapid

   a. **Supratentorial** ICH presents with symptoms referable to the site of bleeding. With rebleeding or development of vasogenic edema or hydrocephalus, often worsening of symptoms and a decline in arousal occur. Transtentorial herniation is the mode of death in massive hemorrhage.

   b. **Infratentorial** hemorrhage with **midline** lesions produces only disequilibrium on standing, walking, and sometimes sitting. The Romberg test is negative because balance with eyes open is already impaired. If gait is not tested, this lesion will not be detected until other cerebellar signs emerge secondary to brain swelling. **Lateral** hemispheric lesions always produce symptoms ipsilateral to the lesion. Patients complain of limb discoordination and demonstrate ataxia with falling toward the side of the lesion, dysmetria (overshoot) on pointing to finger-nose-finger, dysdiadokinesia (inaccuracy on rapid alternating movements), intention tremor (exaggerates approaching target), and nystagmus (worse looking toward the lesion). Speech can be dysarthric (slurred) or explosive.

2. **Acute evaluation** consists of brain imaging. Both CT and MR are sensitive for ICH. A toxicology screen, PT, aPTT, and platelet count should be checked, and signs and symptoms of occult malignancy excluded. Subacute evaluation should identify the cause by imaging and history. MR imaging with magnetic susceptibility may identify areas of prior occult cortical hemorrhage and suggest a diagnosis of amyloid angiopathy in patients with lobar ICH. Repeat MR in 3 to 6 weeks may also detect lesions (e.g.,tumor) masked by acute hemorrhage. Rarely, aneurysmal hemorrhage can result in primary parenchymal hematoma, mimicking ICH. Angiography is indicated in any suspicious cases. Prognosis is based on clinical presentation and imaging findings. Lesions in the posterior fossa that are less than 2 cm in diameter with self-limited cerebellar signs do well. Those with 3 cm lesions or progressive drowsiness will do poorly without intervention. Twenty percent of patients have lesions larger than 3 cm and a poor prognosis regardless of treatment.

3. **Acute treatment** consists largely of supportive care with surgical resection in selected cases.

    a. **Coagulopathies** should be rapidly corrected (Chapter 12).

    b. **Neurosurgical consultation** should be obtained early, especially in cerebellar hemorrhage of 2 cm or greater in maximal diameter. Decompression of posterior fossa hemorrhage can be lifesaving and outcomes are excellent if herniation is prevented. Resection of lobar or basal ganglia ICH can also be lifesaving, but the effect on outcome has not been well established.

    c. Reduction of systolic blood pressure has been advocated to prevent rebleeding. Rates of rebleeding in hypertensive hemorrhage are thought to be low, however, and overly aggressive reductions in blood pressure may precipitate cerebral ischemia.

    d. **Obstructive or communicating hydrocephalus** can develop and usually requires external ventricular drainage.

    e. **Corticosteroids** do not appear to be of benefit in ICH unless deterioration occurs specifically from vasogenic edema.

    f. **Anticonvulsant therapy** (e.g.,phenytoin) is indicated for seizures when the hematoma extends to the cortex or if the consequences of a seizure would be deleterious (e.g., refractory intracranial hypertension, unstable fractures).

    g. **Mortality** remains at 50% to 65% and as high as 90% for patients initially in coma.

  C. **Subarachnoid hemorrhage (SAH)** can be traumatic or nontraumatic. Most aneurysms arise from the carotid circulation, most commonly the ACA and less frequently the posterior cerebral arteries (PCA) or middle cerebral arteries. Posterior circulation aneurysms commonly arise from the basilar tip. Aneurysms can exist on a congenital basis, arise in the setting of atherosclerosis, or more rarely occur from infection (mycotic) or emboli (e.g., atrial myxoma). Rupture of cerebral aneurysms releases blood into the subarachnoid space and causes up to 30% mortality in the first 24 hours. Rebleeding of untreated aneurysms occurs in up to 30% of patients in the first 28 days, with 70% mortality. Hypotension, aspiration pneumonia, neurogenic pulmonary edema, seizures, obstructive hydrocephalus, or ischemia from vasospasm can produce secondary brain injury. Serial examination and brain imaging can identify symptoms suggestive of most of these complications, but separate techniques are necessary to distinguish vasospasm.

    1. **Clinical presentation.** The "worst headache of my life" complaint should raise suspicion of SAH. Nausea, vomiting, altered sensorium, and focal cranial nerve defects (especially third nerve palsy) are associated with SAH. A warning headache may occur, from a "sentinel bleed" in which blood may be confined to the aneurysm wall without true SAH. Clinical grading (Table 29-1) predicts outcome and risk of vasospasm.

    2. **Acute evaluation.** The CT scan—the best initial test for SAH—will detect SAH in approximately

Table 29-1. Classification of patients with intracranial aneurysms according to surgical risk (Hunt and Hess classification)

Grade	Characteristics
I	Asymptomatic or minimal headache and slight nuchal rigidity
II	Moderate to severe headache; nuchal rigidity; no neurologic deficit other than cranial nerve palsy
III	Drowsiness; confusion; mild focal deficit
IV	Stupor; moderate to severe hemiparesis; possibly early decerebrate rigidity; vegetative disturbances
V	Deep coma; decerebrate rigidity; moribund

95% of cases. Lumbar puncture shou formed in cases where SAH is suspected , is negative. Angiography should be perfc gently if SAH is diagnosed. A small prop   . of SAH cases will have normal angiography. Followup imaging is needed in most cases. Attention should be given to arteriovenous fistulas at the base of the skull and aneurysms compressed by hematoma. Magnetic resonance or CT angiography may also reveal aneurysms, and CT angiography can help with surgical planning. Advances in surgical and anesthetic technique currently favor early angiography to identify the culprit aneurysm and early surgery before vasospasm develops. Concerns that angiography itself might lead to aneurysmal rebleeding are unwarranted.

3. **Subacute evaluation.** Transfemoral angiography remains the standard for documenting vasospasm; however, it is invasive and carries some risk. Vasospasm can develop at anytime, but is most frequent between days 4 to 12 postrupture. Many centers perform serial transcranial Doppler ultrasound examinations to detect presymptomatic narrowing of cerebral vessels at the base of the brain. Risk of vasospasm can be predicted by grading of blood collections around the basal arteries on the 24-hour CT scan.

4. **Acute treatment** consists of definitive obliteration of the culprit aneurysm (clipping or endovascular therapy) and prevention of delayed ischemic deficits.

   a. **Blood pressure** is strictly controlled until the aneurysm is secured.

   b. **Surgery, endovascular therapy,** or **both** are performed urgently.

   c. **Nimodipine,** a calcium channel antagonist (60 mg orally every 4 hours for 21 days), was reported to reduce ischemic symptoms from 33% to 22%. **Tirilizad,** a free radical scavenger (6 mg/kg/d), may reduce the risk of vasospasm.

   d. **Release of natriuretic factors** causes cerebral salt wasting and at least 3 L/d of normal saline is often required to prevent hypovolemia. Intravascular volume expansion with albumin solutions often is used to keep central venous pressures above 8 to 10 mm Hg and prevent hypotension. Hemodilution to a hematocrit of approximately 30% provides adequate oxygen-carrying capacity with minimal blood viscosity.

   e. **Induced hypertension** with α-adrenergic agonists (e.g., phenylephrine) is safe and effective at reversing ischemic symptoms caused by decreased cerebral blood flow in patients

with vasospasm. Some patients require inotropic support as well.

    f. **Prophylactic anticonvulsants** may be
helpful in the first 2 weeks, especially in those
patients in whom seizure would be deleterious. In refractory vasospasm or patients who
cannot tolerate induced hypertension, intraarterial vasodilators (e.g.,papaverine) or balloon angioplasty can alleviate ischemia and,
despite higher initial risk, are a mainstay of
therapy.

    g. **Corticosteroids** have no beneficial effect
on vasospasm, but can reduce postoperative
cerebral edema.

D. **Cortical venous sinus thrombosis** causes occlusion
of a cerebral venous sinus, most commonly the saggital,
transverse, or straight sinus, although clot can extend
into the vein of Galen or internal cerebral vein. It can
occur in the setting of infection, tumor, hypovolemia,
coagulation disorders, systemic inflammatory diseases,
oral contraceptive use, pregnancy, and the puerperium.
Despite a thorough diagnostic evaluation, however,
nearly 25% of cases will be deemed idiopathic.

    1. **Clinical presentation** includes signs of increased
ICP (e.g., headache, nausea, and vomiting) often
more pronounced after prolonged recumbency. Focal neurologic signs or seizures may be seen in the
setting of vasogenic edema or venous infarction.
Without recanalization, altered sensorium can progress to coma. If the diagnosis of cortical venous
sinus thrombosis is not considered, it is often overlooked until hemorrhage has occurred.

    2. **Acute evaluation** relies on an imaging diagnosis.
CT with contrast media may demonstrate filling
defects in the superior sagittal sinus ("empty delta"
sign) in up to one third of patients, parenchymal
abnormalities suggestive of deranged venous drainage in up to 60% of patients, small ventricles from
increased ICP, or contrast enhancement of the
falx and tentorium from venous hypertension. MR
imaging and MR venography are sensitive and
specific. Transfemoral angiography is diagnostic if
MR is inconclusive. Lumbar puncture may demonstrate an elevated opening pressure, increased
protein, red cells and mild pleocytosis.

    3. **Acute treatment** is effective, if initiated early, but
prognosis for recovery worsens without treatment.
Treatment with urgent antithrombotic therapy is
widely accepted. Continuous IV unfractionated
heparin titrated to an aPTT two to two and a half
times control should be maintained until the patient stabilizes or improves. Hemorrhagic infarction is not a contraindication to heparin treatment
in this setting. In certain cases of extensive thrombosis or rapid deterioration in patient condition,

chemical **thrombolysis** or **mechanical clot disruption** should be considered. Measures to control ICP elevation and prophylaxis for seizures are undertaken, and factors that exacerbate thrombosis (e.g., dehydration) avoided.

II. **Encephalopathy**

A. **Toxic-metabolic injury** to the CNS, a frequent cause of impaired cognitive performance in critically ill patients, always remains a diagnosis of exclusion. Frequent causes include the effects of medication; perturbations in electrolyte (e.g., sodium), water, glucose, or urea homeostasis; and renal or hepatic failure. CNS depressants, such as anticholinergics, neuroleptic-class antiemetics, benzodiazepines, narcotic analgesics, and anesthetics should be administered with caution. "Short-acting" agents can become "never-ending" agents in critically ill patients because of impaired drug metabolism, drug clearance, or unpredictable pharmacokinetics during continuous infusions. Treatment is supportive with removal of the offending agent when possible.

B. **Hypertensive encephalopathy** is caused by sustained, severe hypertension with associated neurologic abnormalities. Early, reversible symptoms are likely caused by blood–brain barrier disruption and vasogenic edema. Cerebral hemorrhage and irreversible injury can occur with sustained hypertension. Because acute blood pressure elevations are common in many types of brain injury in which antihypertensive therapy could be deleterious (e.g., ischemic stroke, traumatic brain injury), accurate diagnosis is essential.

1. **Clinical manifestations** range from headache and visual scotoma to confusion, seizures, and coma. The likelihood of recovery depends on the extent of injury prior to treatment. Cranial CT is insensitive, but often reveals bilateral posterior subcortical hypodensities. MR imaging typically reveals posterior T2 hyperintensities and echoplanar apparent diffusion coefficient (ADC) images may be diagnostic. Abnormalities, which may diffusely involve subcortical white matter, cortical gray matter, and cerebellum, often include microscopic petechial hemorrhages.

2. **Management** includes arterial pressure monitoring and administration of IV labetalol, nitroprusside, or both for rapid control of blood pressure. Oral calcium channel blockers should be avoided because of the risk of precipitous hypotension.

3. Most patients with hypertensive encephalopathy have underlying **chronic hypertension,** which increases the upper and lower limits of cerebrovascular autoregulation. A rapid reduction in blood pressure in a chronically hypertensive patient can produce acute global ischemia at a pressure that would usually be well tolerated in a normotensive patient.

4. **In patients with eclampsia, cyclosporine toxicity, and tumors,** a similar type of hypertensive encephalopathy may be produced by "relative" hypertension in the setting of an abnormal blood–brain barrier.

C. **Infectious and inflammatory causes**

1. The only treatable form of **viral encephalitis** is that caused by acute herpes simplex viral infection. Patients present with headaches, fever, and cognitive impairments referable to the mesial temporal lobes. Early in the course, a cerebrospinal fluid (CSF) lymphocytosis occurs with a normal glucose concentration and mild increases in protein. Later the CSF becomes bloody because of hemorrhagic necrosis. The electroencephalogram (EEG) shows characteristic bursts of periodic high voltage slow waves. MR imaging reveals temporal and inferior frontal lobe involvement. Brain biopsy is the standard for diagnosis, but polymerase chain reaction (PCR) testing on the CSF is becoming more available and reliable. Because therapy with **acyclovir** (10 mg/kg every 8 hours) is relatively nontoxic and reduces mortality and morbidity from 70% to 20%, it should be instituted whenever the diagnosis of viral encephalitis is suspected. **Other encephalitides** (e.g., Eastern Equine, California, or St. Louis) do not respond to acyclovir but they can have similar initial presentations. Vasogenic edema, seizures, and increased ICP occur in all of these disorders.

2. **Bacterial meningitis** must be diagnosed and treated rapidly, although in the early hours it can be clinically indistinguishable from viral meningoencephalitis. Acute onset of headache, meningeal signs (neck stiffness, photophobia), fever, and altered sensorium should suggest the diagnosis of acute bacterial meningitis. Common causes include *Streptococcus pneumoniae, Neisseria meningiditis,* and *Haemophilus influenzae,* but enteric gram-negative rods should be considered in alcoholics and *Listeria monocytogenes* in the immunosuppressed and elderly. Most bacterial meningitis is community acquired, but important secondary causes include parameningeal infectious foci from otitis, sinusitis, bacteremic contamination, occult skull fractures, and external ventricular drains. Brain imaging with contrast to exclude a mass lesion should be performed prior to lumbar puncture; however, empiric antibiotic therapy is indicated if imaging is delayed or unavailable. Broad initial coverage may include **ceftriaxone** (1–2 g IV every 12 hours), with **ampicillin** if *L. monocytogenes* is a concern and **vancomycin** in populations with penicillin-resistant *S. pneumoniae.* Penicillin monotherapy should be used if a suscep-

tible organism is isolated. **High-dose dexa-methasone** may be of some benefit in children with meningitis, but no definitive benefit has been documented for its use in adults.

III. **Seizures.** Uncontrolled generalized motor seizures that persist longer than 60 minutes are associated with significant neuronal injury and mortality. **Status epilepticus** can be defined as continuous convulsions, or as intermittent convulsions without interictal restoration of premorbid cognitive function. The most common causes of status epilepticus are abrupt cessation of anticonvulsants, meningitis, encephalitis, subdural hematoma, ischemic or hemorrhagic infarction, brain tumor, traumatic brain injury, anoxia, and metabolic disorders.

A. **The clinical presentation** is usually convulsions with unresponsiveness, but seizures with subtle motor manifestations can go unrecognized in critically ill patients. Other causes of jerking limb movements not associated with seizure include myoclonus, pontine ischemia, tremor, and spasticity.

B. **Acute evaluation.** An EEG is often necessary to exclude seizures in the encephalopathic patient.

1. **Laboratory evaluation** includes complete blood count, electrolytes, blood urea nitrogen (BUN), creatinine, glucose, calcium, magnesium, phosphorus, liver function tests, anticonvulsant levels, **toxicology screen,** and, when indicated, pregnancy test and arterial blood gas analysis.

2. **Physical examination** should be performed to exclude occult head trauma, substance abuse, fever, meningismus, and diabetes. Always check for a Medical Alert bracelet or wallet information, and try to contact relatives or neighbors to determine prior medical and seizure history. Cranial CT scan and lumbar puncture may be necessary to establish the diagnosis once seizures are controlled.

3. Neuromuscular blocking drugs in the absence of EEG monitoring have **no role** in the initial management of uncontrolled seizures.

C. **Acute treatment** consists of safely aborting seizures with the appropriate degree of intervention.

1. **Most patients require no intervention** and will spontaneously recover after one or two seizures, and deciding who is truly in status epilepticus is the challenge. Some patients require benzodiazepines and phenytoin without airway protection, whereas others require pentobarbital anesthesia. Management by defined protocol is the best method for assuring that patients are treated promptly, and a thorough evaluation that usually includes brain imaging and lumbar puncture must be completed as soon as the patient is stabilized.

2. Because phenytoin (DPH) is largely albumin bound and renally excreted, correction for hypoalbumine-

mia or acute renal failure is necessary: $DPH_{corrected}$ = $DPH_{total}/[(0.2 \times albumin) + 0.1]$ for low albumin and $DPH_{corrected}$ = $DPH_{total}/[(0.1 \times albumin) + 0.1]$ for low albumin and acute renal failure.

3. **Intravenous phenytoin** can cause bradycardia, hypotension, and cardiovascular collapse and must be given in a monitored setting.

4. **A standard protocol approach** is:

    a. **At 0 to 5 minutes,** assess and perform basic life support. Start supplemental oxygen. Obtain seizure history. Look for evidence of head trauma or toxic ingestion or injections. Send urine and blood toxicology screen, electrolytes, BUN, creatinine, glucose, calcium, magnesium, and osmolality. Check arterial blood gas tensions and perform endotracheal intubation if necessary.

    b. **At 6 to 9 minutes,** begin normal saline IV, administer **thiamine** (100 mg) IV and **dextrose** (25–50 g) IV. Treat fever with acetaminophen and ice packs.

    c. **At 10 to 30 minutes, administer diazepam** (5–20 mg) IV or **lorazepam** (0.1 mg/kg) IV at ≤ 2 mg/min up to 4 to 8 mg. Immediately start **phenytoin** (18–20 mg/kg) IV (load at ≤ 50 mg/min). Administer 10 mg/kg to a patient with epilepsy presumed to be taking phenytoin while awaiting drug levels. Alternatively, **fosphenytoin** (18 mg/kg) IV (load at ≤ 150 mg/min) can be used. Repeat benzodiazepines every 15 minutes for continued motor seizures during the phenytoin load. Send phenytoin levels 20 minutes after the loading dose in patients who are still seizing. **Develop** a hypothesis for a presumptive pathophysiologic mechanism of the seizure.

    d. **At 31 to 60 minutes, administer phenobarbital** (10–20 mg/kg) IV (load at ≤ 70 mg/min). Call for urgent continuous EEG monitoring and obtain expert consultation. Many patients require endotracheal intubation and mechanical ventilation at this point in the protocol.

    e. **At ≥ 60 minutes, administer pentobarbital** (3–5 mg/kg) IV to induce burst suppression. Prepare an infusion of α-adrenergic agonist (e.g., phenylephrine) for treatment of anticipated hypotension. In most adults, a pentobarbital bolus of 400 mg over 15 minutes, followed by 100 mg every 15 to 30 minutes until burst suppression appears, is reasonably well tolerated. This is followed by an infusion at 0.5 to 5.0 mg/kg/h to maintain burst suppression (Fig. 29-1). Decrease the infusion periodically to check the underlying EEG and always de-

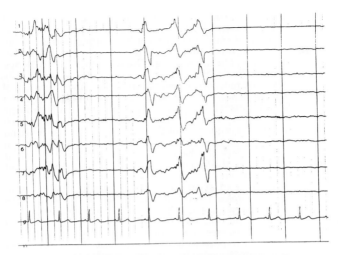

Fig. 29-1. Burst suppression during electroencephalographic monitoring. Bottom line is a tracing from an electrocardiographic lead.

crease by 25 mg/h if electrocerebral silence ("flatline") is present. **Alternative** agents to induce burst suppression include **midazolam** (200 μg/kg) IV slowly followed by 0.75 to 10 μg/kg/min (may produce less hypotension); **lidocaine** (1–2 mg/kg) IV bolus with a 1 to 4 mg/min infusion (unproved); **propofol** (1–2 mg/kg) IV load followed by 30 to 150 μg/kg/min (unproved). **Valproate** (15 mg/kg) IV load may be useful as an adjunctive agent (unproved).

IV. **Traumatic brain injury (TBI) and treatment of cerebral edema**

A. **Motor vehicle accidents and firearms missile injuries** remain the top causes of TBI in the United States, with firearms recently supplanting motor vehicles as the most common cause of fatal brain injury with an incidence of 8.5/100,000 population/year. When the brain (within the skull) is moving and strikes a stationary object (e.g., skull vs. dashboard), the predominant site of brain injury is contracoup. When the brain is stationary and is struck by a moving object (e.g., brain vs. baseball bat), the predominant injury is coup. These events transfer mechanical and thermal energy to the brain and spine, causing primary brain injury. In addition, they can produce immediate mass lesions (e.g., hematoma or foreign body) that further injure the brain. Secondary homeostatic and pathologic responses are initiated which include changes in cerebral blood flow (CBF), cerebral blood volume (CBV), respiratory pattern, systemic circulating volume, and mean arterial pressures. In addition, inflammatory and cytotoxic cascades that can lead to further brain injury are initiated.

B.   The diagnosis of TBI is established by clinical examination and brain imaging. **The Glasgow Coma Score (GCS)** (Table 29-2) is a simple, reproducible, and widely accepted measure of brain dysfunction. Any alteration of consciousness in the setting of even minor trauma should raise the suspicion of TBI and prompt neurologic evaluation, especially in the elderly or anticoagulated patient. Frequent reevaluation of neurologic function is essential, because early detection of secondary brain injury offers the best hope of preventing permanent neurologic dysfunction and should guide subsequent management.

C.   The clinical syndrome can include headache, agitation, decreased level of consciousness, third or sixth nerve palsy, gaze deviation, respiratory variation, papilledema, pupillary changes, or a variety of abnormal motor responses (flexion or extension posturing, clonus). Systemic hypertension occurs as part of the overall vasopressor response to intracranial hypertension mediated by the posterolateral medulla to maintain cerebral perfusion. The **"Cushing reflex"** of hypertension and bradycardia reflects a failure of medullary function seen

Table 29-2.   The Glasgow Coma Scale

Category	Score
Best motor response	
Obeys	6
Localizes	5
Withdraws	4
Abnormal flexion	3
Extensor response	2
None	1
Verbal response	
Oriented	5
Confused	4
Inappropriate words	3
Incomprehensible sounds	2
None	1
Eye opening	
Spontaneously	4
To speech	3
To pain	2
None	1

The Glasgow Coma Score expresses a patient's level of consciousness by assessing motor response, verbal response, and eye opening. The individual scores for each of the three components are added to obtain a summary score. A fully alert and oriented patient would receive a score of 15. A flaccid patient with no eye opening or verbal response would receive a score of 3.

during brainstem herniation. Atrial tachydysrhythmias and ventricular ectopy can occur, especially when ICH is present. Pulmonary edema can occur, probably because of pulmonary capillary fracture during the intense sympathetic outflow induced by intracranial hypertension. A variety of respiratory pattern disturbances can evolve, including changes in rate (bradypnea, tachypnea), rhythm (apneustic, ataxic, agonal, Cheyne-Stokes, apnea), or effective ventilation (hyperventilation, hypoventilation).

D. **Brain imaging** has revolutionized management of TBI. It is useful to divide patients on presentation into three categories: those who require (a) immediate neurosurgical intervention, (b) intensive care management, or (c) focused observation. Availability of CT in the emergency department permits rapid diagnosis of ICH, subdural hematoma (SDH), epidural hematoma (EDH), subarachnoid hemorrhage (SAH), hydrocephalus, depressed skull fracture, and focal contusions; it shortens the time to necessary neurosurgical intervention. In addition, newer techniques, which allow for noninvasive measures of CBF, CBV, and early ischemic tissue changes, are helping to increase understanding of the pathophysiology of TBI.

E. **Increased ICP,** a frequent sequel of TBI, greatly increases morbidity and mortality. Several different approaches are available to permit continuous monitoring of ICP (Fig. 29-2).

    1. **Indications for ICP monitoring** include decreasing level of consciousness, risk of undetectable rise in ICP (e.g., paralyzed patient, intraoperative setting), or need to perform maneuvers that will

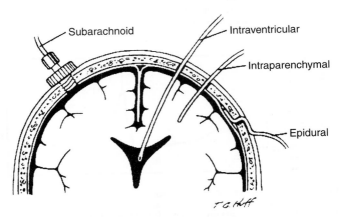

Fig. 29-2. Illustration of four different methods for transducing intracranial pressure. From Lee KR, Hoff JT. Intracranial pressure. In: Youmans JR, ed. *Neurological Surgery,* 4th ed. Philadelphia: WB Saunders, 1996:505, with permission.

likely increase ICP in vulnerable patients (e.g., clearance of pulmonary secretions, medications, positioning). As with all invasive monitoring, ICP monitoring should be initiated only if rational management decisions will be made based on the ICP data.

2. **Interpretation of ICP measurements.** Elevation of ICP, which is generally due to mass lesions, hydrocephalus, brain edema, or increased cerebral blood volume, should prompt urgent evaluation. The ICP waveform typically shows pressure variations within each cardiac and respiratory cycle (Fig. 29-3). The amplitude of the ICP waveform associated with cardiac pulsation normally is 1 mm Hg and increases with increasing ICP. Heterogeneity of intracranial pressure can exist within the cranial vault, especially above and below the tentorium.

3. **Pressure waves** are rhythmic variations in ICP described as **A, B,** and **C** waves (Figure 29-4) Only the **A** waves are clinically significant. **A** waves are 50 to 100 mm Hg waves lasting 5 to 20 minutes. When sustained, they are called **"plateau waves"**; they are often associated with clinical deterioration. Plateau waves can arise spontaneously or be precipitated by hemodynamic fluctuations or nursing procedures. **B** waves are sharper (50 mm Hg) waves occurring at about 1-minute intervals. They can be associated with normal sleep or pathologically decreased levels of consciousness occurring at both high and normal ICP. **C** waves are less than 20 mm Hg waves, occurring about six times per minute, and they may indicate a decreased intracranial compliance. They usually occur in the presence of elevated ICP.

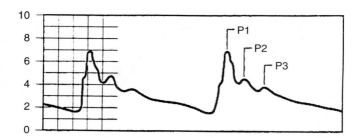

Fig. 29-3. Morphology of the intracranial pressure (ICP) waveform in the setting of normal intracranial pressure and compliance. The ICP waveform shows pressure variations within each cardiac and respiratory cycle. P1, P2, and P3 are cardiac pulsations. The units of measurement are millimeters of mercury. From Lee KR, Hoff JT. Intracranial pressure. In: Youmans JR, ed. *Neurological Surgery,* 4th ed. Philadelphia: WB Saunders, 1996, 497, with permission.

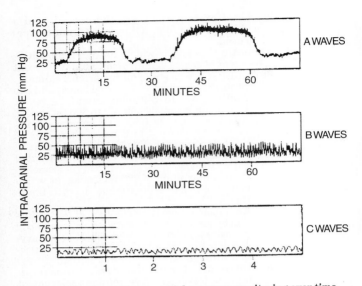

Fig. 29-4. Tracings of intracranial pressure monitoring over time. A waves, also described as "plateau waves," occur in the setting of very poor intracranial compliance. From Lee KR, Hoff JT. Intracranial pressure. In: Youmans JR, ed. *Neurological Surgery*, 4th ed. Philadelphia: WB Saunders, 1996:508, with permission.

F. **Impaired autoregulation of CBF in TBI.** In the early hours after injury, CBF falls to critically low levels and is uncoupled from metabolic demand, which remains normal or elevated. This can cause widespread ischemic infarction and contribute to subsequent cytotoxic edema and increasing ICP, resulting in a poor outcome. Autoregulation of CBF responds to changes in pressure, blood viscosity, and probably some markers of metabolic activity to keep blood flow constant. Cerebrovascular reactivity is a different mechanism by which changes in cerebrovascular resistance (CVR) occur in response to changes in P_{CO_2}. This reactivity is often disordered in TBI, and can be heterogeneously distributed in different brain regions, with areas of both increased and decreased reactivity. Because the degree of vasoconstriction to hypocapnia is highly variable and perhaps also regional within the injured brain, it is possible to increase regional ischemia through excessive vasoconstriction even at relatively modest reductions in P_{CO_2}. This can occur in the setting of seemingly beneficial reductions in ICP. No easy method exists to monitor the adequacy of CBF at the bedside during hyperventilation, but indirect assessment of cerebral oxygenation can provide some information.

G. **Therapy in TBI** is targeted at reducing ICP while maintaining cerebral perfusion pressure (CPP) vigilantly. Serial examinations are the crucial, and a reproducible, method (e.g., **Glasgow Coma Score**) should be used.

1. **Osmotic therapy** is widely used to reduce ICP. The agent of choice is **mannitol,** although recent literature suggests a role for hypertonic saline.

   a. **Mannitol** is given as an initial bolus of 0.25 to 1.50 g/kg over 15 to 30 minutes with the goal of increasing serum osmolality to 300 mOsm/kg. Additional 0.25 to 0.50 g/kg boluses are administered every 4 to 6 hours thereafter as needed to maintain this level of osmolality.

   b. **Further elevations in ICP** can be treated with stepwise increases in target osmolality to a maximum of 320 mOsm/kg, at which point the risk of acute tubular necrosis limits therapy.

   c. An important early mechanism of ICP reduction by mannitol may be its reduction of blood viscosity and increase in cerebral tissue oxygen delivery, stimulating reflex vasoconstriction through cerebral autoregulation.

   d. **Intravascular volume depletion** is inevitable unless aggressive volume replacement is initiated, and urine output must be monitored hourly. Normal saline is the preferred crystalloid because it has an osmolality of ~310 mOsm/kg. Because mannitol is an active osmotic agent, renal function and "trough" osmolality should be checked prior to each dosing interval.

   e. Mannitol can cause acute congestive heart failure, and most patients require central pressure monitoring and bladder catheterization. Repeated dosing can exceed renal excretion capacity and cause inadvertent free water retention and hyponatremia. In this circumstance, intermittent low-dose loop diuretics may be helpful. Fluid restrictions should prohibit all oral intake rather than only "free water" because this term is misleading and often permits hypotonic juices or broths to be consumed.

   f. **Hypotension** is a much more likely complication of osmotic therapy than the theoretical complication of "reverse osmotic shift," in which the osmotic agent crosses the injured blood-brain barrier and draws fluid into the parenchyma.

2. **Loop diuretics** such as **furosemide** (10–20 mg IV every 4 to 6 hours) may be useful for the subacute treatment of intracranial hypertension, possibly by decreasing vasogenic edema and CSF production. Potential adverse effects include hypovolemia, azotemia, metabolic alkalosis, electrolyte abnormalities, nephrotoxicity, and ototoxicity.

3. **Hyperventilation** can provide brief control of ICP but is only a bridging strategy, because homeostatic mechanisms adjust to the new pH rapidly. It can be useful in the treatment of plateau waves. Overly aggressive hypocapnia can cause diffuse cerebral ischemia because of profound vasoconstriction or it can cause seizures.

4. **Corticosteroids** generally have no role in isolated head injury and intracranial hypertension per se, although short courses may be helpful in reducing vasogenic edema associated with injury or with surgical retraction.

5. **Temperature. Fever** increases cerebral metabolic rate by 5% to 7% per degree centigrade and should be treated vigorously with acetaminophen and, if necessary, external cooling. Shivering should be avoided because it increases temperature and CO_2 production. **Hypothermia** lowers cerebral metabolism and may be beneficial in severe head injury. Modest hypothermia is reasonably well tolerated. A recent large-scale clinical trial reported improved outcomes, compared with normothermic patients, in patients with moderately severe traumatic brain injury (GCS 5–7) randomized to hypothermia (32°C to 33°C). More severely injured patients were not benefited. Because of physical discomfort and shivering, patients required paralysis and sedation, greatly complicating neurologic evaluation during hypothermia. **Excessive hypothermia** can be associated with hyperglycemia, increased peripheral vascular resistance, decreased cardiac output, ventricular fibrillation, increased blood viscosity, blunting of the febrile response to infection, increased affinity of hemoglobin for oxygen, acid base abnormalities, decreased gastric motility, and a rebound ICP increase during rewarming.

6. **Ventricular drainage** via ventriculostomy catheter can reduce ICP, especially in situations of outflow obstruction or malabsorption of CSF. Usually, however, drainage is of limited value because the ventricles are already collapsed by increased ICP. Several different approaches are available for continuous monitoring of ICP (Fig. 29-2). **Ventricular catheters** permit therapeutic CSF drainage; they are highly accurate and reproducible and permit CSF sampling for analysis and culture. They pose some risk of infection and require greater skill to place, particularly in patients with increased ICP and ventricular compression or shift. **Subarachnoid and fiberoptic intraparenchymal catheters** are less accurate and more expensive, but provide essential information about ICP with very low risk.

7. **Barbiturate** coma remains a treatment option for increased ICP that is refractory to other med-

ical therapy; although it reduces mortality, it may not improve functional outcome. Refractory elevations in ICP occur in approximately 10% of patients with severe head injury. Barbiturates are effective in lowering ICP in some of these patients, but cause low peripheral vascular tone, hypothermia, ileus, and myocardial depression; obliterate the neurologic examination; and obscure early signs of infection (such as fever). Systemic hypotension results, which requires prolonged vasopressor support. **Pentobarbital,** a short-acting barbiturate without active metabolites, rapidly suppresses neuronal metabolic activity. In patients with preserved autoregulation, reductions in metabolism lead to reductions in CBV and ICP. Lack of response to barbiturate therapy is a poor prognostic sign. Pentobarbital is initiated with a bolus of 3 to 7 mg/kg IV (typically 300–400 mg) and followed by intermittent boluses based on ICP goals or by maintenance IV infusion at 1 to 5 mg/kg/h. **Thiopental** (1–4 mg/kg IV) can be used repeatedly as needed to control ICP, or subsequently infused (4 mg/ml infusion mix) and titrated to desired effects on ICP and blood pressure. Maximal metabolic depression is correlated with a pattern of burst suppression on EEG, and only further toxicity is gained by achieving electrocerebral silence. Maintenance infusions may need to be adjusted frequently, because the pharmacokinetics rely on the volume of distribution into body lipid stores. The benefits of pentobarbital therapy are eliminated if sustained episodes of hypotension occur, and pulmonary artery catheters are often required to properly assess hemodynamics. No benefit has been shown for prophylactic barbiturate therapy. **Lidocaine,** generally at doses of 0.5 to 1.5 mg/kg IV, may be useful acutely to control intracranial hypertension in cases of hemodynamic instability and when barbiturate use is too risky.

8. **Head positioning** can influence ICP. Elevation at 30° to 45° improves cerebral venous drainage and may produce small reductions in ICP. Elevation also causes reductions in cerebral mean arterial pressure (MAP) and may actually lower CPP. Because of this, systemic arterial pressure transducers should be zeroed at the level of the external auditory meatus whenever CPP is being controlled and the patient's head is elevated. Rotation of the head can impede venous drainage and increase ICP.

9. **Positive end-expiratory pressure (PEEP)** may increase ICP in patients with very compliant lungs. The hemodynamic effects of PEEP depend on the developed transpulmonary pressure, which is a function of lung compliance. Pulmonary parenchy-

mal disease (e.g., pneumonia, aspiration, or acute respiratory distress syndrome) decreases pulmonary compliance and reduces the transmission of airway pressure. Consequently, the hemodynamic effects are relatively minimal at moderate levels (≤ 15 cm H_2O) of PEEP. Lungs with normal or increased compliance (e.g., emphysema) readily transmit airway pressure to the thorax. Peripheral venous return and cardiac output can decrease when PEEP is applied. Intravascular pressures that are referenced to atmospheric pressure do not account for the increased intrathoracic pressure and may overestimate ventricular filling. In such cases, the response of left ventricular stroke volume to a volume challenge may prove a better measure of adequate preload. Positive airway pressure also can produce minimal elevations in ICP because of transmission of pressure to the thoracic intervertebral spaces and the vena cava. Because the primary goal of hemodynamic management is to provide adequate tissue oxygenation and cerebral perfusion, however, PEEP should be applied as needed to maintain oxygenation, and compensatory measures (e.g., osmotic therapy) can be initiated if necessary.

10. **Sedation and, rarely, neuromuscular blockade** (Chapters 5 and 7) are required in some patients in whom spontaneous agitation or routine nursing care is associated with unacceptable elevations in ICP, which can be caused by coughing, Valsalva maneuvers, hiccups, discoordination with the ventilator, or sympathetic overactivity. The need for these agents should be continually reassessed; agents such as thiopental, propofol, or morphine sometimes can be used to premedicate patients prior to provocative procedures.

11. **Gastric hyperacidity.** The risk of upper gastrointestinal bleeding is increased by stress and corticosteroid use. Prophylaxis for upper gastrointestinal bleeding should be used in all cases (Chapter 25).

12. **Craniectomy** with duroplasty and resection of necrotic brain plays a limited, but critical, role in the management of refractory ICP. The risk of infection and the generally poor outcome in these patients require that the intervention be considered on a case-by-case basis. Postoperative ICP values can be unreliable and should be measured from the contralateral side or via ventriculostomy catheter. The reduction in ICP occurs to some extent because of extracranial herniation of brain through the skull defect. Some animal studies have suggested improved tissue perfusion following hemicraniectomy, presumably from alleviation of tissue and vascular compression.

13. **Pharmacotherapy** targeted against the secondary ischemic cascade may lead to improved outcomes in brain injury. Free radical scavengers, excitatory amino acid antagonists, growth factors, and opiate peptide antagonists are under investigation in the laboratory and in clinical trials. Results from randomized clinical trials may guide strategies for neuroprotection in the near future.

V. **Determination of death using brain criteria**

A. The medical and legal communities have indicated that locally acceptable guidelines are to be used for the diagnosis of death. Cardiac criteria for determination of death are well established. **Brain death** is defined as the irreversible loss of the clinical function of the whole brain, including the brainstem. Brain death from primary neurologic disease usually is caused by severe head injury or aneurysmal subarachnoid hemorrhage. Hypoxic-ischemic brain insults and fulminant hepatic failure also can result in irreversible loss of brain function. Brain death must be understood to be no different than a diagnosis of death made by other criteria. Guidelines do not replace the physician's judgment in individual cases, because brain death is a clinical diagnosis. It is imperative to distinguish brain death from a persistent vegetative state (i.e., absence of cerebral function with preserved vital functions); brain death is a diagnosis and not a prognostic statement. Diagnostic criteria for the **clinical diagnosis** of brain death in adults, adapted from those used at the Massachusetts General Hospital, are listed below. Other institutions may have different criteria.

B. Brain death is the absence of clinical whole brain function when the proximate cause is known and demonstrably irreversible. **Prerequisites** include:

1. Clinical or neuroimaging evidence of an acute CNS catastrophe that is compatible with the clinical diagnosis of brain death.

2. Exclusion of complicating medical conditions that can confound clinical assessment (e.g., severe electrolyte, acid-base or endocrine disturbance).

3. Toxicology screening with demonstrated barbiturate level less than 10 μg/ml and no evidence of drug intoxication or poisoning.

4. Demonstrated absence of neuromuscular blockade if the patient has had recent or prolonged use of neuromuscular blocking drugs.

5. Core temperature 32°C (90°F) or higher.

6. In the presence of confounding variables, brain death can still be determined with the aid of **ancillary tests** (see below). A period of observation of at least 24 hours without clinical neurologic change is necessary if the cause of the coma is unknown.

C. **Clinical syndrome.** The three cardinal findings in brain death are coma or unresponsiveness, absence of brainstem reflexes, and apnea.

1. **Coma or unresponsiveness** as determined by the absence of any cerebrally mediated motor response to pain in all extremities (nail-bed pressure and supraorbital pressure).
2. **Absence of brainstem reflexes** (all those listed below):
    a. **Pupils**
        (1) No response to bright light.
        (2) Size: from midposition (4 mm) to dilated (9 mm).
    b. **Ocular movement**
        (1) No oculocephalic reflex (tested only when fractures and instability of the cervical spine are absent).
        (2) No deviation of the eyes to irrigation in each ear with 30 to 50 ml of ice water. (Observe for 1 minute after each irrigation and at least 5 minutes between testing on each side).
    c. **Facial motor response to stimulation**
        (1) No corneal reflex to touch with a cotton swab.
        (2) No jaw reflex.
        (3) No facial grimacing to deep pressure on nail bed, supraorbital ridge, or temporomandibular joint.
    d. **Pharyngeal and tracheal reflexes.**
        (1) No response to stimulation of the posterior pharynx with tongue blade.
        (2) No coughing or significant bradyarrhythmia to bronchial suctioning.
3. **Apnea.** Apnea testing can be performed as follows:
    a. **Prerequisites:**
        (1) Core temperature 36.5°C or 97°F or higher, if possible.
        (2) Systolic blood pressure 90 mm Hg or greater, if possible.
        (3) Corrected diabetes insipidus or positive fluid balance in the past 6 hours.
        (4) $PaCO_2$ normal or 40 mm Hg or greater.
        (5) Arterial pH normal (7.35–7.45), if possible. Adjusting the ventilator to obtain a normal arterial pH and $PaCO_2$ prior to initiating the test minimizes time off the ventilator and decreases the risk of hypoxia or severe acidosis.
        (6) Preoxygenation with 100% FIO_2 for 5 minutes or to PaO_2 200 mm Hg or greater, if possible.
    b. **Connect a pulse oximeter.** Attach a catheter to an oxygen source and deliver 100% O_2 at 8 to 10 L/min via the endotracheal tube or tracheostomy to the level of the carina immediately after disconnecting the ventilator. Because most ventilators do not supply a steady flow of oxygen unless the ventilator is cycling,

in general, it is not adequate to leave the patient attached to the ventilator during the test.

   c.   **Observe closely for respiratory movements** (defined as abdominal or chest excursions that produce adequate tidal volumes). Chest wall excursions secondary to cardiac pulsations are not considered respiratory efforts. Arterial pH usually decreases by 0.02 units/min of apnea.

   d.   **Measure Pao_2, $Paco_2$, and arterial pH** after approximately 8 minutes and reconnect the ventilator. The apnea test must be terminated if the patient becomes cyanotic or hypotensive (see below).

   e.   **If respiratory movements are absent** and the final arterial blood gas analysis shows:

   (1)   Arterial pH 7.30 or less (from a patient with pretest pH of 7.4 or greater), **or**

   (2) $Paco_2$ greater than 60 mm Hg, **or**

   (3) $Paco_2$ increasing 20 mm Hg over the pretest baseline, **then apnea** has been demonstrated, supporting the diagnosis of brain death.

   f.   **If respiratory movements are observed or the blood gas criteria are not met, the apnea test result is negative.** Apnea has not been demonstrated and this does **not** support the clinical diagnosis of brain death. If during testing the patient becomes cyanotic, systolic blood pressure becomes 90 mm Hg or less, the pulse oximeter indicates significant oxygen desaturation or cardiac dysrhythmias develop, then immediately draw an arterial blood sample and reconnect the ventilator. If the blood gas values meet the criteria above (see section **V.C.3.e.**), then apnea has been demonstrated. If the blood gas values do not meet the criteria, the apnea test is indeterminate and additional confirmatory testing is necessary.

D.   **Pitfalls in the diagnosis of brain death.** The following conditions can interfere with the clinical diagnosis of brain death, so that the diagnosis cannot be made with certainty on clinical grounds alone. In such cases, confirmatory tests are recommended.

   1.   Severe facial trauma.

   2.   Preexisting pupillary abnormalities.

   3.   Toxic levels of any sedative drugs, aminoglycosides, tricyclic antidepressants, anticholinergics, antiepileptic drugs, chemotherapeutic agents, or neuromuscular blocking drugs.

   4.   Sleep apnea or severe pulmonary disease resulting in severe chronic retention of CO_2.

E.   **Clinical observations still compatible with the diagnosis of brain death.** These manifestations are seen occasionally and should not be misinterpreted as evidence for brainstem function.

1. Spontaneous "spinal" movements of limbs (not to be confused with pathologic flexion or extension response).
2. Respiratorylike movements (shoulder elevation and adduction, back arching, intercostal expansion without significant tidal volumes).
3. Sweating, blushing, tachycardia.
4. Normal blood pressure in the absence of pharmacologic support.
5. Absence of diabetes insipidus (i.e., normal osmolar control mechanism).
6. Deep tendon reflexes, triple flexion responses, or Babinski's reflex.

F. **Confirmatory laboratory tests supporting the diagnosis of brain death.** Brain death is a clinical diagnosis. Consider repeat clinical evaluation 6 hours later, but this interval is arbitrary. A confirmatory test is not mandatory but can be used as supportive data in those patients in whom specific components of clinical testing cannot be reliably performed or evaluated. Remember to write down the name of the physician interpreting the ancillary tests, as this will be needed in the Declaration of Death Note.

1. **Conventional angiography.** No intracerebral filling at the level of the carotid bifurcation or circle of Willis is observed. The external carotid circulation is patent, and filling of the superior sagittal sinus may be delayed.
2. **Electroencephalography.** No electrocerebral activity is present during at least 30 minutes of recording that adheres to the minimal technical criteria for EEG recording in suspected brain death as adopted by the American Electroencephalographic Society, including 16-channel EEG instruments. It should include the absence of nonartifactual activity, and no change should occur with auditory, visual, or painful stimulation. Electrocardiographic artifact should be visible. No need is seen for the patient to be normothermic, but core body temperature should be above 90°F. If an EEG is obtained, the absence of EEG activity should be confirmed by a neurologist prior to the declaration of brain death. This should be noted in the patient's medical record.
3. **Transcranial Doppler ultrasonography:**
   a. Small systolic peaks in early systole occurring without diastolic flow or with reverberating flow are indicative of very high vascular resistance associated with greatly increased intracranial pressure and lack of tissue blood flow.
   b. Previously documented Doppler signals are lost. Because 10% of patients may not have temporal windows that permit insonation, however, the **initial** absence of Doppler sig-

nals cannot be interpreted as consistent with brain death.

4. **Technetium-**99^m hexamethylpropyleneamine-oxime (HMPAO) brain scan: No uptake of isotope in brain parenchyma ("hollow skull phenomenon") occurs, as interpreted by a nuclear medicine physician.

5. **Somatosensory-evoked potentials.** The N20-P22 response with median nerve stimulation is absent bilaterally. The recordings should adhere to the minimal technical criteria for somatosensory evoked potentials recording in suspected brain death as adopted by the American Electroencephalographic Society.

G. **Medical record documentation.** The declaration of death by brain criteria should be documented in the medical record in a manner similar to any other declaration of death and include the following:

1. The time of declaration and name of the attending neurosurgeon or neurologist declaring brain death.

2. Cause and irreversibility of condition.

3. Absence of brainstem reflexes.

4. Absence of motor response to pain.

5. Absence of respiration by Paco$_2$ or pH criteria.

6. Justification for confirmatory testing if indicated, and results of confirmatory test(s) if performed with the name of the physician responsible for interpretation.

7. Results of repeat neurologic examinations, if performed.

8. Indication that the medical examiner was contacted, if appropriate.

SELECTED REFERENCES

An appraisal of the criteria of cerebral death:a summary statement: a collaborative study. *JAMA* 1977;237:982–986.

Chesnut RM, Prough DS. Critical care of severe head injury. *New Horizons* 1995;3:365–581.

Fisher CM, Kistler JP, Davis JM. Relation of cerebral vasospasm to subarachnoid hemorrhage visualized by computed tomographic scanning. *Neurosurgery* 1980;6:1–9.

Grady PA, Blaumanis OR. Physiologic parameters of the Cushing reflex. *Surg Neurol* 1988;29:454–461.

Lundberg N, Troupp H, Lorin H. Continuous recording and control of ventricular fluid pressure in neurosurgical practice. *Acta Psychiatr Neurol Scand* 1960;36(Suppl 149):1–193.

Marion DW, Penrod LE, Kelsey SF, et al. Treatment of traumatic brain injury with moderate hypothermia. *N Eng J Med* 1997;336:540–546.

Mayberg MR, Batjer HH, Dacey R, et al. Guidelines for the management of aneurysmal subarachnoid hemorrhage. A statement for healthcare professionals from a special writing group of the Stroke Council, American Heart Association. *Circulation* 1994;90:2592–2605.

President's Commission for the Study of Ethical Problems in Medicine and Biomedical and Behavioral Research. Guidelines for the determination of death. *JAMA* 1981;246:2184–2186.

Rordorf G, Cramer SC, Efird JT, et al. Pharmacological elevation of blood pressure in acute stroke. Clinical effects and safety. *Stroke* 1997;28:2133–2138.

Rosner MJ, Becker DP. Origin and evolution of plateau waves. *J Neurosurg* 1984;60:312–324.

Rosner MJ, Coley I. Cerebral perfusion pressure, intracranial pressure and head elevation. *J Neurosurg* 1986;65:636–641.

Rosner MJ, Coley I. Cerebral perfusion pressure: a hemodynamic mechanism of mannitol and the postmannitol hemogram. *J Neurosurg* 1987;21:147–156.

Rosner MJ, Daughton S. Cerebral perfusion pressure management in head injury. *J Trauma* 1990;30:933–941.

Schwamm LH, Finklestein S. Infratentorial ischemic syndromes. In: Batjer HH, Caplan LR, Friberg L, et al, eds. *Cerebrovascular disease.* New York: Lippincott-Raven, 1997:347–377.

Acute Neuromuscular Weakness, Spinal Cord Injuries, and Brain Tumors

David Greer, Mustapha Ezzeddine, and Lee H. Schwamm

I. **Weakness**
   A. **Disorders of muscle** typically cause weakness in proximal muscle groups. Defects at the **neuromuscular junction** affect the cranial, limb girdle, and proximal muscles, and can disproportionately affect respiratory muscles. When the lesion is presynaptic, a postexertional increase in strength (e.g., Eaton-Lambert) may arise, whereas when the lesion is postsynaptic, postexertional fatigue (e.g., myasthenia) occurs. **Peripheral nerve** lesions can cause weakness, sensory symptoms, dysautonomia, and depressed deep tendon reflexes. Focal symptoms (nerve compression) or distal symmetric symptoms (toxic neuropathies) may be seen.
   1. **Lower motor neuron and acute upper motor neuron injuries** cause flaccidity and areflexia, whereas **chronic upper motor neuron injury** causes spasticity and hyperreflexia.
   2. **A focused history** should review preexisting neuromuscular or systemic diseases, current medications, illicit drug use, travel, potential envenomations or neurotoxin exposures, and accompanying sensory or autonomic symptoms.
   3. **Laboratory evaluation** should include complete blood count with eosinophil count, erythrocyte sedimentation rate (to aid in diagnosis of vasculitis and myositis), liver function tests, blood urea nitrogen, creatinine, urinalysis, electrolytes, calcium, magnesium, phosphorus, creatine phosphokinase, antiacetylcholine receptor antibody (to diagnose myasthenia), chest radiography (to detect paraneoplastic small cell lung cancer), and electrophysiologic studies, if needed to localize the lesion.
   B. **Myopathy.** Hypokalemia, hyperkalemia, alcohol, chronic steroid use, mechanical or thermal trauma (rhabdomyolysis), immobility, connective tissue disease (dermatomyositis, polymyositis), infection (trichinosis), and critical illness can cause acute muscle injury or dysfunction. Electromyography (EMG) and muscle biopsy are often needed to establish the correct diagnosis and treatment plan. **Critical care myopathy,** which occurs in the setting of sepsis, neuromuscular blockade, and corticosteroids, produces a

selective loss of myosin filaments without focal muscle cell necrosis. Electromyography is characterized by excitation–contraction uncoupling in muscle, without widespread spontaneous activity (fibrillation potentials), and with preserved sensory conduction. Recovery generally occurs in 6 to 12 weeks. A **necrotic myopathy variant** with severe paralysis and diffuse fibrillation potentials and an **axonal sensorimotor neuropathy** variant of critical illness weakness have been described, both with a considerably poorer prognosis. Both immobility and corticosteroid use can produce weakness associated with muscle atrophy (predominantly type II fiber loss) and preserved EMG and nerve conduction. These respond well to discontinuation of steroids and aggressive mobilization.

C. **Neuropathy** can be **axonal** or **demyelinating.** Causes include Guillian-Barré syndrome (GBS), tick bite, diphtheria, porphyria, hypophosphatemia, critical illness, rapid sodium correction (central pontine myelinolysis), and arsenic or shellfish poisoning.

1. **Axonal neuropathy** is a diffuse, symmetric sensorimotor polyneuropathy prominently affecting the most distant axons (stocking and glove distribution). Common causes include diabetes mellitus, neurotoxins, sepsis, chemotherapy (oncologic agents, metronidazole, antituberculous agents), vitamin deficiencies (B_{12}, niacin, E), heavy metals (arsenic, thallium), uremia, dysproteinemias, leprosy, and sarcoidosis. With the exception of critical illness polyneuropathy, these rarely reflect acute neuronal injury and have little impact on critical care management. Delayed blink responses on EMG with preserved ventilatory muscle function are suggestive of a demyelinating component.

2. **Motor neuronopathy** usually results from **amyotrophic lateral sclerosis** or **poliomyelitis** [mostly in the developing world or in patients infected with the human immunodeficiency virus (HIV) with inadvertent exposure to shed liveattenuated polio vaccine].

   a. **ALS** presents with generalized weakness, atrophy, brisk reflexes, and fasciculations. Symptoms may be asymmetric. Oropharyngeal weakness and ventilatory failure inevitably occur. The EMG shows fibrillation potentials in two or more limbs in a pattern inconsistent with peripheral nerve or cord injury. Differential diagnosis includes severe cervical myelopathy, base of skull lesions, heavy metal poisoning, and autoimmune neuropathy. Treatment is supportive.

   b. **Poliomyelitis** presents as an acute febrile illness with asymmetric flaccid paralysis of the limbs, trunk and lower cranial nerves, and occasionally with respiratory failure, pain, and paresthesias. It can produce aseptic meningitis with cerebrospinal fluid (CSF) mononuclear pleocytosis. Treatment is supportive.

3. **Demyelinating neuropathy** is most often caused by **Guillain Barré syndrome** (acute inflammatory demyelinating polyneuropathy). It occurs 1 to 3 weeks after viral respiratory or diarrheal illnesses or immunization; it is characterized by progressive ascending paraparesis, areflexia, distal paresthesias, and low back pain. In severe cases, bulbar and respiratory weakness may be seen, which is maximal at 3 weeks after onset and requires mechanical ventilation in 20% of cases. Autonomic involvement is common and patients may require cardiac monitoring. Infection with *Campylobacter jejuni* may be present in 25% of cases. Segmental demyelination produces slowing and conduction block on electrodiagnostic studies and acellular CSF with elevated protein.

a. **Treatment with plasmapheresis** reduces the duration of mechanical ventilation and intensive care unit (ICU) care. This is the treatment preferred in the United States over intravenous (IV) gamma globulin. Standard therapy is five exchanges, each of 2 to 4 L over 90 to 120 minutes with 5% albumin repletion, over alternate days. Contraindications to plasma exchange include sepsis, myocardial infarction within the last 6 months, marked dysautonomia, and active bleeding. Side effects from treatment include vasovagal reactions, hypovolemia, anaphylaxis, hemolysis, air embolism, hematoma, hypocalcemia, thrombocytopenia, postpheresis infection, hypothermia, and hypokalemia.

b. **IV gamma globulin** (IVIG) treatment does not require the placement of central access; it does not produce hemodynamic instability and is less expensive than plasmapheresis. The dose is 0.4 g/kg/d for 5 days. Potential complications include aseptic meningitis, anaphylaxis (especially in IgA-deficient individuals), acute renal failure, and thromboembolic events (including ischemic stroke). Some studies have suggested a higher relapse rate with IVIG in comparison with plasmapheresis.

c. **Corticosteroids have no role** in the treatment of GBS.

d. **Nonpulmonary causes for ICU admission** include dysautonomia with cardiac dysrhythmia or fluctuations in blood pressure, chest pain or hypotension with plasma exchange, pulmonary embolism, or anaphylaxis. **Dysautonomia** is one of the most frequent causes of morbidity and mortality in patients with

GBS. Dysautonomia is manifested as supraventricular cardiac dysrhythmias and rapidly fluctuating blood pressure. Most fluctuations are best left untreated, but volume resuscitation may be needed. As with all weak patients, early attention to patient positioning and use of splints and braces help prevent bedsores and contractures. Acute pain is managed with nonsteroidal antiinflammatory drugs and narcotics (Chapter 6). Neuropathic pain during the recovery phase can be treated with amitriptyline or mexiletine, although mexiletine is contraindicated in patients with dysautonomia. All patients should receive subcutaneous heparin prophylaxis for deep venous thrombosis, ulcer protection with acid suppression, and aggressive clearance of pulmonary secretions. An Asiatic epidemic variant is also associated with *Campylobacter* organisms, but it causes purely axonal injury. A chronic inflammatory demyelinating polyneuropathy variant is also recognized, which can present more gradually and responds well to immunotherapy.

4. **Central pontine myelinolysis** is a rare disorder seen after rapid correction of hyponatremia that has been present for at least 48 hours. It is likely caused by osmotically mediated intracellular injury in oligodendroglia that had excreted osmotically active particles to maintain their cell volume during the hyponatremic (and hypoosmolar) state. Electromyographic and nerve conduction studies are normal. Lesions are best seen on magnetic resonance (MR) imaging, and patients appear to be "locked in" or deafferented. Prognosis is poor.

D. **Neuromuscular junction (NMJ)** transmission can be inhibited by myasthenic syndromes, botulism, hypermagnesemia, organophosphate poisoning, and prolonged effects of paralytic agents.

1. **Myasthenia gravis** is an autoimmune disease with autoantibodies directed against the acetylcholine receptor (in approximately 80% of cases). Typically, symptoms increase in severity within the first 3 years of onset, and are punctuated by spontaneous, brief remissions. Common presenting signs include ophthalmoparesis, ptosis, jaw weakness, limb weakness, and progressive respiratory failure. The most common reason for ICU admission is **myasthenic crisis** with respiratory decompensation, usually triggered by viral infection, surgery, childbirth, or exacerbating medication. The EMG demonstrates a 10% or greater reduction of the compound muscle action potential amplitude between the first and the fourth responses with supramaximal stimulation and increased jitter and

blocking on single-fiber analysis. The anticholinergic drug, **pyridostigmine,** usually provides symptomatic improvement. **Cholinergic excess** must be excluded whenever clinical decompensation occurs. Signs of cholinergic excess include miosis (myasthenic crisis produces *mydriasis*), thick pulmonary secretions, muscle fasciculations, abdominal cramping, diarrhea, sweating and lacrimation, and symptomatic worsening with Tensilon (edrophonium) challenge. Cholinergic crisis can increase oral and bronchial secretions, which can complicate airway management.

2. **Medications that impair NMJ transmission** should be avoided whenever possible, including particular antibiotics (clindamycin, colistin, kanamycin, neomycin, streptomycin, tobramycin, tetracycline, gentamicin, polymyxin B, bacitracin, trimethoprim–sulfamethoxazole), hormones (corticotropin, thyroid hormone, oral contraceptives), cardiovascular agents (quinidine, propranolol, procainamide, practolol, lidocaine, verapamil, nifedipine, diltiazem), psychotropic agents (chlorpromazine, promazine, phenelzine, lithium, diazepam), anticonvulsants (phenytoin, trimethadione, carbamazepine), paralytics, and miscellaneous agents (penicillamine, chloroquine).

3. **Treatment of serious exacerbations** can include a continuous IV infusion of **pyridostigmine, plasmapheresis** (10–20 L exchange over 1–2 weeks) or **immunoglobulin therapy.** High-dose corticosteroids, although effective in the longer term, can cause acute worsening in the short term. Endotracheal intubation and mechanical ventilation usually are required when vital capacity falls below 15 ml/kg, is decreasing rapidly, or airway protection is compromised.

II. **Traumatic spinal cord injury.** More than 90% of patients with traumatic spinal cord injury (SCI) survive the initial hospitalization. Respiratory complications account for half the nonacute deaths of patients with complete quadriplegia. Of the 10,000 patients seen annually with SCI, 82% are male (mean age 31). Of these, 45% are caused by motor vehicle crashes, 22% by falls, and 16% by acts of violence. Associated trauma to the head and chest is common. Life-threatening complications can occur immediately or secondary to progression of the lesion; they include acute respiratory failure, hemodynamic shock, cardiac dysrhythmias, hypothermia and poikilothermia, infection, and skin ulceration.

A. **Cervical spine stabilization** (Chapter 33)
1. Spine stabilization is achieved through immobilization by first responders and stabilization by orthopedic devices such as a Halo thoracic vest or Gardner, Wells, or Crutchfield tongs. A cervical hard collar does not fully immobilize the neck and

should be treated as a reminder of the potential for cervical cord injury. Emergent surgical decompression is indicated in the early hours after SCI when hematoma or bone fragments impinge on viable spinal cord tissue despite maximal traction or immobilization procedures. Anterior or posterior surgical fusion of the spine and external fixation (e.g., Philadelphia collar, Halo thoracic vest) may be indicated in the acute or subacute setting.

2. Spine stabilization is monitored in the ICU. The traction forces are often reduced when neck muscle spasm secondary to the injury decreases and alignment is satisfactory. On rare occasions, quadriparesis resolves with adequate realignment. While the patient is in traction, the head, neck, and thorax are **log-rolled** or moved as a unit. A rotating platform bed can be used to maintain stable alignment while reducing the risk of decubitus ulcers and improving clearance of pulmonary secretions.

B. **Neuroprotection**
   1. **Serial neurologic assessment with accurate charting of the motor and sensory levels** of function is essential to distinguish nerve root damage from SCI. Neurologic examinations should be performed hourly for the first 24 hours. If the level of the lesion is stable, assessment frequency can be decreased progressively. Any worsening in the examination mandates an immediate investigation of the cause.

   2. **High-dose corticosteroids** may improve the functional outcome of some patients with acute spinal cord injury. For patients presenting within 8 hours of the injury, **methylprednisolone** (30 mg/kg IV) over 15 minutes is administered, followed 45 minutes later by an infusion (5.4 mg/kg IV) for 23 hours. If the patient presents within 3 hours of the injury, additional benefit may be obtained by continuing the infusion for a total of 48 hours. If subacute or acute spinal cord dysfunction is thought to be secondary to neoplastic involvement of the cord rather than trauma, **dexamethasone** (100 mg) IV bolus should be given initially, followed by 10 mg IV every 6 hours.

   3. **Spinal shock,** which refers to dysfunction of spinal cord elements remote to the site of injury, is characterized by flaccid paralysis, areflexia, and bowel and bladder atony. Resolution is accompanied by return of spinal reflexes (e.g., spasticity, muscle spasm, and autonomic dysreflexia) below the level of injury. The simplest example of this is the loss of sacral reflexes (controlled by sacral neurons) in the setting of severe cervical SCI. In acute SCI patients with an absent bulbocavernosus reflex, the level of permanent neurologic

dysfunction cannot be determined and may be better than suggested by the initial examination. If any strength or sensation is present below the level of the bony lesion on initial examination, then the spinal cord is only partially injured and considerable recovery can be expected. Conversely, in the absence of strength or sensation, return of reflex activity below the level of the cord lesion is not a good prognostic sign.

4. **Root and plexus injury** can coexist with SCI and produce overlapping deficits. By comparing the level of vertebral bony injury with the level of sensorimotor dysfunction, the contributions from nerve root or plexus damage can sometimes be separated from those of cord damage. Electrophysiologic studies are useful in the subacute period to distinguish cord, root, plexus, and peripheral nerve contributions.

C. **Respiratory management**
   1. **Respiratory muscle weakness.** With complete cervical cord lesions at or below C6 and in the absence of pulmonary contusions, respiratory function is usually unaffected. With lesions at or above C4, diaphragmatic function (roots C3, C4, C5) is impaired. Clinical signs include paradoxical breathing with enhanced excursions of the abdomen, paradoxical inspiratory retraction of the rib cage, and loss of all active expiratory muscular function. This loss of diaphragmatic and intercostal muscle function causes loss of all expiratory reserve capacity and decreases vital capacity, functional residual capacity, thoracopulmonary compliance, and strength for coughing and secretion clearance. The absence of dyspnea should not be reassuring, because it usually occurs only when forced vital capacity (FVC) falls below 1 L (15 ml/kg). Atelectasis can produce hypoxemia in the acute postinjury period.

   2. **Chest physical therapy** should be instituted early to prevent respiratory complications. A rotating kinetic bed can be useful, safely providing postural drainage. If a Stryker frame is used, a nurse should be at the bedside to observe for respiratory insufficiency while the patient is prone. In this position, the upper chest and pubis should be on pads to minimize abdominal pressure, thereby allowing diaphragmatic excursion. Assisted abdominal compression cough maneuvers (quad coughing) and postural drainage may assist in clearing secretions. Therapeutic fiberoptic bronchoscopy can be invaluable if conservative measures are ineffective.

   3. **The spinal cord lesion can ascend** from below C4 to above C4, producing progressive ventilatory dysfunction and respiratory failure. Thus, the

unintubated acute quadriplegic requires close monitoring. Serial assessments of ventilatory rate, tidal volume, FVC, maximal negative inspiratory force, and arterial blood gas tensions are useful to assess deterioration. Vital capacity is initially checked hourly. If the trend suggests deterioration or if secretion clearance becomes problematic, endotracheal intubation should be performed prior to overt respiratory failure (see Chapter 3, Airway Management; Chapter 4, Mechanical Ventilation).

4. **Pulmonary embolism (PE),** with a peak incidence at 7 to 10 days following injury, is a significant risk and cause of death. Risk factors include venous stasis, immobilization, and hypercoagulability. Prophylactic heparin treatment (5,000 U subcutaneously every 12 hours or an equivalent dose of low molecular weight heparin) should be used for 8 to 12 weeks unless contraindicated by other injuries (Chapters 12 and 21).

5. **Infection.** Early diagnosis of infection can be challenging, because the traditional signs and symptoms can be distorted. Poikilothermia, blunted hemodynamic reflexes, decreased venous vascular resistance, and borderline hypotension from sympathetic dysfunction cloak the signs of early sepsis. Corticosteroid therapy often produces striking elevations in peripheral leukocyte counts, although delayed elevations can signify occult infection. Surveillance sputum Gram's stains and cultures may identify bacterial colonization and provide data for preliminary empiric antibiotic therapy when chest radiographs suggest consolidation.

D. **Cardiovascular management**
1. **Compromise of sympathetic outflow** from T1 to L2 spinal segments occurs in complete cervical SCI.
   a. The acute injury causes massive sympathetic discharge and produces a brief period of hypertension, widened pulse pressure, and tachycardia. Pulmonary capillary stress fractures can occur during this time, producing pulmonary edema that persists after resolution of the sympathetic state. Interruption of descending fibers in the intermediolateral cell column that activate the preganglionic sympathetic nerves can produce **hemodynamic shock secondary to SCI,** with hypotension, bradycardia, and peripheral vasodilation. Without sympathetically mediated venoconstriction, hypotension can occur with as little as a 5% reduction in central venous volume. **Monitoring** of urine output, arterial blood pressure, cardiac rhythm, and central venous pressure (CVP) is essential.

b. **Hypotension should always be investigated,** although it is usually caused by decreased left ventricular end-diastolic volume associated with increased venous capacitance. With pulmonary edema or when the cause of the hypotension is unclear, pulmonary artery catheterization and measurement of cardiac output and stroke volume are indicated. The patient should be kept supine. The goal for blood pressure management is to avoid hypotension, which can exacerbate ischemic injury, and, as in treatment of brain injury, maintain a mean arterial pressure (or cerebral perfusion pressure, as appropriate) of at least 60 mm Hg (Chapter 11).

c. **Fluid resuscitation.** Initially, CVP rises little in response to volume (because of fully dilated capacitance vessels), but then it can rise abruptly. Hypotension unresponsive to fluids necessitates the use of vasopressors.

d. **Adrenergic agonists** commonly are used to treat spinal shock. Alpha agonists (e.g., **phenylephrine**) increase systemic vascular resistance, but can produce reflex bradycardia. Agonists with both α and β activity (e.g., **norepinephrine, dopamine**) increase systemic vascular resistance while providing inotropic and chronotropic support.

2. **Bradycardia** is expected in severe cervical SCI; it is most prevalent in the first 10 days and usually resolves after 2 to 6 weeks. It is rare in lower or incomplete lesions. Significant hypotension and even asystole can occur, particularly during unopposed vagal stimuli such as tracheal suctioning, chest physiotherapy, or rectal care. Pretreatment with atropine (0.4–2.0 mg) IV may prevent hypotension, although it can exacerbate paralytic ileus. With bradycardia refractory to vagolytics, an infusion of isoproterenol or dopamine, or temporary cardiac pacing should be considered. Most bradydysrythmias resolve spontaneously. Permanent pacemakers are rarely indicated and may interfere with future attempts at diaphragmatic pacing for assisted ventilation.

3. **Autonomic dysreflexia** is characterized by paroxysmal severe hypertension, sweating, facial flushing, nasal congestion, and headache in response to visceral autonomic stimulation. The hypertension is refractory to treatment, and hypertensive crisis can occur if the viscus is not decompressed. Autonomic dysreflexia seldom occurs before spinal shock has resolved. Regular bladder and bowel care (including intermittent catheterization and laxatives) and muscle relaxants help prevent these crises.

E. **Temperature regulation.** Disordered temperature regulation, which results from sympathetic dysfunction, is most common with lesions at T8 or above. With the interruption of normal homeothermic mechanisms of sweating and vasodilation, poikilothermia ensues. Close attention to routes of heat loss and conservation (e.g., room temperature, blankets, use of forced air warmers) is usually sufficient to control body temperature.

F. **Gastrointestinal management**
   1. **Undiagnosed abdominal catastrophes**—the third leading cause of death in quadriplegic patients after the acute phase—are responsible for 10% of fatalities. Assessment of abdominal injury is difficult, as sensory loss or cognitive impairment can obscure signs of peritonitis. Intraabdominal pathology may be signaled by autonomic signs (e.g., persistent nausea, vomiting, tachycardia, bradycardia) or diaphragmatic pain referred to the shoulders or cervical region.
   2. **Ileus** is frequently present with cervical or thoracic spine lesions. Ileus can predispose to aspiration and reduce functional residual capacity (FRC), especially in the supine position. Nasogastric decompression reduces the risk of aspiration and gastric distention. With resolution of the ileus, the nasogastric tube can be used for nutrition support, which should begin as soon as possible.
   3. **Fecal impaction** is a major cause of autonomic dysreflexia. It should be prevented with regular use of stool softeners and judicious use of rectal suppositories and enemas. The aim of bowel care is to obtain patient-controlled reflex evacuation. Rectal care in the acute phase can precipitate bradycardia and hypotension.
   4. **Gastrointestinal hemorrhage** caused by **stress ulceration** is a major complication in quadriplegic patients, typically occurring 10 to 14 days postinjury. It is caused in part by unopposed parasympathetic activity, which enhances glandular acid secretion. It may be more common in patients who receive corticosteroids. The risk of hemorrhage is reduced by the prophylactic use of antacids, H_2 blockers, sucralfate, or omeprazole.

G. **Bladder care.** Urinary retention occurs after spinal injury and can cause autonomic dysreflexia. Bladder catheterization should be done to avoid retention and to monitor urine output. Intermittent bladder catheterization, initially every 4 to 6 hours, can be performed once the patient is stable.

H. **Skin care.** The position of paralyzed or anesthetic body parts should be changed at least every 2 hours. A rotating kinetic bed can be used to turn a patient automatically. Specialized foam mattresses, horizontally rotating frames, or sheepskin (clean and dry) also can be used. Heels and elbows should be well padded. Meticulous skin care is essential, especially in perineal and sacral areas. Vulnerable skin (e.g., under the edge of a cast or brace) must be checked frequently.

I. **Rehabilitation.** Physical, occupational, and psychological or cognitive rehabilitation efforts involving the patient, family, and friends (when appropriate) are started in the acute phase. Range-of-motion extremity exercises are begun soon after admission; after sufficient spinal stability has been achieved, upper extremity resistance exercises are begun. Splinting should be instituted early to prevent development of contractures.

III. **Brain tumors.** Intracranial tumors can arise anywhere inside the cranial vault, and can be primary to the brain or meninges or metastatic from cancer elsewhere.

A. **Epidemiology.** Brain tumors are second only to stroke as a cause of death from neurologic disease. The incidence is estimated at 15/100,000 population per year. In adults, most primary brain tumors are supratentorial, including low- to high-grade gliomas (50%), meningiomas (25%, higher in women), primary central nervous system (CNS) lymphoma, and others. In children, most primary brain tumors are infratentorial, including cerebellar astrocytomas (20%), medulloblastomas (20%), brainstem gliomas (15%), and ependymomas (10%). Metastatic intracranial tumors are found in 25% of cancer patients who come to autopsy. Commonly, metastasizing tumors include those from lung, breast, gastrointestinal tract, and melanoma.

B. **Clinical symptoms** are determined by the location of the lesion, presence of hemorrhage or seizure, and degree of edema or ventricular obstruction. Patients can present with focal symptoms, generalized symptoms, or false localizing symptoms when tissue shifts produce focal symptoms at a distance. Low-grade supratentorial tumors are more likely to present with seizures, whereas high-grade gliomas are more likely to present with focal (e.g., hemiparesis) or generalized signs (e.g., headache, lethargy, decreased level of consciousness). Lymphomas typically cause more behavioral changes, given their predilection for the limbic structures. Slowly growing tumors (e.g., meningiomas) are more likely to cause falsely localizing symptoms. Posterior fossa tumors often cause cranial nerve or cerebellar signs, but can also cause headache, nausea, vomiting, and papilledema because of early obstruction of the ventricular system. Headaches are more common in those patients with rapidly growing tumors, especially those that cause hydrocephalus. Compression or traction on pain-sensitive structures (e.g., blood vessels) most likely causes the pain of the headaches, which are often bifrontal or bitemporal and nonthrobbing. Focal or generalized seizures occur in

20% to 50% of patients with brain tumors. When focal, the seizure localizes the tumor. Seizures can cause secondary brain injury if the associated increase in blood flow increases intracranial pressure leading to herniation. Status epilepticus is a common cause of death in brain tumor patients.

C. **Acute evaluation.** Computed tomography (CT) and MR imaging with contrast agents are used to identify brain tumors. Screening for occult deep venous thrombosis is necessary because of increased risk in brain tumor patients.

D. **Acute treatment.** Most intracranial tumors initially are treated with surgery. Exceptions include brainstem gliomas, primary CNS lymphomas, and multiple metastases, which usually are treated with radiation therapy, chemotherapy, or both.

1. **Prophylactic anticonvulsants** should be used in the preoperative period. **Mass effect** should be treated immediately with corticosteroids (e.g., dexamethasone), except if primary CNS lymphoma is suspected. Corticosteroids can alter the lymphoma pathology and can obscure up to 40% of tumors on radiography. In any patient at risk of **herniation**, large doses of dexamethasone (10–100 mg IV in adults) should be given in addition to osmotic therapy with mannitol (50–100 g IV over 15 minutes in the adult). In the setting of imminent herniation and coma, hyperventilation should be performed as a temporary measure until other therapies are instituted.

2. **Complications of steroid therapy** include steroid-induced hyperglycemia, gastric ulceration, infection, adrenocortical insufficiency, myopathy, insomnia, hallucinations, psychosis, seizures, and avascular necrosis of the hip. **Surgical complications** include air embolism (25% in patients operated on in the sitting position), blood loss, disseminated intravascular coagulation, tension pneumocephalus, arterial or venous injury, and cranial nerve injury. **Air embolism** can cause right ventricular failure and cardiogenic shock. Aspiration of air from a pulmonary artery or central venous catheter is diagnostic and often therapeutic, but not always possible. Acute treatment includes stopping further entrainment of air, administration of 100% oxygen, use of inotropes such as norepinephrine to maintain blood pressure, and, if possible, placement of the patient in the left lateral decubitus position. Pulmonary infarction can occur, as can cerebral infarction if a patent foramen ovale is present and paradoxical embolization occurs. Hyperbaric oxygenation treatment may be useful if symptoms persist.

E. **Subacute therapy**

1. The head usually is elevated to 15° from horizontal in the immediate postoperative period. This position reduces intracranial pressure (ICP) without significantly decreasing cerebral perfusion pressure.

2. Postoperative **hematomas** are associated with tumor type (more common with meningiomas), subtotal resection, and hypertension. Blood pressure control must always occur in the context of management of cerebral perfusion pressure (Chapter 11). Postoperative **cerebral edema** starts hours after surgery and peaks at 36 to 72 hours after surgery. It presents as a delayed clinical deterioration following resection. Edema may be secondary to brain traction, ischemic injury, peritumoral inflammation, or fluid shifts.

3. **Venous infarction** occurs after acute occlusion of the superior sagittal sinus or from sacrifice of a major draining vein. If the sinus is occluded by tumor, it can usually be ligated because collateral circulation has usually developed. MR venography is useful to detect thrombosis of the cerebral venous circulation.

4. **Fluid and electrolyte abnormalities** can occur from inappropriate secretion of antidiuretic hormone (SIADH) or neurogenic diabetes insipidus. Patients, particularly those at risk for diabetes insipidus, include those having surgery of the hypothalamic-pituitary axis or with diffuse axonal injury to the brain. Pitressin is the treatment of choice, but patients with prolonged diabetes insipidus can be started on intranasal desmopressin (DDAVP) (see Chapter 26 for diagnosis and management).

5. **Deep venous thrombosis and pulmonary embolism** are major causes of morbidity and mortality in brain tumor patients, especially in the immediate postoperative period when they are immobile (see Chapter 22 for diagnosis and management).

6. **Fever** is associated with increased brain edema and must be treated aggressively in brain tumor patients.

7. **Surgical infections** are typically caused by *Staphylococcus aureus* and *Staphylococcus epidermidis*. Prophylactic antibiotics such as nafcillin, cefazolin, and vancomycin are effective.

8. **Persistent CSF leaks** typically cause fever and headache, and increase the risk for bacterial meningitis. No proven role for prophylactic antibiotics is seen in these cases. It is more common with surgery at the base of the skull or transsphenoidal resection of pituitary tumors. Fluid draining from the nose or ears should be tested for glucose,

because only CSF (and not mucus) contains glucose. Treatment is via passive closure after placement of a lumbar CSF drain, but surgical reclosure of the dura may be required.

SELECTED REFERENCES

Albert TJ, Levine MJ, Balderston RA, et al. Gastrointestinal complications in spinal cord injury. *Spine* 1991;16:S522–S525.

Atkinson PP, Atkinson JL. Spinal shock. *Mayo Clin Proc* 1996;71: 384–389.

Bergofsky EH. Mechanism for respiratory insufficiency after cervical cord injury. *Am Rev Respir Dis* 1964;61:435–447.

Bergofsky EH. Respiratory failure in disorders of the thoracic cage. *Am Rev Respir Dis* 1979;119:643–669.

Black PM. Brain tumors (2 parts). *N Engl J Med* 1991;324:1471– 1476; 1555–1564.

Bracken MB, Shepard MJ, Collins WF, et al. A randomized, controlled trial of methylprednisolone or naloxone in the treatment of acute spinal-cord injury. Results of the Second National Acute Spinal Cord Injury Study. *N Eng J Med* 1990;322:1405–1411.

Bracken MB, Shepard MJ, Holford TR, et al. Administration of methylprednisolone for 24 or 48 hours or tirilazad mesylate for 48 hours in the treatment of acute spinal cord injury. Results of the Third National Acute Spinal Cord Injury Randomized Controlled Trial. National Acute Spinal Cord Injury Study. *JAMA* 1997;277: 1597–1604.

Case records of the Massachusetts General Hospital. Weekly clinicopathological exercises. Case 11-1997. A 51-year-old man with chronic obstructive pulmonary disease and generalized muscle weakness. *N Engl J Med* 1997;336:1079–1088.

Chiles BW, Cooper PR. Acute spinal injury. *N Eng J Med* 1996;334: 514–520.

Ditunno Jr JF, Formal CS. Chronic spinal cord injury. *N Engl J Med* 1994;330:550–556.

Epstein N, Hood DC, Ransohoff J. Gastrointestinal bleeding in patients with spinal cord trauma. Effects of steroids, cimetidine, and minidose heparin. *J Neurosurg* 1981;54:16–20.

Green D, Hull RD, Mammen EF, et al. Deep vein thrombosis in spinal cord injury. Summary and recommendations. *Chest* 1992;102: 633S–635S.

Green D. Prophylaxis of thromboembolism in spinal cord injured patients. *Chest* 1992;102:649S–651S.

Krieger D, Adams HP, Schwarz S, et al. Prognostic and clinical relevance of pupillary responses, intracranial pressure monitoring, and brainstem auditory evoked potentials in comatose patients with acute supratentorial mass lesions. *Crit Care Med* 1993;21: 1944–1950.

Ledsome JR, Sharp JM. Pulmonary function in acute cervical cord injury. *Am Rev Respir Dis* 1981;124:41–44.

Lehmann KG, Lane JG, Piepmeier JM, et al. Cardiovascular abnormalities accompanying acute spinal cord injury in humans: incidence, time course and severity. *J Am Coll Cardiol* 1987;10:46–52.

Mathias CJ, Christensen NJ, Corbett JL, et al. Plasma catecholamines during paroxysmal neurogenic hypertension in quadriplegic man. *Circ Res* 1976;39:204–208.

Ropper A. *Neurological and neurosurgical intensive care,* 3rd ed. New York: Raven Press, 1993.

Soderstrom CA, McArdle DQ, Ducker TB, et al. The diagnosis of intraabdominal injury in patients with cervical cord trauma. *J Trauma* 1983;23:1061–1065.

Zipnick RI, Scalea TM, Trooskin SZ, et al. Hemodynamic responses to penetrating spinal cord injuries. *J Trauma* 1993;35:578–583.

Drug Overdose, Poisoning, and Adverse Drug Reactions

Richard M. Pino

I. Introduction

A. **Drug overdosed or poisoned** patients are frequently cared for in the intensive care unit (ICU). Although an overdose of prescription or nonprescription drugs might poison (i.e., injure or kill cells), "poisoning" is reserved for compounds not used for therapy and for animal toxins. Drug overdose and poisoning might be iatrogenic (e.g., coagulopathy secondary to warfarin during adjustment), secondary to intentional (e.g., suicide attempt) or unintentional (e.g., a child taking his grandmother's digitalis) ingestion of a drug, an animal bite (e.g., rattle snake), inhalation (e.g., carbon monoxide), or as a result of substance abuse (e.g., cocaine). This chapter presents the most common intoxications and how they are treated in the ICU.

B. **Initial treatment and stabilization** might include cardiopulmonary support, administration of an antidote, beginning the elimination of an ingested drug by gastrointestinal (GI) decontamination with activated charcoal, and the initial correction of acid-base alterations. The intensivist needs to understand the sequelae of each drug taken in overdose.

C. In viewing the innumerable drugs and poisonous substances, the physician should be familiar with reference resources in each institution and the telephone number of the area **poison control center.** Hospitals often have readily available texts and on-line drug and toxicology information. A recent survey of hospitals in Massachusetts, however, revealed that only 8 of 82 hospitals sampled stocked all 14 commonly used antidotes.

D. Each overdose should be approached in a systematic manner to determine the following:
   1. The substance(s) taken.
   2. The last dose of the drug and its dosing frequency.
   3. The reason for the medication.
   4. Other medications usually taken.
   5. Coexisting disease.
   6. The effects of the overdose (i.e., hypotension, respiratory failure, life-threatening dysrhythmias).
   7. Can the effects of the drug be reversed or the drug eliminated without further harm to the patient?

II. Overdose and adverse effects of prescription and nonprescription drugs

A. **Acetaminophen (APAP, N-acetyl-p-aminophenol),** the most commonly overdosed medication in the world, is a leading cause of hepatic failure.

1. Most APAP is metabolized by glucuronization and sulfation to inactive compounds. Less than 10% is converted by a cytochrome P-450 mixed-function oxidase to *N*-acetyl-p-benzoquinoneimine (NAPQI) that has a half-life of nanoseconds. If NAPQI is not neutralized by conjugation with glutathione, it injures the bilipid membrane of the hepatocyte. APAP overdose (7.5 g for adult, 150 mg/kg for children) overwhelms the hepatic glutathione stores and results in cell death.

2. **Baseline and daily laboratory tests** include the prothrombin time (PT), alanine leucine aminotransferase (ALT), aspartate serine transferase (AST), and bilirubin.

3. **Treatment** is the enteral administration of *N*-acetylcysteine (NAC). NAC serves as a glutathione substitute, enhances glutathione synthesis, and increases the amount of APAP that is conjugated by sulfation. If the elapsed time after APAP ingestion is 4 or fewer hours or additional overdosed drugs are suspected, activated charcoal is given and an APAP level is drawn. The serum APAP level is then plotted on a nomogram as a function of time after ingestion. The nomogram has three lines indicating lower limits for possible, probable, and high-risk groups. Individuals who have APAP levels above the possible line are treated with an NAC loading dose of 140 mg/kg orally, diluted in a fruit juice or carbonated beverage. Because of its objectionable taste, it is often administered via a gastric lavage or nasogastric tube [the intravenous (IV) preparation of NAC is under investigation.] Aggressive antiemetic therapy may be needed when the elapsed time is 8 or more hours; the initial loading dose is given prior to obtaining an APAP level. Additional doses are 70 mg/kg every 4 hours for 17 doses or until the APAP levels are in the nontoxic range. Doses are repeated when a patient vomits an NAC dose within 1 hour of administration.

4. **Severe hepatotoxicity** secondary to the overdose of APAP is indicated by an ALT or AST greater than 1,000 IU/L. This hepatotoxicity can progress to fulminant hepatic failure and eventually require liver transplantation or lead to death secondary to sepsis, cerebral edema, hepatorenal syndrome, and metabolic acidosis (72–96 hours). Complete resolution of hepatic dysfunction occurs (4–14 days) in survivors.

B. Antipsychotic agents are derived from several classes of compounds in addition to the classic phenothiazines. They are used (a) to treat acute and chronic psychiatric disease; (b) to control acute agitation; (c) to treat migraine headaches; (d) as antiemetics (e.g., droperidol, promethazine, prochlorperazine); (e) to promote gastrokinesis (e.g., metoclopramide; and (f) as part of some anesthetic regimens (e.g., droperidol).

1. **Haloperidol,** because it does not suppress ventilation, is frequently used to treat delirium. These drugs work via dopamine (D_2) receptor blockade but also have variable affinity for α_2-adrenergic, M_1-muscarinic, H_1-histamine, and $5HT_{2A}$-serotonin receptors.

2. **Phenothiazines** have antidysrhythmic effects similar to quinidine. Metabolism is mostly hepatic. The elimination half-lives of many of these drugs administered orally or intramuscularly are long (10–40 hours) and extended—up to 3 weeks for depot preparations.

3. **Toxic manifestations** of antipsychotics include seizures; hypotension; cardiac conduction delays manifested by prolonged QT intervals; ventricular dysrhythmias, especially torsades de pointes; extrapyramidal symptoms; and the neuroleptic malignant syndrome. The judicious use of IV haloperidol in the ICU is not usually associated with any of these manifestations. However, because of its long half-life, prolonged sedation can occur, especially in the elderly, after sequential escalated doses.

4. **Treatment** of antipsychotic overdose is supportive. Gastrointestinal decontamination is employed.

    a. **Seizures** can be treated initially with benzodiazepines, progressing to barbiturate therapy if needed. As for any patient with seizures, other causes (e.g., hypoxemia, cerebral hemorrhage, embolic disease, other drugs) should be ruled out.

    b. **Hypotension** can be treated with phenylephrine or norepinephrine. Epinephrine in lower doses and dopamine can further decrease blood pressure secondary to unopposed β_2-receptor stimulation. The α effects of dopamine might not be present secondary to the reduction in postsynaptic norepinephrine stores.

    c. **Lidocaine** may be more useful for the treatment of ventricular dysrhythmias than agents that prolong intraventricular conduction.

    d. **Physostigmine** (1–2 mg IV for adults, 0.2 mg/kg for children) with repeated doses as needed every 0.5 to 1.5 hours is used to treat an anticholinergic syndrome.

    e. **Dystonic reactions** can be treated with diphenhydramine (25–50 mg).

5. **Neuroleptic malignant syndrome (NMS)** is a relatively rare life-threatening reaction to antipsychotics within 24 to 72 hours after administration. It is characterized by an altered mental status (that may initially be attributed to a treat-

ment failure) prior to the development of fever, muscle rigidity, and autonomic dysfunction.

    a.   **Fever** occurs from an imbalance of dopamine in the hypothalamus, which causes a change in the mechanisms for temperature homeostasis, and centrally mediated muscle rigidity. This is in contrast to the accelerated calcium-associated skeletal muscle metabolism in **malignant hyperthermia** (MH) (section **VII**). The onset of NMS is slower with less severe symptoms compared with MH. The postoperative patient usually has a common reason (e.g., atelectasis, wound infection) for an increase in temperature before MH and NMS are considered. NMS has been seen after the use of prochlorperazine and promethazine as antiemetics and should be considered as a source of fever in patients in the ICU receiving haloperidol, metoclopramide, or droperidol. Initial treatment is the discontinuation of the drug in question and cardiopulmonary support followed by cooling.

    b.   **Dantrolene** (initial IV dose of 1–2.5 mg/kg every 6 hours, followed by an oral dose of 100–300 mg/d or 1 mg/kg IV every 6 hours for 24–72 hours) is used to control skeletal muscle rigidity and hypermetabolism. At these doses, profound muscle weakness occurs that might necessitate endotracheal intubation and mechanical ventilation. The mannitol in dantrolene will create a brisk diuresis as treatment for myoglobin-induced renal failure secondary to rhabdomyolysis.

    c.   **Bromocriptine** (2.5 mg three times daily), a dopamine agonist, is given to offset the action of the antipsychotic on the dopamine receptor.

    d.   **Amantidine** (100–200 mg enterally, twice daily) and **levodopa/carbidopa** (25/250 enterally four times daily) have also been used.

    e.   Laboratory studies include creatinine phosphokinase levels (CK), urinary myoglobin, and electrolytes.

C.   **Beta-adrenergic-blockers** inhibit the pathway of G-protein $\rightarrow$ cyclic adenosine monophosphate (cAMP) production $\rightarrow$ myocyte protein kinase $\rightarrow$ calcium release $\rightarrow$ excitation-contraction coupling. The more lipid soluble β-blockers (e.g., propranolol, metoprolol, and labetalol) also have a membrane stabilizing function. These agents are used to decrease myocardial contractility, the automaticity of pacemaker cells, and the conduction velocity through the atrioventricular node. Beta blockers are divided into β_1 and β_2 classes, based on actions at therapeutic doses. With *therapeutic* doses in susceptible patients or with increased drug levels of a β-selective agent, both β_1 and β_2 effects can be present [e.g., bronchospasm (β_2 blockade) induced with esmolol (β_1-selective)].

1. **Lipophilic β-blockers** are metabolized by the liver, with their bioavailability increased in hepatic disease or by inhibitors of hepatic enzymes such as cimetidine and erythromycin. **Nonlipophilic β-blockers** are eliminated by the kidney. Renal insufficiency or the use of drugs affecting renal perfusion [e.g., nonsteroidal antiinflammatory drugs (NSAIDs)] increases blood levels. Most patients with β-blocker toxicity have symptoms within 4 hours and resolution within 72 hours. The toxic effects of sotalol may not be noticed for several days after ingestion because of its long half-life.

2. **Hypotension** secondary to decreased myocardial contractility can occur even in the absence of a severe bradycardia. **Bradydysrhythmias** [sinus, junctional rhythm, atrioventricular (AV) block, and idioventricular rhythm], widening of the QRS complex, widening of the QT interval, and asystole have been associated with β-blocker toxicity, especially for the lipophilic agents. Lipophilic β-blocker overdose has been associated with **central nervous system (CNS) symptoms,** ranging from a decreased level of consciousness to seizures and coma.

3. **Electrocardiography** is essential in the diagnosis of β-blocker toxicity. Digitalis and calcium channel blocker toxicity (see below) should be considered because these drugs are often given with β-blockers to control heart rate. As for any patient with neurologic symptoms, electrolytes and a serum glucose should be checked. A computerized tomography (CT) scan of the head is useful to eliminate the possibility of an intracranial process (e.g., neoplasm, hematoma, aneurysm) as a basis for these symptoms.

4. **The initial treatment** of β-blocker toxicity is cardiopulmonary support, GI decontamination with activated charcoal, and correction of hypoglycemia and electrolytes as needed.

   a. **Glucagon** is the pharmacologic agent of choice because the myocardial receptor for glucagon is not affected by β-antagonists. The increase in cAMP via stimulation of adenylate cyclase by glucagon increases myocardial contractility and heart rate, thereby overcoming the effects of the β-blockade. The initial dose of glucagon is 50 to 150 µg/kg (up to a total dose of 10 mg if needed) followed by an infusion of 0.07 mg/kg.

   b. The use of **phosphodiesterase inhibitors** for β-blocker overdose treatment has been reported. Although it would seem logical that the administration of β-agonists would readily reverse bradycardia and hypotension, in reality the response is extremely variable even at more than five times the usual maximal dose.

   c.   **Epinephrine** is the β-agonist of choice. Atropine and pacing are not usually effective except for sotalol.

   d.   **Sotalol-induced dysrhythmias** can be treated with overdrive pacing in addition to lidocaine and magnesium.

D.   **Calcium channel antagonists** comprise one of the largest leading classes of antihypertensives and antidysrhythmics. The antihypertensive effect is by inhibiting the influx of extracellular calcium through slow voltage-gated, slow membrane channels in vascular smooth muscle. This is the sole action of the dihydropyridine family (nifedipine, amlodipine, and felodipine). Myocardial depression can also occur in some compromised individuals and in overdose secondary to the effects on atrial and ventricular myocytes.

   1.   **Calcium channel antagonists** are highly protein bound with variable bioavailability and half-lives. Metabolism is hepatic. Verapamil and diltiazem are converted to active metabolites. They are also potent inhibitors of microsomal metabolizing enzymes and can increase the concentration of drugs that are metabolized by this pathway (e.g., phenytoin and theophylline). Conversely, the elimination of calcium channel antagonists is decreased by inhibitors of these hepatic enzymes (e.g., cimetidine).

   2.   **Bradycardia, conduction defects** (e.g., asystole, idioventricular rhythms, bundle branch blocks), and **hypotension** are the hallmarks of verapamil and diltiazem toxicity. Overdose of the dihydropyridines results in hypotension with reflex tachycardia. A common finding with calcium channel blocker excess is an **ileus** in a patient who had been tolerating enteral nutrition. Other symptoms are related to hypotension (e.g., stroke, lethargy, coma).

   3.   **Treatment** initially consists of cardiovascular support. **Calcium chloride** (1 g) or **calcium gluconate** (3 g) is repeated as needed until the blood pressure rises, the heart rate increases, or no effect is seen after four to five administrations. As with β-blockade overdose, **glucagon** (see section II.C.4.a.) administration might be effective.

      a.   **Cardiac pacing and vasopressor inotropes** (norepinephrine, dopamine) should be considered if the heart rate or blood pressure do not respond to the former treatments.

      b.   **Nonabsorbed drug** should be removed via GI decontamination with activated charcoal. This might require several doses because many of the calcium channel antagonists are taken in extended release forms.

E. **Digitalis** preparations (digoxin, digitoxin) are widely used for the treatment of cardiomyopathies and for ventricular rate control in atrial fibrillation and atrial flutter. Because of a narrow therapeutic window, renal dysfunction, and changes in bioavailability secondary to drug interactions, mild digitalis toxicity is relatively common. Through the inhibition of the Na^+/K^+ ATPase pump by digitalis, cardiac myocytes gain intracellular Ca^{2+}, a positive inotrope especially in the failing heart. Digitalis has a chronotropic effect by several mechanisms. An increase in CNS vagal tone decreases the rate of sinoatrial (SA) node depolarization and prolongs the refractory period of the bundle of His. With the exception of the SA node, the increase of $[Na^+]$ increases phase 4 depolarization and increases excitability as well as delayed afterpotentials.

1. **Digoxin,** the most commonly administered form of the drug, is eliminated by renal clearance after an enterohepatic circulation. **Digitoxin** is cleared by hepatic metabolism. The therapeutic index of digitalis is narrow and plasma levels can be affected by several factors. The addition of quinidine, amiodarone, and verapamil to a therapeutic regimen will significantly increase established digitalis levels. Increased levels may also be seen in patients given antibiotics, which alter the GI flora and lead to decreased metabolism. Hypokalemia, hypocalcemia, and hypomagnesemia will increase the sensitivity of the myocardium to digitalis.

2. **Initial symptoms** of digitalis toxicity are **gastrointestinal:** anorexia, nausea, and vomiting. Toxicity may not be readily diagnosed because these symptoms can stem from a variety of causes other than digitalis. **Dysrhythmias,** especially in patients with compromised hearts, are more common indicators of toxicity when other reasons have been excluded. Digitalis toxicity can be manifested by almost any rhythm or conduction disturbance. The most common are premature ventricular contractions (PVCs), first degree AV block, and atrial fibrillation. A characteristic ST depression is seen on the electrocardiogram (ECG). Serum digitalis levels can be influenced by a variety of factors and are secondary in the diagnosis of expected toxicity.

3. **Treatment** of digitalis toxicity can be difficult. **Atropine, cardiac pacing, or both** can effectively treat bradydysrhythmias. The administration of **magnesium, lidocaine, or phenytoin** will often treat ectopy. With a significant overdose, the inhibition of the Na^+/K^+-ATPase will result in significant hyperkalemia that may be refractive to most treatments. This will eventually result in a loss of total body potassium that must be repleted when the overdose is treated. The

most effective method of digitalis overdose treatment is the removal of free digitalis by **Fab fragments of antidigitalis IgG** (Digibind). This enhances the clearance of digitalis from the circulation by renal elimination. The removal of digitalis at tissue sites is also accelerated. The drug dose is calculated from a formula based on the body load of digitalis. This calculation requires a digoxin level that may not be available. It is simpler to administer Digibind (40 mg/vial) until the dysrhythmias are effectively treated or until the maximal dose of 800 mg (20 vials) is reached. Digoxin levels, although elevated, will reflect both the drug bound to the Fab fragments and the unbound drug.

F. **Lithium** is used to treat manic-depression. Lithium toxicity can be the result of a suicide attempt, increased levels during chronic treatment, or increased levels after the new administration of a thiazide diuretic or placement on a low sodium diet. The exact mechanism of lithium's action is unknown, but it may increase hippocampal serotonin release, enhance norepinephrine reuptake, or inhibit adenylate cyclase. Gastrointestinal absorption is rapid; the element is distributed in whole body water and renal elimination occurs with significant reabsorption. The half-life of lithium is 30 hours.

1. **Serious toxicity** is present at serum lithium levels of 2.5 to 3.5 mEq/L, with life-threatening complications at levels greater than 3.5 mEq/L. A change in renal function that permits increased resorption of lithium in the proximal convoluted tubule (e.g., hypovolemia, hyponatremia, NSAIDs) will increase serum lithium levels. **Nephrogenic diabetes insipidus** is the most common toxicity seen. Dysrhythmias and circulatory collapse have been reported.

2. **Treatment** is GI decontamination if an intentional overdose is suspected. Half-normal saline (0.45%) should initially be given to restore euvolemia because the patient usually has a high serum osmolality. The administration of a thiazide diuretic or amiloride may help to control the polyuria. Hemodialysis is required for a life-threatening lithium overdose.

G. **Salicylates. Acetylsalicylic acid (aspirin, ASA),** the most commonly known salicylate, has traditionally been the agent of salicylate overdose. With the advent of child-proof containers, the restriction of child aspirin to 81 mg/tablet, 36 tablets per container, the awareness of **Reye's syndrome,** and the availability of nonsalicylate analgesics, the incidence of salicylate overdose secondary to ASA has markedly diminished. **Methylsalicylate** is found in topical formulations used to treat musculoskeletal pain and in oil of wintergreen. Chronic use on excoriated skin may result in salicylism. **Bismuth subsalicylate** is found in antidiarrheal preparations.

1. **ASA is absorbed** in ionized form in the stomach and in enteric form in the distal small intestine. Hydrolysis of ASA to salicylic acid with elimination by renal filtration and excretion is the major metabolic pathway. Several secondary metabolic pathways exist for salicylic acid. In severe overdose, these pathways become overwhelmed and the elimination half-life of salicylic acid is prolonged—up to 30 hours. A toxic salicylate concentration is greater than 30 mg/dl. Initially, hyperventilation, via direct CNS stimulation by the drug, produces a respiratory alkalosis. Bicarbonate is renally excreted and hypokalemia ensues in a compensatory fashion. An anion gap metabolic acidosis occurs secondary to the uncoupling of oxidative phosphorylation and inhibition of the tricarboxylic acid cycle in the liver. Patients may be agitated and have tinnitus. Hyperglycemia or hypoglycemia may be present. Often, hypernatremia with dehydration exists that is related to large, insensible losses during hyperventilation. Uncommon events are pulmonary edema, coma, hyperpyrexia, and GI bleeding.

2. **Laboratory tests** include plasma salicylate levels until the peak level is defined, electrolytes, blood urea nitrogen (BUN), creatinine, glucose, liver function tests, and arterial blood gas tensions and pH as needed.

3. **Initial treatment** is GI decontamination with activated charcoal; cardiovascular and respiratory support; the replacement of electrolytes, glucose, and fluids; and alkalization of the urine to "ion trap" salicylic acid and prevent reabsorption by the proximal convoluted tubules. Hemodialysis should be considered in cases of renal dysfunction or when salicylate levels are greater than 80 mg/dl.

H. **Theophylline** is a central respiratory stimulant, a smooth muscle relaxant (decreased peripheral vascular resistance, bronchodilation, relaxation of the gastroesophageal sphincter), a positive chronotrope and inotrope, and a diuretic. An increase in cAMP-mediated actions via inhibition of the breakdown of adenylate cyclase by phosphodiesterase is the "classic" mechanism of theophylline. It is now thought that this does not occur at therapeutic levels, and theophylline's actions may be through an increase in catecholamines, competitive antagonism of adenosine, and a direct action on intracellular transport.

1. **Metabolism** is by hepatic cytochrome P-450 to 3-methylxanthine (active) and an inactive hydroxylated compound. Although few drugs enhance the elimination of theophylline (barbiturates, pheny-

toin, carbamazepine, cigarette smoking), plasma theophylline concentrations can be increased by many commonly used drugs that are inhibitors of the cytochrome P-450 system (including macrolides, fluoroquinolones, cimetidine), primary hepatic disease, and a reduction of hepatic blood flow during congestive heart failure.

2. **Toxicity** is dependent on the duration of intoxication. Overdose is often the result of a dose miscalculation or administration error.

    a. **Symptoms** include nausea, vomiting, diarrhea, hypotension, cardiac dysrhythmias (usually sinus tachycardia, but a supraventricular tachycardia, ventricular tachycardia or ventricular fibrillation may occur), agitation or anxiety, seizures, and muscle tremors. A relative hypokalemia with normal total body potassium stores may be present.

    b. **Acute toxicity** produces minor symptoms at 20 to 40 µg/ml, moderate at 40 to 80 µg/ml, severe at 70 to 80 µg/ml, and death at 100 µg/ml or greater. Increasing age, comorbid disease, and decreasing age in children increase the severity of a chronic intoxication for a given plasma level. It is more difficult to predict the effects of acute-on-chronic intoxication.

3. **Initial treatment** is cardiopulmonary support as needed. Theophylline levels and serum electrolytes should be obtained on a periodic basis, especially for acute intoxications. A relative hypokalemia may exacerbate theophylline-induced tachydysrhythmias.

    a. Supraventricular tachycardias can be treated with **adenosine,** an antagonist of theophylline. Hypotension, tachycardia, and hypokalemia may be reversed with **propranolol** unless the patient has a history of bronchospastic disease. **Lidocaine** has been shown to be effective for ventricular dysrhythmias. **Benzodiazepines** have been effective for the treatment of seizures.

    b. Theophylline will readily diffuse from the circulation and adsorb to **activated charcoal** in the lumen of the GI tract. Activated charcoal (1 g/kg) should be administered every 4 hours with aggressive antiemetic therapy to prevent theophylline-induced vomiting. Repeated administration of activated charcoal to remove theophylline has been associated with an ileus. Sustained release preparations can form bezoars that might be difficult to remove.

    c. **Charcoal hemoperfusion** has been the gold standard for removal of theophylline. With the advent of more efficient membranes, **hemodialysis** is now considered equivalent to hemoperfusion. Hemodialysis should be considered for patients who cannot tolerate repeated doses of activated charcoal, have levels greater than 60 µg/ml after activated charcoal, or for initial serum theophylline concentrations greater than 80 µg/ml.

I. **Tricyclic antidepressant (TCA)** toxicity, the most common cause of prescription-related drug deaths, usually occurs within 24 hours of ingestion. The onset of toxic symptoms occurs within hours. In general, TCAs decrease the neuronal reuptake of epinephrine and norepinephrine by inhibiting fast sodium channels and blocking cholinergic, histamine, and γ-aminobuteric acid (GABA) channels. **Trazodone** does not block the reuptake of norepinephrine, but does block adrenergic receptors. **Amoxapine** blocks dopamine receptors.

1. TCAs are quickly absorbed from the GI tract and are rapidly distributed to tissue sites. Elimination is by hepatic hydroxylation and demethylation. The enzymes responsible for hydroxylation are saturated at high concentrations of substrate, resulting in a prolonged elimination. TCAs have half-lives of 8 to 30 hours in therapeutic concentrations that can be prolonged to 81 hours in an overdose.

2. **Initial signs of TCA toxicity** are anticholinergic: tachycardia, hyperthermia, ileus, mydriasis, urinary retention, dry mucous membranes and skin, and altered mental status.

   a. **Manifestations of serious TCA toxicity** are dysrhythmias, hypotension, respiratory depression, pulmonary edema, self-limited seizures, and coma. Life-threatening toxicity is present with serum concentrations of more than 1 µg/ml, with fatality at more than 3 µg/ml.

   b. **The ECG** in an overdose usually demonstrates a sinus tachycardia with a first degree AV block, nonspecific intraventricular conduction delay (secondary to an inhibition of phase 0 depolarization), and rightward axis. An atrial ECG with an esophageal lead might be useful to distinguish this pattern from ventricular tachycardia which is also common with TCA overdose.

   c. **Hypotension** is caused by decreased myocardial contractility (caused by blockade of the fast sodium channels), depletion of norepinephrine reserves in neurons, and vasodilation (from α blockade). The usual cause of death is refractive hypotension.

   d. **Treatment** consists of initial GI decontamination with activated charcoal and cardiopulmonary support as needed. Refractive hypotension should be treated by repletion of intravascular volume and administration of norepinephrine. Sodium bicarbonate also effectively treats TCA cardiotoxicity, either through the alkalization of the blood (to pH 7.5) or through supplementing [Na^+], but not by drug trapping because of minimal renal elimination.

III. Alcohols

A. **Ethanol (EtOH)** is the most extensively used non-prescription drug. It is also present in a variety of cough and cold preparations, mouthwashes, and perfumes.

1. **Ethanol is absorbed** from all levels of the GI tract, but primarily in the stomach and small intestine, with blood levels achieved within 60 minutes of ingestion. It is initially metabolized to acetaldehyde by alcohol dehydrogenase in the liver. A cytochrome P-450–dependent pathway is used for less than 10% of metabolism, but is increased in chronic drinkers. Acetaldehyde is metabolized to acetate via acetaldehyde dehydrogenase. Ethanol elimination can be as low as 120 µg/ml/h in nondrinkers to 500 µg/ml/h in chronic alcoholics. The blood alcohol level will reflect the peak amount of ethanol ingested.

2. **The effects of ethanol intoxication** depend on whether there is chronic or acute use and the amount ingested. The standard values for blood alcohol levels are only valid for the nondependent person.

    a. **Acute intoxication** in the "nonalcoholic" may be manifested by symptoms ranging from euphoria to total circulatory and respiratory collapse. A frequent cause of morbidity is hypoxemia secondary to **aspiration** of gastric contents after loss of airway reflexes. **Dehydration** may be present from an ethanol-induced depression of antidiuretic hormone. A "holiday heart" syndrome of **atrial fibrillation or flutter** that corrects with cessation of use is associated with ethanol ingestion in nonalcoholics.

    b. **Chronic intoxication** is a spectrum of comorbid conditions. Many patients have no symptoms other than an increased tolerance for ethanol. Malnutrition, peptic ulcer disease, bone marrow suppression, and immunosuppression may be subtle. Pulmonary complications secondary to concomitant tobacco and ethanol use are common. More severe forms of chronic ethanol intoxication include cardiomyopathy, dysrhythmias, Wernicke's encephalopathy, Korsakoff's psychosis, cerebellar ataxia, ketoacidosis, hepatic cirrhosis, and GI hemorrhage.

3. **Treatment** of the ethanol intoxicated patient in the ICU is initially focused on the reason for admission (e.g., subdural hematoma, aspiration, musculoskeletal trauma, co-ingestion) in addition to cardiopulmonary support.

   a. **Other causes for altered mental status** (e.g., sepsis, encephalopathy, hypoglycemia, or head trauma) should be ruled out. The emergence of focal neurologic signs should prompt a detailed workup (For example, an acute subdural hematoma might not be evident on an admission CT scan but may be evident several hours later).

   b. **Fluid losses** secondary to alcohol-induced diuresis, decreased oral intake, and vomiting need to be repleted. Cardiovascular support will depend on the level of intravascular volume depletion and degree of cardiomyopathy.

   c. **Attention to pulmonary function** and secretion clearance is important, in view of the high probability of pulmonary dysfunction secondary to tobacco use. Although antibiotic coverage for aspiration of community-acquired flora is usually not needed, empiric administration of a broad-spectrum antibiotic (e.g., ampicillin–sulbactam) may be prudent in the initial stages of treatment if malnutrition or immunosuppression is suspected.

   d. **Vitamin therapy** with thiamin and folate and repletion of electrolytes should be initiated. Alcoholic ketoacidosis requires volume resuscitation and glucose administration in a manner similar to resuscitation for diabetic ketoacidosis.

   e. **The altered coagulation profile** of patients with cirrhosis, including the thrombocytopenia of splenomegaly, does not require treatment unless clinically indicated. Bleeding esophageal varices may require endoscopic or surgical intervention.

4. **Ethanol withdrawal** is often seen following elective surgery or an emergent admission. Symptoms include anxiety, tremors, irritability, hypertension, and hallucinations that generally peak approximately 24 hours after cessation of ethanol but can appear within 10 hours. These symptoms might easily be attributed to a mild postoperative effect of drugs or disorientation in a "pleasantly confused" elderly patient.

   a. **Denial** and underestimation of one's ethanol daily consumption is commonplace. Clearly, some elderly patients who have had "one glass of wine a night" for years will exhibit signs of withdrawal. A tactful and nonjudgmental approach often elicits a more accurate history in such situations.

    b. **Tonic-clonic seizures** can occur within 48 hours after a decrease in ethanol use.

    c. **Delirium tremens (DTs)** is a life-threatening syndrome marked by autonomic instability (hypertension, tachycardia, hyperpyrexia, tremors, and diaphoresis) that may be present 3 to 5 days following the cessation of ethanol.

  5. **Benzodiazepines**, through their binding to GABA receptors, are cross tolerant with ethanol. All benzodiazepines have been used with success. Intravenous or enteral **diazepam** or **lorazepam** can be administered in a dosage schedule that is appropriate for the patient's age, size, and physical condition. The long activity of diazepam secondary to its active metabolite nor-diazepam should be considered in subsequent dosing schedules.

    a. For the treatment of seizures and severe DTs, the IV route is used with escalating doses.

    b. Tracheal intubation and mechanical ventilation may be required if respiratory depression occurs because of the need for high doses of benzodiazepines.

    c. Immediately following a seizure, an arterial blood gas measurement will usually exhibit metabolic acidosis with a pH sometimes lower than 7.0. Measurement is not indicated in this setting, because the acidosis will spontaneously correct after the seizure.

  6. **Haloperidol** is useful for the psychotic reactions accompanied with ethanol withdrawal. It can be given intravenously beginning at 1 mg, with doubling of the dose after each intervention. Because of the long half-life, prolonged sedation (but without respiratory depression) can occur after sequential administrations. The QT-segment on the ECG should be checked for prolongation during haloperidol treatment (Chapter 5).

B. **Methanol (MtOH)** (wood alcohol) is a commonly used solvent. It is often ingested after synthesis in home distilleries (i.e., moonshine) or by alcoholics seeking any form of alcohol. Peak levels are reached within 90 minutes of ingestion. The fatal dose can be as little as 60 ml. Most of the MtOH is initially converted by alcohol dehydrogenase to formaldehyde, followed by oxidation by several enzymes to formic acid.

  1. **Signs and symptoms** include blurred vision or blindness, GI reactions (nausea, vomiting, severe abdominal pain, diarrhea), a severe anion gap metabolic acidosis, and respiratory depression.

  2. **Treatment** of MtOH poisoning, in addition to cardiopulmonary support, is the administration of **intravenous ethanol** to achieve a blood level of

100 mg/dl. Start with a loading dose of 0.6 g/kg followed by 66 mg/kg to 154 mg/kg, depending on the past ethanol use pattern of the patient. The ethanol will compete with MtOH for metabolism by alcohol dehydrogenase and reduce the production of formaldehyde. **Hemodialysis** is initiated to remove nonmetabolized MtOH. Recently, fomepizole has been available as an inhibitor of alcohol dehydrogenase for the treatment of ethylene glycol toxicity (see below). Although it is not indicated for MtOH poisoning, its mechanism of action suggests that it may be efficacious for this purpose.

C. **Ethylene glycol,** commonly used as antifreeze but also found in other solvents, is usually lethal after an ingestion of 100 ml if not treated swiftly. As with ethanol and MtOH, ethylene glycol is initially metabolized by alcohol dehydrogenase. Subsequent metabolic products are lactic acid, aldehydes, glycolate, and oxalic acid.

1. **Intoxication** is marked by a severe anion gap metabolic acidosis, a large osmolal gap (increased osmolality not accounted for by glucose, sodium, or BUN), and tissue damage secondary to the deposition of oxalate crystals. Hypocalcemia results from the chelation of calcium by the oxalate. Patients may be admitted in coma; they may have seizures, neuromuscular dysfunction secondary to hypocalcemia (myoclonic activity, loss of deep tendon reflexes, tetany), acute renal failure, congestive heart failure, and pulmonary edema (both related to deposition of oxalate).

2. **Treatment** of ethylene glycol toxicity includes cardiopulmonary support, treatment of the metabolic acidosis, IV ethanol administration, as for MtOH poisoning (see above), and hemodialysis. **Fomepizole** (Antizol), a competitive inhibitor of alcohol dehydrogenase, has recently been approved for ethylene glycol poisoning. The initial dose is 15 mg/kg, followed by 10 mg/kg every 12 hours for four doses, and then 15 mg/kg every 12 hours (all given as infusions over 30 minutes) until the ethylene glycol levels are less than 20 mg/dl.

IV. **Substance abuse**

A. **Amphetamine and cocaine intoxications** can be the primary reason for admission or comorbidities after trauma. **Amphetamines** are indirect sympathomimetics that increase postsynaptic catecholamines by inhibiting the presynaptic uptake and storage of catecholamines as well as their destruction by oxidase. **Cocaine** works in a similar fashion and also binds to the dopamine reuptake transporter. Both have been associated with seizures, intracerebral hemorrhage, ischemic strokes, hypertension, tachycardia, myocardial ischemia and infarctions, dysrhythmias, hyperpyrexia, rhabdomyolysis, acute renal failure, disseminated intravascular coagulation, and pulmonary edema. Pulmonary edema can occur several days after drug use, and initially appears as acute respiratory distress with hypoxemia followed by a noncardiogenic pulmonary edema. Treatment is supportive care for the organ systems involved and aggressive control of hyperpyrexia, if present. Unopposed β blockade should be avoided because it worsens outcome. Hyperadrenergic symptoms can be treated with benzodiazepine administration.

B.   **Barbiturates** are used to treat seizure disorders, induce general anesthesia, and produce conscious sedation in children. They are a source of substance abuse and have been implicated in suicides. Co-ingestion of other substances must be considered. These highly lipid, soluble drugs are absorbed rapidly from the GI tract and rapidly distributed to the brain. Barbiturates are oxidized by enzymes in the smooth endoplasmic reticulum of hepatocytes and are cleared to a variable extent by the kidney. Induction of the oxidative enzymes can increase elimination of compounds metabolized by the same pathways and also produce tolerance to barbiturates.

1.   **Severe acute barbiturate overdose** is manifested by coma, hypoventilation, hypothermia, and hypotension (secondary to cardiovascular depression).

2.   **Treatment** includes cardiopulmonary support and the removal of barbiturate by alkaline diuresis and GI decontamination with activated charcoal. Neurologic status is assessed with frequent physical examinations, CT scans to determine the presence of focal lesions, and lumbar puncture to rule out meningitis. An **isoelectric electroencephalogram** may indicate suppression of neuronal activity by the barbiturate rather than brain death.

C.   **Benzodiazepines** have sedative, anxiolytic, anticonvulsant, and hypnotic actions and high abuse potential. They enhance the binding of GABA to its receptor and potentiate neuronal inhibition through hyperpolarization of the plasma membrane.

1.   Oral formulations are easily absorbed from the GI tract and appear in the systemic circulation within 30 minutes. The metabolism of all benzodiazepines is by hepatic cytochrome P-450 with transformation to secondary products and conjugation to inactive compounds that are cleared by the kidney. The metabolic products (desalkylflurazepam, desmethyldiazepam) of some benzodiazepines retain the affinity for the GABA receptor and have half-lives greatly exceeding their parent compounds. As for other drugs that use the cytochrome P-450 pathway, their metabolism can be increased by age, hepatic disease, and inducers

(e.g., EtOH, barbiturates) or decreased by inhibitors (e.g., cimetidine, erythromycin).

2. **The toxicity** of benzodiazepines taken in overdose is minimal because of a high therapeutic index. Patients will exhibit CNS depression marked by drowsiness, stupor, or ataxia. Coma, respiratory depression, and death are rare. If co-ingested with EtOH, barbiturates, TCAs, or antipsychotics, however, the safety margin of benzodiazepines is markedly diminished. Profound CNS depression, cardiovascular instability, and respiratory failure may be present.

3. **Diazepam** is frequently used for sedation in concert with opiates to facilitate mechanical ventilation (Chapter 5). Toxicity caused by elevated diazepam and desmethyldiazepam levels may be seen if the initial dose is not decreased after a few days, especially for elderly patients. Profound sedation can confound the physical examination to the point of requiring an invasive and expensive neurologic investigation (e.g., lumbar puncture, CT).

4. **Treatment** is supportive after GI decontamination with activated charcoal. **Flumazenil** (0.5–5 mg IV) is a benzodiazepine antagonist that will reverse the effects of an overdose. Because the half-life is almost 1 hour, redosing after 1 to 2 hours is required to prevent resedation. Seizures from co-ingested drugs (e.g., TCAs, ethanol) can occur when flumazenil reverses the therapeutic effects of the benzodiazepine.

D. **Opioid overdose** in the ICU is often iatrogenic. Manifestations include somnolence, decreased respiratory drive with hypercarbia, and, rarely, apnea. Symptoms are treated by temporarily stopping or reducing the source of the opiate, administration of naloxone in 40 μg increments to reverse the respiratory depression without compromising pain control, and ventilatory support as needed.

1. Patients admitted to the ICU after illicit use of opioids may have had respiratory depression reversed by naloxone or nalmefene in the emergency department, need further monitoring for respiratory depression and continued treatment with naloxone, have a requirement for mechanical ventilation, or need treatment for an overdose of co-ingested substances.

2. **Heroin** can cause the rapid onset of noncardiogenic pulmonary edema, similar to neurogenic pulmonary edema. This can occur several days after heroin use and is often initially diagnosed as acute respiratory distress syndrome (ARDS). Resolution follows ventilatory support with positive end-expiratory pressure and appropriate diuresis.

3. **Withdrawal** of therapeutic or abused opiates is often associated with an abrupt increase in sym-

pathetic output. Agitation, severe hypertension, tachycardia, and pulmonary edema can result. α_2-adrenergic agonism with **clonidine** (0.1–0.3 mg/d, by mouth or by a weekly patch) will relieve some of the symptoms. Benzodiazepines can be used to treat anxiety and concomitant ethanol withdrawal. **Early consultation** with specialists in substance abuse facilitates continuity of treatment.

E. **Designer drugs** are "recreational" drugs that are produced through small modifications of the chemical structure of a variety of compounds. Because of these structural changes, the drugs may fall outside current classifications of illicit compounds. The designer drugs used in a community and their precise effects vary, but are usually well known to law enforcement agencies and emergency room personnel. Treatment is usually supportive.

V. **Poisonings**

A. **Carbon monoxide** (CO) is a common cause of poisoning because CO is undetectable and ubiquitous wherever incomplete oxidation of propane, natural gas, kerosene, or gasoline occurs. It is a frequent prehospital cause of death following smoke inhalation (Chapter 34). An unappreciated source is through the metabolism of methylene chloride that is inhaled or absorbed from commercial paint products. Carbon monoxide binds to any hemeprotein and cuproprotein with an affinity much greater than oxygen.

1. Mild symptoms include headache and nausea. The signs and symptoms of more serious exposures may reflect tissue hypoxia and reperfusion injury: ataxia, dyspnea, myocardial ischemia, dysrhythmias, hypotension, lactic acidosis, seizures, and coma. The diagnosis is made on clinical suspicion and the level of arterial or venous carboxyhemoglobin (COHb) measured spectrophotometrically with a CO-oximeter. Because oxyhemoglobin and COHb absorb light at the same wavelength, pulse oximetry cannot be used as an indicator of CO poisoning.

2. **Treatment** of CO poisoning is 100% O_2 to compete with CO bound to hemoglobin. The half-life of CO is 2 to 7 hours. It is reduced to an average of 90 minutes with 100% O_2 via face mask, 60 minutes by endotracheal administration, and 23 minutes with hyperbaric O_2 (HBO) at 2.8 to 3 atmospheres absolute (2128–2280 mm Hg) (Chapter 34).

B. **Cyanide**-containing compounds are widely used in industry and found in many synthetic compounds, insecticides, and cleaning solutions.

1. **Cyanide** can be released from many burning plastics during structure fires (Chapter 34).

2. **Amygdalin,** a supposed herbal antineoplastic remedy from apricot pits, and similar plant com-

pounds will release cyanide when degraded in the GI tract.

3. **Sodium nitroprusside (SNP)** is metabolized to nitric oxide and cyanide. In the liver, the cyanide reacts with thiosulfates via the enzyme rhodanase to form thiocyanates that are cleared by the kidney. Both cyanide and thiocyanates bind to the ferric iron of mitochondrial cytochrome oxidase, uncouple oxidative phosphorylation, and cause histotoxic hypoxia. Cyanide toxicity can occur when SNP is used at high doses, over periods usually longer than 3 to 4 days, in patients with renal insufficiency (decreased elimination of thiocyanate), and in hepatic insufficiency (increased cyanide levels secondary to decreased thiocyanate formation).

4. **Symptoms** of mild cyanide toxicity, as seen with SNP use, include lethargy, confusion, agitation, increasing tachycardia, tachyphylaxis, and a lactic acidosis. In the appropriate clinical scenario, lactate levels have been considered one of the best markers for cyanide toxicity because cyanide levels are usually not readily available. The difference between the arterial and mixed venous SpO_2 increases to more than 70% because tissues cannot use oxygen. Severe poisoning produces coma, seizures, cardiac collapse, and respiratory failure.

5. **Treatment** of SNP-induced toxicity is supportive after discontinuation of the drug. Gastrointestinal decontamination with activated charcoal is used for ingested cyanide compounds. **Sodium nitrite** (300 mg IV over more than 5 minutes in a volume of 100 ml 5% dextrose) can be administered. Rapid administration of sodium nitrite will cause hypotension. The nitrite reacts with hemoglobin to form methemoglobin. The cyanide complexed to cytochrome oxidase will then form methemoglobin-cyanide, thereby restoring active enzyme. In severe toxicity, inhaled **amyl nitrite** has been used as a quick source of nitrite. Subsequent treatment with **sodium thiosulfate** (12.5 g) leads to the formation of thiocyanate that can be removed by the kidney. If needed, additional half doses of sodium nitrite and sodium thiosulfate can be given.

VI. **Envenomations**
  A. **Snake bite** rates from *Elapidae* (coral snakes) and *Crotalidae* (pit vipers) are highest in the southern and southwestern regions of the United States. The *Crotalidae* are in virtually every state and every climate. Coral snake bites are relatively rare.
  B. **Crotalid venom** nonenzymatically damages microvascular endothelial cells, producing transudation of intravascular fluid.
    1. Symptoms occur within 12 hours of the envenomation.

    a. With severe bites, **hypovolemic shock** secondary to intravascular depletion, hemoconcentration, and hypoproteinemia are produced. An enzymatic degradation of the subendothelial tissues worsens shock via the extravasation of erythrocytes.

    b. An enzyme-mediated **disseminated intravascular coagulopathy (DIC)-like process** occurs by primary fibrinogenolysis. Unlike true DIC, some hemostasis is maintained because thrombin formation is maintained; the D-dimer is not positive because the venom does not activate factor XIII to cross-link fibrin. The administration of procoagulant blood products will not be useful because this is not a consumptive coagulation process. Thrombocytopenia is caused by a loss of platelets at the disrupted envenomation site.

    c. **Destruction of muscle** by digestive enzymes or from a compartment syndrome at the site of the bite is possible with the sequel of acute renal failure secondary to myoglobinuria.

    d. With the exception of the Mojave rattlesnake, neuromuscular blockade is not produced.

  2. **Treatment** includes fluid resuscitation and cardiopulmonary support.

    a. **Compartment pressures** in the region of the bite should be monitored and fasciotomies and debridements performed if indicated.

    b. **Crotalid antivenin** is administered according to the supplier's recommendations. Because the antivenin is in serum of equine origin, skin testing should be performed to determine if the patient has an immune reaction to horse antigens. If the test is positive and the antivenin is required, the patient should be pretreated with diphenhydramine and an H_2 blocker. Be prepared to treat an anaphylactoid reaction (see section **VIII**) to the antivenin. Serum sickness can develop.

    c. **Laboratory tests** every 4 hours include a complete blood count with platelets, PT, partial thromboplastin time, fibrinogen, and activated fibrin split products. Because the antivenin contains horse proteins, blood samples for typing and cross-matching should be obtained prior to its administration.

C. **Coral snake venom** contains polypeptides that bind to the postsynaptic receptors of the neuromuscular junction. The result is a competitive, nondepolarizing **neuromuscular blockade** characterized by a slow onset (> 10 hours), precipitous manifestation, and prolonged duration (up to 2 months). Little local tissue damage occurs.

1. Patients are observed for at least 24 to 48 hours. The bite area should be vigorously scrubbed with soap to remove residual venom on the skin that can enter the circulation through breaks in the integument.

2. An infusion of **coral snake antivenin** should be administered according to the guidelines of the manufacturer. Because the antivenin is in serum of equine origin, skin testing should be performed as described above to determine if the patient has an immune reaction to horse antigens.

3. Patients who develop neuromuscular blockade should be treated with mechanical ventilation and supportive care until resolution.

VII. **Malignant hyperthermia (MH)** is an inherited, hypermetabolic state, caused by the inability of skeletal muscle sarcoplasmic reticulum to reuptake calcium after exposure to volatile anesthetics or succinylcholine. The precise pathophysiologic mechanism of MH is not known. It usually occurs immediately after induction of anesthesia, especially if succinylcholine is administered, or at some time during the anesthetic. Malignant hyperthermia can also occur several hours into the postoperative period.

A. **Signs** of MH reflect its hypermetabolic state: severe hypercarbia that is difficult to correct with increased ventilation, metabolic acidosis, tachycardia, and a temperature increase of 1°C to 2°C every 5 minutes. Initially, signs of MH may be considered mild and mistaken for atelectasis or infection. The true extent of hypercarbia and metabolic acidosis is best measured in a sample of central venous blood, which may reveal a P_{CO_2} of 90 mm Hg in contrast to an arterial P_{CO_2} of 60 mm Hg. Also seen are hyperkalemia, hypertension, hypercalcemia, a creatinine phosphokinase (CPK) increasing to 20,000 U/L or more within the first 12 to 24 hours, and myoglobinuria. Dysrhythmias stem from the hypercarbia and the combined metabolic and respiratory acidosis. Disseminated intravascular coagulation can occur from the release of tissue thromboplastin from damaged muscle tissue.

B. **Initial treatment** of MH hinges on the administration of **dantrolene** to inhibit the release of calcium from the sarcoplasmic reticulum and decrease the intracellular calcium concentration. The initial dose is 2.5 mg/kg with doses repeated until the hypercarbia, tachycardia, temperature, and acidosis resolve. A total initial dose greater than the recommended maximum of 10 mg/kg is sometimes required. A dose of 1 mg/kg IV or orally can be repeated every 6 hours for 48 to 72 hours to prevent the recrudescence of MH.

1. **Metabolic acidosis** requires treatment with sodium bicarbonate if respiratory compensation is inadequate.

2. **Persistent dysrhythmias** are controlled with procainamide.

3. **Hyperthermia** can be treated with external cold packs and gastric and rectal lavage with cold saline.

4. **Myoglobinuria** is initially treated with the mannitol that is admixed with the IV preparation of dantrolene [Each ampule of dantrolene (20 mg) contains 3 g of mannitol].

5. **Hypokalemia and hypocalcemia** are common after treatment of the crisis.

C. Therapy for MH is often begun prior to the knowledge of CPK and blood gas measurements. **In the face of a normal value** or an incomplete clinical picture, the use of dantrolene should be discontinued because it can produce muscle weakness so severe that mechanical ventilation will be required.

VIII. **Anaphylaxis and anaphylactoid reactions**

A. **Anaphylaxis** is a life-threatening immunologic response to an antigenic stimulus usually occurring within a few minutes after exposure.

1. **Common drugs** known to cause anaphylaxis in susceptible individuals are the thiobarbiturates, penicillins, cephalosporins, protamine in patients receiving NPH insulin, and IV contrast dye for radiology procedures. Many patients have a known anaphylaxis to bee stings and foods such as shellfish, peanuts, soybeans, and eggs. Allergy to **latex products** (e.g., balloons, surgical gloves, urinary catheters, IV tubing, and many other products) is increasingly common and may produce anaphylaxis. Simplistically, following an initial sensitization, some individuals synthesize high titers of IgE. On reexposure, the antigen binds to specific IgEs on the surfaces of mast cells and basophils, initiating activation of the cells. A rapid, massive release of mediators of the immune response (e.g., histamine, prostaglandins, leukotrienes, kinins) subsequently occurs.

2. **Signs and symptoms.** The "classic" cutaneous manifestations of urticaria and flushing may not be evident prior to life-threatening symptoms of respiratory distress, hypotension, hypovolemia, pulmonary hypertension, and dysrhythmias.

3. **Treatment** for a severe reaction includes endotracheal intubation before airway edema becomes severe, rapid infusion of crystalloid to replete the lost intravascular volume (liters will be needed), and the parenteral administration of epinephrine (begin with 300–500 µg IV).

a. **Epinephrine** will increase blood pressure through effects on vascular tone (α_1), augmentation of cardiac output (β_1), and will inhibit the release of mediators (β_2), and it is a potent bronchodilator (β_2). Bronchodilation can be maintained with an infusion of epinephrine titrated to effect ($\sim$ 1–2 µg/min) with the caveat that lower doses (0.5–1 μg/min) can cause vasodilation through β_2 activity on vascular smooth muscle.

    b. Secondary treatment includes the blockade of H_1 and H_2 receptors with **diphenhydramine** (0.5–1.0 mg/kg, IV) and the administration of **corticosteroids** (1–2 g methylprednisolone) to further inhibit the immune response.

    c. Subsequent management includes immunologic testing as needed and the standard intensive care management of resolving respiratory and cardiovascular sequelae of the anaphylaxis and resuscitation. The choice of invasive monitors will depend on the comorbidity and severity of the reaction in a given patient.

B. Anaphylactoid reactions, in contrast to anaphylaxis, do not involve presensitized IgE. Anaphylactoid reactions can involve the IgG- or complement-mediated release of immunologic mediators or be the result of an idiosyncratic interaction of the drug with mast cells or basophils.

    1. Many drugs that can cause anaphylaxis in some individuals will cause an anaphylactoid reaction in others (e.g., thiobarbiturates, protamine).

    2. Mild anaphylactoid reactions caused by drug-induced histamine release produce transient hypotension, flushing, and urticaria. Such reactions are frequently noted with atracurium (but not *cis*-atracurium), *d*-tubocurarine, morphine, and vancomycin. These are easily treated with crystalloid administration, low doses of ephedrine, and time.

    3. Severe anaphylactoid reactions are clinically indistinguishable from anaphylaxis and are treated in the same manner.

SELECTED REFERENCES

Haddad LM, Shannon MW, Winchester JF, eds. *Clinical management of poisoning and drug overdose,* 3rd ed. Philadelphia: WB Saunders, 1998.

Litovitz TL, Klein-Schwartz W, Dyer KS, et al. 1997 Annual report of the American Association of Poison Control Centers toxic exposure surveillance system. *Toxicology* 1998;16:443–497.

Mowry JB, Furbee RB, Chyka PA. Poisoning. In: Chernow B, ed. *The pharmacologic approach to the critically ill patient,* 3rd ed. Baltimore: Williams & Wilkins, 1994:975–1008.

Woolf AD, Chrisanthus K. On-site availability of selected antidotes: results of a survey of Massachusetts hospitals. *Am J Emerg Med* 1997;15:62–66.

Wright RO, Wang RY. Poison antidotes: guidelines for rational use in the emergency department. *Emergency Medicine Reports* 1995;16:201–212.

Dermatologic Considerations

Bonnie T. Mackool

I. **Purpura**
   A. The descriptive term, **purpura,** defined as nonblanching erythema, encompasses many of the most serious cutaneous disorders that will be encountered in the intensive care unit (ICU) setting. Purpura results from either dysfunction of the blood vessel or hematologic disturbances. **Palpable purpura** represents vasculitis, excepting perhaps a traumatized lesion into which an individual has bled, in which case there is not a primary inflammatory process around the vessels causing the palpable purpura. Vascular tumors are also purpuric.
   B. **Vasculitis** implies damage to blood vessels by an inflammatory infiltrate, which can result from a primary vasculitic process such as **Wegener's granulomatosis, polyarteritis nodosa,** and **Churg-Strauss syndrome.** In the infectious vasculitides, an infectious organism may lodge itself in the smallest vessels, causing an inflammatory response and damaging vessels, such as in **meningococcemia, gonococcemia, yeast, deep fungal infections, or endocarditis.**
      1. **Inflammatory vasculitis**
         a. Skin findings occur in nearly one half of patients with **Wegener's granulomatosis.** Palpable purpura of the lower extremities is the most common presentation. Ulcers, papules, and nodules can occur. Oral ulcerations occur frequently and may be the initial presentation. Laryngeal, pulmonary, neurologic, renal, or ocular disease often is present. The latter symptoms include conjunctivitis and scleritis. Skin or tissue biopsy shows necrotizing vasculitis, although skin biopsy alone may show only a leukocytoclastic vasculitis. An antineutrophil cytoplasmic antibody (ANCA) test is often positive.
         b. In **polyarteritis nodosa,** a livedo or netlike pattern of purpura is often present with papules, nodules, or ulcers in a linear distribution. Palpable purpura of the lower extremities is another presentation. Polyarteritis nodosa can be associated with hepatitis B surface antibody as well as with a positive ANCA.
         c. **Churg-Strauss syndrome** occurs in patients with a history of asthma and eosinophilia. Skin findings consist of palpable purpura on the lower extremities. Skin biopsy shows a leukocytoclastic vasculitis.

2. **Infectious vasculitis**

   a. **Endocarditis** can produce characteristic purpuric macules or papules on the palms (**Janeway lesions,** or when more prominent, **Osler's nodes**), **petechiae** (often scant in number), and **splinter hemorrhages** on the nails (a more reliable sign when present on multiple fingers and the proximal nailbed). Purpuric pustules or, in sepsis, large areas of purpura and necrosis can occur. Red blood cells may be present in the urine. Blood cultures confirm infection. Necrotizing vasculitis may be present on skin biopsy.

   b. Both **meningococcemia and gonococcemia** are characterized by small pustules on a purpuric base. In gonococcemia, the lesions are scant in number and located over joints. In meningococcemia, petechiae may be numerous or scant. Lesions can range in size with no characteristic distribution and can vary in number. Prompt diagnosis and treatment for meningococcemia is crucial (Chapter 27).

   c. **Rocky Mountain spotted fever** initially presents with small, lightly erythematous macules or papules on the wrist and palms. The papules then spread up the arms centrally on the trunk and concomitantly become purpuric. The lack of purpura with the initial lesions often causes the physician to overlook the possibility of the diagnosis of Rocky Mountain spotted fever. Prior to or accompanying the rash of Rocky Mountain spotted fever, the patient appears abruptly ill with fevers, headaches, and often abdominal pain, which can mimic an acute abdomen. If these symptoms occur before the rash, exploratory abdominal surgery can ensue with suspicions of an acute abdominal process. The fatality rate is high. Any suspicion necessitates prompt antibiotic therapy [e.g., doxycycline (except in pregnancy or for children), chloramphenicol (for children)]. Laboratory tests, which should not delay treatment, include serology for *Rickettsia* in acute and convalescent serum, and immunofluorescent staining of the antigen in skin biopsies (not offered at most centers).

3. **Hypersensitivity vasculitis.** Apart from palpable purpura as a sign of vasculitis, petechiae combined with larger areas of purpura can represent the hypersensitivity vasculitis known as **Henoch-Schönlein purpura (HSP)** in patients aged less than 21 years. In older patients, it is simply called **hypersensitivity vasculitis.** It is characterized by petechiae on the lower legs with larger purpuric papules or plaques. Lesions can extend from the

lower legs to the upper thighs on to the buttocks. Skin lesions often are preceded or accompanied by abdominal pain, diarrhea, hematochezia, renal failure, and elevated liver function tests. Monitoring of hepatic and renal function is imperative. If cutaneous lesions are absent, the initial abdominal pain may precipitate exploratory abdominal surgery for an acute abdomen. Attacks are often recurrent. Skin biopsy shows a leukocytoclastic vasculitis and, if performed within 12 to 24 hours of lesion onset, may demonstrate staining of perivascular IgA. Eosinophilia and anemia may be present. The antigen is often a drug or infection. In addition to supportive treatment and eliminating the offending organism, prednisone sometimes in combination with cytotoxic immunosuppressive agents can be used in severe cases.

C. **Depositional disorders.** These disorders represent damage to the blood vessels, with resultant extravasation of blood and resultant purpura.

   1. In depositional disorders such as **systemic amyloidosis,** material is deposited within the vessel, which causes the vessel to be fragile. The production of purpura by pinching a thin-skinned area such as the eyelid is very suggestive of amyloidosis. Macroglossia and smooth erythematous or purpuric papules can occur.

   2. In **cryoglobulinemia,** cryoglobulin deposition within the wall of the blood vessel renders the blood vessel susceptible to trauma. Purpuric lesions in cryoglobulinemia occur most distally in cooler areas (e.g., fingers, toes, hands, feet, and ears).

   3. **Cholesterol emboli** characteristically manifest on the distal skin, mainly hands and feet. A livedo or netlike pattern is characteristic. A patient with cholesterol emboli may present with ulceration. Renal failure can ensue days to months later. Early onset of renal failure indicates a poor prognosis.

D. **Purpura from hematologic disorders** not caused by an inherent blood vessel deficiency, but rather from a hematologic disorder that results in purpura.

   1. **Disseminated intravascular coagulation (DIC).** Large stellate-shaped purpuric macules appear in an asymmetric fashion on the body. Lesions can appear at any location and can be several centimeters in diameter. Petechia may also be present.

   2. **Protein C and protein S deficiency.** Patients with abnormal or deficient protein C or protein S may present with large areas of purpura that can subsequently undergo necrosis. Patients with one of these deficiencies are most at risk for cutaneous infarction when warfarin or heparin therapy is initiated or when doses are loaded. In warfarin-induced necrosis, fatty areas such as the breast and the calves are most susceptible.

3. **Heparin-related thrombosis.** Distal purpura and even necrosis can result from heparin-induced antibodies.

E. **Purpura with pain and induration. Calciphylaxis** is a poorly understood disorder that occurs most frequently in patients with renal failure and secondary hyperparathyroidism. Massive amounts of calcium precipitate with phosphate and are deposited in the skin. It appears that dysfunctional protein C or S plays a role in precipitating the depositional process. At the time of symptom onset with pain and induration, the calcium–phosphate product may be normal. Purpura ensues as vessels become more damaged, and ulceration follows. Death frequently follows. Partial or total parathyroidectomy appears to decrease or halt progression in some cases. Debridement of ulcers or affected areas and intravenous (IV) antibiotics may be necessary. Warfarin or heparin loading should be avoided, if possible, in patients at risk. Low molecular weight heparin should be substituted, when possible, in patients with calciphylaxis necessitating anticoagulation. Early diagnosis is critical. **Skin biopsy is imperative for the diagnosis,** and is distinguishable from calcinosis cutis or dystrophic calicification.

II. **Erythema**

A. **Erythema** is caused by dilation of the dermal blood vessels. Epidermal change is signified by scale. Patients with widespread erythema, covering almost the entire body surface, are termed **erythrodermic.** The differential diagnosis of erythroderma is broad and includes previous existing skin disorders (e.g., psoriasis, atopic dermatitis, pityriasis rubra pilaris, contact dermatitis), drug eruption, erythema multiforme major, cutaneous T-cell lymphoma, Norwegian scabies, toxic shock syndrome, graft-versus-host disease, and *Staphylococcal* scalded skin syndrome.

B. **Diagnosis.** A skin biopsy of a characteristic area should be done to determine the cause of the erythroderma. Morphologic and other clues are often lost with disease progression.

1. **Psoriasis** is characterized by symmetrically distributed plaques with coarse silvery scale. It may involve the scalp and intergluteal cleft. Nail changes with yellowish discoloration of the nail plate, pitting, and onycholysis (i.e., lifting up of the nail plate from the nail bed) are common features. Pustular psoriasis has small white pustules that can coalesce into lakes. The patient is often febrile, appearing very ill, often with joint pain and an elevated white blood cell count.

2. **Erythema multiforme** is characterized by erythematous macules or papules with a variety of hues of erythema, eventually creating target lesions with three hues of erythema. Erythema multiforme minor has a limited distribution of target lesions. Erythema multiforme major is characterized by mucosal mem-

brane erythema and erosiveness, and large areas of cutaneous involvement.

a. **Stevens Johnson syndrome (SJS)** refers to large areas of involvement with target lesions and mucosal membrane involvement that can include ocular involvement in the form of conjunctivitis.

b. **Toxic epidermal necrolysis** is the most feared form of erythema multiforme major, involving death and subsequent necrosis and sloughing of the epidermis. It is often characterized by its flaccid bullae, which when compressed, extend beyond the visible boundaries of the bullae, creating the so-called positive Nikolsky sign.

c. **Potential causes of erythema multiforme** apart from medications are herpes simplex and *Mycoplasma pneumoniae.* Skin biopsy will help confirm the diagnosis of erythema multiforme. Any erosive mucosa areas should be cultured for herpes simplex and a chest radiograph should be performed to look for pneumonia. For a very quick diagnosis, rolling dead elevated skin around a swab and submitting this for pathology study is another method of diagnosing toxic epidermal necrolysis.

d. **Treatment** is only considered palliative in erythema multiforme. If the patient's skin has begun to slough, which suggests evolving toxic epidermal necrolysis, steroids are not advised because of the risk of infection. With suspicion of toxic epidermal necrolysis, immediate transfer to a burn unit is advised (Chapter 34). Observation for any signs of pneumonia are important because all visceral mucosa, including pulmonary and gastrointestinal mucosa, may shed with the skin.

3. **Atopic dermatitis** generally is characterized by a light intensity, diffuse erythema with scale. Areas may be impetiginized with a characteristic yellow crusting appearance. Systemic antibiotics are indicated.

4. **Pityriasis rubra pilaris (PRP)** is characterized by orange discoloration, prominent hair follicles, and islands of sparing, particularly in the periumbilical area. Palms and soles often pass through a brief period of orange or yellow discoloration. Pityriasis rubra pilaris often is misdiagnosed as psoriasis.

5. **Cutaneous T-cell lymphoma** is characterized by papules, plaques, and nodules. Erythrodermic patients with cutaneous T-cell lymphoma, by definition, have an advanced stage of T-cell lymphoma. The intensity of erythema often is deep as opposed to atopic dermatitis, which has light intensity erythema.

6. **Staphylococcal scalded-skin syndrome (SSSS)** is characterized by painful erythema that can be localized or generalized, with or without flaccid bullae. Erythema is periorifical and in intertriginous areas initially and becomes generalized. Bullae can lead to erosions. Because the disease is toxin-mediated, the bullae do not contain *Staphylococcus* organisms unless it is the site of inoculum. Children and individuals with renal failure are at increased risk because of their inability to eliminate the toxin.

7. **Toxic shock syndrome (TSS)** is another toxin-mediated illness that can cause generalized erythema from *Staphylococcus aureus*. Fever, hypotension, and multiorgan symptoms, including weakness, diarrhea, dyspnea and seizures, can have an abrupt onset. The rash has a variety of presentations including widespread erythema or a scarlet feverlike eruption with small rough papules. Mucosal membrane involvement, including a strawberry tongue, other oral findings, and ocular involvement, is common. The rash is often more prominent around the infected site.

C. **Laboratory data.** Patients with erythroderma often are hypokalemic, hypoalbuminemic, and dehydrated. Patients with pustular psoriasis may have white blood cell counts in the range of 20,000 cells/μl. Erythrocyte sedimentation rates often are elevated in all forms of erythroderma. Pustules in pustular psoriasis are usually negative on culture. *S. aureus* is sometimes cultured, because patients can be colonized from prior hospitalizations or from contact with other people.

D. **Treatment.** The patient who is erythrodermic is generally very cold, shivering, and highly uncomfortable. Initial treatment is aimed at alleviating these symptoms.

1. **Topical steroids** with occlusion are used in a noninfectious, inflammatory process (e.g., psoriasis, atopic dermatitis) because they are vasoconstrictive. In pustular psoriasis, topical steroids without occlusion are suggested. Plastic wraps or occlusive suits are applied over a medium potency topical steroid such as 0.025% fluocinolone acetonide twice daily. The areas are occluded for 2 hours twice a day. Topical steroids, especially over large areas or under occlusions, as with systemic steroids, will decrease serum potassium concentration and increase blood glucose levels in predisposed patients. In addition, the erythroderma by itself predisposes to hypokalemia.

2. Treatment after the short-term use of topical steroids is directed toward the underlying cause of the erythroderma. For a drug eruption, a period of 2 to 3 weeks leads to improvement and care is supportive. In psoriatic patients, systemic immunosuppressive therapy for a severe flare and phototherapy are options. If phototherapy is anti-

cipated, additional lubrication and topical steroid treatments are administered to decrease scale and allow for the penetration of light therapy. Systemic steroids are *not* a treatment for psoriasis.

3. The patient with an erythrodermic pustular psoriatic condition with blood cultures positive for *S. aureus* should be treated with IV antibiotics.

4. **Norwegian scabies** is treated overnight with an antiscabetic agent such as a permethrin cream (Elimite), rinsed off 8 hours after application. The drug is reapplied approximately 7 days later to treat any remaining eggs. Sheets should be cleaned before and after treatment. Clothing worn prior to treatment should only be worn again after washing or after 3 days have elapsed since wearing.

5. In **SSSS or TSS**, IV antibiotic therapy and fluid resuscitation should be instituted immediately.

III. **Generalized erythema without erythroderma**

A. Generalized erythema can present as a **drug eruption** or as another **hypersensitivity reaction** to an antigen such as a virus or parasite. A decreased inflammatory response imposed by steroids may allow a parasite to proliferate and a hypersensitivity response will then worsen. In the event that pruritus or erythema is worsened with systemic steroid administration, a search for parasitic infection should be pursued.

B. **Viral infections** that can cause such eruptions include **parvovirus** B19 (associated with erythema infectiosum or fifth disease), **measles (rubeola),** and **German measles (rubella).**

1. In **rubeola,** small, bright red lesions on the buccal mucosa, called Koplik's spots, can precede the rash and become less distinct with rash progression. Coryza is prominent. An erythematous rash consisting of macules and papules begins in the posterior auricular areas and in the forehead and extend inferiorly over the face, neck, trunk, and extremities.

2. The rash of **rubella** begins on the face and progresses rapidly to the neck, arms, trunk, and legs. The rash usually disappears at the end of 2 or 3 days. Erythematous macules and papules are discrete and become coalescent to the trunk. Lymphadenopathy may be prominent. Petechiae on the soft palate may be seen during the prodrome.

3. **Acute human immunodeficiency virus (HIV) conversion** also can cause a generalized macular or papular erythematous eruption.

C. **Scarlet fever** caused by group A *Streptococcus* (and occasionally *S. aureus*) is characterized by light intensity erythema, often consisting of fine papules. The papules give the skin a "sandpaperlike" feel, which can generalize and be accentuated in skin folds (Pastia's lines).

IV. **Vesicular and pustular disorders**

A. **Herpes simplex (HSV) infections** are commonly seen in critically ill patients (Chapter 28). These infections are characterized by vesicles or pustules that may be hemorrhagic and which are grouped on the nose, lips, or other areas. Traumatic procedures to these areas, such as endotracheal intubation and nasogastric tube placement, tend to predispose individuals to outbreaks of herpes simplex. Genital herpetic lesions when cleansed or traumatized, especially in patients who have any type of urinary or bowel incontinence or diarrhea, can spread from inoculation of herpes simplex to irritated areas. Monomorphic erosions, papules, vesicles, or pustules, and pain in any erythematous or scaly area should raise the possibility of herpes simplex.

1. Uncomplicated HSV infections in adults can be treated with **acyclovir** (200 mg) orally, five times daily, or **famciclovir** (125 mg; 250 mg for initial infection) orally twice daily for 5 to 10 days.

2. In immunocompromised adults, HSV can be treated with IV **acyclovir** (5 mg/kg; the dose must be decreased in renal insufficiency) every 8 hours for 3 to 10 days. With improvement, drug administration can be switched to the oral route.

B. **Herpes zoster** is characterized by grouped vesicles or pustules in a dermatomal distribution. In immunosuppressed patients, lesions of herpes zoster can be atypically papular or nodular. Herpes zoster frequently begins with pain, absence of skin findings, and localized erythema, initially without any vesiculation. In these cases, the erythema may be misdiagnosed as cellulitis. Likewise, preeruptive zoster, depending on the location of pain, can be misdiagnosed as nephrolithiasis, angina, or an acute abdomen. Herpes zoster in the perianal area can lead to diarrhea and temporary bowel incontinence. At the time that erythema presents, it is useful to perform a complete skin examination to look for isolated vesicles outside of the dermatome. A small number of isolated vesicles occur outside of involved dermatomes.

C. **Varicella zoster infection** is characterized by fever, malaise, and light intensity erythematous plaques with a central vesicle. Lesions can be scant or numerous. Small erosive lesions can occur on the buccal mucosa or on the tongue. Lesions of varicella zoster can become impetiginized, especially in children with atopic dermatitis. When this occurs, isolated bullae with yellow crust occupy the sites of previous vesicles.

1. Varicella zoster can be treated in adults with **acyclovir** (800 mg) orally five times a day or **famciclovir** (500 mg) orally three times daily.

2. In immunocompromised adults, varicella zoster can be treated with **acyclovir** (10 mg/kg) every 8 hours (the dose must be decreased in renal insufficiency).

D. **Vesicular and pustular drug eruptions.** Any drug can cause a vesicular or pustular drug reaction. Vesicles can become pustular or pustules, which may occur as the primary lesion. Initial vesiculation should also raise the possibility of evolving bullous erythema multiforme or toxic epidermal necrolysis.

1. **Pustular drug reaction (early).** Pustules can represent infectious causes such as cutaneous candidiasis and staphylococcal infections. On the feet, superficial fungal infections can manifest themselves as either vesicles or pustules.

2. **Sweet's syndrome and pyoderma gangrenosum (PG).** Lesions frequently start as a small pustule on an erythematous base and enlarge into a nodule, which can be several centimeters in diameter. Patients often exhibit high white blood cell counts and fevers during eruptive periods. The surface is described as having a hint of vesiculation, but the lesions do not produce fluid. Lesions are often painful. The most common associated diagnosis is acute myelogenous leukemia with Sweet's syndrome and ulcerative colitis with pyoderma gangrenosum. Both are histopathologically characterized by a neutrophilic infiltrate in the dermis and epidermis.

   a. **Avoid debridement.** Sweet's syndrome and pyoderma gangrenosum commonly are misdiagnosed as bacterial infections and subsequently debrided. It is important to avoid debridement until a biopsy is performed and the results known because Sweet's syndrome and PG exhibit pathergy. Trauma elicits further manifestation of disease activity, most commonly exhibited as progressive ulceration. Lesions, therefore, often occur at IV sites and other sites of trauma.

   b. **Treatment** for Sweet's syndrome and PG is with high-dose **systemic steroids,** usually beginning with IV Solu-Medrol and later replaced by oral prednisone with a minimal strength dose beginning at 60 mg daily. **Intralesional steroid injections** of the expanding rim is another treatment option, given alone in mild cases or in combination with systemic steroids in more severe cases. The application of **cromolyn solution,** a mast cell inhibitor, is complementary therapy.

V. **Ulcerative processes**

   A. **Skin breakdown on the heels and sacrum, as well as the posterior scalp and scapular area** can occur in the ICU setting where patients are immobile for long periods. A patient with **vascular disease** is even more susceptible to ulceration from pressure and trauma. **Herpes simplex** is common in perianal and hip areas, and ulcer edges should be examined for a scalloped shape characteristic of previously coalescent vesicles. A Tzanck preparation or viral culture should be performed as needed. Ulcers should be cultured for bacteria and yeast, if such are suspected. Treatment of pressure ulcers involves frequent side-to-side turning and placement of padding under pressure areas such as the heels. Wet-to-dry dressings are preferable if lesions are infected, and occlusive dressings should be avoided in these areas other than to avoid infection from fecal incontinence. Systemic antibiotics may be necessary.

B. **Cancers** that metastasize to the skin can cause ulceration. Frequently, the surface of the ulcer is nodular or undulating. Metastatic carcinomas can cause deep induration around the ulcer.

C. **Infectious causes** of ulcerative processes include the initially nodular entities of **eccthmya gangrenosum and eccthyma. Meleney's ulcer** is an insidious process in which synergistic staphylococcal and streptococcal infections result in an aggressive ulcerative process that responds only to debridement and IV antibiotics.

D. **Warfarin-induced necrosis** is characterized by ulceration of fatty areas such as the breasts, abdomen, calves, or buttocks. Purpura often borders these areas and the initial lesion often is a purpuric plaque. Many individuals with warfarin-induced necrosis have low levels of protein.

E. **Calciphylaxis** is discussed above (see section **I.E.**).

F. Lesions of pyoderma gangrenosum and Sweet's syndrome frequently ulcerate (see section **IV.D.2.**).

VI. **Bullae** may begin as vesicles and enlarge.

A. **Bullous hypersensitivity reactions** can result from any drug. A skin biopsy is necessary to distinguish them from **bullous pemphigoid, bullous erythema multiforme, or toxic epidermal necrolysis.**

B. Bullae also can be caused by local ischemia (e.g., in DIC or in cholesterol emboli). In these cases, bullae are generally preceded by purpura.

C. **Contact dermatitis** can present with bullae on an erythematous and scaly base, often in a geometric pattern. Bullae also can result from peripheral edema, which commonly occurs on the lower extremities.

D. **Toxic epidermal necrolysis and pemphigus vulgaris** are characterized by short-lived, flaccid bullae. The skin sloughs easily, and both diseases demonstrate mucosal ulceration that is diffuse. The Nikolsky sign is positive, meaning that the bullae expand when compressed. All mucosa including ocular, oral, anal, and genital mucosa should be examined.

E. Intact bullae, often tense, are seen in **bullous impetigo, bullous lupus erythematosus, bullous pemphigoid,** and **bullous diabeticorum.** When compressed, the bullae do not expand, thereby exhibiting **a negative Nikolsky sign. Bullous lupus erythematosus** and **bullous pemphigoid** are diagnosed by skin biopsy. The lesions of bullous diabeticorum are nonspecific. In bullous impetigo, the bullous fluid grows *S. aureus* or *Streptococcus* spp.

F. **Treatment guidelines.** The area should be cleaned with sterile saline and then dried. A moist covering with a dressing such as xeroform is optional. Lesions susceptible to breakage can be drained by piercing the edge of the lesion once or twice with a sterile needle. In inflammatory processes, it is advisable that the bullae remain intact to provide a protective covering of the dermis. The underlying causes of **bullous pemphigoid** and **bullous lupus erythematosus** frequently require systemic immunosuppressive therapy.

SELECTED REFERENCES

Champion RH, ed. *Rook / Wilkinson / Ebling textbook of dermatology,* 6th edition. London: Blackwell Science, 1998.

Fitzpatrick TB, Johnson RA, Wolff K. *Color atlas and synopsis of clinical dermatology,* 3rd ed. New York: McGraw-Hill, 1997.

Freedberg IM, Eisen AZ, Wolff K. *Fitzpatrick's dermatology in general medicine,* 5th ed. New York: McGraw Hill, 1999.

Surgical Considerations

Special Considerations in Trauma Patients

Ralph L. Warren

I. **Introduction**
   A. One of the important developments in the care of trauma patients has been the widespread acceptance of a philosophical and strategic operative approach termed "**damage control.**" This strategy consists of rapid temporary measures to control bleeding and to stop intestinal leakage. This is followed by rapid abdominal closure and transport of the patient to the intensive care unit (ICU), rather than proceeding immediately with definitive repair of multiple severe injuries in an unstable patient. Early admission to the ICU allows for correction (or even prevention) of the "lethal triad" of hypothermia, acidosis, and coagulopathy. After stabilization in the ICU, the patient is returned to the operating room for definitive reconstruction in a controlled situation.
   B. **The principles of resuscitation** for trauma victims are the same as for any other patient.
      1. **Acidosis** is corrected by restoration of adequate circulation (Chapters 2, 9, and 10).
      2. **Coagulopathy** is corrected by transfusion of blood products, especially fresh frozen plasma and platelets (Chapter 12).
      3. **Hypothermia** can be lethal, rendering the myocardium susceptible to dysfunction and dysrhythmias, and producing severe coagulopathies when the core temperature is below 34°C. Hypothermia is an insidious consequence of massive volume resuscitation and the need for complete exposure of the patient to ambient temperature for evaluation and management. Trauma patients start to lose heat at the scene, but heat loss is greatly accelerated in the emergency department, the operating room, and the ICU, unless preventive measures are taken.
         a. **Resuscitation fluids** should all be warmed to at least 42°C (it is probably safe to heat even blood to as high as 49°C), preferably using a high-volume warmer.
         b. **Inspired gases** from the ventilator can also be heated to 42°C.
         c. **Warming blankets** should be used and the **room temperature** increased. Forced warm air blankets, such as the "Bair Hugger," are effective and should cover all parts of the patient not needed to be exposed for examination or treatment.

II. **Blunt myocardial injury**
   A. **Blunt cardiac injury** is the currently accepted term that encompasses a variety of injuries to the heart and

its components secondary to blunt chest trauma. Included are valvular disruption and coronary artery dissection and thrombosis, as well as *blunt myocardial injury,* which is commonly known as "myocardial contusion." The diagnosis of blunt myocardial injury, short of pathologic examination, remains controversial.

B.   Complications of blunt myocardial injury include dysrhythmias, complete heart block, congestive heart failure, myocardial ischemia, pericarditis, tamponade, cardiogenic shock, and late constrictive pericarditis. In one study, 25% of patients with cardiac complications had no external stigmata of chest injury.

C.   Diagnosis

1.   Electrocardiogram (ECG). Over the first few hours after injury serial ECGs are important *screening* tools in patients with blunt chest trauma. Although an abnormal ECG is significant, a normal admission ECG alone cannot rule out a myocardial injury. Approximately one third of patients with blunt myocardial injury who initially had normal ECGs subsequently develop ventricular dysrhythmias. Myocardial contusions also have been documented at autopsy in patients who had a normal admission ECG.

a.   A 24-hour period is a reasonable upper limit for cardiac monitoring if the ECG is normal. Although some later ECG changes may occur, they are not significant. They are not associated with complications and do not require treatment.

b.   Sinus tachycardia is the most common ECG abnormality associated with blunt myocardial injury. Premature atrial and ventricular contractions are the next most common signs, but are generally of little clinical significance.

c.   Significant ECG findings, which may portend future dangerous dysrhythmias, include ST-T wave changes suggestive of myocardial ischemia, intraventricular conduction defects, multifocal premature vascular contractions (PVCs), ventricular tachycardia or fibrillation, and new atrial fibrillation or flutter.

2.   Creatine phosphokinase (CPK)-MB measurements are of little value in blunt myocardial injury. They do not correlate with ECG changes, wall motion abnormalities seen on echocardiogram, or with subsequent development of cardiac complications. The value of serum **troponin** levels remains under investigation.

3.   Radionuclide imaging studies, such as gated blood pool scintigraphy (GBPS), indium-111 antimyosin scintigraphy, and single photon emission computed tomography (SPECT), have been evaluated in patients with chest trauma. Blood pool scanning is neither sensitive nor specific and antimyosin scintigraphy and SPECT, although perhaps more accurate, are too expensive to be useful screening tools.

4. **Echocardiography** is the current procedure of choice to assess the heart for possible blunt injury. Because of its immediate substernal location, the right ventricle is the chamber most frequently and most severely damaged by blunt chest trauma. Not only can wall motion abnormalities be visualized, but the valves and the pericardium can be evaluated.

   a. Whether **transthoracic** echo (TTE) or **transesophageal** echocardiography (TEE) is preferred depends mostly on local expertise and availability. Visualization of the right ventricle is often superior with a transesophageal approach.

   b. **The correlation** between echocardiographic wall motion abnormalities and the subsequent occurrence of important dysrhythmias is poor. Consequently, echocardiography should not be used as a *screening* tool to "rule out myocardial contusion" in everyone with blunt chest trauma. Rather, it should be used to answer a specific question or evaluate a specific problem.

   c. **A reasonable approach** is to use echocardiography only in those patients with a new murmur (to evaluate the valves), hemodynamic instability or insufficiency (to evaluate the pericardium, the valves, and ventricular wall motion), and possibly in those patients with significant ECG abnormalities.

5. **Sternal fractures** are associated with seatbelt use, but not necessarily with blunt myocardial injury. It is likely that the seat belt and the fractured sternum absorb a substantial portion of the energy in an accident and may prevent more serious injuries. Isolated sternal fractures (i.e., without other evident chest injuries) do not mandate ECG monitoring, unless other risk factors are present, including age more than 55 years, a history of ischemic heart disease, or abnormal ECG findings.

D. **A reasonable strategy for management** includes:

   1. **ICU admission** if hemodynamics are unstable or an important dysrhythmia or conduction defect is present.

   2. **Cardiac monitoring** in the hospital and serial 12-lead ECGs over 24 hours if hemodynamics and initial ECG are normal.

   3. **Echocardiography** only if hemodynamically unstable or if a new murmur is present.

   4. **Operations for other injuries** should be performed as needed. Additional monitoring (e.g., peripheral and pulmonary arterial catheters) may be necessary in those patients with dysrhythmias or hemodynamic instability.

III.   Traumatic disruption of the thoracic aorta

A.   Disruption of the thoracic aorta secondary to blunt trauma is the most common injury of the great vessels. Of the 50,000 traffic accident fatalities in the United States each year, approximately 15% (7,500) are caused by rupture of the thoracic aorta. Injuries consist of transverse, usually circumferential, tears of the intima and varying amounts of media and adventitia. If the full thickness of media and adventitia are torn, as is the case in 85% of those with the injury, immediate death from exsanguination into the pleural cavity occurs. In the remaining 15%, at least the outer layers of the adventitia and mediastinal pleura are intact, and the patient can survive to reach a hospital. The tear is most often a well-localized lesion; actual dissection of the aortic wall rarely occurs in the absence of preexisting degenerative changes.

B.   Location. Approximately 90% of tears occur at the **aortic isthmus,** which is the most proximal portion of the descending thoracic aorta just distal to the origin of the left subclavian artery. This part of the aorta is relatively fixed to the main pulmonary artery by the ligamentum arteriosum. The aortic arch and more distal descending aorta are free to move during rapid accelerations or decelerations. Approximately 5% of tears occur in the **ascending aorta** a few centimeters above the aortic annulus (This is also the site of most intimal tears in cases of spontaneous aortic dissection.) This lesion is immediately fatal in 95% of victims. A few tears occur in the more distal thoracic aorta (and even fewer in the abdominal aorta), most often adjacent to a spinal fracture. A few occur at the origins of the great vessels, and up to 5% of patients have more than one tear.

C.   The diagnosis of traumatic aortic disruption requires a high index of suspicion. Most patients have other more obvious injuries. No pathognomonic symptoms or signs are present, and, if treatment is not instituted expeditiously, sudden death is likely.

1. Most aortic tears occur secondary to high speed (greater than 20 miles/h) motor vehicle accidents. The incidence is higher in car occupants if they are driving, if they are unbelted, and if they are ejected. Both head-on and side-impact collisions can disrupt the aorta. Aortic tears occur in all age groups, although they are relatively rare in children.

2. **Symptoms** are nonspecific and most often overshadowed by associated injuries. Chest or upper back pain and dyspnea are frequent, but they are usually attributable to overlying chest wall injury. Symptoms suggestive of a mediastinal mass (e.g., stridor or wheezing, dysphagia, hoarseness, or superior vena cava obstruction) are rarely present. Some patients with aortic disruption are completely asymptomatic.

3. **Physical findings** are usually nonspecific: external evidence of chest wall injury is present in 70% to 90%. Less than a third of patients have a "pseudo-coarctation" syndrome: unequal arm blood pressures, upper extremity hypertension with diminished femoral pulses, or both, and decreased lower extremity blood pressure. A precordial or interscapular systolic murmur is found in 10% to 20%. Importantly, 2% to 5% will present with paraplegia, caused by either concomitant direct cord trauma or spinal cord ischemia secondary to the aortic disruption.

4. **The chest radiograph (CXR),** the single most helpful initial test, shows evidence of mediastinal bleeding (mediastinal widening) in 90% to 95% of those with disrupted aortas. Eighty percent of mediastinal bleeding in victims of blunt trauma is caused by injuries other than aortic disruption, and up to 5% of patients with an aortic tear have a normal CXR.

5. Several factors complicate the interpretation of mediastinal widening:
   a. Most mediastinal widening is caused by bleeding from small vessels rather than from the aorta or its large branches.
   b. Anteroposterior (AP) portable CXRs will display an apparent widening of the mediastinum because of geometry alone.
   c. The definition of "widened" is problematic; 8 cm is usually considered the upper limit of normal for the width of the mediastinum at the level of the aortic knob. Alternatively, a ratio of the mediastinal width to the internal width of the chest at the level of the aortic knob greater than 0.25 is considered abnormal.

6. **Other chest radiographic signs** of thoracic aortic injury include obscuring of the normally quite distinct "aortic knob," obliteration of the notch between the aortic knob and the left main pulmonary artery, rightward deviation of the trachea or a nasogastric tube in the esophagus, depression of the left main bronchus to an angle of more than 140° from the trachea, fluid in the left pleural cavity, widening of the right paratracheal or paraspinous stripes, and a left "apical cap," which is a result of blood dissecting from the mediastinum up over the dome of the hemithorax.

7. **Definitive diagnosis** can be made by contrast angiography, computed tomography (CT), transesophageal echocardiography, or magnetic resonance imaging (MRI).
   a. **Angiography** is the "gold standard," with nearly 100% sensitivity and specificity. Angiography also provides a complete view of the aorta, its branches, and the extent of the injury. Disadvantages of angiography include the need

for potentially nephrotoxic intravenous (IV) contrast agents and the time it takes to assemble the vascular radiology team and perform the procedure.

b. **Computed tomography** of the chest is increasingly useful because of the increasing sophistication of CT scanners. To maintain high sensitivity, the criteria used to properly interpret the CT scans must be strictly followed (Table 33-1). Unless all five criteria for a negative scan are fulfilled, the study cannot reliably exclude aortic injury, and aortography is mandated. Most cardiac surgical groups require aortography to confirm positive findings and provide detailed anatomic images.

c. **Transesophageal echocardiography** offers several advantages over aortography. It is less invasive, the injured aorta is not directly instrumented, it is usually less time-consuming, it can be done in remote locations, no nephrotoxic contrast agents are required, and the heart can be examined at the same time. TEE, however, cannot always adequately visualize the aortic arch and its main branches. Injuries to the other great vessels can be missed. In addition, few operators currently have sufficient experience with traumatic aortic injuries to perform a reliable examination.

d. **Magnetic resonance imaging** is an excellent modality to visualize the thoracic aorta, but is not yet readily available in most emergency trauma situations. It also remains extremely

Table 33-1.   Criteria for interpreting CT scans in aortic injury

Negative CT scans in patients with suspected aortic injury
Good contrast enhancement of aorta
No interfering artifacts
A complete study
Film read by an experienced CT radiologist
Absence of "positive" criteria
Positive CT scans in patients with suspected aortic injury
Mediastinal hematoma contiguous with the aorta
False aneurysm
Irregular aortic contour
Divided aortic lumen
Intimal flap

CT, computed tomography.
Adapted from Agee CK, Metzler MH, Churchill RJ, et al. Computed tomographic evaluation to exclude traumatic aortic disruption. *J Trauma* 1992;33: 876–881.

difficult to closely monitor and continue to resuscitate unstable patients while they are in the scanner.

D. Treatment

1. **Initial resuscitation.** (Chapters 1, 9, and 10)

    a. Place large gauge IV lines and begin fluid resuscitation with Ringer's lactate or normal saline solution.

    b. Place chest tubes (36 French) when blood pressure and pain can be controlled. Blood drained from the chest tubes can be autotransfused.

    c. Place a nasogastric tube prior to performing a peritoneal lavage. Otherwise, wait until hypertension is under control.

    d. If severe hypotension is persistent, do not perform an angiogram and proceed directly to the operating room.

2. As soon as the diagnosis is suggested, begin pharmacologic therapy in hemodynamically stable patients. The goal is to decrease the force of the blood pressure pulse (**dP/dt**) on the injured aorta with β-adrenergic blockers, calcium channel blockers, or both. **Hemodynamic goals** generally are a heart rate in the 60 bpm range, a systolic blood pressure of 90 to 110 mm Hg, and a mean arterial blood pressure of 65 to 70 mm Hg. Higher limits may be necessary if the patient develops oliguria, myocardial ischemia, or mental status changes.

    a. Place radial arterial line, preferably on the right side.

    b. Administer **propranolol,** starting at 1 mg IV every 2 to 5 minutes.

    c. **Labetalol** 5–10 mg IV every 5 to 10 minutes and IV infusions of **esmolol** are acceptable alternatives.

    d. Do not use nifedipine because it has little effect on decreasing dP/dt.

    e. **Nitroprusside** should be used only when the lower limit of heart rate (55–65 bpm) has been reached, such that further β-blockade will lead to atrioventricular (AV) conduction problems.

    f. Adequate analgesia and sedation are important adjuncts for blood pressure control (Chapters 5 and 6).

E. Emergency surgery for aortic disruption

1. Only two injuries take precedence:

    a. Operative head injury (e.g., epidural hematoma).

    b. Massive intraabdominal hemorrhage (i.e., grossly positive abdominal tap with hemodynamic instability).

2. Prolonged medical treatment can be considered for patients with:

    a. Severe central nervous system injury.

    b. Sepsis.

        c. Extensive burns.

        d. Severe right lung injury, which precludes a left thoracotomy.

    3. For prolonged medical management, antihypertensive therapy is continued until the time of operation, slowly changing from parenteral to enteral medications. Tight control of heart rate and blood pressure must be maintained at all times.

IV. Nonoperative management of blunt hepatic injuries

  A. The liver is the organ most frequently injured by blunt torso trauma. Nonoperative management is successful in up to one half to two thirds of all adult patients with liver injuries, and up to three fourths of patients who are stable enough to undergo abdominal CT. The benefits of avoiding an operation include eliminating the short- and long-term morbidity of laparotomy (The risk of mechanical small bowel obstruction from adhesions is estimated to be ≈ 8% to 10% over 20 years.) and the exacerbation of extraabdominal injuries (e.g, closed head injury, pulmonary contusion) during anesthesia and surgery.

  B. **Indications** for nonoperative management of hepatic trauma include:

    1. **Absence of other indications for laparotomy** (e.g., peritoneal signs on physical examination, CT evidence of other operative injury).

    2. **No need for prolonged nonabdominal surgery** (e.g. craniotomy), which will limit repeated physical examinations of the abdomen.

    3. **Adequate mental status** to reliably report symptoms during repeated abdominal examinations.

    4. **Hemodynamically stable** and without requirements for intravascular volume expansion. A hemodynamically unstable patient is defined as having a blood pressure lower or heart rate higher than that expected for the patient's age, or demonstrating signs of poor peripheral perfusion (e.g., clammy skin, cool extremities).

    5. **The appearance of the liver on CT** (Table 33-2) and the amount of hemoperitoneum can help guide the decision to operate, but the CT grade correlates poorly with operative and pathologic findings and is *not* predictive of those who can receive successful nonoperative management. Nevertheless, 90% of grade V injuries and all grade VI injures will be associated with hemodynamic instability.

    6. **Some injuries** are well-suited to nonoperative management (e.g., posterior right hepatic injuries, "split liver").

    7. **Pooling of IV contrast** in the liver parenchyma indicates active bleeding, which can be embolized in the interventional radiology suite.

  C. **Complications** of nonoperative management include:

    1. **Blood transfusions;** however, in many series, operative management has a higher transfusion risk.

Table 33-2. AAST hepatic injury scale

Grade		Injury description
I	Hematoma	Subcapsular, nonexpanding, <10% surface area
	Laceration	Capsular, nonbleeding, <1 cm depth
II	Hematoma	Subcapsular, nonexpanding, 10% to 50% surface area
		Intraparenchymal, nonexpanding, <2 cm diameter
	Laceration	Capsular, active bleeding, 1–3 cm depth, <10 cm length
III	Hematoma	Subcapsular, expanding or >50% surface area
		Ruptured subcapsular with active bleeding
		Intraparenchymal >2 cm diameter or expanding
	Laceration	>3 cm depth
IV	Hematoma	Ruptured central hematoma with active bleeding
	Laceration	25% to 50% of lobe parenchymal disruption
V	Hematoma	>50% of lobe parenchymal disruption
	Laceration	Venous disruption: major hepatic veins, retrohepatic inferior vena cava
VI		Hepatic avulsion

AAST, American Association for the Surgery of Trauma.

2. **Missed injuries.** Some injuries are not well demonstrated by CT, especially hollow viscus injuries. The incidence of such missed injuries is estimated to be between 2% and 15% (probably closer to 2%).
3. **Delayed bleeding** is uncommon (< 10%) and usually occurs in the first 10 days, but has been reported up to 4 weeks following injury. Most bleeding can be treated nonoperatively with angiographic embolization.
4. **Bilomas, hemobilia, and abscesses** are rare and will be evident by physical signs and symptoms. Most can be treated nonoperatively.

D. **Details of nonoperative management**
   1. **Length of ICU stay** is determined by the overall condition of the patient and perhaps by the CT grade of the hepatic injury. The minimal safe length of stay in the ICU has not been determined, but a prolonged stay (> 24 hours) is probably not warranted in the absence of hemodynamic instability.
   2. **The required duration of bedrest** and limited activity has not been determined. It is likely that more than 2 to 3 days of bedrest are not necessary for the hepatic injury *per se,* and that full activity can be

resumed in 4 months at most. The necessity for bedrest was probably best summarized by Meredith in 1994: "If the Oldsmobile Delta 88 striking the patient did not stimulate sufficient hemorrhage to warrant surgery, then it is unlikely that walking to the bathroom will."

3. **Time for resolution** of the injury correlates with injury severity. The worst injuries are completely healed in 4 months.

4. **Follow-up CT scans** should be obtained only to investigate persistent or new symptoms or signs. A late scan in an asymptomatic patient may be useful to demonstrate complete resolution in order to return the patient to full activity before 4 months.

V. **Abdominal compartment syndrome**

A. **Normal intraabdominal pressure** is zero (equal to ambient atmospheric pressure) or less. Many pathologic conditions produce elevated intraabdominal pressure, ranging from intestinal obstruction to hemorrhagic pancreatitis.

B. **Excessive intraabdominal pressure** has several physiologic effects.

1. Starting at pressures as low as 10 to 15 mm Hg, **stroke volume and cardiac output are decreased** through effects on both preload and afterload. Venous return via the inferior vena cava is impaired. Ventricular diastolic filling is impaired because of increased extracardiac intrathoracic pressure. Systemic vascular resistance is increased, not only because of elevated periaortic intrathoracic pressure, but also because of mechanical compression of extrathoracic capillary beds. The result is a pericardial tamponadelike state. Measured intracardiac pressures appear high and the patient appears hypovolemic. Tachycardia, oliguria, and excessive respiratory variation in the arterial pressure trace are present. The left ventricle is small and hyperdynamic on gated blood pool scans or echocardiography. Cardiac output and stroke volume are low. They *do* increase with a volume challenge, but at the expense of further increases in filling pressures. All these abnormalities disappear immediately on relief of high intraabdominal pressure.

2. **The lungs are compressed** by the elevated hemidiaphragms. Thoracopulmonary compliance is reduced and airway pressures during mechanical ventilation may be greatly elevated. Hypoxemia occurs from a mismatch of ventilation to perfusion, and is sometimes worsened by increasing positive end-expiratory pressure (PEEP).

3. **Urine output** is particularly sensitive to increased intraabdominal pressure. Renal perfusion is decreased, glomerular filtration is impaired, and renal venous outflow is obstructed. Plasma renin and aldosterone levels rise and oliguria appears with intraabdominal pressure as low as 10 mm Hg.

Glomerular filtration rate is only 25% of normal with an intraabdominal pressure of 20 mm Hg. A reversal of normal cortical-medullary blood flow occurs, and elevated levels of circulating antidiuretic hormone (ADH) and renin-angiotensin further contribute to low urine output.

4. **Perfusion of all abdominal viscera** is compromised by intraabdominal hypertension. Gut ischemia can be sufficiently severe to cause obvious sepsis from necrotic intestine, or be less overt, contributing to the development of systemic inflammation.

5. **Intracranial pressure is increased** and cerebral perfusion pressure decreased in response to intraabdominal hypertension. These effects can occur even with the low (< 15 mm Hg) pressures used for abdominal laparoscopic procedures.

C. **Diagnosis of intraabdominal hypertension** is straightforward. Both gastric and bladder pressures accurately reflect pressures measured via inferior vena caval catheters and intraabdominal transducers. Because of ease and cost, the method of choice for clinical measurements is to instill 100 to 200 ml sterile saline into the bladder via a urinary catheter, clamp the catheter, and transduce the intravesical pressure by placing a needle connected to a pressure transducer through the sampling port of the urinary catheter. The patient should be supine and the abdominal muscles relaxed. Acceptable pressures are below 20 mm Hg; above 20 mm Hg, deleterious effects start to appear. A pressure above 40 mm Hg usually mandates prompt intervention.

D. **Treatment of intraabdominal hypertension** consists of either reducing the mass of the intraabdominal contents [e.g., removal of fluid (blood, ascites, edema), tissue (tumor, nonviable viscus), or foreign bodies (packs)], or by simply opening the container (i.e., laparotomy). Relief of elevated pressure produces immediate improvement in all cardiopulmonary derangements. The renal and visceral impairments are corrected as long as irreversible ischemic injury has not occurred. The abdomen must either be closed without tension or left open until it can. In most cases, complete closure cannot be accomplished until the primary intraabdominal problems have resolved. In such instances, skin can be closed without the fascia or, better, be closed using synthetic material, such as a silastic sheet, to bridge the fascial gap. As the intraabdominal swelling resolves, the sheet can be reefed gently to bring the fascial edges of the wound together. The aim should be to close the fascia within a week to reduce the likelihood of wound infection.

VI. **Guidelines for the evaluation of the cervical spine in adult and pediatric patients with blunt trauma**

A. **Cervical spine injuries** occur in a minority of blunt trauma patients, but the consequences of a missed or untreated spine injury are so devastating that an extremely high index of suspicion is required. Cervical spine injury should be assumed to be present until it is ruled out.

B. Clinical evaluation. To rule out a cervical spine injury clinically, the following criteria *all* need to be met:

1. Normal mental status.
2. No neck pain.
3. No distracting injury (i.e., a source of significant pain that may overshadow any neck pain).
4. No neurologic symptoms or neurologic physical findings.
5. No neck tenderness on palpation.
6. No neck pain on gentle active (by the patient) range of motion, first side-to-side, then flexion and extension.

C. Radiologic evaluation. When cervical spine injury cannot be ruled out clinically, radiologic evaluation should be carried out with either plain films or spiral CT.

1. A complete **plain film series** consists of six films: cross-table lateral with the collar on, cross-table lateral with the collar off, AP, open-mouth odontoid, and two oblique views. Occasionally a "swimmer's view" is needed to visualize C7 and T1.
2. **Spiral CT** of the entire cervical spine can replace plain films in those patients who are undergoing CT of another body region (e.g., cranial, chest, abdomen, and pelvis). A plain film cross-table lateral view with the collar on, as part of the three-film "trauma series" on major trauma patients, should precede the spiral CT. A plain film cross-table lateral view with the collar off after the CT completes the evaluation.
3. The cervical collar should be replaced after the films are performed. The treating physician should then assess the patient for persistent significant pain, tenderness, and neurologic symptoms and signs. If these are absent (and the radiologic examination is normal), then a significant cervical spine injury has been excluded and the collar can be removed. If the patient has significant neck pain or neurologic signs and symptoms, the hard collar should be left on despite the negative radiologic evaluation, and the patient should undergo plain films with active flexion and extension (i.e., the patient moves his or her own head) in 1 to 3 weeks (to allow muscle spasm to subside) to rule out ligamentous injury (section **VI.D.3.**).
4. For comatose patients, leaving the collar on until ligamentous injury can be ruled out is not generally necessary if the plain film series or the helical CT is normal, except for the rare case in which the treating physicians deem the possibility of ligamentous injury to be high (section **VI.D.3.**).

D. Special considerations
1. **Patients transferred** from another hospital after blunt trauma should continue to have their cervical spines immobilized until an evaluation has been repeated at the receiving hospital. Any films from the referring facility should be reviewed by the receiving hospital, and additional studies performed if necessary.
2. **Patients with isolated gunshot wounds of the head** (no blunt injury) generally do not require radiologic evaluation of the cervical spine.
3. **Ligamentous injury** can be ruled out by either flexion and extension films (preferable) or by MRI. Flexion and extension films are done only with the patient providing active range of motion, up to but not beyond the point of pain. The neck is never moved by another person.
4. **Patients should not be left on backboards for more than 2 hours,** regardless of the presence of a spine injury. The backboard should be removed at the time the patient is log-rolled to assess the back during the secondary trauma survey, or when the patient is transferred to the x-ray or operating table, even if spine injury has not been ruled out.

SELECTED REFERENCES

Damage Control/Hypothermia
Brasel KJ, Ku J, Baker CC, et al. Damage control in the critically ill and injured patient. *New Horizons* 1999;7:73–86.
Ku J, Brasel KJ, Baker CC, et al. Triangle of death: hypothermia, acidosis, and coagulopathy. *New Horizons* 1999;7:61–72.
Porter JM, Ivatury RR, Nassoura ZE. Extending the horizons of "damage control" in unstable trauma patients beyond the abdomen and gastrointestinal tract. *J Trauma* 1997;42:559–561.
Watts DD, Trask A, Soeken K, et al. Hypothermic coagulopathy in trauma: effect of varying levels of hypothermia on enzyme speed, platelet function, and fibrinolytic activity. *J Trauma* 1998;44: 846–854.

Blunt Myocardial Injury
Cachecho R, Grindlinger GA, Lee VW. The clinical significance of myocardial contusion. *J Trauma* 1992;33:68–73.
Fabian TC, Cicala RS, Croce MA, et al. A prospective evaluation of myocardial contusion: correlation of significant arrhythmias and cardiac output with CPK-MB measurements. *J Trauma* 1991;31: 653–660.
Isenberg JS, Ozuner G, Girgis I, et al. A rational approach to the diagnosis of cardiac contusion. *Contemporary Surgery* 1991;38:47–54.
Jones JW, Hewitt RL, Drapanas T. Cardiac contusion: a capricious syndrome. *Ann Surg* 1975;181:567–574.
Mattox KL, Flint LM, Carrico CJ, et al. Blunt cardiac injury [Editorial]. *J Trauma* 1992;33:649–650.
McLean RF, Devitt JH, McLellan BA, et al. Significance of myocardial contusion following blunt chest trauma. *J Trauma* 1992;33: 240–243.

Reif J, Justice JL, Olsen WR, et al. Selective monitoring of patients with suspected blunt cardiac injury. *Ann Thorac Surg* 1990;50:530–533.

Aortic Disruption

Agee CK, Metzler MH, Churchill RJ, et al. Computed tomographic evaluation to exclude traumatic aortic disruption. *J Trauma* 1992; 33:876–881.

Akins CW, Buckley MJ, Daggett WM, et al. Acute traumatic disruption of the thoracic aorta: a ten-year experience. *Ann Thorac Surg* 1981;31:305–309.

Eddy AC, Rusch VW, Fligner CL, et al. The epidemiology of traumatic rupture of the thoracic aorta in children: a 13-year review. *J Trauma* 1990;30:989–991.

Lee RB, Stahlamn GC, Sharp KW. Treatment priorities in patients with traumatic rupture of the thoracic aorta. *Am Surg* 1992;58:37–43.

Miller FB, Richardson D, Thomas HA, et al. Role of CT in diagnosis of major arterial injury after blunt thoracic trauma. *Surgery* 1989;106:596–603.

Warren RL, Akins CW, Conn AK, et al. Acute traumatic disruption of the thoracic aorta: emergency department management. *Ann Emerg Med* 1992;21:391–396.

Wheat MW, Palmer RF, Bartley TD, et al. Treatment of dissecting aneurysms of the aorta without surgery. *J Thorac Cardiovasc Surg* 1965;50:364–373.

Nonoperative Management of Hepatic Trauma

Boone DC, Federle M, Billiar TR, et al. Evolution of management of major hepatic trauma: identification of patterns of injury. *J Trauma* 1995;39:344–350.

Bynoe RP, Bell RM, Miles WS, et al. Complications of nonoperative management of blunt hepatic injuries. *J Trauma* 1992;32:308–315.

Cogbill TH, Moore EE, Jurkovich GJ, et al. Severe hepatic trauma: a multi-center experience with 1,335 liver injuries. *J Trauma* 1988; 28:1433–1438.

Gates JD. Delayed hemorrhage with free rupture complicating the nonsurgical management of blunt hepatic trauma: a case report and review of the literature. *J Trauma* 1994;36:572–575.

Hiatt JR, Harrier HD, Koenig BV, et al. Nonoperative management of major blunt liver injury with hemoperitoneum. *Arch Surg* 1990;125:101–103.

Knudson MM, Lim Jr RC, Oakes DD, et al. Nonoperative management of blunt liver injuries in adults: the need for continuing surveillance. *J Trauma* 1990;30:1494–1500.

Meredith JW, Young J, Bowling J, et al. Nonoperative management of blunt hepatic trauma: the exception or the rule? *J Trauma* 1994;36:529–535.

Mirvis SE, Whitley NO, Vainwright JR, et al. Blunt hepatic trauma in adults: CT-based classification in correlation with prognosis and treatment. *Radiology* 1989;171:27–32.

Pachter HL, Knudson MM, Esrig B, et al. Status of nonoperative management of blunt hepatic injuries in 1995: a multicenter experience with 404 patients. *J Trauma* 1996;40:31–38.

Sherman HF, Savage BA, Jones LM, et al. Nonoperative management of blunt hepatic injuries: safe at any grade? *J Trauma* 1994;37: 616–621.

Abdominal Compartment Syndrome

Bloomfield GL, Ridings PC, Blocher CR. A proposed relationship between increased intra-abdominal, intrathoracic, and intracranial pressure. *Crit Care Med* 1997;25:496–503.

Burdick JF, Warshaw AL, Abbott WM. External counterpressure to control postoperative intra-abdominal hemorrhage. *Am J Surg* 1975;129:369–373.

Caldwell CB, Ricotta JJ. Changes in visceral blood flow with elevated intraabdominal pressure. *J Surg Res* 1987;43:14–20.

Cullen DJ, Coyle JP, Teplick R, et al. Cardiovascular, pulmonary, and renal effects of massively increased intra-abdominal pressure in critically ill patients. *Crit Care Med* 1989;17:118–121.

Diebel LN, Dulchavsky SA, Brown WJ. Splancnic ischemia and bacterial translocation in the abdominal compartment syndrome. *J Trauma* 1997;43:852–855.

Iberti TJ, Lieber CE, Benjamin E. Determination of intra-abdominal pressure using a transurethral bladder catheter: clinical validation of the technique. *Anesthesiology* 1989;70:47–50.

Schein M, Ivatury R. Intra-abdominal hypertension and the abdominal compartment syndrome. *Br J Surg* 1998;85:1027–1028.

Evaluation of the Cervical Spine

Pasquale M, Fabian TC. Practice management guidelines for trauma from the Eastern Association for the Surgery of Trauma. *J Trauma* 1998;44:941–956 and available on the World Wide Web at http://www.east.org.

The Burned Patient

Robert L. Sheridan

I. **Introduction**
   A. **Background.** The prognosis for burn patients, both for survival and for quality of life, has changed dramatically over the past 20 years. This change began with a realization that the natural history of burns can be changed by prompt surgery, the objective of which is to remove deep wounds and achieve immediate biologic closure prior to the otherwise inevitable development of wound sepsis. To support a patient with a serious burn through the physiologic trial of staged wound closure requires sophisticated critical care; many aspects are unique to the burn unit. This chapter presents these techniques in a concise format.
   B. **The role of intensive care in management of burns** is to bring a patient from a tragic injury to the optimal outcome—total reintegration into family, community, school, and productive work.
   C. **Overall management strategy.** Patients with large burns typically present with a deep wound, associated with pain, impending sepsis, and potentially progressive multiorgan dysfunction. Immediate needs must be met, but a specific overall plan of care must also be generated. An organized plan of care can be viewed as having four phases (Table 34-1). The **initial evaluation and resuscitation phase,** from days 1 though 3, requires that an accurate fluid resuscitation be performed while the patient is thoroughly evaluated for other injuries and comorbid conditions. The second phase, **initial wound excision and biologic closure,** describes the maneuver that so profoundly changes the natural history of the disease. Typically, a series of staged operations are completed during the first few days after injury. The third phase, **definitive wound closure,** involves replacement of temporary wound covers with definitive covers, and closure and acute reconstruction of areas of small surface area, but high complexity, such as the face and hands. The final stage of care is **rehabilitation.** Although rehabilitation begins early—even during resuscitation—it becomes involved and time consuming toward the end of the acute hospital stay. Ideally, patients are ready to return home when they are discharged from the burn unit.

II. **Physiologic implications of burn injury**
   A. **Predictable physiologic changes.** Successfully resuscitated burn patients manifest a sequence of predictable physiologic changes (Table 34-2). Anticipation of these changes is possible:

Table 34-1. Phases of burn care

Phase	Objectives	Time period
Initial evaluation and resuscitation	Accurate fluid resuscitation and thorough evaluation	0–72 hours
Initial wound excision and biologic closure	Exactly identify and remove all full thickness wounds and achieve biologic closure	Days 1–7
Definitive wound closure	Replace temporary with definitive covers and close small complex wounds	Day 7– week 6
Rehabilitation, reconstruction, and reintegration	Initially, to maintain range of motion; reduce edema; subsequently to strengthen and facilitate return to home, work, school	Day 1 through discharge

1. **Early ebb phase and later hyperdynamic phase.** Cuthbertson first described the ebb and flow phases of injury. The ebb phase relates to a period of hours to a day after injury in which is seen a relative hypodynamic state, which needs to be supported in the resuscitation period. The flow phase relates to the subsequent predictable development of high cardiac output, reduced peripheral vascular tone, fever, and muscle catabolism that becomes particularly exaggerated in patients with large burns.

2. **Physiology of the resuscitation period.** Unique to a patient suffering a serious burn is a massive diffuse capillary leak, believed to be secondary to wound-released mediators, that results in the extravasation of fluids, electrolytes, and even moderate-sized colloid molecules. Burn patients initially require a massive fluid resuscitation. Formulas have been developed over the past 40 years that attempt to predict resuscitation volume requirements based on body weight or body surface area and burn size. Multiple other variables, however, affect resuscitation requirements, including delay until resuscitation, inhalation injury, and the depth and vapor transmission characteristics of the wound itself. No two injuries are exactly alike and no formula has yet been developed that accurately predicts volume requirements in all patients. Inaccurate volume administration is associated with substantial morbidity. Therefore, it is essential that burn resuscitations be guided by hourly reevaluation of resuscitation endpoints, the formula serving only to help determine initial volume infusion rates and to roughly predict overall requirements.

Table 34-2.   Predictable physiologic changes in burn patients

Period	Physiologic changes	Clinical implications
Resuscitation period (day 0 to 3)	Massive capillary leak	Closely monitor fluid resuscitation
Postresuscitation period (day 3 until 95% wound definitive wound closure)	Hyperdynamic and catabolic state with high risk of infection	Remove and close wounds to avoid sepsis; nutritional support is essential
Recovery period (95% wound closure until 1 year after injury)	Continued catabolic state and risk of nonwound septic events	Accurate nutritional support essential; anticipate and treat complications

3. **Postresuscitation physiology.** In those successfully resuscitated, volume requirements abruptly decline 18 to 24 hours after injury, as the diffuse capillary leak predictably abates. Subsequently, a diffuse inflammatory state evolves that is characterized by a hyperdynamic circulation, fever, and massively increased protein catabolism. Release of poorly characterized inflammatory mediators; the counterregulatory hormones, cortisol, catecholamines, and glucagon; bacteria and their by-products from the wound and a compromised gastrointestinal barrier; pain; and infection are thought responsible for these changes.

B. **Physiologic support.** The metabolic stress associated with a large burn is enormous. Support includes accurate fluid repletion, provision of an adequate quantity and quality of substrate, control of environmental temperature, prompt removal of nonviable tissue with physiologic wound closure, support of the gastrointestinal barrier, and proper management of pain and anxiety. A critical component is support of **body temperature.** Burn patients have enormous evaporative water and energy losses if they are maintained in the typical cool, dry air of a general hospital. Burn units and operating rooms need to be engineered to maintain high ambient temperatures and humidity to avoid hypothermia.

III. **Initial evaluation.** The initial management of a seriously burned patient is usually not completed prior to arrival in the intensive care unit (ICU). All of these patients should be approached as a potential polytrauma patient. The evaluation follows the primary and secondary survey format of Advanced Trauma Life Support (ATLS).

A. **The primary survey** encompasses the first few seconds and minutes of the initial evaluation of the burn patient. Points of emphasis include:

1. **Airway evaluation and protection.** The patency and security of the airway must be established, realizing that progressive mucosal edema can compromise airway patency over the first few postinjury hours. This is especially true of young children, as airway resistance varies inversely with the fourth power of the airway radius. Endotracheal intubation should be performed if progressive airway edema is suspected. Do not wait until edema is symptomatic and intubation must be performed emergently. Facial and airway edema makes the burn patient's airway among the most challenging to intubate. Proper tube security is critical, because inadvertent extubation in the patient with a burned, swollen face and airway is potentially lethal. A harness system using umbilical ties is recommended.

2. **Vascular access and initial fluid support.** Reliable and secure vascular access is essential. This usually requires central venous access, although the placement of central lines is most safely per-

formed after immediate postburn hypovolemia has been corrected by volume administration.

3. **Multiple trauma issues.** All of these patients must be approached as polytrauma patients, because other injuries are common. Key issues in the trauma patient are outlined in Chapter 32.

B. **Burn-specific secondary survey.** In parallel with the trauma secondary survey, a number of burn-specific issues must be considered during the initial evaluation (Table 34-3).

1. **History.** The initial evaluation is the best time to elicit important points of medical history and mechanism of injury. These data should be actively sought from emergency personnel and family members, because access to these individuals and their information often is transient. Important points include details of the injury mechanism, initial neurologic status, extrication time, and tetanus immune status.

2. **Burn-specific systematic physical examination.** Burn and trauma patients require a comprehensive physical assessment at the time of their initial admission. Several aspects of this physical assessment are unique to burn patients.

a. **Head, eyes, ears, nose, and throat.** The head should be inspected for trauma. Pressure on the burned occiput should be avoided. The globes should be inspected prior to the development of massive adnexal edema that can severely limit an adequate examination. Serious burns of the globe are generally apparent by a clouded appearance of the cornea. More subtle injuries are detectable after fluorescein staining. Adnexal burns are noted, but acute tarsorrhaphy is virtually never indicated. Ear burns are noted; pressure is avoided on the burned auricle and topical mafenide acetate is applied. Finally, signs of inhalation injury (e.g., carbonaceous debris and singed vibrissae) are noted on examination of the nose and throat. Devices used to secure the nasogastric and endotracheal tubes are adjusted so that they do not apply pressure on the nasal septum.

b. **Neurologic.** Assess the patient for central nervous system trauma. Imaging of the head and axial spine is indicated, depending on the mechanism of injury (Chapter 32). Pain and anxiety management is ideally begun during the initial evaluation. In paralyzed or obtunded patients, it is important to ensure no pressure on peripheral nerves exists, so that neuropathies are avoided. Finally, those burned in structural fires should be assessed for carbon monoxide exposure by history, neurologic examination, and carboxyhemoglobin level,

**Table 34-3. Important aspects
of the burn-specific secondary survey**

System	Important considerations
History	1. Important points include the mechanism of injury, closed space exposure, extrication time, delay in seeking attention, fluid given during transport, and prior illnesses and injuries.
HEENT	1. The globes should be examined and corneal epithelium stained with fluroscein before adnexal swelling makes examination difficult. Adnexal swelling provides excellent coverage and protection of the globe during the first days after injury. Tarsorrhaphy is virtually never indicated acutely.
	2. Corneal epithelial loss can be overt, giving a clouded appearance to the cornea, but is more often subtle, requiring fluorescein staining for documentation. Topical ophthalmic antibiotics constitute optimal initial treatment.
	3. Signs of airway involvement include perioral and intraoral burns or carbonaceous material and progressive hoarseness.
	4. Hot liquid can be aspirated in conjunction with a facial scald injury and result in acute airway compromise requiring urgent intubation.
	5. Endotracheal tube security is crucial and is best maintained with an umbilical tape harness, rather than adhesive tape, on the burned face.
Neck	1. The radiographic evaluation is driven by the mechanism of injury.
	2. Rarely, in patients with very deep burns, neck escharotomies are needed to facilitate venous drainage of the head.
Cardiac	1. The cardiac rhythm should be monitored for 24–72 h in those with electrical injury.
	2. Although elderly patients can develop transient atrial fibrillation if modestly over resuscitated, significant dysrhythmias are unusual if intravascular volume and oxygenation are adequately supported.
	3. Those with a prior history of myocardial infarction may reinfarct with the hemodynamic stress associated with the injury and should be appropriately monitored.
Pulmonary	1. Ensure inflating pressures are <40 cm H_2O by performing chest escharotomies when needed.
	2. Severe inhalation injury can lead to sloughing of endobronchial mucosa and thick bronchial secretions that can occlude the endotracheal tube; be prepared for sudden endotracheal tube occlusions.

(continued)

Table 34-3. *Continued*

System	Important considerations
Vascular	1. The perfusion of burned extremities should be vigilantly monitored by serial examinations. Indications for escharotomy include decreasing temperature, increasing consistency, slowed capillary refill and diminished Doppler flow in the digital vessels. Do not wait until flow in named vessels is compromised to decompress the extremity. 2. Fasciotomy is indicated after electrical or deep thermal injury when distal flow is compromised on clinical examination. Compartment pressures can be helpful, but clinically worrisome extremities should be decompressed regardless of compartment pressure readings.
Abdomen	1. Nasogastric tubes should be in place and their function verified, particularly prior to air transport in unpressurized helicopters. 2. An inappropriate resuscitative volume requirement can be a sign of an occult intraabdominal injury. 3. Torso escharotomies may be required to facilitate ventilation in cases of deep circumferential abdominal wall burns. 4. Immediate ulcer prophylaxis with histamine receptor blockers and antacids is indicated in all patients with serious burns.
Genitourinary	1. Bladder catheterization facilitates using urinary output as a resuscitation endpoint and is appropriate in all who require a fluid resuscitation. 2. It is important to ensure that the foreskin is reduced over the bladder catheter after insertion, as progressive swelling can otherwise result in paraphimosis.
Neurologic	1. An early neurologic evaluation is important, as the patient's sensorium is often progressively compromised by medication or hemodynamic instability during the hours after injury. This may require computed tomography scanning in those with a mechanism of injury consistent with head trauma. 2. Patients who require neuromuscular blockade for transport should also receive adequate sedation and analgesia.
Extremities	1. Extremities that are at risk for ischemia, particularly those with circumferential thermal burns or those with electrical injury, should be promptly decompressed by escharotomy or fasciotomy when clinical examination reveals

(continued)

Table 34-3. *Continued*

System	Important considerations
	increasing consistency, decreasing temperature, and diminished Doppler flow in digital vessels. Limbs at risk should be dressed so they can be frequently examined.
	2. The need for escharotomy usually becomes evident during the early hours of resuscitation. Many escharotomies can be delayed until transport has been effected if transport times will not extend beyond 6 h postinjury.
	3. Burned extremities should be elevated and splinted in a position of function.
Wound	1. Wounds, although often underestimated in depth and overestimated in size on initial examination, should be evaluated for size, depth, and circumferential components.
Laboratory	1. Arterial blood gas analysis is important when airway compromise or inhalation injury is present.
	2. A normal admission carboxyhemoglobin concentration does not eliminate the possibility of a significant exposure as the half-life of carboxyhemoglobin is 30–40 min in those effectively ventilated with 100% oxygen.
	3. Baseline hemoglobin and electrolytes can be helpful later during resuscitation.
	4. Urinalysis for occult blood should be done in those with deep thermal or electrical injuries.
Radiograph	1. The radiographic evaluation is driven by the mechanism of injury and the need to document placement of supportive cannulae.
Electric	1. Monitor cardiac rhythm in high (>1000 V) or intermediate (>220 V) voltage exposures for 24 to 72 h.
	2. Low and intermediate voltage exposures can cause locally destructive injuries, but uncommonly result in systemic sequelae.
	3. After high voltage exposures, delayed neurologic and ocular sequelae can occur, so a carefully documented neurologic and ocular examination is an important part of the initial assessment.
	4. Injured extremities should be serially evaluated for intracompartmental edema and promptly decompressed when it develops.
	5. Bladder catheters should be placed in all patients suffering high voltage exposure to document the presence or absence of pigmenturia, which is treated adequately with volume loading in most patients.

(continued)

Table 34-3. *Continued*

System	Important considerations
Chemical	1. Irrigate wounds with tap water for at least 30 min. Irrigate the globe with isotonic crystalloid solution. Blepharospasm may require ocular anesthetic administration.
	2. Exposures to hydrofluoric acid can be complicated by life-threatening hypocalcemia, particularly exposures to concentrated or anhydrous solutions. Such patients should have serum calcium closely monitored and supplemented. Subeschar injection of 10% calcium gluconate solution is appropriate after exposure to highly concentrated or anhydrous solutions.
Tar	1. Tar should be initially cooled with tap water irrigation and later removed with a lipophilic solvent.

HEENT, head, eye, ear, nose, throat.
Adapted from Sheridan RL. Burns. In: Greenfield LJ, Mulholland MW, Oldham KT, Zelenock GB, eds. *Surgery: scientific principles and practice.* Philadelphia: JB Lippincott, 1996;12:422–438.

because selected patients with significant exposures can benefit from hyperbaric oxygen treatment.

  c. **The neck** should be assessed for trauma, based on mechanism of injury. This is particularly important in those suffering high voltage injuries. Extremely deep circumferential neck burns may require escharotomy to facilitate normal venous drainage of the head.

  d. **The chest** should be assessed for compliance and deep eschar should be sectioned if it interferes with ventilation. Escharotomy is best done, bilaterally if needed, along the anterolateral chest wall. The presence of bilateral air movement should be verified.

  e. **Cardiovascular system.** Most patients initially are hypovolemic and respond favorably to volume administration. Occasionally, patients with massive burns will have an element of primary myocardial dysfunction. These patients, identified with invasive monitoring, will benefit from the administration of β-adrenergic agonists, such as dobutamine.

  f. **Genitourinary system.** In males, foreskin retracted over the glans should be reduced after catheterization of the bladder so that progressive edema does not result in acute paraphimosis. Occasionally, a deeply burned foreskin must be sectioned to permit bladder catheterization.

    g. Musculoskeletal system. Burned extremities must be assessed for other trauma and monitored for adequacy of perfusion. It can sometimes be difficult to identify fractures in this setting, so liberal use of radiography is appropriate. Fractured and burned extremities are initially stabilized with external splints. Progressive edema during resuscitation can result in the late development of profound limb ischemia, secondary to swelling within circumferential eschar or inelastic muscle compartments. Extremity perfusion should be monitored throughout the resuscitation period.

3. Initial wound evaluation and management. Wounds are assessed for extent, using a Lund-Browder or other burn diagram (Fig. 34-1); depth, using the practiced examiner's eye; and the presence of circumferential components, which may require decompression to assure adequate perfusion.

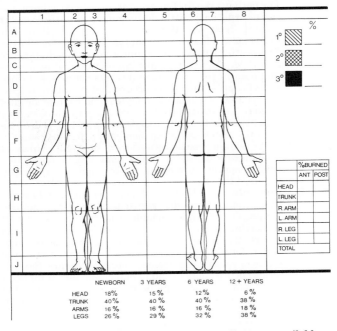

Fig. 34-1.   There are many age-specific burn diagrams available to facilitate accurate estimation of the extent of a burn, compensating for the varying anthropometrics between age groups.

4. **Laboratory and radiographs.** Little laboratory evaluation is required beyond routine electrolyte and hematologic testing except for carboxyhemoglobin and arterial blood gas determinations in the proper clinical setting. Chest radiographs are appropriate to ensure proper placement of resuscitative cannulas and the absence of chest trauma. Inhalation injuries rarely cause early radiographic changes. The mechanism of injury will dictate the need for other radiographs.

5. **Possibility of abuse.** All patients should be screened for abuse as the injury mechanism. Approximately 20% of burns in young children are reported to state authorities for investigation, but abuse occurs in all age groups. Often this determination is not made until the patient has been admitted into the ICU. The entire team must consider this possibility and file any suspicious case with appropriate state agencies. Careful and complete documentation of the circumstances and physical characteristics of the injury is essential. Photographic documentation is ideal.

IV. **Resuscitation**

A. **Physiology of the immediate postburn period.** For perhaps the first hour after an extensive burn, patients experience little derangement in intravascular volume, explaining the common observation that after even massive injuries patients can be quite alert for the first postinjury hour. As wound-released mediators are absorbed into the systemic circulation and as stress- and pain-triggered hormonal release occurs, a diffuse loss of capillary integrity occurs that results in the extravasation of fluids, electrolytes, and even moderate-sized colloid molecules. For reasons yet unknown, this leak abates between 18 and 24 hours later in those successfully resuscitated. An increased leak can be seen in those whose resuscitations are delayed, which is thought to be caused by the systemic release of reactive oxygen species formed on reperfusion of marginally perfused tissues

B. **Formulas** have been developed over the past 40 years that attempt to predict resuscitation volume requirements. The multiple variables that have an impact on resuscitation requirements render all such formulas inherently inaccurate. No two injuries are exactly alike and no formula has yet been developed that accurately predicts volume requirements in all patients. Several formulas are widely used to determine initial infusion rates and to roughly guide resuscitation efforts. One such consensus formula is the modified Brooke, which is summarized in Table 34-4.

C. **Monitoring.** Inaccurate volume administration is associated with substantial morbidity. Burn resuscitations must be guided by hourly reevaluation of resuscitation endpoints, which are summarized in Table 34-5.

Table 34-4.   The Modified Brooke formula for resuscitation

First 24 hours
Adults and children >20–30 kg:
  Ringers lactate: 2–4 ml/kg/%burn/24 h (first half in first 8 h)
  Colloid: None

Children <20 kg:
  Ringers lactate: 2–3 ml/kg/%burn/24 h (first half in first 8 h)
  Ringers lactate with 5% dextrose: maintenance rate
  Colloid: None

Second 24 hours
All patients:
  Crystalloid: To maintain urine output. If silver nitrate is used,
    sodium leeching mandates continued isotonic crystalloid. If
    other topical is used, free water requirement is significant.
    Serum sodium should be monitored closely. Nutritional support
    should begin, ideally by the enteral route.
  Colloid: (5% albumin in Ringers lactate):
    0–30% burn: None
    30–50% burn: 0.3 ml/kg/%burn/24 h
    50–70% burn: 0.4 ml/kg/%burn/24 h
    >70% burn: 0.5 ml/kg/%burn/24 h

Adapted from Sheridan RL. Burns. In: Greenfield LJ, Mulholland MW, Oldham KT, et al, eds. *Surgery: scientific principles and practice.* Philadelphia: JB Lippincott, 1996;12:422–438.

Table 34-5.   Age-specific resuscitation endpoints[a]

Endpoint	Target
Sensorium	Comfortable, arousable
Urine output	Infants: 1–2 ml/kg/h Children: 0.5–1 ml/kg/h All others: 0.5 ml/kg/h
Base deficit	Less than 2
Systolic pressure	Infants: 60 to 70 mm Hg Children: 70 to 90+ (twice age in years) mm Hg Adolescents and adults: 90–120 mm Hg

[a] Should be assessed regularly throughout burn resuscitation and infusions adjusted up or down in 10 to 20% increments to meet the needs of the individual patient.
Adapted from Sheridan RL. Burns. In: Greenfield LJ, Mulholland MW, Oldham KT, et al, eds. *Surgery: scientific principles and practice.* Philadelphia: JB Lippincott, 1996;12:422–438.

Oxygen delivery and consumption determinations have been advocated as guides to the adequacy of burn resuscitation, but no compelling data suggest such information provides clinically relevant guidance in this setting.

D. Recognition and management of resuscitation problems. The volume of infusate required by patients with large injuries can be enormous. It is essential to promptly recognize when a resuscitation is not proceeding as it should, and to know what to do in such cases. At any point during a resuscitation, the total 24-hour volume can be predicted based on the known volume infused so far and the current rate of infusion. If this number exceeds 6 ml/kg per percent burn/24 hours, it is likely that the resuscitation is not proceeding optimally. At this point, consider the use of low-dose dopamine, colloid administration, or the placement of a pulmonary artery catheter to gather additional information regarding the adequacy of ventricular filling and myocardial contractility. This is particularly important in older patients whose underlying cardiac disease is unmasked by the stress of burn resuscitation.

V. Neurologic issues that must be commonly addressed are pain and anxiety management, the exposed globe, and peripheral neuropathies.

A. Uncontrolled pain and anxiety have adverse physiologic, as well as psychologic, sequalae. Both can contribute to the development of posttraumatic stress syndrome. Inadequate pain and anxiety management is a legacy that burn intensivists must correct.

   1. In the past, inadequate pain management occurred because the extraordinary opioid doses required to adequately address pain in the seriously burned inspired fear of respiratory depression, addiction, and litigation among providers of burn care.

   2. The opioid tolerance that rapidly develops in patients with large open wounds can be remarkable. Despite this, addiction is rare; opioid requirements rapidly decrease after wound closure. In fact, the best way to manage pain in burn patients is with prompt biologic closure of their wounds.

   3. Successful management is greatly aided by an organized pharmacologic guideline supplemented with nonpharmacologic measures. A combination of benzodiazepines and opiates can be used to decrease overall dosage requirements (Chapters 5 and 6).

B. Ocular exposure. Commonly, progressive contraction of the burned eyelids and periocular skin results in exposure of the globe. This predictably results in desiccation of the globe, which is followed by keratitis, ulceration, and globe-threatening infection. Frequent lubrication of the exposed globe with hourly application of ocular lubricants and surgically releasing the eyelid in those who do not rapidly respond help prevent these sequalae.

C. **Peripheral neuropathies** can be seen in burn patients because of direct thermal damage to peripheral nerves or because of one of the many metabolic derangements that these patients can suffer. Many peripheral neuropathies can be avoided. Diligent monitoring of extremity perfusion will avoid the morbidity of constricting eschar and missed compartment syndromes. Proper application of well-fitting splints will avoid pressure-induced neuropathies. Careful positioning of deeply sedated or anesthetized patients will avoid traction and pressure injuries.

D. **Delirium** often is seen in burn patients. When anoxia and head injury are excluded, increased doses of anxiolytics or haloperidol may be useful (Chapter 5).

VI. **Pulmonary issues**
   A. **Airway issues.** The critical importance of initial airway evaluation and proper control has already been reviewed. This need continues throughout the period of intubation. The security of the endotracheal tube should be regularly verified and ICU personnel should be trained and equipped to deal with sudden airway emergencies.

   B. **Inhalation injury**
      1. **Diagnosis of inhalation injury.** Inhalation injury is a clinical diagnosis based on a history of closed spaced exposure, presence of singed nasal vibrissae, and carbonaceous sputum. Fiberoptic bronchoscopy, which facilitates diagnosis in equivocal cases, can help document laryngeal edema. Such information is useful when making decisions regarding preemptive intubation for evolving upper airway edema.

      2. **Clinical consequences and management.** Five events with major clinical implications occur predictably in patients with inhalation injury.
         a. **Acute upper airway obstruction** is anticipated and managed with endotracheal intubation.
         b. **Bronchospasm** from aerosolized irritants is a common occurrence during the first 24 to 48 hours, particularly in young children. This is managed with inhaled β_2-adrenergic agonists (**Chapter 21**). Some children will require intravenous bronchodilators such as terbutaline or low dose epinephrine infusions and occasionally steroids. Ventilatory strategies should be designed to minimize auto-PEEP (intrinsic positive end-expiratory pressure).
         c. **Small airway obstruction** occurs as necrotic endobronchial debris sloughs and complicates clearance of secretions. Small endotracheal tubes can become suddenly occluded; it is important to be prepared to evaluate and respond to a sudden deterioration of the patient–ventilator unit (Table 34-6). Therapeutic bronchoscopy facilitates clearance of the airways.

**Table 34-6.   How to address sudden deterioration
of the patient–ventilator unit—a predictable emergency**

When a sudden deterioration of the patient–ventilator unit occurs,
act quickly to see which of the 4 possibilities [(a) = mechanical ventilator problem, (b) = obstruction, (c) = displacement out (c1) or into
mainstem (c2), (d) = pneumothorax] is present:

1. *Disconnect* from ventilator and ventilate with self-inflating
   bag (remember pop-off valve) and maximal FIO_2. This eliminates and treats possibility (a). If this is not the immediate
   solution . . .
2. *Manually ventilate;* if ventilation is not successful, you have
   possibility (b). If the patient is "stable," suction the tube. If it
   cannot be quickly cleared, extubate, mask ventilate, and reacquire the airway.
3. *If the ventilations are successful,* you have either (c) or (d).
   Auscultate in the axillae. If there are R ≫ L sided sounds,
   you probably have (c2). *Back tube out cautiously and re-
   assess.* If you hear gurgling in the hypopharynx, you probably have (c1). *Extubate, mask ventilate, and reacquire the
   airway.*
4. *If you hear unilateral breath sounds* you may have (d). This
   can be difficult to differentiate from (c2) at times, but is often
   accompanied by hemodynamic deterioration or hyperresonance (or a recent subclavian line insertion attempt). If you
   suspect (d), *place a 14 or 16 g catheter* in the 2nd interspace,
   midclavicular line, and later place a chest tube.
5. The final common pathway if things are not going right is *extubation, mask ventilation, and reacquisition of the airway.*
   Remember: oxygen buys you time.

If you cannot reintubate (or if you cannot effectively mask ventilate),
options include laryngeal mask airway, needle cricothyroidotomy,
surgical cricothyroidotomy or tracheostomy, percutaneous cricothyroidotomy.

    d.   Pulmonary infection develops in between
30% and 50% of patients with inhalation injury. Differentiating between pneumonia and
tracheobronchitis (purulent infection of the de-
nuded tracheobronchial tree) is often difficult,
but generally of little clinical consequence. A
patient with newly purulent sputum, fever,
and impaired gas exchange should be treated;
the antibiotic coverage is adjusted according to
the results of sputum Gram's stain and culture. Secretion clearance is a particularly important component of management, because
inhalation injury to bronchial mucosa greatly
impairs mucocilliary clearance.

    e.   Respiratory failure is common in those
sustaining inhalation injury, and is managed
as outlined in Chapters 4 and 20. These patients do well with a pressure-limited venti-

lation strategy based on permissive hypercapnia. Patients who fail this approach should be considered for innovative methods of support, such as inhaled nitric oxide.

3. **Carbon monoxide (CO)** exposure is common in patients injured in structural fires. Many are obtunded from a combination of CO, anoxia, and hypotension. Hyperbaric oxygen has been proposed as a means of improving the prognosis of those suffering serious CO exposures, but its use remains controversial. The question of whom to treat in the hyperbaric chamber commonly arises on a busy burn service.

   a. **Physiology.** Carbon monoxide avidly binds and inactivates heme-containing enzymes, particularly hemoglobin and the cytochromes. The formation of carboxyhemoglobin results in an acute physiologic anemia, much like an isovolemic hemodilution. As a carboxyhemoglobin concentration of 50% is physiologically similar to a 50% isovolemic hemodilution, the routine occurrence of unconsciousness at this level of carboxyhemoglobin makes it clear that other mechanisms are involved in the pathophysiology of CO injury. It is likely that CO binding to the cytochrome system in the mitochondria, which interferes with oxygen utilization, is more toxic than CO binding to hemoglobin. For unknown reasons, between 5% and 20% of patients with serious CO exposures have been reported to develop delayed neurologic sequelae.

   b. **Management options.** These patients can be managed with 100% isobaric oxygen or with hyperbaric oxygen. If serious exposure has occurred, manifested by overt neurologic impairment or a high carboxyhemoglobin level, then hyperbaric oxygen (HBO) treatment is probably warranted if it can be administered safely.

   c. **HBO treatment** regimens vary, but an exposure to 3 atm for 90 minutes, with three 10-minute "air breaks" is typical. An air break refers to the breathing of pressurized room air rather than pressurized oxygen, which decreases the incidence of seizures from oxygen toxicity. Because treatment is generally in a monoplace chamber, unstable patients should not be treated. Other contraindications are wheezing or air trapping, which increases the risk of pneumothorax, and high fever, which increases the risk of seizures. Prior to placement in the chamber, endotracheal tube balloons should be filled with saline to avoid balloon compression and associated air leaks. Upper body central venous cannulation should be avoided, if possible, to reduce the chance of a pneumothorax that can enlarge suddenly during decompression. Myringotomies are required in intubated patients.

d. **Cyanide exposure** is often detectable in patients extricated from structural fires, but is rarely of a severity to justify the risk of treatment with amyl nitrate and sodium thiosulfate.

VII. Gastrointestinal issues

A. **Ulcer prophylaxis.** Until the routine use of prophylactic therapies, burn patients had a virulent ulcer diathesis ("Curling's ulcer") that was a common cause of death. Ulceration is believed to be secondary to periods of reduced splanchnic flow. At present, it is advisable to treat most patients with serious burns with empiric histamine receptor blockers and antacids (Chapter 25). Although it is unclear when to stop prophylactic therapy, most would agree that patients with closed wounds who are tolerating tube feedings are at low enough risk that this therapy can be stopped.

B. **Nutritional support.** Burn patients have predictable and protracted needs for supplemental protein and caloric support, which needs to be accurate because both under- and overfeeding have adverse sequelae (Chapter 8).

1. **Route and timing.** Intragastric continuous tube feedings are ideal and usually successful. Tube feedings are begun at a low rate during resuscitation. Initially, a sump nasogastric tube is used so that gastric residuals can be used to help determine feeding tolerance. Parenteral nutrition is used if tube feedings are not tolerated. Highly catabolic burn patients tolerate prolonged periods of fasting very poorly.

2. **Nutritional targets** in severely injured burned patients remain controversial. The many formulas propagated to predict these requirements vary widely in their predictions. The current consensus is that protein needs are approximately 2.5 gm/kg/d, and caloric needs are between 1.5 and 1.7 times a calculated basal metabolic rate, or 1.3 to 1.5 times a measured resting energy expenditure.

3. **Monitoring.** Substrate support needs to be titrated to nutritional endpoints during a lengthy burn hospitalization if the complications of over- or underfeeding are to be avoided. Regular physical examination, quality of wound healing, nitrogen balance, and indirect calorimetry are all useful in this regard. The combination of a highly catabolic state, the critical need to heal extensive wounds, and the length of time that support is required make monitoring and adjustment of nutritional support particularly important in patients with extensive burns.

VIII. Infectious disease issues

A. **Wound topical care.** The best way to avoid wound sepsis is through prompt excision and successful closure of deep wounds. Topical agents are an adjunct in this regard, slowing the inevitable occurrence of wound sepsis in deep wounds and minimizing desiccation and colonization of healing wounds. Several agents in wide general use are available; the most common are itemized in Table 34-7.

B. Antibiotic use. Antibiotics are double-edged swords in this clinical setting. Burn physiology includes the routine occurrence of moderate fever, which is not necessarily a sign of infection. When unexpected fever occurs, a complete physical assessment is done, wounds are inspected for evidence of sepsis, directed laboratory studies and radiographs are done, and cultures of blood, urine, and sputum are sent for evaluation. If the patient appears unstable, empiric broad-spectrum coverage is reasonable pending return of culture data (Chapters 27 and 28). If no infectious focus is identified, then antibiotics are stopped. It is critically important that deteriorating burn patients be thoroughly evaluated for occult foci of infection to allow prompt treatment prior to the development of systemic sepsis.

C. Infection control issues. Patients referred from other facilities often bring highly resistant bacterial species with them. Proper infection control practices are of particular importance to avoid cross-contamination of vulnerable patients with these organisms. Universal precautions are essential components of practice.

D. Recognition and management of burn complications. Successful management requires that a predictable series of complications (Table 34-8), mostly infectious, are successfully treated as the wound is progressively closed. Compulsive attention to changes in clinical status will facilitate early detection and successful intervention.

IX. Rehabilitation efforts in the burn ICU. Rehabilitation efforts begin with resuscitation and proceed throughout critical illness.

Table 34-7. Common topical agents used as adjuncts in wound management[a]

Silver sulfadiazine	Painless on application, fair to poor eschar penetration, no metabolic side effects, broad antibacterial spectrum
Mafenide acetate	Painful on application, excellent eschar penetration, carbonic anhydrase inhibitor, broad antibacterial spectrum
Silver nitrate (0.5%)	Painless on application, poor eschar penetration, leeches electrolytes, broad spectrum (including fungi)

[a] These agents slow the inevitable occurrence of wound sepsis in deep wounds, minimizing desiccation and colonization of healing wounds.

**Table 34-8.   Systematic reassessment
of seriously ill burn patients**

System	Complication
Neurologic	1. *Transient delirium* occurs in up to 30% of patients; it generally resolves with supportive therapy when the possibility of anoxia, metabolic disturbance, and structural lesions are eliminated by appropriate studies. 2. *Seizures* most commonly result from hyponatremia or abrupt benzodiazepine withdrawal. 3. *Peripheral nerve injuries* occur from direct thermal injury, compression from compartment syndrome; or from overlying inelastic eschar, major metabolic disturbances, or improper splinting techniques. 4. *Delayed peripheral nerve and spinal cord deficits* develop weeks or months after high voltage injury secondary to small vessel injury and demyelinization.
Renal	1. *Early acute renal failure* follows inadequate perfusion during resuscitation or myoglobinuria. 2. *Late renal failure* complicates sepsis and multiorgan failure or the use of nephrotoxic agents.
Adrenal	1. *Acute adrenal insufficiency* secondary to hemorrhage into the gland presents with hypotension, fever, hyponatremia, and hyperkalemia.
Cardiovascular	1. *Endocarditis and suppurative thrombophlebitis* are intravascular infections that typically present with fever and bacteremia without signs of local infection. 2. *Hypertension* occurs in up to 20% of children and is best managed with β-adrenergic blockers. 3. *Venous thromboembolic complications* are infrequent in patients with large burns. 4. *Iatrogenic catheter insertion complications* are minimized by meticulous technique.
Pulmonary	1. *Carbon monoxide intoxication,* which is best managed acutely with effective ventilation with pure oxygen, can be associated with delayed neurologic sequelae. 2. *Pneumonia* can occur with or without antecedent inhalation injury and is treated with pulmonary toilet and antibiotics. 3. *Respiratory failure* can occur early postinjury, secondary to inhalation of noxious chemicals, or later in the course, secondary to sepsis or pneumonia.

(continued)

Table 34-8. *Continued*

System	Complication
Hematologic	1. *Neutropenia and thrombocytopenia,* as well as *disseminated intravascular coagulation,* are common indicators of impending sepsis and should prompt appropriate investigations.
	2. *Global immunologic deficits* associated with burn injury contribute to a high rate of infectious complications.
Otologic	1. *Auricular chondritis* secondary to bacterial invasion of cartilage results in rapid loss of viable tissue; it is prevented by the routine use of topical mafenide acetate on all burned ears.
	2. *Sinusitis and otitis media* can be caused by transnasal instrumentation; they are treated by relocation of tubes, antibiotics, and judicious surgical drainage.
	3. *Complications of endotracheal intubation* include nasal alar and septal necrosis, vocal cord erosions and ulcerations, tracheal stenosis and tracheoesophageal and tracheoinnominate artery fistulae. The occurrence of such complications is minimized by meticulous attention to tube position, avoidance of oversized tubes, and attention to cuff pressures.
Enteric	1. *Hepatic dysfunction,* secondary to transient hepatic blood flow deficits and manifested as transaminase elevations, is extremely common during resuscitation from large burns and it resolves with volume restitution. Late hepatic failure, beginning with elevations of cholestatic chemistries and progressing through coagulopathy and frank failure, complicates sepsis and multiorgan failure.
	2. *Pancreatitis,* beginning with amylase and lipase elevations and ileus and progressing through hemorrhagic pancreatitis, is generally coincident with splanchnic flow deficits early and sepsis-induced organ failures later in the hospital course.
	3. *Acalculous cholecystitis* can present as sepsis without localized symptoms or signs accompanied by rising cholestatic chemistries. A standard radiographic evaluation can be followed by bedside percutaneous cholecystostomy in unstable patients.
	4. *Gastroduodenal ulceration,* secondary to splanchnic flow deficits that degrade mucosal defenses, is extremely common and often life threatening if routine histamine receptor blockers and antacids are not administered.

(continued)

Table 34-8. *Continued*

System	Complication
	5. *Intestinal ischemia,* which can progress to infarction, is secondary to inadequate resuscitation and splanchnic flow deficits.
Ophthalmic	1. *Ectropia,* from progressive contraction of burned ocular adnexae, results in exposure of the globe. This requires acute eyelid release. Tarsorrhaphy is rarely helpful, more often resulting in injury to the tarsal plate as contraction forces pull out tarsorrhaphy sutures.
	2. *Corneal ulceration,* which develops after initial epithelial injury or later exposure secondary to ectropion, can progress to full thickness corneal destruction if secondary infection occurs. This is prevented by careful globe lubrication with topical antibiotics in the former case and acute lid release in the latter.
	3. *Symblepharon,* or scarring of the lid to the denuded conjunctiva following chemical burns or corneal epithelial defects complicating TENS, are prevented by daily examination and adhesion disruption with a fine glass rod.
Genitourinary	1. *Urinary tract infections* are minimized by maintaining indwelling bladder catheters only when absolutely required; they are treated with appropriate antibiotics. Neither catheterization nor colonic diversion is necessarily required for management of perineal and genital burns.
	2. *Candidal cystitis* occurs in those patients treated with bladder catheters and broad-spectrum antibiotics. Catheter change and amphotericin irrigation for 5 days is generally successful. If infections are recurrent, the upper urinary tracts should be screened ultrasonographically.
Musculoskeletal	1. *Burned exposed bone* is generally debrided with a dental drill until viable cortical bone is reached, which is then allowed to granulate and is autografted. Patients whose overall condition and wounds are appropriate are managed with local or distant flaps.
	2. *Fractured and burned extremities* are best immobilized with external fixators, whereas overlying burns are grafted. Burn patients with coincident fractures in unburned extremities benefit from prompt internal fixation.

(continued)

Table 34-8. *Continued*

System	Complication
	3. *Heterotopic ossification* develops weeks after injury; it is seen most commonly around deeply burned major joints such as the triceps tendon and presents with pain and decreased range of motion. Most patients respond to physical therapy, but some require excision of heterotopic bone to achieve full function.
Soft Tissue	1. *Hypertrophic scar formation* is a major cause of long-term functional and cosmetic deformities seen in burn patients. This poorly understood process is heralded by a secondary increase in neovascularity between 9 and 13 weeks after epithelialization. Management options include grafting of deep dermal and full thickness wounds, compression garments, judicious steroid injections, topical silicone products, and scar release and resurfacing procedures.

TENS, topical epidermal necrolysis.
Adapted from Sheridan RL. Burns. In: Greenfield LJ, Mulholland MW, Oldham KT, et al, eds. *Surgery: scientific principles and practice.* Philadelphia: JB Lippincott, 1996;12:422–438.

A. **Physical and occupational therapists** play important roles in the burn ICU. Initially, twice-daily passive ranging of all joints and static antideformity positioning is begun to prevent the development of contractures.

B. **Perioperative therapy.** Physical and occupational therapists should be informed of the sequence of planned operations and the modifications of therapy plans that these imply. Therapists should be encouraged to range patients under anesthesia in conjunction with planned operations and to fabricate custom face molds and splints in the operating room, particularly in children who often poorly tolerate these activities when awake.

X. **Intraoperative support.** Burn patients must undergo staged excision and closure of their wounds even if they are critically ill; not to do so will render them even sicker. Close communication between the ICU and operating room teams is essential.

A. **Environmental considerations.** Transport to and from the operating room must be carefully planned and properly attended. Operating rooms must be maintained hot and humid to minimize the occurrence of hypothermia in exposed burn patients. Intraoperative hypothermia is poorly tolerated; it causes coagulo-pathies and increases bleeding.

B. Intraoperative critical care and communication. Critical care must proceed during surgery. The surgical and anesthesia teams must be in constant communication so that each knows what the other is doing, blood replacement can be appropriate, and extension of the operation can be thoughtfully considered.

XI. Special considerations

A. Electrical injury

1. Patients exposed to low and intermediate voltages may have severe local wounds, but rarely suffer systemic consequences.

2. Those exposed to high voltages commonly suffer compartment syndromes, myocardial injury, fractures of the long bones and axial spine, and free pigment in the plasma that can cause renal failure if not promptly cleared.

3. Those suffering high-voltage injuries should receive cardiac monitoring, radiographic clearance of the spine, and examination of the urine for myoglobin. Fluid resuscitation initially is based on burn size, but this generally does not correlate well with deep tissue injury, so resuscitations need to be closely monitored and adjusted. Muscle compartments at risk should be closely monitored by serial physical examinations; they should be decompressed in the operating room when an evolving compartment syndrome is suspected. Wounds are debrided and closed with a combination of skin grafts and flaps.

B. Tar injury

1. Numerous thermoplastic road materials are the source of occupational injury. They are highly viscous and heated to between 300°F and 700°F.

2. The wounds should be immediately cooled by tap water irrigation. Resuscitation is based on burn size and monitored. Wounds are dressed in a lipophilic solvent and then debrided, excised, and grafted. The underlying wounds are generally quite deep.

C. Cold injury

1. Soft tissue necrosis from cold injury is often managed in the burn unit. Wound care is conservative until the extent of irreversible soft tissue necrosis is apparent; this often requires several weeks if not months. When definitely demarcated, surgical debridement, excision, and reconstruction or closure is carried out, if needed, with lesser injuries often healing without need for surgery.

2. Cold-injured patients can manifest all the problems of systemic **hypothermia** when they present, and should be managed accordingly (Chapter 32).

D. Chemical injury

1. Patients can be exposed to thousands of chemicals, which are often heated. It is important to consider

the thermal, local chemical, and systemic chemical effects.

2. Liberal consultation with **poison control information centers** for guidance regarding systemic effects is extremely useful. Most agents can be washed off with tap water.

   a. **Alkaline substances** can take longer to remove than the traditional 30 minutes. When the soapy feel that these alkalis typically impart to the gloved finger is gone or when litmus paper applied to the wound shows a neutral pH, irrigation can be stopped.

   b. Concentrated **hydrofluoric acid** exposure will cause dangerous hypocalcemia, and subeschar injection of 10% calcium gluconate and emergent wound excision may be appropriate.

   c. **Elemental metals** should be covered with oil, and **white phosphorus** should be covered in saline to prevent secondary ignition.

E. **Toxic epidermal necrolysis (TENS)**

   1. TENS is a diffuse process of unknown pathophysiology in which epidermal-dermal bonding is acutely compromised. Patients commonly present with a drug exposure preceding the illness, and have both a cutaneous and visceral wound.

   2. This disease is similar in presentation to a total-body second-degree burn. With good wound care, most patients will heal the cutaneous wound without the need for surgery. Involvement of the aerodigestive tract mucosa can lead to sepsis and organ failures, particularly if septic complications are not promptly recognized and treated.

F. **Purpura fulminans (PF)**

   1. PF is a complication of meningococcal sepsis in which extensive soft tissue necrosis and, commonly, organ failures, occur. It is believed to be secondary to a transient hypercoagulable state that occurs early in the primary septicemic event.

   2. These patients often present with sepsis-associated organ failures and extensive deep wounds. Both should be managed concurrently, because the wounds are susceptible to infection if not promptly excised and closed.

G. **Soft tissue infections**

   1. Patients with soft tissue infections share many characteristics of burn patients. Accurate classification of serious soft tissue infections is difficult, but all are approached in the same general fashion.

   2. These patients need to go directly to the operating room. Operative goals are exposure of the infection so that its anatomic extent can be accurately described and its microbiology determined by culture, Gram's stain, and biopsy. Debridement under general anesthesia is repeated until infection is controlled and the wounds are then closed or grafted. Broad-spectrum, then focused antibiotics are im-

**Table 34-9.   Burn polytrauma patients:
conflicting priorities that require thoughtful compromise**

Area of conflict	Consensus resolution
Neurologic	
Patients with burns and head injuries must have cerebral edema controlled during resuscitation; pressure monitors increase risk of infection.	A very tightly controlled resuscitation with short-term placement of indicated pressure monitors with antibiotic coverage.
Chest	
Patients with blunt chest injuries and overlying burns may require chest tubes through burned areas with risk of empyema, and difficulty closing the tract.	Use a long subcutaneous tunnel to decrease difficulty closing the tract and remove tubes as soon as possible to decrease empyema risk.
Abdomen	
Blunt abdominal injuries may be hard to detect if there is an overlying burn. A high incidence of wound dehiscence if operating through a burned abdominal wall.	Liberal use of imaging to detect occult injuries. Routine use of retention sutures after laparotomy.
Orthopedic	
Optimal management of a fracture can be compromised by an overlying burn.	Most such extremities are best managed with prompt excision and grafting of the wound with external fracture fixation.

portant adjuncts. Some patients, particularly those with clostridial infection may benefit from adjunctive HBO, but prompt surgery is the primary therapeutic modality.

   H.   The burned polytrauma patient. Burn care priorities frequently conflict with orthopedic, neurosurgical, and other priorities. Thoughtful resolution of these differences is an important part of successful management (Table 34-9).

XII.   Conclusion. Seriously burned patients can do extremely well in the long term; skillful critical care is essential to patient salvage. Thoughtful and diligent effort in the ICU not only enhances rates of survival, but also directly has an impact on the quality of life of those who survive serious burns.

SELECTED REFERENCES

Goldstein AM, Weber JM, Sheridan RL. Femoral venous catheterization is safe in burned children: an analysis of 224 catheters. *J Pediatrics* 1997;3:442–446.

Prelack K, Cunningham J, Sheridan RL, et al. Energy provided and protein provisions for thermally injured children revisited: an outcome-based approach for determining requirements. *J Burn Care Rehabil* 1997;10:177–182.

Sheridan RL. The seriously burned child: resuscitation through reintegration. Part I and Part II. *Curr Probl Pediatr* 1998;28:105–127.

Sheridan RL, Gagnon SW, Tompkins RG, et al. The burn unit as a resource for the management of acute nonburn conditions in children. *J Burn Care Rehabil* 1995;16:62–64.

Sheridan RL, Hinson M, Blanquierre M, et al. Development of a pediatric burn pain and anxiety management program. *J Burn Care Rehabil* 1997;18:455–459.

Sheridan RL, Hinson MM, Liang, MM, et al. Long term outcome of children surviving massive burns. *JAMA* 2000;281:69–73.

Sheridan RL, Hurford WE, Kacmarek RM, et al. Inhaled nitric oxide in burn patients with respiratory failure. *J Trauma* 1997;42:641–646.

Sheridan RL, Kacmarek RM, McEttrick MM, et al. Permissive hypercapnia as a ventilatory strategy in burned children: effects on barotrauma, pneumonia and mortality. *J Trauma* 1995;39:854–859.

Sheridan RL, Prelack K, Cunningham JJ. Physiologic hypoalbuminemia is well tolerated by severely burned children. *J Trauma* 1997;43:448–452.

Sheridan RL, Shank E. Hyperbaric oxygen treatments: a brief overview of a contraversial topic. *J Trauma* 1999;47:426–435.

Sheridan RL, Tompkins RG, Burke JF. Management of burn wounds with prompt excision and immediate closure. *Journal of Intensive Care Medicine* 1994;9:6–19.

Sheridan RL, Weber JM, Benjamin J, et al. Control of methicillin resistant *Staphylococcus aureus* in a pediatric burn unit. *Am J Infect Control* 1994;22:340–345.

Thoracic Surgery

William E. Hurford

I. **Bronchoscopy**
   A. **Flexible bronchoscopy** can be performed in the awake patient under local anesthesia with supplemental intravenous (IV) sedation, if needed.
   B. **Common indications** for bronchoscopy include:
      1. Assistance with endotracheal intubation and confirmation of endotracheal tube position.
      2. Assessment of the upper airway for edema, obstruction, disruption, or other pathology.
      3. Examination of the tracheobronchial tree.
      4. Clearance of pulmonary secretions and assistance with pulmonary hygiene.
      5. Bronchoalveolar lavage and sampling for pulmonary infection.
      6. Performance of lung biopsy to diagnose malignancy or other pulmonary disease.
   C. **Anesthesia** for flexible bronchoscopy in the awake patient without an artificial airway most commonly is achieved by the topical application of 4% lidocaine (spray or nebulized) to the oropharynx or nasopharynx, larynx, vocal cords, and trachea. If this is done patiently, no further anesthesia is required. Premedication with atropine or glycopyrrolate will limit salivary dilution of the anesthetic, providing quicker and more predictable anesthesia. Nerve blocks are rarely needed. Intravenous sedation can be used as well (Chapter 5).
   D. **If an endotracheal tube is in place,** a sufficient lumen to permit ventilation must be maintained during the bronchoscopy. Many adult operating bronchoscopes require at least a 7.5-mm inner diameter (ID) tube, although pediatric bronchoscopes can pass through tubes as small as 4.5 mm. With any question of incompatibility, the fit of the bronchoscope within a specific endotracheal tube should be checked prior to insertion of the bronchoscope into the patient's airway.
   E. **Rigid bronchoscopy** may be needed in cases of massive hemoptysis or an obstructing airway lesion. Rigid bronchoscopy permits superior visualization and control of the airway compared with fiberoptic bronchoscopy, but it also requires general anesthesia for adequate operating conditions.
   F. **Complications**
      1. **Hypercarbia** secondary to inadequate ventilation is the most common complication during bronchoscopy; it frequently results in ventricular dysrhythmias. Lidocaine should be available for

immediate use. Most dysrhythmias are best treated by withdrawing the bronchoscope and increasing ventilation.

2. **Hypoxemia** secondary to intermittent and un-
even ventilation can be minimized by using controlled ventilation with 100% oxygen. The tidal
volume delivered to the patient during pressure-
limited modes of mechanical ventilation can decrease dramatically because of increased airway
resistance of the bronchoscope within the airway.

3. **Other complications** of bronchoscopy include
dental and laryngeal damage from intubation, injuries to the eyes or lips, airway rupture, pneumothorax, and hemorrhage. Airway obstruction
can occur from excessive bleeding or obstruction
by a foreign body or dislodged mass.

II. Lung isolation

A. **Placement of a double-lumen endotracheal tube**
may be indicated for differential lung ventilation (i.e.,
separate ventilators providing different levels or patterns of positive pressure to each lung in cases of
bronchopleural fistulas, giant emphysematous blebs,
asymmetric lung disease such as following single-
lung transplantation), airway protection (e.g., hemoptysis), or bronchoalveolar lavage (e.g., pulmonary
alveolar proteinosis).

1. **Double-lumen endobronchial tubes** range in
size from 28 to 41 French (in general 39–41
French for men; 35–37 French for women) and
are designed to conform to either the right or left
mainstem bronchus, providing separate channels
for ventilation of the distal bronchus and the trachea. The right-sided tube has a separate opening
for ventilation of the right upper lobe.

2. **Insertion**

a. The endobronchial tube, including both cuffs
and all necessary connectors, should be carefully checked before placement. The tube can
be lubricated, and a stylet should be placed in
the bronchial lumen.

b. Following laryngoscopy, the endobronchial
tube is inserted initially with the distal curve
facing anteriorly. Once into the trachea, the
stylet should be removed and the tube rotated
so that the bronchial lumen faces toward the
appropriate side. Turning the patient's head
away from the side of insertion aids placement
of the tube into the appropriate bronchus. The
tube is advanced to an average depth of 29 cm
or less if resistance is met.

c. The tube also can be guided into position with
a fiberoptic bronchoscope. In any event, proper positioning of the tube should be confirmed by both physical signs and fiberoptic
bronchoscopy. The most common error is posi-

tioning the tube too far into the bronchus so that the distal lumen ventilates a single lobe. Severe barotrauma can result.

B. **Univent tubes** (Vitaid, Ltd., Lewiston, NY) are large-caliber endotracheal tubes encompassing a small integrated channel for a built-in bronchial blocker. Although single- or double-lung ventilation is possible, differential lung ventilation is not. The Univent tube is inserted into the trachea in the usual fashion and rotated toward the appropriate bronchus. Following inflation of the tracheal cuff, the bronchial blocker is advanced into the selected mainstem bronchus under fiberoptic guidance and the cuff is inflated. Collapse of the blocked lung occurs through both the small distal opening in the blocker and absorption of oxygen from the lung.

C. **Bronchial blockers** can be used in situations in which it is not possible to place an endobronchial tube, typically in pediatric patients, in those with difficult airway anatomy, or in cases of massive hemoptysis in which the amount of hemorrhage would obstruct a double-lumen tube. Differential lung ventilation is not possible with this technique.

   1. **Insertion.** An appropriately sized Fogarty catheter (e.g., for an adult, an 8–14 French venous occlusion catheter with a 10-ml balloon) is placed into the trachea under direct vision prior to endotracheal intubation. Following intubation, the balloon tip is positioned in the appropriate mainstem bronchus with a fiberoptic bronchoscope and inflated.

   2. **Placement of a blocker after endotracheal intubation** can be difficult, because the blocker can be displaced easily by the bronchoscope and it is difficult to fix in position. A bronchoscope adapter can be used to help hold the blocker in position.

D. As with any technique for lung isolation, it is necessary to carefully and continuously monitor the position of the tube and blocker, if present. Lung isolation can be lost with even small movements of the patient or tube. Usually, deep sedation and, occasionally, neuromuscular blockade are necessary.

E. **Complications** of lung isolation techniques include collapse of obstructed segments of the lung, airway trauma, bleeding, and aspiration during prolonged efforts at intubation. Hypoxia and hypoventilation can occur during placement efforts because of malpositioning, or from single or differential lung ventilation.

F. **Differential lung ventilation** can be performed if a double-lumen tube is in place. Separate mechanical ventilators are used to provide positive pressure to each lung. The degree of positive end-expiratory pressure (PEEP), inflating pressure, ventilatory pattern, and F_{IO_2} can be individually set for each lung. The respiratory rate and pattern need not be identical for both lungs. Successful ventilator settings vary greatly with the underlying mechanical characteristics of each lung.

III. **Chest tubes** are inserted to drain the pleural cavity, promote lung expansion following pneumothorax, or provide a route for administering sclerosing agents to treat recurrent pleural effusions.

A. **Insertion.** Chest tubes commonly are inserted using an **anterior** approach (second or third intercostal space in the midclavicular line), to evacuate a pneumothorax, or a **lateral** approach (sixth or seventh intercostal space in the midaxillary line), to evacuate either fluid or air. The lateral approach usually is easier, safer, and more cosmetic.

B. **Technique (Fig. 35-1)**

1. The patient is advised what to expect during the chest tube insertion, including the burning sensation of the local anesthetic, the transient discomfort at the moment of pleural penetration, and cough as air or fluid is evacuated.

2. The skin over the site is sterilized and draped.

3. The planned site of pleural entry is identified. Approximately 2 to 3 cm inferior to this site, a skin wheal is produced with 1% to 2% lidocaine. Infiltration of local anesthetic is continued through all layers of the chest wall, directing the needle cephalad toward the selected interspace. Local anesthetic (3 ml) is injected just inferior to the rib to block the intercostal nerve bundle.

4. The pleura also is infiltrated with local anesthetic and can be penetrated with the needle to confirm pneumothorax.

5. A linear skin incision is made at the site of the skin wheal. The subcutaneous tissues and intercostal muscles are spread bluntly with a curved clamp, creating a subcutaneous tunnel from the skin to the site of pleural entry.

6. The curved clamp is grasped with the palm of the hand such that the index finger will serve as a stop to prevent excessive penetration. The parietal pleura then is penetrated with the closed clamp, which is inserted immediately over the **upper border** of the rib. Perforation of the parietal pleura is transiently painful for the patient. The clamp is spread to widen the hole.

7. The pleural space is explored with a gloved finger to assure that the space is open and free of adhesions.

8. The end of the chest tube is grasped with the curved clamp and inserted into the pleural space. The tube is advanced toward the apex of the lung, making certain that all the side holes of the chest tube lie within the pleural cavity.

9. The chest tube is connected to a "three bottle" suction apparatus (Fig. 35-2), the insertion site sutured, and the chest tube secured with a silk suture.

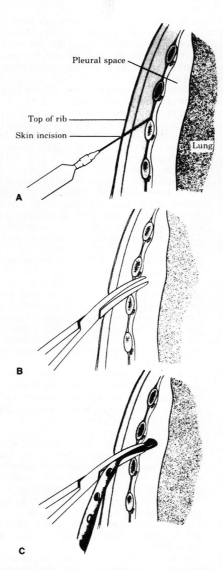

Fig. 35-1.   Chest tube insertion technique. A. Infiltration with local anesthetic. B. Perforation of the parietal pleura with a blunt, curved clamp. C. Insertion of the chest tube with the curved clamp.

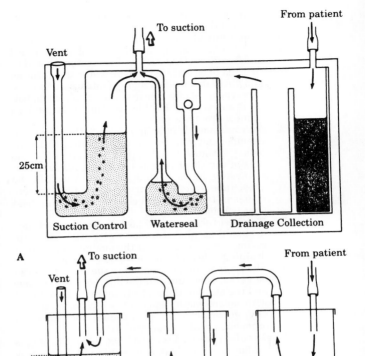

Fig. 35-2. Chest tube drainage system. A. Commercial apparatus equivalent to a "three-bottle" system. The proximal chamber is for pleural drainage; the middle chamber (water seal) prevents air or fluid from being drawn into the pleural space; and the distal chamber regulates the level of suction by the adjusted depth of water filling the chamber. B. A traditional "three-bottle" system is shown for comparison.

      10. A chest radiograph is obtained to confirm the position of the chest tube.

  C. Management of chest tubes

    1. Chest tubes usually are placed under water seal and 0 to 20 cm H_2O suction. The system should be checked to be certain that the water seal is intact and fluctuates with changes of intrathoracic pressure, the level of water in the suction control bottle is correct and bubbles continuously, and all connections are secure.

    2. Air continuously bubbling through the water seal chamber can indicate an ongoing intrapleural air leak. Continuous bubbling also can occur if a side port of the chest tube is outside the pleura or a connection to the system is loose. A leak in the chest tube system is suggested if bubbling continues in the water seal chamber after the chest tube is briefly clamped.

    3. If a chest tube is used following pneumonectomy, it should be placed under water seal only. Applying suction could shift the mediastinum to the draining side and reduce venous return.

    4. The level of suction applied to the chest tube can be varied depending on the degree of air leakage and the state of the underlying lung. In patients with severe emphysema, a low level of suction (if any) generally is used to reduce the chance of bronchopleural fistula formation.

  D. Chest tube removal is considered when the lung is fully inflated, no air leak is present, and drainage is less than 150 ml over 24 hours.

    1. Cut the retaining suture.

    2. While intrathoracic pressure is positive (have the patient hold a deep breath and perform a Valsalva maneuver), hold a petrolatum gauze dressing over the insertion site while rapidly withdrawing the tube.

    3. Apply an occlusive dressing and obtain a chest radiograph to check for the presence of a residual pneumothorax.

  E. Complications of chest tube placement include hemorrhage from laceration of intercostal or internal mammary vessels, lung laceration, and subcutaneous emphysema.

IV. Thoracentesis

  A. Indications include drainage of a pneumothorax or pleural effusion for either diagnosis or therapy.

  B. Pleural effusions can be free-flowing or loculated. Thoracentesis can be performed under ultrasonic guidance or during computed tomography (CT) scanning.

    1. Drainage of a pleural effusion usually is accomplished with the patient in a sitting position. A posterior or midaxillary approach can be used. The level of the pleural effusion can be determined by percussion or, preferably, by ultrasound examination. Generally, the planned insertion site should not be lower than the eighth intercostal space.

2. After sterile preparation and draping of the planned insertion site, the skin, subcutaneous fat, underlying muscles, and pleura are infiltrated with 1% to 2% lidocaine. The upper border of the rib is identified with the anesthetizing needle. The needle then is slid off the upper border of the rib, and the parietal pleura penetrated and aspirated to confirm intrapleural placement and the presence of pleural fluid.

3. A thoracentesis needle attached to a stopcock and syringe is inserted along the same route as the anesthetizing needle. As the needle is constantly aspirated, it is slid over the upper border of the rib, penetrating the pleura. Pleural fluid can then be aspirated while maintaining a constant depth of insertion.

4. Alternatively, a flexible intravenous catheter can be placed through an introducing needle [e.g., 14-gauge Intracath (Becton, Dickenson and Co., Franklin Lakes, NJ)] placed as described above. A stopcock is placed on the catheter and fluid aspirated with a 50-ml syringe or a vacuum bottle. Large volumes of fluid can be removed in this manner.

5. **Complications** include pneumothorax, laceration of intercostal vessels or lung, and penetration of abdominal organs.

C. **Tension pneumothorax** is a progressive accumulation of intrapleural air that significantly increases intrapleural pressure and shifts the mediastinum and trachea away from the side of the pneumothorax. Increased intrathoracic pressure can decrease venous return and cause hypotension.

1. **Signs and symptoms** include dyspnea, decreased breath sounds over the side with the pneumothorax, hyperresonance to percussion, and a hyperinflated but poorly moving hemithorax. Hypoxemia and hypotension may be present. A chest radiograph, ideally taken at end-expiration, is usually diagnostic.

2. **Immediate treatment** is by **emergent thoracentesis.** A large-bore needle or IV catheter is inserted in the second intercostal space in the midclavicular line and air is aspirated. A chest tube (see above) is inserted following emergent decompression of the pneumothorax.

V. **The thoracotomy patient**

A. **Patients should be awake,** comfortable, and breathing spontaneously at the end of most thoracic surgical procedures. Postoperative endotracheal intubation and mechanical ventilation should rarely be necessary following most common thoracic surgical procedures (except for lung transplantation). Prompt extubation avoids the potential disruptive effects of endotracheal intubation and positive-pressure ventilation on fresh suture lines. If postoperative ventilation is required, inspiratory pressures should be kept as low as possible.

B. **Excellent analgesia** is critically important following a thoracotomy.

  1. **Thoracic epidural analgesia** is currently considered the best available method for pain management following thoracotomy. **Thoracic epidural catheters** often are inserted at the time of operation and used to provide continuous intraoperative and postoperative analgesia. Combinations of local anesthetics (e.g., 0.1% bupivacaine) and opioids (typically, dihydromorphone or fentanyl) usually provide adequate analgesia (Chapter 6).

   a. **Complications** include systemic hypotension from sympathetic blockade, pruritus from the epidural administration of opioids, and, rarely, complications of catheter insertion (e.g., epidural hematoma, infection, trauma to nerves).

   b. The continuous infusion of an α-adrenergic agent (e.g., phenylephrine) or increased infusion of IV fluids may be required to maintain adequate blood pressure.

  2. **Intercostal nerve blocks** can be used in situations where epidural analgesia is impractical or ineffective (Chapter 6).

  3. **Nonsteroidal antiinflammatory agents.** Ketorolac has proved effective as a supplemental analgesic, but should be used with caution in elderly patients with renal insufficiency or a history of gastric bleeding.

  4. **Parenteral opiods,** if required, should be administered with caution. **Patient-controlled analgesia (PCA)** can be used and combined with a continuous epidural infusion of local anesthetic to titrate each agent separately.

C. **Atrial dysrhythmias** are common following a pulmonary resection. They are more frequent with more extensive lung resections (e.g., pneumonectomy) and their incidence peaks on the second to fourth postoperative days.

  1. **Supraventricular tachycardias, premature atrial contractions, and atrial fibrillation** are the most common dysrhythmias occurring in this setting.

  2. **Potential causes** of atrial dysrhythmias in this setting include volume overload, myocardial ischemia, pulmonary embolism, hypoxemia, infection, empyema, and electrolyte imbalances. The dysrhythmias usually are self-limited, but can be a sign of more serious complications (e.g., a pulmonary embolism), which must be carefully considered. Prophylactic administration of digoxin, commonly used in the past, is ineffective in preventing atrial dysrhythmias.

3. **The rate of ventricular response** can be controlled with a β-adrenergic blocker such as propranolol or a calcium channel blocker such as verapamil or diltiazem. Refractory dysrhythmias may respond to procainamide or amiodarone. (Chapters 15 and 17 contain additional information concerning treatment.) Many practitioners administer digoxin, but the other therapies listed generally are more effective. Cardioversion is rarely necessary or effective.

D. **Acute respiratory distress syndrome (ARDS),** which sometimes occurs following a pulmonary resection, is often fatal. It is more common with more extensive lung resections such as pneumonectomy.

1. **The cause of ARDS following pulmonary resection is unknown.** Pathologically, the hallmarks of the disease are those of ARDS (i.e., inflammation and subsequent fibrosis) rather than simply pulmonary edema. ARDS following pulmonary resection appears best treated in the same manner as ARDS arising from other causes (Chapter 20).

2. **Treatment** generally includes endotracheal intubation, pressure-limited mechanical ventilation, bronchoscopy to clear secretions, empiric antibiotic therapy (until the results of sputum cultures are known), fluid restriction, and diuretic administration. Prone or lateral positioning, inhaled nitric oxide, and high-dose systemic steroid administration may be useful in selected cases.

VI. **Tracheal resection and reconstruction**

A. **The surgical approach** depends on the location and extent of the lesion. Lesions of the cervical trachea are approached through a transverse neck incision. Lower lesions necessitate a manubrial split. Lesions of the distal trachea and carina may require a median sternotomy or a single or bilateral thoracotomy.

B. **Postoperative endotracheal intubation and mechanical ventilation are to be avoided,** if possible, because of the increased pressure placed on the fresh anastomosis. A small tracheostomy can be placed below the tracheal repair in patients with tenuous anatomy, copious secretions, or respiratory failure.

C. **Maintenance of neck flexion** helps minimize tension on the tracheal suture line. A single large "guardian" suture is placed from chin to anterior chest to help preserve neck flexion.

D. If tracheomalacia, edema, or secretions cause respiratory distress after extubation, the airway should be intubated with a small, uncuffed endotracheal tube under fiberoptic guidance, preferably with the head maintained in forward flexion.

      E. Frequent bedside bronchoscopies may be required in the postoperative period to remove secretions from the lungs.

VII. **Tracheal disruption** can be caused by airway instrumentation or thoracic trauma.

      A. **Clinical presentation** includes hypoxia, dyspnea, subcutaneous emphysema, pneumomediastinum, and pneumothorax.

      B. **The membranous portion of the trachea** is most commonly involved. Increased external pressure to the chest in the setting of a closed glottis, as can occur in motor vehicle accidents, can overpressurize the trachea and "blow out" the membranous wall.

      C. **Positive-pressure ventilation** will exacerbate the air leak and rapidly worsen symptoms from pneumothorax or pneumomediastinum. If possible, the patient should be allowed to breathe spontaneously.

      D. The airway can be secured initially by advancing a small endotracheal tube past the point of injury. This is best done over a fiberoptic bronchoscope. A tracheostomy may be required in the case of a difficult airway. Once the tracheal disruption is excluded by the endotracheal tube, controlled positive-pressure ventilation can begin. Operative repair of the tracheal injury is usually necessary.

VIII. **Intrapulmonary hemorrhage**

      A. **Massive hemoptysis** can be caused by trauma, pulmonary artery rupture secondary to catheterization, or erosion into a vessel by a tracheostomy, abscess, or tumor.

      B. **The airway must be immediately suctioned,** the trachea intubated, and ventilation begun with 100% oxygen. **Rigid bronchoscopy** may be necessary to adequately clear the airway of blood and clots.

      C. **If a unilateral source is identified,** lung isolation (see above) can be undertaken to protect the uninvolved lung and facilitate corrective surgery. Obstruction of the endotracheal tube is an ever-present danger and frequent suctioning may be necessary.

          1. Placement of an **endobronchial blocker** (Fogarty catheter) provides the best isolation. Placement of a double-lumen tube may be technically difficult and is reserved for patients who will immediately undergo thoracotomy and repair.

          2. **In an emergency,** the existing endotracheal tube can be advanced into the bronchus of the uninvolved lung and the cuff inflated.

          3. **Fiberoptic bronchoscopy** is essential for suctioning blood and confirming isolation of the bleeding lung.

          4. **Definitive treatment** may require angiographic embolization or surgical repair.

IX. **Lung transplantation**

      A. **Common indications** include emphysema, cystic fibrosis, and idiopathic pulmonary hypertension. Techniques include living donor single lobe, single and double lung, sequential single lung, and combined heart–lung transplantation. Cardiopulmonary bypass may be necessary during the procedure. (Chapter 36 contains information on perioperative considerations.)

B. Because the patient will be immunosuppressed, **sterile technique** for all procedures is paramount. Special considerations for immunosuppression are similar to patients receiving solid organ transplants (Chapters 27 and 38).

C. The patient remains sedated and endotracheal intubation and mechanical ventilation are continued in the immediate postoperative period until the transplanted lung begins to function well and symptoms of reperfusion edema and acute rejection are controlled.

    1. **Serial measurements of arterial blood gas tensions** document the function of the transplanted lung. Acute rejection can manifest as decreasing compliance with worsening arterial oxygenation.

    2. The patient must be monitored for signs of toxicity from the immunosuppressive regimen (Chapter 38).

    3. Repeated bronchoscopies and biopsies of the transplanted lung, which are necessary following surgery, are managed under local anesthesia with IV sedation.

X. **Lung volume reduction surgery** is sometimes performed on patients with chronic obstructive pulmonary disease (COPD) who experience incapacitating dyspnea despite maximal medical therapy.

A. **The goal** of the surgery is to relieve thoracic distention and improve ventilation. Patients are selected under strict criteria and undergo a period of cardiopulmonary conditioning prior to surgery.

B. **Surgical procedure**

    1. The surgical approach is via bilateral thoracotomies, median sternotomy, or bilateral, video-assisted thoracoscopies.

    2. The least functional parts of the lung as determined by ventilation and perfusion scintigraphy and intraoperative observation are resected.

C. **Postoperative course**

    1. Postoperative mechanical ventilation is to be avoided, as severe ventilator dyssynchrony is common in such patients. Increased airway pressure may contribute to the development of air leaks.

    2. **Excellent analgesia,** most commonly provided by a thoracic epidural catheter, is essential to maintaining adequate postoperative pulmonary function.

    3. **Common postoperative problems** include air-trapping, difficulty clearing secretions, persistent air leaks, anxiety, and hypercapnic respiratory failure. **Noninvasive ventilation** can be useful in selected patients (Chapter 4).

XI. **Esophageal surgery** includes procedures for resection of esophageal neoplasms, antireflux procedures, and repair of traumatic or congenital lesions.

    A. Patients may be **malnourished,** from both systemic illness (carcinoma) and anatomic interference with swallowing.

    B. Both esophageal carcinoma and traumatic disruption of the distal esophagus are associated with **ethanol abuse;** patients may have impaired liver function, elevated portal pressures, anemia, cardiomyopathy, and bleeding disorders (Chapter 24).

    C. Patients who have had difficulty swallowing may be **hypovolemic.** Cardiovascular instability can be further exacerbated by preoperative chemotherapy.

    D. Following esophageal resection, patients are at continued risk of pulmonary **aspiration** of gastric contents. Prophylactic measures include minimizing oversedation, elevating the head of the bed, appropriate drainage of the gastric remnant, and administration of H_2 blockers (e.g., ranitidine).

    E. Endotracheal intubation and mechanical ventilation often are continued in the early postoperative period. Mechanical ventilation can be discontinued and the trachea extubated once the patient is awake, comfortable, breathing adequately (Chapter 4), normothermic, and hemodynamically stable.

SELECTED REFERENCES

Adoumie R, Shennib H, Brown R, et al. Differential lung ventilation. Applications beyond the operating room. *J Thorac Cardiovasc Surg* 1993;105:229–233.

Baehrendtz S, Hedenstierna G. Differential ventilation and selective positive end-expiratory pressure: effects on patients with acute bilateral lung disease. *Anesthesiology* 1984;61:511–517.

Ballantyne JC, Carr DB, deFerranti S, et al. The comparative effects of postoperative analgesic therapies on pulmonary outcome: cumulative meta-analyses of randomized, controlled trials. *Anesth Analg* 1998;86:598–612.

Cooper JD, Patterson GA, Sundaresan RS, et al. Results of 150 consecutive bilateral lung volume reduction procedures in patients with severe emphysema. *J Thorac Cardiovasc Surg* 1996;112:1319–1329.

Frist WH. Perioperative procedures. In: Hoffman WJ, Wasnick JD, Kofke WA, et al, eds. *Postoperative critical care of the Massachusetts General Hospital,* 2nd ed. Boston: Little, Brown and Company, 1992:469–490.

Kaplan JA, ed. *Thoracic anesthesia,* 2nd ed. New York: Churchill Livingstone, 1991.

Kopec SE, Irwin RS, Umali-Torres CB, et al. The postpneumonectomy state. *Chest* 1998;114:1158–1184.

Mathisen DJ, Kuo EY, Hahn C, et al. Inhaled nitric oxide for adult respiratory distress syndrome after pulmonary resection. *Ann Thorac Surg* 1998;66:1894–1902.

Sabiston DC, Spencer FC, eds. *Surgery of the chest,* 5th ed. Philadelphia: WB Saunders, 1990.

Slinger PD. Perioperative fluid management for thoracic surgery: the puzzle of postpneumonectomy pulmonary edema. *J Cardiothorac Vasc Anesth* 1995;9:442–451.

Slinger PD. Pro: every postthoracotomy patient deserves thoracic epidural analgesia. *J Cardiothorac Vasc Anesth* 1999;13:350–354.

Tagliavia AA, Cowan GA. Anesthesia for thoracic surgery. In: Hurford WE, Bailin MT, Davison JK, et al, eds. *Clinical anesthesia procedures of the Massachusetts General Hospital,* 5th ed. Philadelphia: Lippincott-Raven, 1998:347–368.

Cardiac Surgery

Brian J. Poore

I. **Approach to the postoperative management of the cardiac surgery patient.** The intensive care unit (ICU) care of the patient following cardiac surgery begins with the report received from the anesthesiologist when the patient arrives. Many postoperative problems evolve from preoperative or intraoperative events.

A. **Preoperative** identification of individuals who will suffer perioperative morbidity or mortality remains difficult. Several patient characteristics, however, define a group at increased risk of having a difficult postoperative course.

1. **Myocardial dysfunction.** The lower the preoperative ejection fraction (EF), the higher the probability of perioperative problems.

2. **Renal dysfunction.**

3. **Older age.** Beyond the age of 50, morbidity appears to increase with age.

4. **Prior coronary artery bypass** (CAB) surgery.

5. **Emergency surgery.** Increased surgical priority is consistently associated with poorer outcomes.

6. **Type of surgery.** Mortality increases as the complexity of the operation increases. CAB < Valve < CAB and Valve

B. **Intraoperative** events, although not usually included in outcome predictions, often foretell the problems a patient will manifest in the ICU. These events include:

1. **Myocardial ischemia.** At some point during most cardiac operations myocardial ischemia occurs, which places the heart at risk for further injury. This usually occurs during aortic cross-clamping. As the length of **ischemic time** increases, so does predicted mortality. Effective myocardial protection techniques make it difficult to individualize this prediction. An important point is that cardiopulmonary bypass (CPB) causes biventricular dysfunction in most patients. Those who begin with reasonable ventricular function tolerate the insult better than those with poor ventricular function. The magnitude of the insult should be evident immediately on attempting separation from CPB. Stroke volume will be reduced despite higher-than-baseline filling pressures [i.e., pulmonary artery occlusion pressure (PAOP), central venous pressure (CVP), or left atrial pressure (LAP)]. The anesthesiologist should report a visual interpretation of cardiac function and relate if the filling pressures correlated with the heart's appearance. (i.e., with a

PAOP of 18 mm Hg, did the heart appear over-filled? What happened to the filling pressures when the thorax was closed?)

2. **Dysrhythmias** can be the most frustrating problem encountered after bypass. Any rhythm difficulties should be recounted to the ICU team, as well as the treatments that improved the situation.

3. **Bleeding.** The quality of intraoperative hemostasis is important information to be shared with the ICU team. In addition, recent laboratory results (e.g., hematocrit, platelet count, coagulation parameters) and therapeutic interventions should be communicated.

II. **Postoperative care of the routine cardiac surgical patient.** Cardiac surgery lends itself to standardization of postoperative care. The different procedures are usually followed by a typical pattern of recovery. Patients who have isolated coronary disease and few other medical problems can be managed using a "**fast track**" approach. Their anesthetic is tailored for early awakening so that rapid extubation (< 4 hours) may be possible. This should translate into shorter ICU stays, faster initiation of cardiac rehabilitation, earlier hospital discharge, and reduced costs. This approach appears to be safe for selected patients and does not appear to increase morbidity or mortality for patients who fail. This chapter discusses the ICU course of a patient undergoing a standard CAB. Many of the principles are applicable to other cardiac operations.

A. **ICU admission.** Several activities must take place when the patient arrives from the operating room. The anesthesiology team is responsible for the patient throughout this transition until a full report is given to the ICU team.

1. **Monitoring.** During the arrival of the patient in the ICU, it is important to prevent any gaps in monitoring of the cardiac rhythm. The arterial and pulmonary artery transducers should be connected to the ICU monitor and re-zeroed. Then the electrocardiogram (ECG) cables can be switched to the ICU monitor. If pacing, the pacemaker should be examined to assure capture and that the mode of pacing is correct. Preferably, the pacemaker should be set in an inhibited mode. The chest tube reservoirs should be marked for a baseline drainage fluid level and connected to suction.

2. **Mechanical ventilation.** Airway patency and bilateral breath sounds should be assured, followed by transfer of the patient to the ICU ventilator.

3. **Infusions.** The vasoactive infusions that the patient is receiving and their infusion sites are noted. The hemodynamic goals should be discussed with the ICU team, as well as which infusions to use to achieve these goals.

4. **Data.** Blood samples should be sent for arterial blood gas (ABG) analysis, electrolytes, hematocrit,

and platelet count, prothrombin time (PT), and partial thromboplastin time (aPTT) if the patient is bleeding. A portable chest radiograph and an ECG should be obtained. Baseline hemodynamics and vitals signs should be measured, including cardiac output (CO), mean arterial pressure (MAP), pulmonary artery (PA) pressures, CVP, heart rate, temperature, ventilatory pressures, and oxygen saturation (SpO_2).

5. **Report.** A thorough report includes medical history, outpatient medications, preoperative events with pertinent cardiac data, intraoperative events, vasoactive drugs, last dose of muscle relaxant, anticipated time of emergence from anesthesia, and an active problem list.

B. **Cardiovascular function and weaning support measures.** On arrival, most routine CAB patients are hypothermic and receiving an antihypertensive, usually sodium nitroprusside (SNP). Their CO usually will be adequate [cardiac index (CI) > 2.5 L/min/m^2], if ventricular function was good preoperatively and no significant ischemic insults occurred. Active warming, using a forced air system, may be necessary if the patient is to be extubated early. This often causes a temperature-overshoot that produces hyperthermia 6 to 12 hours later. As patients warm, they will vasodilate, their SNP requirement will decrease, and they will usually require intravascular volume replacement.

C. **Pulmonary function and ventilator weaning.** Most patients arrive intubated and fully ventilated (i.e., controlled mechanical ventilation). As the anesthetics and muscle relaxants clear, spontaneous breathing returns. A few patients may require additional sedation and mechanical ventilation until hypothermia, shivering, bleeding, or hemodynamic instability resolve. Most cardiac ICUs have a standardized approach to ventilator weaning and determining if the patient is ready for extubation. Regardless of how this point is approached, it is important for the cardiac patient to have a trial of unassisted ventilation prior to tracheal extubation (Chapters 4 and 21). Once extubated and hemodynamically stable, the patient is mobilized to a bedside chair.

1. The patient with marginal ventricular function may not tolerate the elimination of positive intrathoracic pressure, which decreases venous return and left ventricular afterload. Central hemodynamics and cardiac output must be followed carefully during ventilator weaning.

2. If a patient fails a breathing trial or requires re-intubation, an aggressive search for the cause of respiratory failure should be undertaken. It is not acceptable to simply allow the patient another "day of rest" on the ventilator. Many patients with marginal ventricular function will require aggressive diuresis prior to the withdrawal of positive-pressure ventilation.

D. **Renal function, fluids, and electrolytes.** Most healthy CAB patients will initially be intravascularly hypovolemic but also will have increased extravascular fluid. Intravascular volume can be challenging to maintain if the patient received intraoperative diuretics.

1. Packed red blood cells (PRBC) are excellent for fluid replacement if the hematocrit warrants transfusion. Otherwise, a balanced crystalloid solution (e.g., lactated Ringer's) is appropriate. The fluid of choice in cardiothoracic ICUs had been colloid (e.g., albumin or plasma). Current literature does not support the routine use of colloid solutions, and the difference in cost is substantial.

2. During the early period after bypass, urinary sodium excretion is very low and potassium excretion is high. Serum potassium levels should be monitored and repleted to maintain serum levels greater than 4.0 mEq/L. Many units replace K^+ continuously (~10 mEq/h).

3. By postoperative day (POD) 1, the routine CAB patient will be relatively volume overloaded as evidenced by an increasing CVP, a decreasing PaO_2, and possibly oliguria. Diuretic therapy is appropriate.

E. **Lines and drains.** The chest radiograph (CXR) should be reviewed to assess proper line placement, position of the endotracheal tube, proper chest tube placement, and to check the pleural spaces for collections of fluid or air. The chest tubes should be "milked" hourly to prevent clots from obstructing drainage. Drainage of more than 100 ml/h should prompt an investigation (see section **III.A**).

1. On POD 1, the chest tubes can be removed if the drainage is less than 150 ml for the previous 8 hours, and no air leak is present.
   Note: If the patient has a left atrial line in place, it should be removed prior to removal of the drainage tubes.

2. The central lines can be removed prior to the patient leaving the ICU. Introducers for pulmonary artery catheters should be removed with the patient supine to prevent venous air embolism. The bladder catheter can be discontinued. The epicardial pacing wires will remain, and be removed immediately prior to hospital discharge. The patient will proceed to the floor with only a peripheral intravenous (IV) line in place. Prophylactic antibiotics are routinely continued until the chest tubes are removed.

III. **Postoperative complications**

A. **Bleeding** is a common problem following cardiac surgery. The common causes include:

1. **Surgical.** What constitutes brisk bleeding for one surgeon might be normal for another. Usually, more than 100 ml/h of bleeding should trigger an inter-

vention [e. g., tighter blood pressure control, empiric additional protamine, positive end-expiratory pressure (PEEP), patient warming, rechecking coagulation parameters, and CXR to rule out pleural accumulation of blood]. Reoperation is usually indicated if bleeding exceeds 400 ml in any hour or is more than 200 ml/h for 4 consecutive hours. In addition, evidence of cardiac tamponade should prompt exploration (see section **III. H.**).

2. **Anticoagulant.** Elevated activated clotting time (ACT), aPTT, or quantitative heparin assay suggests inadequate heparin neutralization and is treated by the slow administration of additional protamine (1 mg/kg IV).

3. **Platelet abnormalities.** Qualitative or quantitative platelet problems often contribute to bleeding. Although platelets may be present in sufficient number to begin hemostasis, they may not be properly functioning. Platelet transfusion should be considered even with a count greater than $100,000/mm^3$ in a patient who continues to bleed after correcting or ruling out anatomic, anticoagulant, or clotting factor abnormalities. Platelet counts below $70,000/mm^3$ warrant replacement in an actively bleeding patient. **Bleeding time** measurements should *not* be used to guide blood component therapy in the ICU.

4. **Clotting factors.** Clotting factor levels fall rapidly during CPB. Most levels remain above 30% of normal and do not contribute significantly to increased bleeding. Plasma products are often empirically transfused in the operating room. In the ICU, however, fresh frozen plasma (FFP) and cryoprecipitate transfusions should be guided by appropriate coagulation studies.

5. **Other considerations**

   a. **Desmopressin acetate (DDAVP)** in a dose of 0.3 µg/kg has been used with varying success in cardiac surgery. DDAVP administration may be useful in postoperative patients with excessive blood loss of obscure origin and in uremic patients.

   b. **Positive end-expiratory pressure** is believed to decrease blood loss in post-CAB patients. The proposed mechanism of action is tamponade of venous bleeding by the expanded lung. Although PEEP is still used by many surgeons, most studies have not shown its benefit.

   c. **Antifibrinolytics,** including **aprotinin** (Trasylol) and **aminocaproic acid** (Amicar), have been shown to decrease blood loss when administered prior to initiation of CPB. The utility of postoperative administration is questionable, unless ongoing fibrinolysis is documented.

      d. Blood pressure control, to prevent hypertensive episodes, is very important to prevent bleeding in the postoperative cardiac patient. Deliberate reduction of a patient's blood pressure, below normal baseline, is done in an attempt to decrease bleeding from arterial sites. This practice carries a substantial risk of unrecognized hypoperfusion of other organs (e.g., brain, kidneys, gut).

B. Dysrhythmias are frequently encountered in the cardiac surgery patient. Although many are benign, they often contribute to a reduced cardiac output and can limit the effectiveness of other therapies [e.g., lack of an adequate trigger for intraaortic blood pump (IABP)]. See Chapters 15 and 17 for additional discussion of dysrhythmias and their pharmacologic treatment.

    1. Common causes of dysrhythmias in the cardiac ICU include:

      a. Electrolyte abnormalities. Hypokalemia is frequently encountered on POD 1. It is best to maintain the serum potassium level greater than 4.0 mEq/L. Hypomagnesemia can be associated with several cardiovascular abnormalities. Magnesium levels should be repleted (2 g MgSO$_4$ IV over 30 minutes, repeated every 4 hours up to four times) until greater than 2.0 mEq/L.

      b. Surgical trauma. Injury to the conduction system may present as heart block. Local inflammation can produce atrial fibrillation. These rhythm disturbances are usually transient (hours to days).

      c. Myocardial ischemia. Any type of dysrhythmia may be seen in conjunction with ischemia. A trial of increased perfusion pressure (e.g., vasopressors, IABP) is warranted for refractory dysrhythmias.

      d. Medications. Exogenous catecholamines (e.g., dobutamine, dopamine, inhaled albuterol) frequently contribute to dysrhythmias. Digoxin toxicity should be suspected in anyone receiving digoxin (Chapter 30). Drugs that can precipitate a physiologic rebound (e.g., clonidine, β-blockers) should be continued perioperatively.

    2. Epicardial pacing wires are extremely useful in the diagnosis and treatment of postoperative dysrhythmias. Nearly every cardiac surgical patient will arrive with pacing wires in place. The atrial wires usually exit the thorax on the patient's right and the ventricular wires exit on the left.

    3. Dysrhythmias can be categorized according to their location. (See Chapters 15 and 17 for pharmacologic treatment.)

      a. Ventricular. Premature ventricular contractions (PVCs) are the most common dysrhythmia encountered in the cardiac patient. Although often benign, they warrant treatment when they occur more frequently than 6/min, are multifocal, or they occur in salvos of three or more consecutive beats. The easiest treatment for PVCs is atrial pacing at a rate faster than the patient's baseline (as long as the patient's intrinsic rate is less than 100). PVCs that occur during atrioventricular (AV) sequential pacing can be eliminated by shortening the AV interval to 100 to 150 msec (despite the fact that a longer AV interval may produce a better CO).

b. **Supraventricular** tachycardias are the second most common dysrhythmia in the postcardiac surgery patient. **Atrial fibrillation** (AF) still affects 25% of postoperative CAB patients regardless of prophylactic regimen used. **Atrial flutter** is treated similarly to AF, with the addition of rapid atrial pacing as an alternative therapy. Using the atrial epicardial electrodes, the atrium is captured (usually at rates of 350–400 bpm) and then the rate is either slowly decreased or the pacing is abruptly stopped. Diagnosis of atrial flutter can be aided by an atrial-wire ECG, which is performed by connecting the atrial electrode to a precordial (or limb) lead of the electrocardiograph. **Paroxysmal supraventricular tachycardia** is a reentrant rhythm with atrial and ventricular rates of 150 to 200 bpm.

c. **Nodal rhythms and heart block.** Therapy for these rhythms is dictated by the hemodynamic response to the loss of atrial-ventricular synchrony. Most **nodal** rhythms are transient and well tolerated. In some patients, however, atrial contraction contributes significantly to CO by increasing ventricular end-diastolic volume (EDV). The best and easiest treatment of nodal rhythms is atrial pacing at a rate above the nodal rate. β-blockade is useful to restore sinus rhythm and to slow a rapid nodal rhythm, which permits atrial pacing to occur. **Third degree heart block** following cardiac surgery is uncommon. It generally occurs in the setting of aortic or mitral valve or ventricular septal defect repairs. The injury to the conduction system is often transient. Allow at least 4 postoperative days to regain native AV conduction before considering placement of a permanent pacemaker.

C. **Myocardial dysfunction,** as evidenced by a low cardiac output (usually considered as a cardiac index of < 2.5 L/min/m^2) is common in the cardiac surgical patient. Remember, that **cardiac output = stroke vol-**

ume **(SV)** × **heart rate (HR),** and therapy can be directed at either variable.

1. **Heart rate** can be manipulated by atrial or AV sequential pacing. In a patient with an HR of 80 and a SV of 30 ml, increasing the HR to 100 bpm will improve the CO from 2.4 L/min to 3.0 L/min (provided the stroke volume is maintained at 30 ml). Of course, the underlying cardiac function remains unchanged despite the higher output. Maintenance of sinus or AV sequential rhythm is crucial when attempting to optimize cardiac output. When using AV sequential pacing, the optimal AV delay must be determined for each patient (but the best CO is usually obtained with an AV delay ~200 msec).

2. **Stroke volume = ventricular end-diastolic volume − ventricular end-systolic volume.**

    a. **Ventricular end-diastolic volume** is synonymous with preload. Preload is manipulated according to the Frank-Starling relationship (Chapter 1). Measurements of LAP or PAOP are often used as surrogates for EDV. Pressure measurements can be extremely inaccurate and misleading measures of volume, especially in the cardiac surgical patient. The relationship between EDV and PAOP can change, so that the "ideal" filling pressure can change over time. Informal construction of a ventricular function curve should be undertaken every time preload is increased or decreased. This is easily accomplished by plotting stroke volume against PAOP or LAP before and after a volume challenge or a trial of diuresis. The cardiac patient with postischemic ventricular dysfunction is expected to have a relatively flat ventricular function curve. Remember that perfusion pressure to the subendocardium can be approximated by the difference between MAP and left ventricular EDP. Any volume challenge in a patient with depressed ventricular function and coronary inadequacy should proceed cautiously. The aphorism "a small heart is a happy heart" underscores the primary difference in hemodynamic management between cardiac ICU and trauma ICU patients. Decreasing end-systolic volume (ESV) should be considered as the initial therapy in the cardiac patient with poor ventricular function, followed by conservative use of increased EDV.

    b. **Ventricular end-systolic volume** is determined by ventricular afterload and contractility. **Afterload** is a complex concept in the intact heart, and for simplicity will be discussed as the impedance to ventricular ejection, oversimplified as systemic vascular resistance (SVR) or tone. Decreasing afterload by using vasodilators (e.g., nitroprusside) will increase stroke volume by decreasing ESV. This effect becomes more pronounced as ventricular function deteriorates. The goal is an equivalent MAP with a lower SVR and higher CO. **Contractility** is the ability of the heart to perform work, and is simplistically reflected by the **ejection fraction** (EF = SV/EDV). The most common causes of decreased contractility in the cardiac ICU are myocardial ischemia (acute and reversible) and myocardial scar with altered ventricular geometry (chronic and mostly irreversible). The choice of a positive inotropic agent to increase contractility is largely institution-specific. Clinical studies have not demonstrated one clearly superior agent. The first line of inotropic support usually includes a β-adrenergic agonist (e.g., dobutamine, dopamine, epinephrine). These agents can be titrated to increase SV until adverse effects (usually dysrhythmias) occur. When an individual has significant tachycardia or fails to respond appropriately, a cyclic nucleotide phosphodiesterase (PDE) inhibitor (e.g., amrinone, milrinone) may be selected. When initiating therapy with a PDE inhibitor, SVR usually decreases. An agent to increase MAP (e.g., phenylephrine, norepinephrine) should be readily available.

When inotropes and volume titration are unable to improve CO to a reasonable level, **intraaortic balloon counterpulsation** can improve CO, reduce afterload, and increase coronary perfusion (Chapter 13).

c. **Valvular abnormalities** can reduce cardiac output (Chapter 18). **Regurgitant lesions** will increase EDV initially, and eventually increase ESV as chronic volume overload causes decreased contractility. **Aortic stenosis** causes increased afterload, increased ESV, and compensatory concentric hypertrophy. **Mitral stenosis** causes an increase in left atrial pressure (i.e., increased PAOP) with a normal or low left ventricular EDV. A bedside **transthoracic or transesophageal echocardiogram** is invaluable in the diagnosis of low CO of unclear cause.

D. **Pulmonary dysfunction,** defined as mechanical ventilation for more than 48 hours, complicates the postoperative course of 8% of cardiac surgery patients. The incidence of severe ARDS is approximately 1%. The cause of respiratory failure in the postoperative patient is multifactorial:

1. Prolonged atelectasis during CPB contributes to V/Q mismatching and hypoxemia.

2. Complement activation during CPB can cause acute lung injury.

3. Hypoperfusion can produce gut ischemia and endo-toxin translocation, which can contribute to acute lung injury.

4. High filling pressures in the patient with poor cardiac function can cause hydrostatic pulmonary edema.

5. Intraoperative trauma can cause phrenic nerve paralysis.

6. Pleural effusions can decrease respiratory system compliance and increase work of breathing.

E. **Acute renal failure** (ARF) following CPB occurs in approximately 7% of patients, depending on the definition used. The incidence of ARF requiring hemodialysis is probably about 1%. The leading risk factors for postoperative ARF are preoperative chronic renal insufficiency, diabetes mellitus, and postoperative hypotension. ARF following cardiac surgery is an independent risk factor for mortality. Postoperative oliguria (< 0.5 ml/kg/h) should be aggressively evaluated and treated (Chapter 23). Hypoperfusion can contribute to ARF, so it is imperative to maintain MAP near its preoperative value. Early institution of continuous renal replacement therapy is indicated for impending renal failure and volume overload.

F. **Neurologic dysfunction.** Overt neurologic injury occurs in 0.5% to 2% of closed-chamber procedures (CAB). This incidence increases to 4% to 10% with open-chamber procedures (i.e., valve surgery). Subtle neurologic changes, including cognitive dysfunction, ophthalmologic abnormalities, and the appearance of primitive reflexes, are much more frequent—60% at 1 week postoperative, most resolving over the following year. Intraoperative emboli of air, clot, and vascular "debris" to the cerebral circulation are the likely causes of most neurologic injuries. In the ICU, the patient suspected of intraoperative neurologic injury should be treated similarly to other patients with embolic stroke. Hypotension, hypoxemia, hypercarbia, and hyperthermia should be avoided in an attempt to limit secondary cerebral injury.

G. **Gastrointestinal complications** occur with a frequency of 0.5% to 2% following cardiac surgery, with an associated mortality of 15% to 40%. Patients with low CO and other organ system failures are at the highest risk for gastrointestinal complications. The problems most commonly encountered are gastric or duodenal ulceration and bleeding, cholecystitis (often acalculous), pancreatitis, and intestinal ischemia, perforation, or obstruction. These entities can be subtle in presentation and difficult to diagnose. They can occur anytime from 2 days to 4 weeks postoperatively. A high index of suspicion is necessary for rapid diagnosis and treatment of these often-fatal complications (Chapter 25).

H. **Cardiac tamponade** produces a low cardiac output in about 1% of postoperative cardiac patients. Tamponade decreases stroke volume by compression and consequent underfilling of the ventricles. Tamponade can occur with mediastinal drains still in place, even in the patient whose pericardium was left open. The diagnosis of tamponade can be difficult in the postoperative patient. The classic diagnostic signs of tachycardia, low CO, elevation and equalization of filling pressures, exaggerated blood pressure response to positive-pressure ventilation, and widened mediastinum by chest radiograph may not be present, and even classic echocardiographic criteria may be insensitive to postoperative tamponade. Tamponade also has been described to occur as late as several weeks postoperatively. A patient whose condition deteriorates for unclear reasons may require operative exploration of the mediastinum.

   I. **Readmission** to the ICU deserves special mention as a complication. The high mortality rate (~ 35%) of these patients warrants aggressive initial diagnosis and treatment.

SELECTED REFERENCES

Levy JH, Buckley MJ, D'Ambra MN, et al. Symposium: pharmacologic control of bleeding in patients undergoing open heart surgery. *Contemporary Surgery* 1996;48:175–188.

Ryan TA, Rady MY, Bashour CA, et al. Predictors of outcome in cardiac surgical patients with prolonged intensive care stay. *Chest* 1997; 112:1035–1042.

Wijns W, Vatner SF, Camici PG. Hibernating myocardium *N Engl J Med* 1998;339:173–181.

Vascular Surgery

Laura Niklason and David Schinderle

I. **General considerations.** Arteriosclerosis, manifesting as coronary artery and peripheral vascular disease, is the single largest cause of mortality in the United States.

   A. Factors that contribute to the development of arteriosclerotic plaque include hypertension, tobacco use, hyperlipidemia, and diabetes mellitus. Arteriosclerotic disease and its concomitant vessel wall degeneration cause most of the arterial occlusive and aneurysmal complications that require surgical correction.

   B. The postoperative management of vascular surgical patients and the postoperative complications they suffer is largely driven by the underlying arteriosclerotic disease process and its comorbidities. The physician must maintain a high index of suspicion for undiagnosed vascular disease and for vascular complications at locations that are remote from the operative site.

II. **Comorbid diseases** commonly accompany vascular disease and are exacerbated by the stress of surgery.

   A. **Hypertension** is probably the single most common condition affecting vascular surgical patients. Up to 90% of patients with aortic aneurysms are hypertensive, as are 60% of patients with peripheral occlusive vascular disease and claudication. Treatments for hypertension include diuretics, β-adrenergic and α-adrenergic blockers, angiotensin-converting enzyme (ACE)-inhibitors, and calcium channel blockers (Chapter 10). **Renal artery stenosis** leading to excess production of angiotensin can cause renovascular hypertension that can be particularly difficult to control medically.

   B. **Coronary artery disease (CAD),** manifesting as angina, myocardial infarction (MI), or congestive heart failure (CHF), afflicts between 30% and 50% of vascular surgical patients. If those with clinically silent or undiagnosed disease were taken into account, this percentage would increase to 60% to 80% of patients. Perioperative MI occurs in 6% to 13% of vascular surgical patients. Factors increasing the risk of MI include a history of angina, perfusion defects on dipyridamole thallium scanning, and ischemic ST depression during preoperative stress testing. (See Chapter 17 for details concerning diagnosis and management.)

   C. **Chronic obstructive pulmonary disease** (COPD). More than 80% of patients with vascular disease either currently smoke tobacco or have smoked in the past. Many vascular patients are maintained on inhaled bronchodilators for outpatient management of their pulmonary disease. Continued treatment following surgery with bronchodilators provides symptomatic relief.

Pulmonary complications in patients with COPD are common (Chapter 21).

1. Patients undergoing aortic surgery have a 30% incidence of severe COPD (defined as an FEV_1 of less then 50% of predicted), and up to a 40% incidence of significant postoperative pulmonary complications. The postoperative management of aortic surgery patients can be complicated by large intraoperative blood loss and consequent fluid resuscitation, which can lead to pulmonary edema and worsened lung mechanics.

2. The differential diagnosis for wheezing or respiratory decompensation in the vascular surgical patient must always include primary cardiac causes, including acute myocardial ischemia. Fluid shifts that occur 2 to 3 days postoperatively can lead to acute development of CHF, which is poorly tolerated in patients with COPD.

D. Diabetes mellitus (predominantly type II, or adult onset diabetes) is a major contributor to arteriosclerotic disease of both large caliber arteries and the microvasculature. Microvascular disease of the extremities and the heart can cause ischemic symptoms and complications that are not amenable to surgical therapy. Diabetes occurs in 10% to 40% of vascular surgery patients.

1. For diabetic patients undergoing any surgical procedure, control of blood glucose is often more difficult in the postoperative period. Even type II diabetics who usually do not require insulin require frequent measurement of blood glucose levels, and they often need supplemental insulin injections for several days postoperatively (Chapter 26).

2. **Hyperglycemia** can produce an osmotic diuresis and fluid losses that must be taken into account in postoperative fluid management.

3. **Diabetic ketoacidosis** (insulin-dependent, type I diabetics) and **hyperosmolar coma** (non–insulin-dependent, type II diabetics) are rare but preventable complications in these patients (Chapter 26).

E. Chronic renal insufficiency can result from several factors, including advanced age, hypertensive nephrosclerosis, diabetic nephropathy, and renal artery stenosis. Diagnostic procedures using iodinated contrast agents can further worsen renal function, as can aminoglycoside antibiotics and other nephrotoxins that are often administered in the perioperative period (See Chapter 23 for details and management.)

1. Vascular patients who have an elevated creatinine (> 3.0 mg/dl) preoperatively are at increased risk for acute renal dysfunction postoperatively. If renal dysfunction progresses to the point of requiring dialysis, the hospital mortality rate exceeds 50%.

2. Those undergoing repair of suprarenal abdominal or thoracoabdominal aortic aneurysms are at great-

est risk. Up to 25% of these patients present with a baseline creatinine level of 1.5 mg/dl or higher. Renal insults from the aneurysm repair include ischemia during suprarenal cross-clamping, as well as possible showers of atheromatous emboli that occur following reperfusion of the kidneys.

III. **Peripheral vascular procedures** improve either inflow (e.g., aortobifemoral bypass grafts) or outflow (e.g., femoral-popliteal bypass grafts).

A. **A staging scheme** has been developed to grade signs and symptoms. Stage 0: no signs or symptoms; stage I: intermittent claudication but no physical changes; stage II: severe claudication and dependent rubor; stage III: rest pain and cyanosis; stage IV: nonhealing ulcer or gangrene. Surgical intervention is usually indicated for symptoms in stages III and IV.

B. **Monitoring and restoring graft patency.** Following completion of an infrainguinal bypass procedure, a major part of postoperative care is directed at ensuring continued distal perfusion of the limb and patency of the conduit.

1. **To minimize early thrombosis,** many patients are maintained on one of several anticoagulants, including heparin, warfarin, aspirin, or other antiplatelet agents (Chapter 12). Complications secondary to anticoagulation do occasionally occur, including wound hematomas and, rarely, intracerebral hemorrhage.

2. **Postoperative graft thrombosis** occurs in approximately 5% of infrainguinal bypass procedures, but immediate revision is often successful.

3. The most important indicator of graft patency and limb perfusion is a **palpable pulse,** which is best compared with the pulse examined preoperatively or at the conclusion of surgery. Other subjective assessments include limb color and temperature, reports of pain, or motor or sensory impairment.

4. **Semiquantitative measures** such as **pulse volume recordings** (PVRs) or **segmental arterial pressure measurements** such as the ankle-brachial index (ABI) can supplement subjective evaluations. PVRs are measured using a sphygmomanometer cuff that is applied either directly on top of or distal to the bypass graft. The cuff is inflated and the pulsatile volume of flowing blood beneath the cuff is recorded on a stripchart. Serial PVRs provide a useful monitor of graft patency and they are sometimes the first indicator of early graft thrombosis. Serial ABIs, which are ratios of the measured systolic blood pressures at the ankle and forearm, are also useful.

5. **Early graft occlusion** is signaled by a combination of decreased peripheral pulses, a cool or cyanotic limb, and decreased PVRs or ABIs. Although graft kinking can sometimes occur, early graft oc-

clusion is generally caused by thrombosis. When graft occlusion is suspected, prompt surgical evaluation is often followed by reexploration and thrombectomy. Rarely, acute arterial occlusion can be caused by emboli that originate proximal to the graft, in either the aorta or the heart. The likelihood of embolic events is increased in patients with known atrial fibrillation or with aortic aneurysmal disease.

6. **In cases of repeated or idiopathic arterial or graft thrombosis,** an inherited or acquired hypercoagulable state should be considered (Chapter 12).

7. **Late graft thrombosis** is sometimes treated using selective intraarterial thrombolytic therapies (Chapter 12). **Streptokinase** can be administered intraarterially at 5,000 to 10,000 IU/h for 12 to 48 hours via a femoral catheter. A low-grade fever sometimes occurs with treatment; it can be caused by antigen–antibody interactions with preformed antistreptococcal antibodies. **Urokinase** is harvested from human renal cells and is not antigenic, but it is more expensive than streptokinase. Low-dose urokinase is infused intraarterially at 20,000 U/h for 12 to 24 hours. The therapeutic effect of these agents is monitored by physical examination and serial arteriography. The risks of these therapies are localized bleeding at the catheter insertion site and intracranial hemorrhage.

C. **Myocardial complications.** Patients who undergo infrainguinal bypass surgery are generally older and have more advanced CAD than patients undergoing other types of vascular procedures. The 30-day operative mortality for all patients undergoing infrainguinal arterial reconstructions for threatened limbs ranges from 2% to 12%, with the principal cause of death being MI. In addition, the 5-year mortality rates for patients undergoing infrainguinal bypass are higher than for any other type of vascular procedure, approaching 50% in some series. Approximately half of late deaths in these patients are related to cardiac causes. Actuarial studies, however, have shown that the surgery itself imparts minimal long-term cardiac risk.

1. **"Silent" ischemia** without angina can be a common occurrence because a high percentage of these patients are diabetic.

2. **Treatment of ischemia** is by standard measures: oxygen administration, sublingual or intravenous (IV) nitroglycerin (starting at 50 µg/min), IV β-blockers (e.g., propranolol starting at 0.5 mg, or metoprolol starting at 5 mg given slowly), and control of incisional pain with opioids or epidural analgesia (Chapter 17 discusses details and management.)

D. **Analgesia.** Infrainguinal bypass procedures are often performed under regional anesthesia, most commonly using an epidural catheter. This anesthetic is chosen, in part, because of the advanced age and poor clinical status of many of these patients and because of concerns regarding the negative inotropic effects of general anesthetics. In addition, perfusion to the lower extremities can be enhanced by the sympathectomy that is produced by regional anesthesia.

1. **For postoperative analgesia,** continuous infusions of a dilute local anesthetic (e.g., bupivacaine 0.1%, alone or in combination with fentanyl 3–10 μg/ml) provide excellent pain relief (Chapter 6). Occasionally, the concentration of local anesthetic must be decreased to allow a complete sensory and motor examination and ambulation. In elderly patients, the concentration of narcotics can be reduced to decrease the risk of hypoventilation. Epidural catheters are typically left in place for 3 to 7 days postoperatively.

2. **Complications of epidural catheter placement** include spinal headache from inadvertent dural puncture, infection, and epidural hematoma formation, which can cause spinal cord compression and subsequent paraplegia. **Epidural hematoma formation** is somewhat more likely in the vascular surgical patient than in others because of the perioperative administration of anticoagulants. An epidural hematoma must be considered in the differential diagnosis of any patient who complains of back pain near the site of an epidural catheter, or who develops unexplained lower extremity motor deficit. If confirmed by emergent magnetic resonance imaging, immediate surgical decompression is indicated. To reduce the risk of hematoma formation, epidural catheters should not be inserted or removed when patients are receiving anticoagulants.

IV. **Abdominal and thoracic aortic surgery**
   A. **Classification of aortic disease**
      1. **Abdominal aortic aneurysms (AAA)** occur in 5% to 7% of people over age 60. Elective surgical intervention is indicated for most patients with AAAs greater than 5 cm in diameter to prevent rupture; it is associated with 3% to 5% perioperative mortality.

      2. **Thoracoabdominal aortic aneurysms (TAA)** are classified according to their anatomic locations (Crawford classification):
         a. **Type I,** from proximal descending to upper abdominal aorta, ending proximal to the visceral vessels.
         b. **Type II,** from proximal descending aorta to the distal abdominal aorta.
         c. **Type III,** from mid-descending thoracic aorta to the distal abdominal aorta.
         d. **Type IV,** infradiaphragmatic abdominal aorta with the graft carried proximal to the celiac axis.

3. **Repair of thoracoabdominal aneurysms** entails 10% perioperative mortality in most series.
4. **Aortoocclusive disease** is often treated with aortobifemoral reconstruction to improve inflow to the lower extremities.

B. **Paraplegia and spinal cord protection**

1. **Paraplegia** is a rare complication following infrarenal aortic procedures, but occurs at rates of up to 16% following suprarenal AAA or TAA repair. Paraplegia is also a well-recognized complication of acute dissection of the aorta, caused by "stripping off" of the spinal arterial supply.

2. **Pharmacologic agents** that have been investigated for their neuroprotective effects during aortic surgery include barbiturates, steroids, naloxone, free radical scavengers (e.g., superoxide dismutase), and vasodilators. Although many of these agents have shown some beneficial effects in animal models, none has shown clear, consistent benefit in human studies.

3. **Local spinal cord cooling** is used to protect the spinal cord from intraoperative ischemia during TAA repair at the Massachusetts General Hospital. With this technique, the spinal cord is cooled by infusion of iced saline into the epidural space via a 4 French epidural catheter placed at the T10-T12 level. A 4 French single lumen intrathecal catheter is placed at the L3-L4 level to monitor cerebrospinal fluid (CSF) temperature and pressure and to withdraw CSF in case of increased CSF pressure. Approximately 30 to 45 minutes prior to thoracic aortic cross-clamping, local cooling of the spinal cord is initiated using a continuous infusion of 4 to 5 ml/min of epidural iced saline. The target CSF temperature is maintained at 24°C to 26°C. To maintain spinal cord perfusion pressure, the CSF pressure is maintained at least 40 mm Hg less than the mean arterial pressure. After aortic unclamping, the epidural infusion is stopped and the temperature of the spinal cord rapidly returns to normal. By using this local cooling technique, the incidence of postoperative paraplegia after TAA repair has been reduced to approximately 3%.

4. The spinal catheter typically remains in place approximately 24 hours postoperatively, allowing monitoring of CSF pressure and the withdrawal of CSF if the pressure rises above 15 to 20 mm Hg. The spinal catheter is usually removed on the first postoperative day after correction of any postoperative coagulopathy. The epidural catheter usually remains in place for 3 to 7 days to permit continuous epidural analgesia.

5. **Delayed paraplegias** can occur in patients who have undergone TAA repair. Delayed deficits usually are associated with major hypotensive epi-

sodes, illustrating that the circulation to the spinal cord is in a fragile balance for some patients following surgery. Maintenance of adequate systemic arterial pressure and, therefore, adequate spinal cord perfusion pressure is necessary to prevent such late neurologic sequelae.

C. **Cardiac complications,** including infarction, dysrhythmias, CHF, and unstable angina, occur in 5% to 10% of aortic surgical patients.

1. **The overall goals for hemodynamic management** change during the first postoperative days. Care during the first postoperative day focuses on correction of coagulopathies and infusion of blood products or crystalloids to ensure adequate intravascular volume and urine output. This "resuscitation phase" is often bypassed for patients who have suffered minimal operative blood loss. During the next 2 to 3 days, fluid management is directed at removing excess intravascular volume that results from mobilization of "third space" accumulations, avoiding the development of CHF, and improving pulmonary function.

2. **Intraoperative monitoring** for aortic surgical patients typically includes radial artery and pulmonary artery (PA) catheters. The baseline hemodynamic values that were observed at the beginning of the operation provide useful benchmarks for postoperative care. Volume infusion or diuresis can be guided by the value of the central venous pressure (CVP), with a target being the preoperative value. The exception would be the patient with low urine output and intraoperative renal ischemia, who may benefit from sequential volume challenges (bringing the CVP value to 6–10 mm Hg) to improve blood pressure and cardiac output.

3. **Pulmonary capillary occlusion pressures (PAOP),** which reflect the filling pressure of the left ventricle, should be targeted to the preoperative value (Chapter 1).

4. **Cardiac complications,** including dysrhythmias, CHF, and infarction, occur most commonly during the first 3 to 4 postoperative days. Patients who are considered to be at high risk for these complications can benefit from continued cardiac monitoring after leaving the ICU setting.

D. **Pulmonary complications**

1. **The intubated patient** is weaned from the ventilator as soon as safely possible. Patients who have suffered minimal to moderate blood loss and who are not volume overloaded can be extubated in the operating room or soon after arrival in the ICU.

2. Minimizing volume overload and avoiding CHF is important in maintaining adequate pulmonary function in these patients. Targeting the PAOP to the preoperative value (or below) helps minimize

pulmonary blood volume and extravascular lung fluid. Other chapters in this book describe the management of acute respiratory failure (Chapter 20), chronic obstructive disease and bronchospasm (Chapter 21), and pneumonia (Chapters 27 and 28).

E. Renal dysfunction

1. Patients who undergo aortic surgery and have a baseline creatinine level greater than 1.5 mg/dl, an intraoperative renal ischemia time greater than 100 minutes, or prolonged intraoperative hypotension are at increased risk for renal failure.

2. No convincing evidence indicates that any particular postoperative intervention has a significant effect on renal outcome. Diligent efforts to avoid *secondary insults* (e.g., hypotension and exposure to nephrotoxic drugs) are important in postoperative care.

3. **Direct ischemic insult** to the kidneys manifests as acute tubular necrosis (ATN) (Chapter 23). In most cases, ATN is self-limited and resolves without the need for dialysis. If renal injury is compounded by a secondary insult (e.g., sepsis, hypotension, or administration of nephrotoxic drugs), then the progression to complete renal failure is more likely.

4. **Atheroembolic renal injury,** which occurs during unclamping and possibly postoperatively, is characterized by a slowly rising creatinine level and often a maintained urine output. Creatinine levels can rise progressively until reaching a stable peak value that is substantially higher than baseline or until dialysis is required. Treatment for this condition is supportive (Chapter 23).

F. Mesenteric ischemia. The incidence of **ischemic colitis** following aortic reconstruction is approximately 2%. It is more likely to occur following repair of AAA than following reconstruction for aortoocclusive disease, possibly because of ligation of the inferior mesenteric artery. Bloody diarrhea is one of the earliest manifestations of ischemic colitis, occurring within 48 hours of operation. Sigmoidoscopy is helpful in detecting mucosal ischemia and necrosis. Mild mucosal ischemia can be treated conservatively, but evidence of transmural necrosis, peritonitis, or bowel perforation demands urgent operative intervention to resect the compromised bowel (Chapter 25).

G. Bleeding and coagulation disorders. Aortic surgery can be associated with anywhere from minimal (< 500 ml) to massive (> 5 L) blood loss.

1. Resuscitation from hemorrhage can produce **dilutional coagulopathies** and systemic **hypothermia,** which can impair coagulation. In addition, TAA repair has been associated with a fibrinolytic reaction after aortic cross-clamping that is biochemically similar to **disseminated intravascular coagulation.** Caused in part by these coagulo-

pathies, a small percentage of patients require re-exploration for bleeding.

2. **Reversal of hypothermia,** using forced hot air systems, heated blankets, increased room temperature, and warmed IV fluids, is essential.

3. **Coagulopathies** are corrected by appropriate transfusion of blood components as described in Chapter 12. Transfusion of large volumes of blood products may necessitate diuresis, typically with furosemide, to prevent volume overload. Use of starch products such as Hespan for volume expansion should be avoided, because they have been associated with worsened coagulopathy in this setting.

V. **Endovascular stent repair**

A. **Selected aortic aneurysms** can be treated by endovascular stent placement. Stent placement is far less invasive than standard operations, and patients who have undergone this procedure usually bypass the ICU after 4 to 6 hours of observation in the recovery room. Stents, which are typically deployed via the femoral arteries, function to exclude the aneurysm wall from the radial force imposed by arterial blood flow.

B. **Complications** include inadvertent deployment of the stent across the ostia of one or both renal arteries, which can lead to renal failure if blood flow to the kidneys is impaired. Dissection or rupture of the femoral, iliac, or aortic vessels can occur with stent deployment. Failure to achieve complete exclusion of the AAA from the bloodstream can produce "endoleak" at the stent attachment site. This leak permits continued blood flow into the aneurysm sac around the stent, with failure to eliminate pressure on the dilated arterial wall. Alternatively, persistent flow from the inferior mesenteric or lumbar arteries can continue to pressurize the aneurysm. These complications can lead to further aneurysmal dilation and rupture. Symptoms such as abdominal pain and distention, especially when accompanied by hypotension, should trigger suspicion for aneurysm dilation or rupture.

VI. **Carotid endarterectomy** is the most frequently performed noncardiac vascular procedure.

A. Patients who undergo carotid endarterectomy (CEA) usually have no significant sequelae and are transferred to a surgical floor after 4 to 6 hours of observation in the recovery room. Blood pressure is maintained within an acceptable range, typically 120 to 160 mm Hg systolic, and sometimes patients can be maintained on IV infusions of low molecular weight dextran to decrease blood viscosity and platelet clumping.

B. **Neurologic assessments** are routinely performed every hour for the first 4 hours, and then every 4 hours for the next 24 hours. Approximately 5% of CEA patients will have injury to the hypoglossal nerve, which manifests as deviation of the extended tongue to the side of the operation. Facial nerve injury will manifest as drooping of the corner of the mouth to the operated side; unilateral recurrent laryngeal nerve injury can present as hoarseness of voice. Bilateral recurrent laryngeal nerve injury can lead to acute upper airway obstruction and respiratory distress.

C. **Hemodynamic assessment.** The incidence of either hypertensive or hypotensive episodes after CEA is more than 60%. Hypertension is more common than hypotension after CEA, and it occurs more frequently in patients with poorly controlled hypertensive disease. The exacerbation of hypertension after CEA may be related to injury of the carotid baroreceptors by surgical dissection and generally lasts less than 24 to 48 hours. Postoperative hypertension has been correlated with a 10% incidence of neurologic deficits following CEA, versus 3% in normotensive subjects.

1. **Postoperative hypotension** (with systolic blood pressures less than 120 mm Hg) is observed in 5% of CEA patients. It usually responds well to fluids and low-dose IV phenylephrine infusion (starting at 10 µg/min and titrating upward). Hypotension requiring treatment for more than 1 to 2 days postoperatively is unusual. The differential diagnosis of postoperative hypotension in the CEA patient must always include myocardial ischemia.

2. **Hypertension** (with systolic blood pressures less than 180 mm Hg) can usually be controlled with oral medications. If the patient was maintained on antihypertensives preoperatively, then doubling the dose of one medication, or giving doses early, may be sufficient to keep systolic pressures less than 160 mm Hg.

3. If systolic blood pressures are consistently greater than 180 to 200 mm Hg for more than 4 hours after surgery, then invasive monitoring with an arterial catheter is indicated. An IV infusion of nitroglycerin, (starting at 50 µg/min and titrating upward) or sodium nitroprusside (starting at 2 µg/min and titrating upward) is the treatment of choice because of the short half-lives of these agents. Oral agents such as calcium channel blockers or β-blockers can be given after the blood pressure is controlled by IV drugs. The importance of aggressive management of severe hypertension in the CEA patient cannot be overstated, because of the correlation of severe hypertension with catastrophic neurologic complications.

D. **Neurologic complications**

1. **Postendarterectomy hyperperfusion syndrome** occurs in some patients who have had a high-grade carotid stenosis with long-standing hypoperfusion of the ipsilateral cerebral hemisphere prior to operation. This leads to impairment of cerebral autoregulation and a profound increase in

cerebral blood flow following CEA, which can in turn lead to a severe unilateral headache that is improved by upright posture. Cerebral edema and even intracerebral hemorrhage can occur secondary to hyperfusion syndrome. When intracerebral hemorrhage (ICH) occurs, it is catastrophic and often fatal.

2. **ICH** as a complication of CEA generally occurs within several days postoperatively, but can occur as late as 2 to 3 weeks after the operation.

3. **Cerebral ischemic events** generally present on emergence from anesthesia or immediately thereafter. The patient who awakens with a new neurologic deficit or who develops focal neurologic findings in the immediate postoperative period represents a surgical emergency. Reexploration to treat thrombosis of the operated carotid artery may be required. Noninvasive evaluation by carotid ultrasound is often helpful in making the diagnosis of acute carotid thrombosis.

4. **Emboli** to the cerebral circulation can cause focal neurologic deficits and are generally apparent on emergence from anesthesia. Embolic events are generally treated conservatively with anticoagulation.

5. **Seizures** are uncommon. In the absence of cerebral infarction or ICH, they are generally attributed to cerebral hyperperfusion and the early stages of hypertensive encephalopathy.

E. **Wound hematomas** sometimes occur in CEA patients. The neck is a vascular area and the heparin that is given before arterial cross-clamping is generally not reversed. Most wound hematomas can be safely observed. A rapidly expanding neck hematoma, however, can displace the trachea and compress the airway. A rapidly expanding neck wound with tracheal deviation is a surgical emergency. The airway should be secured with an endotracheal tube and the hematoma decompressed. If loss of the airway is imminent, the neck wound should be opened immediately and the hematoma decompressed.

F. **Myocardial infarction** remains the chief cause of death following CEA. The rate of MI in the population undergoing CEA is approximately 6%. Many clinicians advocate continuous ECG monitoring for the first 24 hours following surgery, but most infarctions occur on postoperative day 2 to 3. (Diagnosis and treatment are outlined in Chapter 17.)

VII. **Hemodialysis access procedures**

A. **Types of fistulas for vascular access** in patients with renal failure fall into two groups: autogenous arteriovenous fistulas, referred to here as "Cimino" fistulas; and bridge fistulas, which incorporate either autogenous vein or a prosthetic material such as Teflon.

1. **The Cimino fistula** is a surgical connection between artery and vein constructed directly from the patient's own vessels. Arterial pressure transmitted directly to the veins results in dilation and hypertrophy of the venous walls. This "arterialization" of the veins may take up to 6 weeks before hypertrophy is sufficient for the venous wall to withstand repeated venipuncture, and hemodialysis must be performed by some other route until the fistula matures. Typical sites for placement of Cimino fistulas include the radial artery–cephalic vein, brachial artery–basilic vein, and brachial artery–cephalic vein.

2. **Bridge fistulas** have generally poorer long-term patency than Cimino fistulas, but they can be placed between almost any suitably sized superficial artery and vein in the body. Typical sites include between radial artery and antecubital fossa vein, or the brachial artery and the axillary vein. Because bridge fistulas often use synthetic graft material, they are more susceptible to infectious complications than Cimino fistulas. Newly placed bridge fistulas should not be punctured until approximately 2 weeks after implantation when the graft becomes invested with fibrous tissue to prevent leakage.

B. **Common complications**

1. **Thrombosis** is the most common complication occurring in arteriovenous fistulas. Direct examination of the fistula and the absence of a "thrill" are generally sufficient to establish the diagnosis of thrombosis. Early thrombosis of a Cimino fistula can be treated by conversion to a bridge prosthetic fistula, whereas late thrombosis can be treated with thrombectomy.

2. **Infection** is an important complication of both autogenous and synthetic fistulas. The diagnosis is typically made if erythema and inflammation are seen over the fistula and fever and leukocytosis are present. Organisms most commonly implicated are coagulase negative *Staphylococcus* spp and *Staphylococcus aureus*. An infected graft should be removed, and an interval of 2 to 3 days allowed before a new fistula is placed in a different location after administration of IV antibiotics.

3. **Arterial insufficiency,** or "steal" syndrome, occurs in a small percentage of patients with Cimino and bridge fistulas in the upper extremity. The "steal" phenomenon is caused by an area of very low resistance on the venous portion of the anastomosis. This causes blood to course through the palmar arch from the ulnar to the radial side, thereby reversing flow in the distal radial artery and "stealing" flow from the tissues of the hand. The syndrome is characterized by pain on exertion

of the hand, which often is worsened during dialysis. Treatment is either by surgical narrowing of the fistula or by complete ligation of the fistula if the limb is threatened.

4. **Venous insufficiency** of the forearm is caused by high arterial pressures applied to the venous side of the fistula. If combined with incompetent venous valves, the high pressures impede venous drainage of the forearm, resulting in edema and bluish discoloration of the distal extremity. The correction is surgical, by ligation of the vein immediately distal to the fistula.

5. Rarely, a large arteriovenous fistula can allow a sufficiently high flow rate to provide a substantial increase in venous return to the heart. In patients with CAD or cardiomyopathy and decreased cardiac reserve, this can lead to congestive heart failure. Treatment consists of "banding" of the fistula to decrease the graft flow rate.

SELECTED REFERENCES

Adams MB. Hemodialysis for end-stage renal disease: options and strategies. *Semin Vasc Surg* 1997;10:151–156.

Biller J, Feinberg WM, Castaldo JE, et al. Guidelines for carotid endarterectomy: a statement for healthcare professionals from a Special Writing Group of the Stroke Council, American Heart Association. *Circulation* 1998;97:501–509.

Brewster DC. Current controversies in the management of aortoiliac occlusive disease. *J Vasc Surg* 1997;25:365–379.

Brewster DC, Geller SC, Kaufman JA, et al. Initial experience with endovascular aneurysm repair: comparison of early results with outcome of conventional open repair. *J Vasc Surg* 1998;27:992–1003.

Burkhart HM, Cikrit DF. Arteriovenous fistulae for hemodialysis. *Semin Vasc Surg* 1997;10:162–165.

Cambria RP, Davison JK, Zannetti S, et al. Clinical experience with epidural cooling for spinal cord protection during thoracic and thoracoabdominal aneurysm repair. *J Vasc Surg* 1997;25:234–241.

Cambria RP, Davison JK. Regional hypothermia for prevention of spinal cord ischemic complications after thoracoabdominal aortic surgery: experience with epidural cooling. *Semin Thorac Cardiovasc Surg* 1998;10:61–65.

Gertler JP, Cambria RP, Brewster DC, et al. Coagulation changes during thoracoabdominal aneurysm repair. *J Vasc Surg* 1996;24:936–943.

Kashyap VS, Cambria RP, Davison JK, et al. Renal failure after thoracoabdominal aortic surgery. *J Vasc Surg* 1997;26:949–955.

Lintott P, Hafez HM, Stansby G. Spinal cord complications of thoracoabdominal aneurysm surgery. *Br J Surg* 1998;85:5–15.

L'Italien GJ, Cambria RP, Cutler BS, et al. Comparative early and late cardiac morbidity among patients requiring different vascular surgery procedures. *J Vasc Surg* 1995;21:935–944.

L'Italien GJ, Paul SD, Hendel RC, et al. Development and validation of a Bayesian model for perioperative cardiac risk assessment in a cohort of 1,081 vascular surgical candidates. *J Am Coll Cardiol* 1996;27:779–786.

Moore WS. *Vascular surgery: a comprehensive review.* Philadelphia: WB Saunders, 1993.

Treiman GS, Bernhard VM. Endovascular treatment of abdominal aortic aneurysms. *Ann Rev Med* 1998;49:363–373.

Veith FJ, Hobson R, Williams R, et al. *Vascular surgery: principles and practice,* 2nd ed. New York: McGraw-Hill, Inc, 1994.

Wilke HJ 2nd, Ellis JE, McKinsey JF. Carotid endarterectomy: perioperative and anesthetic considerations. *J Cardiothorac Vasc Anesth* 1996;10:928–949.

Wittgen CM, Brewster DC. Current status of the surgical treatment of patients with carotid artery disease: the surgical management of carotid atherosclerosis. *Annu Rev Med* 1997;48:69–77.

Zannetti S, L'Italien GJ, Cambria RP. Functional outcome after surgical treatment for intermittent claudication. *J Vasc Surg* 1996; 24:65–73.

Liver, Kidney, and Pancreatic Transplantation

John A. Powelson

I. Principles of care for transplant patients

A. **Time course.** The complex clinical picture of transplant patients (Table 38–1) can be simplified by considering time periods that emphasize different issues:

1. **First 48 hours: donor and recipient surgery.** As a rule, the allograft is the organ most affected by hemodynamic perturbations, so that good allograft function will almost always lead to swift clinical improvement. Allograft dysfunction, on the other hand, requires sorting out the contribution of the recipient's preoperative status and intraoperative course, the quality of the donor organ, and the possibility of technical complications.

2. **One week: acute rejection.** Because of the numerous steps in the complex cascade leading to full T-cell differentiation, clinically detectable acute rejection does not usually occur until 1 week after implantation. As long as technical complications have been ruled out, organ dysfunction at that point is usually attributed to rejection, and is treated empirically with increased immunosuppression.

3. **After 6 months: chronic issues.** The risk of opportunistic infections increases with the recipient's total exposure to immunosuppression (Chapter 27). Thus, these unusual infections are more typical in the late postoperative period, especially if repeated bouts of rejection have required multiple courses of heightened immunosuppression. Late allograft dysfunction raises the specters of disease recurrence and chronic rejection, both of which can lead to steadily worsening allograft failure.

B. **Immunosuppression.** Administration of any immunosuppressive agent is invariably limited by side effects. By combining different agents, it is possible to increase immunosuppression while limiting troublesome side effects. For this reason, most patients with whole organ transplant receive either double or triple (two or three drugs) immunosuppression.

1. **Cyclosporin and tacrolimus (FK506)** specifically target T-lymphocytes (the immune cells principally responsible for rejection). These agents form the lynchpin of current immunosuppressive protocols. Either one can be started perioperatively, and then taken orally as long-term maintenance. Both are nephrotoxic and require careful adjustment based on blood levels. Other side effects include

Table 38-1.   Factors affecting the transplant recipient's postoperative course

Underlying preoperative organ failure
Quality of the donor allograft
Intraoperative hemodynamics
Technical complications
Rejection
Immunosuppression
Adverse drug reaction
Disease recurrence

hypertension, hyperkalemia, hyperglycemia (especially in patients on high-dose steroids), neurotoxicity (seizures and tremors), and hyperuricemia (gout).

2. **Antilymphocyte agents (OKT3, ATG)** also target T-cells, but can only be given intravenously (IV). They are usually reserved for treating steroid-resistant acute rejection. Multiple courses are often ineffective and possibly dangerous. In patients with postoperative renal failure, cyclosporin or tacrolimus can be discontinued, with OKT3 or ATG being substituted for equivalent, but non-nephrotoxic, immunosuppression. This simplifies the early postoperative management, but uses up a major weapon that then may not be available to treat subsequent resistant rejection early in the postoperative course.

3. **Antimetabolite agents (mycophenolate or azathioprine)** inhibit DNA or RNA synthesis and, therefore, block lymphocyte proliferation. Dosages may have to be reduced if leukopenia, thrombocytopenia, or anemia occur.

4. **Corticosteroids**
   a. **Corticosteroids** provide nonspecific background immunosuppression. High-dose IV **methylprednisolone** (Solu-Medrol) typically is initiated on the day of transplantation and reduced over the next 4 to 5 days to a maintenance level. When feeding resumes, oral prednisone is substituted. If rejection occurs, high-dosage methylprednisolone boluses (500 mg IV every day for 2 days) are given as initial treatment.
   b. **Stress steroids.** Once receiving corticosteroids, patients require stress dose supplementation for major procedures. Intravenous **hydrocortisone** (Solu-cortef, 100 mg IV every 8 hours) is given on the day of surgery and tapered over 3 days. During this time, maintenance immunosuppression is continued, with either oral prednisone or IV methylpredniso-

lone (same total daily dose as prednisone, given in two divided doses).

   c. Patients on high-dose steroids can develop hyperglycemia and gastrointestinal bleeding, which can be treated prophylactically with H_2-blockers.

   5. Drug interactions. The transplant patient's complex drug regimen should constantly be reevaluated and simplified. This approach improves compliance and avoids potentially catastrophic and sometimes unpredictable drug interactions. In particular, the addition of new medications to an immunosuppressive regimen should be carefully considered. For example, **allopurinol,** if administered in combination with azathioprine, can precipitate life-threatening leukopenia. Numerous medications (e.g., sucralfate, verapamil, and erythromycin) can alter cyclosporin absorption and, thus, precipitate rejection or toxicity.

C. Infections

   1. Prophylactic strategies. Different types of infections occur at predictable times in the postoperative course, leading to corresponding prophylactic strategies (Chapter 27). Long-term, low-dose **trimethoprim-sulfamethoxazole** effectively prevents pneumocystis infections. During periods of heightened immunosuppression, **gancyclovir** or **acyclovir** is added to lower the incidence of cytomegalovirus (CMV) and Epstein-Barr virus (EBV) infections. Because invasive procedures increase the risk of bacterial infections, systemic antibiotics are administered during the perioperative period and prior to cholangiograms or percutaneous biopsies.

   2. Preventative measures include minimizing immunosuppression, avoiding endotracheal intubation and intravascular catheters whenever possible, and correcting malnutrition. Evaluation of possible hematomas, abscesses, or fluid collections should be pursued by serial ultrasound studies or computed tomography (CT), and appropriate drainage expeditiously undertaken. Because immunosuppression blunts the usual signs of inflammation, an aggressive surveillance and diagnostic approach is crucial, with routine cultures (e.g., biweekly cultures of sputum, urine, bile, and wound drainage) and daily chest radiographs while the recipient is receiving mechanical ventilation.

II. Liver transplantation

  A. Indications for transplantation influence ICU course. The indications for liver transplantation include virtually any disease leading to progressive, irreversible liver disease. These numerous disorders can be grouped according to features that will have an impact on the postoperative course:

1. **Chronic and progressive liver scarring (cirrhosis).** Liver fibrosis impedes portal blood flow, with resultant portal hypertension (ascites, bleeding varices, thrombocytopenia from hypersplenism). Multiple venous collaterals develop throughout the abdomen, increasing the likelihood of major perioperative blood loss and hemodynamic instability.

2. **Chronic hepatocyte injury or dysfunction.** Patients eventually develop hepatocyte failure (encephalopathy, fatigue, coagulopathy) and tend to be debilitated and malnourished. Poor healing, susceptibility to infection, and a prolonged recovery can be predicted.

3. **Acute hepatocyte injury (fulminant hepatic failure).** These patients are technically straightforward and do very well with a timely allograft, but can develop fatal cerebral edema, which is a physical disorder, in contrast to encephalopathy, which is a reversible metabolic disturbance. Perioperative intracerebral pressure monitoring is often helpful.

4. **Preserved hepatocyte function.** In these individuals, the pathologic process in the biliary tree is either too diffuse or too complex, or the hepatic reserve too compromised for conventional surgery (e.g., biliary atresia, sclerosing cholangitis, primary biliary cirrhosis, cryptogenic cirrhosis, or hepatoma with cirrhosis from any cause). Transplantation in these patients is technically straightforward and they do very well in the perioperative period.

B. **Donor allograft**

1. **Donor.** The likelihood of early allograft failure is correlated with donor characteristics (obesity, prolonged ICU stay, malnutrition, terminal hypotension, and fatty liver changes). A marginal organ may be selected for a critically ill patient who is likely to die before another organ becomes available.

2. **Cold preservation.** Prolonged ischemia time is also correlated with allograft dysfunction. After recovery, the donor allograft is flushed with University of Wisconsin (UW) solution, and stored on ice until transplantation. This cold ischemia time usually is limited to 12 to 15 hours, but fewer in marginal donor livers.

C. **Recipient operation**

1. **Native hepatectomy.** The coagulopathy of end-stage liver disease and the multiple venous collaterals of portal hypertension can lead to massive intraoperative blood loss, which is directly correlated with postoperative morbidity and mortality. Once the liver is removed, patients often develop metabolic acidosis, requiring correction to prepare for reperfusion. Over-correction with $NaHCO_3$, however, can lead to severe postoperative metabolic al-

kalosis. This phenomenon results from the metabolism of the citrate administered with transfused blood products to bicarbonate by a functioning allograft.

2. **Donor liver implantation** includes the supra- and infrahepatic vena cava and portal vein hepatic artery and bile duct anastomoses (either a choledochocholedochostomy or Roux-en-Y choledochojejunostomy). A biliary stent or a T-tube is placed across the anastomosis and exits percutaneously. Drains are also placed in the supra-and infrahepatic spaces.

3. **Reperfusion of the allograft,** usually within 60 minutes of warm ischemia time, returns a sudden bolus of cold, hyperkalemic, acidotic blood from the lower body and liver; it can cause severe pulmonary artery vasoconstriction with resultant hypotension. Reperfusion of the ischemic liver can also precipitate accelerated fibrinolysis. Aggressive replacement of coagulation factors and administration of antifibrinolytic agents (Chapter 12) may be required to achieve hemostasis.

D. **Posttransplant management**

1. **General care.** In addition to routine invasive monitoring, evaluation includes the physical examination (check mental status, abdomen, wound, and peritoneal and biliary drains), serial laboratory studies, and Doppler ultrasound examination in the first 48 hours to screen for hepatic artery thrombosis (see below). Intravenous fluids should always contain dextrose to avoid depletion of glycogen stores in the liver. Patients often tolerate sips by 24 to 48 hours after surgery, although feeding is resumed cautiously in patients with a Roux-en-Y jejunojejunostomy. On the fifth postoperative day, a cholangiogram is routinely obtained, after which the biliary stent or T-tube is clamped for increasing periods of time so that it is fully clamped by the tenth day.

2. **Cardiovascular**

   a. **Hemodynamics.** The high cardiac output and low peripheral vascular resistance typical of end-stage liver disease commonly persist into the early postoperative period, so that inotropic agents are rarely required in liver transplant recipients.

   b. **Hypotension.** The usual first therapeutic response is volume administration. Excessively high central venous pressures should be avoided, because transmission back to the hepatic sinusoids can exacerbate allograft edema already present from reperfusion injury. If hypotension persists without detectable hypovolemia or cardiac dysfunction, sepsis should be suspected, blood cultures obtained, and empiric antibiotic therapy initiated.

      c. Hypertension. Because of the increased risks of cerebral edema, hemorrhage, and seizures, sustained hypertension requires aggressive treatment.

3. Respiratory. Successful endotracheal extubation usually can be accomplished within 12 to 48 hours, but can be delayed by right diaphragmatic paralysis from intraoperative placement of the suprahepatic vascular clamp and by metabolic alkalosis (see above).

4. Renal

      a. Most liver allograft recipients develop mild postoperative renal dysfunction because of preexisting renal insufficiency, intraoperative caval occlusion, bleeding and hypotension, postimplantation hepatic allograft dysfunction, and nephrotoxic drugs (e.g., cyclosporin and tacrolimus). Other nephrotoxic drugs, such as aminoglycosides, should be avoided. Prostaglandin E_1 can have a beneficial effect on the liver recipient's renal function during the early postoperative period.

      b. If postoperative oliguria persists despite optimized hemodynamics, the non-nephrotoxic immunosuppressant OKT3 is substituted for tacrolimus or cyclosporin. With this approach, dialysis usually can be avoided.

      c. Continuous venovenous hemofiltration is preferred if dialysis is indicated. Dialysis should be used with extreme caution because rapid osmotic shifts can worsen the cerebral edema already present in patients with hepatic failure. In patients whose renal dysfunction progresses to the need for dialysis, mortality rates can be as great as 90%.

5. Hematologic leukopenia and **thrombocytopenia** secondary to hypersplenism typically persist into the early postoperative period. The azathioprine dosage may have to be reduced. If the white blood cell count falls below 1500/mm³, **granulocyte colony-stimulating factor (GCSF)** can be administered to decrease the incidence of postoperative infections. The postoperative hematocrit is maintained in the range of 25% to 30%, because higher values can be associated with hepatic artery thrombosis.

6. Postoperative bleeding. The likelihood of significant postoperative bleeding is related directly to the severity of intraoperative bleeding and the quality of immediate allograft function. If major blood loss persists despite reversal of coagulopathy, urgent surgical reexploration is indicated. Even in patients whose early bleeding stops, reexploration may be indicated to evacuate clot, which may otherwise become secondarily infected.

E. **Allograft dysfunction (Fig. 38-1).**
  1. **Primary graft nonfunction (PGNF),** defined as initial poor hepatic allograft function, occurs in approximately 10% of recipients; it has a greater than 80% mortality without retransplantation.
    a. PGNF must be differentiated from the reversible preservation injury that is frequently noted in the first 2 postoperative days. Preservation injury is typically associated with an aspartate aminotransferase (SGOT) peak below 2,000 U/L and rapid clinical improvement. In contrast, PGNF is associated with a marked elevation of bilirubin and transaminases (e.g., SGOT > 2,000 U/L), persistent hepatic encephalopathy, minimal bile output (< 30–60 ml/d, often colorless or white), uncorrectable coagulopathy, and profound hypoglycemia.
    b. **Treatment** consists of early prostaglandin E_1 infusion, intensive support, and retransplantation.
  2. **Acute rejection.** Both acute rejection and viral hepatitis (B, C, or CMV) may be heralded by a bilirubin and transaminase elevation. Acute rejection often occurs during the first or second postoperative weeks, whereas hepatitis usually occurs later. A percutaneous biopsy may be necessary to establish the correct diagnosis. Approximately two thirds of patients suffer a rejection episode; of these, two thirds respond to steroid boluses. Most

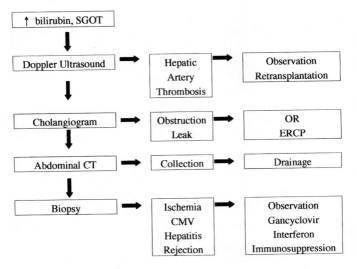

Fig. 38-1. Liver allograft dysfunction.

of the remainder respond to OKT3, but retransplantation is occasionally required because of uncontrolled rejection.

3. **Technical complications**

   a. **Hepatic artery thrombosis (HAT)** occurs more often in pediatric recipients, especially those with small or multiple allograft arteries. Presentation varies: approximately one third of these patients have acute hepatic failure, with marked elevation of transaminases (SGOT 2,000–10,000 U/L), or bile duct leak (the hepatic artery being the only blood supply to the bile ducts); one third have recurrent septic episodes with or without hepatic abscess; and one third have only an asymptomatic incidental finding. Late sequelae of HAT can include biliary dysfunction or ductal stricture. Doppler ultrasound is used liberally to screen for HAT, and an arteriogram may be required to confirm the diagnosis. Treatment options depend on the presentation; they include retransplantation, reoperation, selective urokinase injection, or no treatment.

   b. **Bile duct complications** can be detected by the appearance of bile in a drain or an unexplained rise in serum bilirubin. **Endoscopic retrograde cholangiopancreaticography (ERCP)** or reexploration may be required.

   c. **Other complications,** such as portal vein or vena cava thrombosis, are exceedingly rare. Treatment options usually include medical support, radiologic intervention, or operative correction.

III. **Renal transplantation**

A. **Renal transplant recipients** clearly are at risk for cardiovascular complications, because diabetes is the most common indication for renal transplantation and hypertension and hypercholesterolemia often complicate renal failure. Cardiovascular complications are nevertheless rare in the immediate postoperative period, because aggressive pretransplant screening (and subsequent treatment, if found) of occult coronary artery disease is the rule. On the other hand, long-term recipients are at high risk for cardiovascular complications.

B. **Donor allograft.** Adverse donor characteristics (e.g., advanced age, terminal or prolonged hypotension, and the need for vasopressors) are highly correlated with posttransplant acute tubular necrosis (ATN). Nevertheless, as long as the allograft has reasonable underlying parenchyma (established by biopsy), recovery can be expected. Delayed allograft function is much easier to manage in kidney recipients than in liver recipients because of the availability of dialysis. Acute tubular necrosis is extremely rare in living donor recipients.

C. **Recipient operation.** The allograft is implanted in the pelvis, with the renal artery and vein sewn to the corresponding iliac vessels. If the ureter is implanted into the bladder, a Foley catheter should be left in place for 5 days to prevent bladder distention and resultant anastomotic strain. On the other hand, if an ureteroureterostomy is constructed (after a native nephrectomy), bladder drainage is not required. In either case, a Jackson-Pratt drain is left in place.

D. **Immediate postoperative course**
   1. **Immediate allograft function** is heralded by a massive diuresis necessitating aggressive fluid replacement (e.g., previous hours urine output + 30 ml, but limited to 400 ml/h to prevent an ever-increasing spiral) and electrolyte monitoring.
   2. **Oliguria** in the early postoperative course is usually caused by reversible ATN, but technical complications need to be excluded (Fig. 38-2).

E. **Late course.** An increasing creatinine level (Fig. 38-3) leads to the classical dilemma: should the nephrotoxic immunosuppressant (cyclosporin or tacrolimus) be reduced to lower toxicity or increased to treat rejection? Empiric therapy can be first attempted: for example, an increasing creatinine level 1 week posttransplantation, with a normal cyclosporin level, should be treated as acute rejection; on the other hand, a rising creatinine level, in association with hypertension, hyperkalemia, and tremors (signs of drug toxicity), and a high cyclosporin level should prompt a decreased cyclosporin dosage. A biopsy often is required to clarify the situation.

IV. **Kidney and pancreas transplantation**
   A. **The aim of pancreas transplantation** is to provide a source of insulin that will maintain normal blood glucose values in a diabetic. It is usually performed simultaneously with kidney transplantation in patients with diabetic nephropathy.

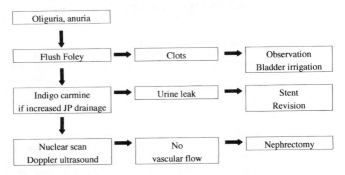

Fig. 38-2. Oliguria in immediate postoperative period.

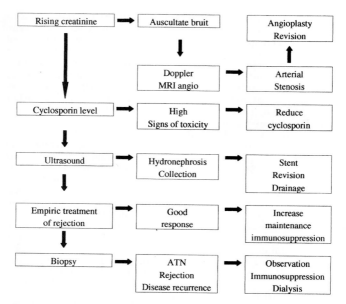

Fig. 38-3.   Rising creatinine in a renal allograft recipient.

B. **Technique**
   1. **The allograft is revascularized** by anastomosing the donor portal vein and superior mesenteric artery to the corresponding (usually right) iliac vessels; the renal allograft is placed in the contralateral pelvis.
   2. **Donor duodenum** is then sewn to recipient bladder to allow exocrine drainage. Because of resultant bicarbonate loss in the urine, most patients exhibit some degree of **metabolic acidosis.** During periods of decreased renal function, this can become quite severe and may require intensive bicarbonate supplementation.
C. **Posttransplant management**
   1. **Thrombotic complications** historically have accounted for up to 25% of pancreatic allograft failures. Low molecular weight dextran and IV heparin are administered intraoperatively and continued for 5 days. Aspirin is started on day 1, and continued for 4 months unless gross hematuria necessitates earlier withdrawal.
   2. **Bladder leak** can occur at the duodenocystostomy and require bladder or percutaneous drainage.
   3. **Renal and pancreatic allograft** functions are monitored primarily by serum creatinine and blood glucose levels. Some indication of pancreatic allo-

graft function is provided by monitoring urine pH (generally > 7.5) and urinary amylase levels (generally > 30,000 U/24 h).

SELECTED REFERENCES

Alexander JW, Vaughn WX. The use of "marginal" donors for organ transplantation. The influence of donor age on outcome. *Transplantation* 1991;51:135–141.

Ascher NL, Lake JR, Emond JC, et al. Liver transplantation for fulminant hepatic failure. *Arch Surg* 1993;128:677–682.

Busutill RW, Klintmaim GB. *Transplantation of the liver,* 1st ed. Philadelphia: WB Saunders Company, 1996.

Busuttil RW, Shaked A, Millis JM, et al. One thousand liver transplants. The lessons learned. *Ann Surg* 1994;219:490–497.

Cosimi AB, Auchincloss H, Delmonico FL, et al. Combined kidney and pancreas transplantation in diabetics. *Arch Surg* 1988;123:621–625.

Dietheim AG, Deierhoi MH, Hudson SL, et al. Progress in renal transplantation. A single center study of 3359 patients over 25 years. *Ann Surg* 1995;221:446–457.

Mor E, Klintmalm GB, Gonwa TA, et al. The use of marginal donors for liver transplantation. A retrospective study of 365 liver donors. *Transplantation* 1992;53:383–386.

Ploeg RJ, D'Alessandro AM, Knechtle SJ, et al. Risk factors for primary dysfunction after liver transplantation—a multivariate analysis. *Transplantation* 1993;55:807–813.

Sollinger HW, Knechtl SJ, Reed A, et al. Experience with 100 consecutive simultaneous kidney-pancreas transplants with bladder drainage. *Ann Surg* 1991;214:703–711.

Starzl TE, Miller C, Broznick B, et al. An improved technique for multiple organ harvesting. *Surg Gynecol Obstet* 1987;165:343–348.

Tolkoff RN, Rubin RH. The infectious disease problems of the diabetic renal transplant recipient. *Infect Dis Clin North Am* 1995;9:117–130.

Tzakis AG, Gordon RD, Shaw Jr BW, et al. Clinical presentation of hepatic artery thrombosis after liver transplantation in the cyclosporin era. *Transplantation* 1985;40:667–671.

Neonatal Intensive Care

Maria M. Zestos, Robert M. Insoft, and
Jesse D. Roberts, Jr.

I. **Human development**
   A. **Organogenesis** is virtually complete after the 12th gestational week.
   B. **Respiratory** development.
      1. **Anatomic**
         a. The lungs begin as a bud on the embryonic gut in the fourth week of gestation.
         b. Failure of separation of the lung bud from the gut later results in the formation of a tracheoesophageal fistula.
         c. The diaphragm forms during the tenth week of gestation, dividing the abdominal and thoracic cavities. If the diaphragm is not completely formed when the midgut reenters the abdomen from the umbilical pouch, the abdominal contents can enter the thorax. The posterior part of the diaphragm is the last part to close; the left side closes after the right. Although the mechanism is incompletely understood, the presence of abdominal contents within the thorax is associated with arrested lung growth. The lungs from patients with **congenital diaphragmatic hernia** show a decreased number of arterioles in the hypoplastic lung. In addition, the pulmonary arteries of both lungs are abnormally thick and reactive, resulting in increased pulmonary vascular resistance.
      2. **Physiologic**
         a. **Lung development** is generally insufficient for survival at less than the 23rd week of gestation. This may be related to an alveolar to pulmonary capillary distance, that is too great for oxygen diffusion to take place.
         b. **Secretion of surfactant,** which reduces alveolar wall surface tension and promotes alveolar aeration, is inadequate until the last month of gestation. Birth prior to 32 weeks gestation is associated with **respiratory distress syndrome (RDS).** Because maternal diabetes can decrease lung maturation, newborns from these mothers can have RDS if born later in gestation.
         c. **Following birth,** the first breath and the onset of postnatal breathing are stimulated by hypoxemia, hypercarbia, tactile stimulation, and a decrease in plasma prostaglandin E_2.

Following aeration and distention of the lung, the pulmonary vascular resistance decreases and pulmonary blood flow increases nearly tenfold. Failure of the pulmonary vascular resistance to decrease following birth is associated with **persistent pulmonary hypertension in the newborn (PPHN).**

C. Cardiovascular development

1. Anatomic

a. **The primitive cardiac tube,** which forms during the first month of gestation, consists of the sinoatrium, the primitive ventricle, the bulbus cordis (primitive right ventricle), and the truncus (primitive main pulmonary artery). During the second month of gestation, a heart with two parallel pumping systems develops out of this initial tubular system. During this process, various structures divide and migrate. Failure of structural maturation at this stage of development causes numerous cardiac malformations, including:

(1) Failure of the sinoatrium to divide into the two atria results in a single atrium. Improper closure results in an **atrial septal defect (ASD).**

(2) Failure of the ventricular septum and atrioventricular valve to migrate between the primitive ventricle and the bulbus cordis results in a **double-outlet left ventricle** (single ventricle). Minor migrational defects result in a **ventriculoseptal defect (VSD).**

(3) Failure of the truncus to divide into the pulmonary artery and the aorta results in **truncus arteriosus.**

b. The aortic arch system initially consists of six pairs of arches; only the *third, fourth,* and *sixth* aortic arches develop further.

(1) **The third arches** form the connections between the external and internal carotid arteries.

(2) **The sixth arches** produce the pulmonary arteries. The ductus arteriosus develops from the distal portion of the right sixth arch. Although the left proximal sixth arch usually degenerates, it can persist and form an aberrant left ductus arteriosus.

(3) **The left fourth arch** becomes the segment of aorta between the left carotid and the subclavian arteries. The **right fourth arch** becomes the proximal subclavian artery.

(4) Failure of various portions of the aorta and arch system to regress can result in

aberrant vessels. For example, failure of regression causes a **double aortic arch**. Regression of the left-sided arches but not the right-sided ones can result in a **right-sided aortic arch**.

2. **Physiologic**
   a. **Fetal circulation.** After the twelfth week, the circulatory system is in its final form. Oxygenated blood from the placenta passes through the umbilical vessels, the ductus venosus, and returns to the heart. Subsequently, most of the blood bypasses the pulmonary circulation by passing from right to left through the foramen ovale and the ductus arteriosus into the aorta.
   b. **At birth,** umbilical placental circulation ceases. The blood flow through the ductus venosus decreases. The ductus venosus closes in 3 to 7 days. The decrease in venous return causes reduced right atrial pressure and functional closure of the foramen ovale. At the same time, the gas exchange is transferred from the placenta to the newly ventilated lungs. Pulmonary resistance decreases as the postnatal pulmonary circulation is established. With increasing PaO_2, the ductus arteriosus constricts. Cessation of ductal blood flow often occurs within several hours.

D. **Body composition**
   1. **Extracellular fluid (ECF)** decreases as the fetus grows. ECF is 90% of total body weight at 30 weeks, 85% at 36 weeks, and 75% at term.
   2. **After birth, a physiologic diuresis occurs,** with the infant losing about 5% to 10% of ECF in the first few days of life. The fluid requirements of a newborn are influenced by prematurity, use of phototherapy, and so on.
   3. Before 32 weeks of gestation, the **neonatal kidney** is immature and less able to concentrate urine or handle solute loads. Renal tubular function improves with postnatal age.

II. **General assessment**
A. **History**
   1. **Prenatal.** The history of the neonate begins in utero. Fetal growth and development are affected by maternal disorders, including hypertension, diabetes, and use of drugs, cigarettes, or alcohol. Polyhydramnios, abnormal α-fetoprotein, maternal infections, and premature labor are often associated with neonatal problems.
   2. **Perinatal history** should include gestational age, time of onset of labor and rupture of membranes, use of tocolytics and fetal monitors, signs of fetal distress, type of anesthesia, mode of the newborn's delivery (spontaneous, forceps assisted,

or cesarean), condition of the infant at delivery, Apgar scores, and immediate resuscitation steps required. Ensure that vitamin K and ocular antibiotic ointment were given.

B. **Physical examination**

1. **General inspection.** A careful, complete, systematic evaluation is needed. No assumptions concerning the development, location, or function of organ systems should be made. An abnormality in one system can be associated with abnormalities in another.

2. **Vital signs** provide a useful physiologic screen of organ function. If cardiac abnormality is suspected, an electrocardiogram (ECG) and upper and lower extremity blood pressure measurements are required. In addition, an ECG and pediatric cardiology consultation should be considered. Normal vital signs are summarized in Table 39-1.

3. **The Apgar score** reflects the degree of intrapartum stress as well as the effectiveness of initial resuscitation (Table 39-2). Points are awarded for each of the five criteria, with the maximal score being 10. Although the Apgar score at 1 minute correlates best with intrauterine conditions, Apgar scores at 5 and 10 minutes correlate best with neonatal outcome.

4. **Gestational age** influences care, management, and survival potential of the neonate. An infant is considered term if the gestational age is 37 to 42 weeks, preterm if it is less than 37 weeks, and postterm if the gestational age is 42 weeks. Although the date of conception and ultrasound examination can be used to predict gestational age, a physical examination and Dubowitz scoring should be done to determine gestational age. The **Dubowitz scoring system** involves evaluation of physical characteristics of the skin, external genitalia, ears, breasts, and neuromuscular behavior to assess gestational age.

5. **Weight determination.** Infants who are **small for gestational age (SGA)** often have had intrauterine growth retardation. This can result from chromosomal defects, maternal hyperten-

Table 39-1. Neonatal vital signs

Vital sign	Term	Preterm
Pulse (beats/min)	110–120	140–180
Respiration (breaths/min)	35–40	50–70
Blood pressure (mm Hg)	60–90/40–60	40–60/20–40
Temperature (°C)	37.5 (rectal)	37.5

Table 39-2. Apgar scores

Sign	0	1	2
Heart rate	Absent	<100 beats/min	100 beats/min
Respiratory effort	Absent	Irregular or slow	Good
Muscle tone	Limp	Some flexion of extremities	Good tone
Reflex irritability	No response	Grimace	Cough
Color	Blue	Pink body, blue extremities	All pink

sion, maternal cigarette or drug use, chronic placental insufficiency, or congenital infection. These infants have a high incidence of hypoglycemia, hypocalcemia, and polycythemia. Infants who are **large for gestational age (LGA)** may have mothers with diabetes. In the immediate postnatal period, LGA newborns should be evaluated for hypoglycemia and polycythemia.

6. **Respiratory.** Signs of respiratory distress include tachypnea, grunting, nasal flaring, intercostal retractions, rales, rhonchi, asymmetry of breath sounds, and apneic periods. **Pulse oximetry** has become a standard noninvasive screen of oxygenation in neonates.

7. **Cardiovascular.** Central cyanosis and capillary refill should be assessed. Distal pulses should be palpated, noting whether they are bounding. A delay between brachial and femoral pulses is suggestive of coarctation of the aorta. Note the character and location of murmurs and splitting of the second heart sound. During the first 48 hours, murmurs may appear as intracardiac pressure gradients change or disappear as the ductus arteriosus closes.

8. **Gastrointestinal.** A scaphoid abdomen suggests diaphragmatic hernia. A normal umbilical cord has two arteries and one vein. Note the location and patency of the anus, the size of the liver, spleen, and kidneys by palpation, as well as the presence of hernias or abdominal masses.

9. **Neurologic.** A thorough examination includes evaluation of motor activity, strength, symmetry, tone, and newborn reflexes (e.g., Moro, tonic neck, grasp, suck, stepping). Full-term newborns should have an upgoing Babinski reflex and brisk deep tendon reflexes.

10. **Genitourinary.** The gonads may be differentiated or ambiguous, and the testes should be pal-

pable. The location of the urethra should be determined.

11. **Musculoskeletal.** Any deformities, unusual posturing, or asymmetric limb movement should be noted, and the hips should be examined for possible dislocation. Clavicles can be fractured during a difficult delivery.

12. **Craniofacial.** Determine head circumference, the location and size of the fontanels, and the presence of hematoma or caput. A No. 8 suction catheter passed through each naris and into the posterior pharynx will rule out choanal atresia.

C. **Laboratory studies.** Routine laboratory studies may include an initial hematocrit and serum glucose. Additional studies should be guided by the individual problem. For example, blood type and Coombs' test may be indicated for infants at risk for hyperbilirubinemia.

D. **Fluids and electrolytes**
1. **Fluids**
   a. **Volume requirements** vary with birthweight.
      (1) Less than 1.0 kg, use 100 ml/kg/d.
      (2) 1.0 to 1.5 kg, use 80 to 70 ml/kg/d.
      (3) More than 1.5 kg, use 80 ml/kg/d.
   b. **Isosmolar solutions** should be used.
      (1) **Electrolyte supplementation** is not required within the first day of life to maintain fluids in full-term infants. For premature infants, check the electrolytes at 12 hours of life and consider adjusting the fluid infusion rate, adding electrolytes, or both.
      (2) Dextrose (5% to 10%) in water (D/W) can be used for babies weighing 1.0 kg and 10% D/W for those weighing more than 1.0 kg.
   c. Additional fluids may be required for **insensible water loss.**
      (1) Fluid requirements increase with lower birthweight, phototherapy, or radiant warmer use.
      (2) Insensible water loss must be replaced, as should water loss from pathologic causes (e.g., omphalocele). The electrolyte composition of the replacement fluid should match that of what is lost.
      (3) Infants who are mechanically ventilated absorb free water from their respiratory system.
   d. Several signs will determine adequacy of fluid infusions:
      (1) Urine output at 0.5 ml/kg/h.
      (2) Only a 1% loss in body weight per day for the first 10 days of life.
      (3) Stable hemodynamics and good perfusion.
      (4) Stable body weight.

2. Electrolytes

    a. The usual electrolyte requirements after the first 12 to 24 hours of life are:

        (1) Na^+, 2 to 4 mEq/kg/d.

        (2) K^+, 1 to 3 mEq/kg/d.

        (3) Ca^{2+}, 150 to 220 mEq/kg/d.

    b. The frequency of laboratory tests for serum electrolyte levels will be determined by the rate of insensible losses.

3. Glucose. Supplemental glucose should be given after birth to keep blood glucose levels 40 to 125 mg/dl.

    a. In most infants, 10% D/W at maintenance fluid rates will provide adequate glucose. This infusion rate provides the 5 to 8 mg/kg/min of glucose required for basal metabolism.

    b. Infants with hyperinsulinism or intrauterine growth retardation will require higher glucose infusion rates or 12 to 15 mg/kg/min.

    c. In peripheral intravenous (IV) lines, up to 12.5% D/W can be infused; 15% to 20% D/W can be infused via central lines.

    d. Hypoglycemia (glucose = 40 mg/dl) is treated with a bolus of glucose and increased glucose infusion rate.

        (1) Glucose (200 mg/kg) is given IV over 1 minute (example: 2 ml/kg of 10% D/W).

        (2) The glucose infusion rate is increased from the current level or started at 8 mg/kg/min IV.

        (3) Serial blood tests are necessary to determine the effectiveness of the increased glucose.

E. Nutrition. The gastrointestinal tract is functional after 28 weeks' gestation but is of limited capacity. Requirements vary with each neonate.

    1. Calories. Requirements are 100 to 130 kcal/kg/d.

    2. Protein. Requirements are 2 to 4 g/kg/d.

    3. Fat. Requirements begin at 1 g/kg/d. Fat should provide 40% of calories.

    4. Vitamins. A, B, D, E, C, and K should be replaced.

    5. Iron. Requirements are 2 mg/kg/d.

        a. The adequacy of iron supplementation can be assessed by measuring the hematocrit and reticulocyte count.

    6. Minerals. Calcium, phosphate, magnesium, zinc, copper, manganese, and iron need to be replaced.

    7. Enteral feedings. A formula that simulates human milk with a high whey:casein ratio is preferred. Preterm infants often have lactose intolerance, for which numerous nonlactose formulas are available. Infants under 32 weeks' gestation often have poor suck and swallow reflexes and require gavage feedings. With all premature infants or ill neonates, small feedings with a slowly advancing schedule should be used.

8. **Parenteral feeding.** When needed, parenteral nutrition should be started as soon as possible to promote positive nitrogen balance and growth. The infant should be followed closely to adjust the solutions to the infant's needs and to identify signs of toxicity from total parenteral nutrition. Usual studies include serum glucose, electrolytes, osmolality, liver function tests, blood urea nitrogen (BUN), creatinine, lipid levels, and platelet count.

III. **Common neonatal problems**
   A. **Respiratory disorders**
      1. **Differential diagnosis.** Many diseases share the same signs and symptoms with pulmonary parenchymal disease and should be considered when evaluating an infant with respiratory distress.
         a. **Airway obstruction.** Choanal atresia, vocal cord palsy, laryngomalacia, tracheal stenosis, and external tracheal masses (e.g., cystic hygroma, hemangioma, and vascular ring) can obstruct the airway.
         b. **Developmental anomalies** include tracheoesophageal fistula, congenital diaphragmatic hernia, congenital emphysema, and lung cysts.
         c. **Nonpulmonary** conditions include cyanotic heart disease, PPHN, congestive heart failure, and metabolic disturbances (e.g., acidosis).
      2. **Laboratory studies** for an infant in respiratory distress should include arterial blood gas tensions and pH, pre- and postductal oxygen saturation by pulse oximetry to evaluate for extrapulmonary shunting of deoxygenated blood at the level of the patent ductus arteriosus (PDA), hematocrit, 12-lead ECG, and chest radiograph. Consider echocardiogram and cardiology consultation.
      3. **Apnea**
         a. **Etiology**
            (1) **Central apnea** is caused by immaturity or depression of the respiratory center (e.g., opioids). It is related to the degree of prematurity and is exacerbated by metabolic disturbances such as hypoglycemia, hypocalcemia, hypothermia, hyperthermia, and sepsis. Central apnea is often treated with **methylxanthines** such as theophylline and caffeine.
            (2) **Obstructive apnea,** which is caused by inconsistent maintenance of a patent airway, can be associated with incomplete maturation and poor coordination of upper airway musculature. This form of apnea may respond to changes in head position, insertion of an oral or nasal

airway, or placing the infant in a prone position. Occasionally, administration of **continuous positive airway pressure (CPAP)** is beneficial.

   (3) **Mixed apnea** represents a combination of both central and obstructive apnea.
   b. **Postoperative apnea** in the neonate.
      (1) **Apnea** can be associated with anesthesia in formerly preterm infants. Although it has been associated with general anesthesia, some reports of apnea have been associated with local anesthesia.
      (2) It is prudent to use **postoperative apnea monitoring** in neonates who undergo anesthesia at less than 45 weeks postconception.

4. **Respiratory distress syndrome (RDS)**
   a. **Pathophysiology.** RDS (formerly referred to as hyaline membrane disease) results from physiologic surfactant deficiency. This leads to decreased lung compliance, alveolar instability, progressive atelectasis, and intrapulmonary shunting. All of these events produce cyanosis, hypoxemia, and respiratory distress.
   b. **Infants at risk for RDS** include premature infants, infants of diabetic mothers, and infants born by cesarean delivery. Infants at risk can be identified prenatally by amniocentesis and evaluation of the amniotic fluid **phospholipid profile.** Lung maturity is associated with a lecithin (phosphatidylcholine):sphingomyelin ratio (L/S ratio) greater than 2, saturated phosphatidylcholine level (SPC) more than 500 µg/dl, or presence of phosphatidylglycerol in the specimen.
   c. **Clinical features** include tachypnea, nasal flaring, grunting, retractions, and cyanosis that appears shortly after birth. Because of intrapulmonary shunt, the infants remain hypoxemic despite breathing at high FIO_2.
   d. **The chest radiograph** will show low lung volumes. A "ground-glass" pattern of the lung fields, and air bronchograms also may be evident.
   e. **Glucocorticoid** (betamethasone) treatment of the mother at least 2 days before delivery decreases the incidence and severity of RDS.
   f. **Initial treatment** includes treating the patient with warmed, humidified oxygen administered by hood. The FIO_2 should be adjusted to maintain the PaO_2 between 50 and 80 mm Hg ($SaO_2 < 96\%$). If a FIO_2 greater than 60% is required to maintain oxygenation, nasal CPAP can be administered. With more severe disease, endotracheal intubation and mechan-

ical ventilation with positive end-expiratory pressure (PEEP) may be required. **High-frequency oscillatory ventilation (HFOV)** decreases the incidence of pneumothorax and chronic lung disease in infants with severe RDS. Endotracheal administration of **exogenous surfactant** decreases the severity, morbidity, and mortality of the disease.

g. Because the clinical signs and chest radiograph of patients with RDS are indistinguishable from pneumonia, **broad-spectrum antibiotics** are begun after appropriate cultures are obtained.

h. Respiratory distress syndrome can be self-limited; clinical improvement after 2 to 3 days can be associated with a spontaneous diuresis.

i. **The morbidity and mortality of patients with RDS** are directly related to the degree of prematurity, the perinatal resuscitation, and the coexistence of other problems (e.g., PDA). Pneumothoraces and pulmonary interstitial emphysema can complicate recovery and can be associated with the evolution to chronic lung disease.

5. **Bronchopulmonary dysplasia (BPD)**

a. **Etiology.** BPD is defined as the continued need for respiratory support with oxygen therapy or mechanical ventilation beyond 36 weeks postconceptual age. Bronchopulmonary dysplasia usually follows severe RDS, and is associated with oxygen toxicity, chronic inflammation, and mechanical injury to the lung. BPD can be worsened by the presence of a PDA and resultant pulmonary edema.

b. **Clinical features** include retractions, rales, and areas of lung hyperinflation and underinflation. Because of inhomogeneous ventilation, intrapulmonary shunt can produce hypoxemia in patients with BPD. Hypoxemia also can be associated with bronchospasm in many patients with severe BPD. Most patients have growth retardation.

c. **Treatment** consists of supportive respiratory care, adequate nutrition, and diuretic therapy. Because patients with BPD may have lung regions with prolonged expiratory time constants, a ventilatory pattern with a low respiratory rate and prolonged expiratory time may decrease gas trapping and improve gas exchange. **Bronchodilator therapy** can be life-saving in patients with BPD and bronchospasm. **Systemic or inhaled steroids** sometimes are used to treat patients with chronic lung disease.

    d. **Prognosis** varies with the severity of the disease. Of severely affected infants, 25% die within the first year. Most infants are asymptomatic by 2 years of age. It is rare for infants to have signs and symptoms of BPD beyond 5 years of age.

6. Pneumothorax

    a. **Etiology.** Pneumothoraces can occur in mechanically ventilated newborns. In addition, nonventilated, otherwise normal full-term infants can have spontaneous pneumothoraces. Although the cause is unknown, uneven ventilation with overdistention of airways and alveoli can be associated with pneumothoraces. The incidence is 2% in patients born by cesarean deliveries, 10% in patients with meconium staining, and 5% to 10% in RDS.

    b. **Clinical features.** The diagnosis should be considered in any neonate with respiratory distress or in the ventilated infant with an acute deterioration in clinical condition (e.g., sudden cyanosis and hypotension). Occasionally, asymmetric chest movement with ventilation and asymmetric breath sounds may be noted. An endobronchial intubation should be excluded.

    c. **Transillumination** of the chest with a strong light usually will show a hyperlucent hemithorax. A chest radiograph will confirm the diagnosis.

    d. **Treatment**

        (1) In an otherwise stable and well-oxygenated infant with minimal respiratory distress, washout of nitrogen by breathing a high concentration of oxygen may resolve the pneumothorax and be the only therapy required.

        (2) In the unstable infant, the pleural space should be aspirated immediately with an IV catheter. Reaccumulation of air after a needle aspiration warrants placement of a chest tube.

7. Meconium aspiration syndrome

    a. **Meconium staining** of amniotic fluid, which occurs in 10% of all births, can be associated with fetal distress and asphyxia.

    b. To decrease the effects of aspiration in infants with meconium-stained fluid observed below the vocal cords, **endotracheal intubation and airway suctioning** are prudent.

    c. **Meconium aspiration** can produce lung air-space disease by mechanical obstruction of the airways and pneumonitis. Complete obstruction of the airways by meconium results in distal atelectasis. Partial obstruction of the airway can overinflate the distal air spaces by a ball-valve effect, leading to pneumothorax. The bile in meconium can cause chemical pneumonitis and airway edema.

d. Meconium aspiration syndrome has also been associated with persistent pulmonary artery hypertension of newborn infants (see section **B.5**).

e. **Respiratory support** for meconium aspiration is dependent on the cause of the poor gas exchange. Obstruction of airways with meconium may require mechanical ventilation with prolonged expiratory times to decrease gas trapping. Pneumothorax is treated by placement of a chest tube. Sometimes high-frequency oscillatory ventilation is useful to recruit closed lung segments and improve gas exchange. Systemic alkalosis and inhaled nitric oxide have been used to decrease pulmonary vasoconstriction in patients with meconium aspiration.

8. **Congenital diaphragmatic hernia**

a. **Congenital diaphragmatic hernia** occurs in 1 of 5,000 live births. It has a high mortality rate, with 50% not surviving infancy; 70% of the defects occur on the left. The embryology and pathophysiology are discussed in section **I.B.**

b. **Clinical features.** The defect often can be seen on prenatal ultrasonographic examination. At birth, a scaphoid abdomen often is noted, and breath sounds are absent on the involved side. Rarely, bowel sounds are heard in the affected hemithorax. Although the clinical spectrum can vary and is probably related to the degree of lung hypoplasia, often patients exhibit severe respiratory distress in the postnatal period.

c. **The diagnosis** is confirmed by chest radiograph. Often the intestine and stomach are observed in the thorax.

d. **Treatment** consists of respiratory and cardiovascular support. Endotracheal intubation and mechanical ventilation often are used to decrease air entry into the stomach and intestines within the thorax. Positive-pressure ventilation by mask is minimized by performing endotracheal intubation while the patient is spontaneously breathing. If the patient is apneic, use the minimal pressure required to ensure lung inflation. Continuous gastric suction also decreases air insufflation. Treatment is often directed toward decreasing pulmonary vascular resistance and facilitating CO_2 elimination. Conventional ventilation or HFOV is used. The main cause of mortality is respiratory insufficiency (section **III.B.5**). Pneumo-thorax in the unaffected lung can occur and is often the cause of death during resuscitation. Hypotension and shock can occur because of prolonged systemic hypoxemia, shifting of the mediastinal contents by the hernia, and gas-trointestinal fluid losses.

e.   **Surgical repair** involves replacing the abdo-minal contents and repairing the diaphragm. In the past, this was performed urgently in the critically ill infant. Currently, many patients are first stabilized with medical and ventila-tory treatment and, often, with extracorporeal membrane oxygenation (ECMO) prior to sur-gery (section **B.6**).

B.   Cardiovascular disorders

1.   **Laboratory studies.** In the infant with signs and symptoms of cardiovascular disease, relevant stud-ies include arterial blood gas tensions and pH, pre- and postductal oxygen saturation, determination of arterial blood gas tensions during inhalation of pure oxygen ("hyperoxia test"), hematocrit, chest radiograph, and ECG. Echocardiography is fre-quently performed to evaluate structured heart lesions.

2.   **Patent ductus arteriosus (PDA)**

a.   **Clinical features.** PDA, which is commonly seen in the premature infant, is characterized by a murmur at the left sternal border radi-ating to the back, bounding pulses, widened pulse pressure difference, evidence of in-creased pulmonary blood flow by chest radi-ograph, and excessive weight gain. In some cases, cardiac dysfunction associated with a PDA can decrease systemic blood pressure, peripheral perfusion, and urine output, and be associated with metabolic acidosis.

b.   Although early treatment of a PDA consists of fluid restriction and diuretic therapy, it is im-portant to maintain systemic perfusion. If the degree of shunt through the ductus arteriosus becomes clinically significant and renal and platelet function are adequate, pharmacologic closure of the ductus with **indomethacin** can be attempted. **Surgical closure** of a PDA is for the infant who has failed indomethacin, has decreased renal or platelet function, or for whom indomethacin is contraindicated. Open ductus arteriosus surgery also can be indi-cated for those with decreased systemic oxy-genation because of associated pulmonary failure.

3.   **Cyanosis**

a.   **Etiology.** Many causes of cyanosis are seen, including pulmonary disorders, intracardiac and extracardiac shunts, and polycythemia.

    b. **Cardiac lesions** can cause systemic hypoxemia by decreasing pulmonary blood flow or causing mixture of systemic and pulmonary venous blood via shunts.

    c. In the fetus and in the immediate postnatal period, the ductus arteriosus may permit pulmonary blood flow in patients with transposition of the great arteries, pulmonic stenosis or atresia, tetralogy of Fallot, and ventricular hypoplasia. Most of these infants become symptomatic as the ductus arteriosus closes at 2 to 3 days of life. If a ductal-dependent lesion exists, **prevention of ductal closure** is critical to maintain pulmonary blood flow. This can be done with a prostaglandin E_1 infusion. Side effects include apnea, hypotension, and seizure activity.

    d. Many patients with septal defects may be asymptomatic during the fetal and neonatal period. With increased pulmonary vascular resistance, however, right-to-left shunting of blood can produce systemic hypoxemia. Later in life, with decreased pulmonary vascular resistance, increased pulmonary blood flow can cause pulmonary vascular disease and pulmonary hypertension.

    e. A chest radiograph and a hyperoxia test can confirm the diagnosis of an intracardiac shunt. The chest radiograph may reveal decreased pulmonary blood flow. The PaO_2 remains less than 150 mm Hg when an infant with a significant shunt breathes 100% oxygen. An echocardiogram is invaluable in determining the etiology of the intracardiac shunt.

4. **Dysrhythmias**

    a. **Paroxysmal atrial tachycardia (PAT)** is the most frequent dysrhythmia seen in neonates. Although PAT is usually self-limited and well tolerated, treatment may be required if hypotension or desaturation occurs.

    b. **Treatment** consists of **vagal maneuvers** such as nasopharyngeal stimulation or placement of cold on the face. Massage of the eye should be avoided, as this can lead to disruption of the lens in neonates. **Adenosine** and **esophageal pacing** also have been used for acute management.

    c. **Digoxin** will usually convert paroxysmal atrial tachycardia to sinus rhythm; maintenance therapy for 1 year sometimes is indicated. **Propranolol** and **quinidine** are second-line medications.

    d. **Cardioversion** is indicated if the patient is hemodynamically unstable.

5. **Persistent pulmonary hypertension of the newborn**
    a. **Pathophysiology.** PPHN, previously referred to as persistent fetal circulation, is manifested by an increase in pulmonary vascular resistance (PVR) with resulting pulmonary arterial hypertension, right-to-left shunting across the foramen ovale and the ductus arteriosus, and profound cyanosis.
    b. **Etiology.** It is suggested that many newborns with PPHN have abnormal pulmonary artery reactivity and structure. Although many infants with PPHN can have asphyxia, meconium aspiration, bacterial pneumonia, and sepsis, the role of these in causing the disease is unknown.
    c. **Clinical features.** Newborns with PPHN have severe systemic hypoxemia unrelieved by breathing high FIO_2. An ECG may reveal right ventricular hypertrophy; a chest radiograph may show decreased pulmonary vascular markings. Echocardiography may show shunting of blood at the level of the PDA, patent foramen ovale (PFO), or both.
    d. **Treatment of severe systemic hypoxemia**
        (1) **Endotracheal intubation and mechanical ventilation with high FIO_2.** Often sedation with opioids (e.g., fentanyl 1–2 µg/kg/h) and neuromuscular blockade will facilitate ventilation.
        (2) **Induced respiratory or metabolic alkalosis.**
        (3) **Inhaled nitric oxide** rapidly decreases pulmonary vasoconstriction and may decrease shunt and increase systemic oxygenation. In many infants, inhaled NO reverses PPHN and decreases the need for ECMO.
        (4) **ECMO** can be life-saving for some patients with PPHN refractory to ventilatory and medical therapy (Chapter 14). Because of its high expense, ECMO is not available at all medical centers.
C. **Hematologic disorders**
    1. **Hemolytic disease of the newborn (erythroblastosis fetalis)**
        a. **Isoimmune hemolytic anemia** in the fetus is caused by the transplacental passage of maternal antibody against fetal erythrocytes into the fetus. Only IgG can cross the placenta.
        b. **Rh hemolytic disease** is usually caused by the anti-D antibody, but can also be caused by antibodies to minor antigens including Kell, Duff, Kidd, or Ss antigens. The absence of D

antigen, which makes an individual Rh negative, occurs in 15% of whites and 5% of blacks. A mother can be sensitized to fetal antigens by leakage of fetal blood into the maternal circulation during pregnancy, delivery, abortion, or amniocentesis. To prevent sensitization, an unsensitized Rh-negative mother is given anti-D immune globulin (RhoGAM) during pregnancy and after delivery. Once a mother is sensitized, immune prophylaxis is of no value. Even if treated with immune globulin, a mother can still be sensitized during pregnancy if a large fetomaternal transfusion occurs.

c. **ABO hemolytic disease** can occur without maternal sensitization, because a mother with group O blood has naturally occurring anti-A and anti-B antibodies in her circulation. These are usually IgM antibodies, but some can be IgG. This disease tends to be milder than Rh disease, with little or no anemia, mild indirect hyperbilirubinemia, and rarely a need for exchange transfusion.

d. **An indirect Coombs' test** on maternal blood can detect the presence of IgG antibodies in her serum.

e. **A direct Coombs' test** on the infant's blood can detect cells already coated with antibody, thus indicating a risk for hemolysis.

f. **Hemolysis** occurs when antibody crosses the placenta, attaches to the corresponding antigen on fetal erythrocytes, and causes hemolysis. Hepatosplenomegaly results from increased hematopoiesis triggered by hemolysis.

g. **Clinical features.** Physical examination may reveal hepatosplenomegaly, edema, pallor, or jaundice.

h. **Laboratory studies** often reveal anemia, thrombocytopenia, a positive direct Coombs' test, indirect hyperbilirubinemia, hypoglycemia, hypoalbuminemia, and an elevated reticulocyte count that increases proportionally with the severity of the disease. Serial hematocrit and indirect bilirubin levels should be followed.

i. **Treatment** consists of phototherapy. An exchange transfusion may be required if the level of bilirubin is high or the rate of rise of bilirubin exceeds 1 mg/dl/h.

2. **Hydrops fetalis**
   a. **Hydrops fetalis,** defined as the excessive accumulation of fluid by the fetus, can range from mild peripheral edema to massive anasarca.
   b. **Etiology.** Hydrops can be seen in hemolytic disease and is thought to be caused by in-

creased capillary permeability secondary to anemia. Other causes of hydrops include anemias (e.g., fetomaternal hemorrhage, donor twin-twin transfusion), cardiac dysrhythmias (e.g., complete heart block, supraventricular tachycardia), congenital heart disease, vascular or lymphatic malformation (e.g., hemangioma of the liver, cystic hygroma), or infection (e.g., viral, toxoplasmosis, syphilis).

    c. Treatment. The main goals of therapy include prevention of intrauterine or extrauterine death from anemia and hypoxia, restoration of intravascular volume, and avoidance of neurotoxicity from hyperbilirubinemia.

        (1) Survival of the unborn infant can be improved by in utero transfusion via the umbilical vein.

        (2) Care of the liveborn infant should include correction of hypovolemia and acidosis, as well as potential exchange transfusion.

        (3) Late complications include anemia; mild graft-versus-host reactions; inspissated bile syndrome (characterized by persistent icterus with elevated direct and indirect bilirubin); and portal vein thrombosis (as a complication of umbilical vein catheterization).

D. Gastrointestinal disorders

  1. Hyperbilirubinemia

    a. Pathophysiology. Bilirubin is formed from the breakdown of heme, then it is bound to albumin, transported to the liver (where it is conjugated with glucuronide), and delivered to the intestine in bile. In the intestine, it is either deconjugated by intestinal bacteria and reabsorbed or converted to excretory urobilinogen.

    b. Etiology. Hyperbilirubinemia results from overproduction (e.g., hemolysis, absorption of sequestered blood, polycythemia), underconjugation (e.g., immature or damaged liver), or underexcretion (e.g., biliary atresia). It is often seen in sepsis, asphyxia, and metabolic disorders (e.g., hypothyroidism, hypoglycemia, and galactosemia) as well as in healthy newborns and breastfed infants.

    c. Toxic effects. Unconjugated (indirect) bilirubin is lipid soluble and is capable of entering the central nervous system. Toxic levels result in bilirubin staining and necrosis of neurons in the basal ganglia, the hippocampus, and the subthalamic nuclei. This process, known as bilirubin encephalopathy or **kernicterus,** can have clinical symptoms ranging from mild lethargy and fever to convulsions. Infants with respiratory distress, sepsis, metabolic acidosis, hypoglycemia, hypoalbuminemia, or severe hemolytic disease are at increased risk for kernicterus. Survivors evaluated in childhood are found to have neurologic sequelae ranging from diminished cognitive function to mental retardation and choreoathetoid cerebral palsy.

d. Physiologic jaundice results from increased red blood cell turnover and an immature hepatic conjugation system. It occurs in 60% of newborns, and peak bilirubin levels occur by day 2 to 4 of life. Premature infants have an increased incidence (80%) and later bilirubin peak (day 5 to 7).

e. Breast milk jaundice develops gradually, occurring in the second or third week of life, with peak bilirubin levels of 15 to 25 mg/dl, which can persist for 2 to 3 months. Other causes should be excluded before making this diagnosis. Interrupting nursing for a few days results in a marked decrease in serum levels, at which time nursing can be restarted. This is a benign type of jaundice without adverse sequelae.

f. Laboratory studies include total and direct bilirubin, direct Coombs' test, reticulocyte count, blood smear for red blood cell morphology, electrolytes, BUN, creatinine, and appropriate cultures if sepsis is suspected.

g. Treatment

(1) Management of physiologic or mild hemolytic jaundice consists of monitoring serial bilirubin levels and starting **early feeding** to reduce enterohepatic cycling of bilirubin.

(2) Phototherapy is used if moderate indirect bilirubin levels or an accelerated rate of rise is noted (e.g., indirect bilirubin level > 5 in a full-term infant on day 1 of life). Light therapy of 420 to 470-nm wavelength results in photoisomerization of bilirubin, which makes it water soluble. Eyes must be shielded to prevent retinal damage.

(3) For severe hyperbilirubinemia, **exchange transfusion** is indicated (e.g., indirect bilirubin > 25 mg/dl in a full-term infant).

2. Esophageal atresia and tracheoesophageal fistula

a. Esophageal atresia is usually associated with a **tracheoesophageal fistula** (TEF). The location of the fistula is variable in these patients.

      b. **Pathophysiology.** The proximal blind esophageal pouch has a small capacity, resulting in overflow aspiration. This leads to the classic clinical triad of coughing, choking, and cyanosis. Occasionally, only drooling that requires frequent suctioning may be noted.

      c. **The diagnosis** is confirmed by the inability to pass a nasogastric tube into the stomach. A chest radiograph with air or water-soluble contrast agents will confirm the existence of esophageal atresia.

      d. **Medical treatment** is directed at reducing aspiration. Neonates should have nothing by mouth. A nasogastric tube is placed on continuous low suction and the head of the bed is elevated. Aspiration pneumonia should be treated with chest physiotherapy, antibiotics, and oxygen as required. Endotracheal intubation and ventilation may be required for severe pneumonia. Ventilation can be difficult when a TEF exists.

      e. **Surgical treatment** depends on the stability of the infant. In newborns with severe pneumonia, it is often prudent to delay surgery until the lungs improve. Nevertheless, a gastrostomy tube can be placed under local anesthesia if required to decompress the stomach. In stable patients, definitive repair of the esophagus and fistula can be performed.

      f. It is sometimes difficult to establish an airway in patients with a TEF. Surgeons should be readily available should emergent decompression of the stomach be required. If the patient already has a gastrostomy tube, it should be placed to water seal. To facilitate placement of the tip of the endotracheal tube between the fistula and the carina, the tube first can be placed into the right mainstem bronchus. The tube can then be slowly withdrawn until breath sounds are heard over the left thorax. Decreased breath sounds and insufflation of the stomach or gas exiting from the gastrostomy tube suggest that the end of the endotracheal tube is above the fistula and that it should be advanced.

3. **Duodenal atresia**

      a. **Clinical features.** Duodenal atresia usually presents with bile-stained emesis, upper abdominal distention, and increased volume of gastric aspirates. It is associated with trisomy 21 (Down's syndrome) and can coexist with other intestinal malformations.

      b. **An abdominal radiograph** often reveals a "double bubble," representing air in the stomach and upper duodenum.

  c. **Medical supportive care** includes avoiding oral feedings, use of nasogastric suction, and ensuring adequate hydration and serum electrolyte levels prior to surgery.

4. **Pyloric stenosis**

  a. Although usually presenting in the second or third week of life, pyloric stenosis can present in the immediate newborn period.

  b. **Clinical features** include persistent nonbilious emesis and a metabolic alkalosis from loss of hydrochloric acid because of prolonged gastric suctioning. With protracted vomiting, the patient may present with metabolic acidosis and shock. An abdominal mass consisting of the hypertrophic pylorus or "olive" is often palpable.

  c. **An abdominal radiograph** usually shows gastric dilation. The diagnosis is confirmed by abdominal ultrasound or by barium swallow.

  d. **Medical supportive care** includes rehydration, correction of metabolic alkalosis, and nasogastric drainage before surgical repair.

5. **Omphalocele and gastroschisis**

  a. An **omphalocele** is caused by failure of the intestine to migrate into the abdomen and subsequent closure of the abdominal wall. The viscera remain outside the abdominal cavity, where they are covered with intact peritoneum. Omphaloceles may be associated with cardiac lesions, exstrophy of the bladder, and Beckwith-Wedeman syndrome.

  b. **Gastroschisis** occurs later in fetal life from interruption of the omphalomesenteric artery. The resulting abdominal wall defect allows exposure of the bowel to the intrauterine environment without peritoneal coverage; bowel loops are often edematous and covered with an inflammatory exudate.

  c. **Medical stabilization** includes nasogastric drainage, IV hydration, and protection of the viscera before imminent surgical repair. If the peritoneal sac is intact, the omphalocele should be covered with sterile, warm, saline-soaked gauze to decrease heat and water loss and the risk of infection. If the sac has ruptured or if the infant has gastroschisis, saline-soaked gauze should be used to wrap the exposed viscera; the infant should then be wrapped in warm sterile towels prior to surgical repair.

6. **Necrotizing enterocolitis**

  a. **Necrotizing enterocolitis (NEC)** is an acquired intestinal necrosis that appears in the absence of functional (e.g., Hirschsprung's) or anatomic (e.g., malrotation) lesions. It occurs predominantly (90%) in premature infants and can be endemic. It usually develops during the first few weeks of life, and almost always occurs after the institution of enteral feedings. Mortality can be as high as 40%.

b. **Pathogenesis** is unclear but involves critical stress of an immature gut by ischemic, infectious, or immunologic insults. Enteral feedings seem to potentiate mucosal injury. Breast milk feedings appear to protect against NEC.

c. **Clinical features** include abdominal distention, ileus, increase in gastric aspirates, abdominal wall erythema, or bloody stool. The infant may demonstrate systemic signs such as temperature instability, lethargy, respiratory and circulatory instability, oliguria, and bleeding diathesis.

d. **Laboratory studies** should include an abdominal radiograph (that may show pneumatosis intestinalis, fixed loops of bowel, portal air, or free intraperitoneal air), complete blood count (revealing leukocytosis, leukopenia, or thrombocytopenia), arterial blood gas tensions and pH (demonstrating acidosis), stool guaiac (often showing occult blood), and stool Clinitest (showing evidence of carbohydrate malabsorption). Because the differential diagnosis includes sepsis, cultures of blood, urine, and stool should be obtained. If the patient is stable and disseminated intravascular coagulation is not evident, cerebrospinal fluid (CSF) should be obtained by lumbar puncture for Gram's stain and culture.

e. **Treatment.** When necrotizing enterocolitis is suspected, enteral feedings are discontinued and the stomach is decompressed with a nasogastric tube. Oral feedings are withheld for at least 2 weeks and the patient is supported with parenteral feedings. Broad-spectrum antibiotics (ampicillin, an aminoglycoside, and if perforation is suspected, clindamycin) are administered empirically.

f. **Surgical consultation** is indicated, although laparotomy is usually reserved for intestinal perforation.

7. **Volvulus**

a. **Volvulus** can occur as a primary lesion or more commonly as the result of intestinal malrotation. If volvulus has occurred in utero, intestinal necrosis may be present at birth and immediate resection is indicated.

b. **Clinical features** include abdominal distention, bilious emesis, and signs of sepsis or shock.

    c. **The diagnosis** of malrotation is made by barium enema, which demonstrates an abnormally positioned ligament of Treitz.

    d. **Treatment** involves volume resuscitation, placement of a nasogastric tube, and surgical repair.

E. Neurologic disorders

  1. Seizures

    a. **Seizures** can be generalized, focal, or subtle. Even jitteriness can be a manifestation of a seizure disorder.

    b. **Etiologies** include birth trauma, intracranial hemorrhage, postasphyxial encephalopathy, metabolic disturbances (hypoglycemia or hypocalcemia), drug withdrawal, and infections.

    c. **Laboratory evaluation** should include:

      (1) Electrolytes, glucose, calcium, magnesium, and arterial blood gas tensions and pH. If a metabolic disease is suspected, serum and urine amino acids should be obtained.

      (2) Appropriate cultures, including CSF.

      (3) Cranial ultrasound, computed tomography (CT) scan, or both.

      (4) Electroencephalogram before and after pyridoxine administration.

    d. **Treatment** includes supportive care. Adequate oxygenation should be assured and underlying problems (e.g., hypoglycemia, hypocalcemia) corrected. Anticonvulsants are started, and, if indicated, a test dose of pyridoxine is administered.

    e. **Anticonvulsants (Chapter 29)**

      (1) Acute medical treatments in order include:

        (a) **Benzodiazepines** (e.g., lorazepam 0.1–0.3 mg/kg IV).

        (b) **Phenobarbital,** 20 mg/kg IV load, over 10 minutes, then 2.5 mg/kg twice daily to maintain a serum level of 20 to 40 μg/ml.

        (c) **Phenytoin** (Dilantin), 15–20 mg/kg IV load over 15 minutes, then 2.5 mg/kg twice daily to maintain a therapeutic level of 15 to 30 μg/ml.

        (d) **Paraldehyde,** 0.2 ml/kg rectally.

      (2) **Chronic treatment** for seizures usually is phenobarbital.

  2. Intracranial hemorrhage

    a. **Intraventricular hemorrhage** occurs in more than 40% of infants with birthweights below 1500 g. Subdural and subarachnoid hemorrhages are much less common.

b. **Clinical features.** Intraventricular hemorrhage is often asymptomatic, although it can present with unexplained lethargy, apnea, and seizures. On examination, the head circumference is increased and the fontanelles may be bulging. Laboratory examination indicates anemia and acidosis. Diagnosis is made by cranial ultrasonography or CT scan.

c. **Grading** of intraventricular hemorrhage.
   (1) **Grade I.** Subependymal bleeding only.
   (2) **Grade II.** Intraventricular bleeding without dilation of ventricles.
   (3) **Grade III.** Intraventricular bleeding with dilation of ventricles.
   (4) **Grade IV.** Grade III with intraparenchymal blood.

d. The **major complication** of intraventricular hemorrhage is CSF obstruction resulting in **hydrocephalus.** This is followed by measuring daily head circumferences and by serial ultrasonography. Intraventricular shunting is often required.

e. **Hypertonic agents** (e.g., 25% dextrose in water for treatment of hypoglycemia) have been implicated in the cause of intraventricular hemorrhage and should be avoided.

3. **Retinopathy of prematurity (ROP)**
   a. **Etiology**
      (1) The risk of ROP is increased in premature neonates requiring oxygen therapy. ROP is seen in infants with birthweights less than 1700 g, with an 80% incidence in infants weighing less than 1000 g. Hyperoxia should be avoided to decrease the incidence of ROP.
      (2) Factors other than hyperoxic exposure and prematurity can produce ROP, as has been demonstrated in full-term infants, infants with cyanotic heart disease, stillborn infants, and infants with no hyperoxic exposure, as well as in a single eye. Factors that can increase risk include anemia, infection, intracranial hemorrhage, acidosis, and PDA.
   b. **Pathophysiology.** ROP begins in the temporal peripheral retina, which is the last part of the retina to vascularize. An elevated ridge demarcating vascularized and nonvascularized retina is seen initially. **Fibrovascular proliferation** from this border extends posteriorly; in 90% of patients, gradual resolution occurs from this stage. These patients can develop strabismus, amblyopia, myopia, or peripheral retinal detachment in later life.

      c. In 10% of patients, fibrovascularization extends into the vitreous, resulting in vitreous hemorrhage, peripheral retinal scarring, temporal dragging of the disk and macula, and partial retinal detachment. In severe disease, extensive fibrovascular proliferation can result in a retrolental white mass (leukokoria), complete retinal detachment, and loss of vision.

      d. All infants at risk are examined with indirect ophthalmoscopy after 1 month of age. If ROP is identified, the infant is reexamined at 2-week intervals until spontaneous resolution occurs. New cases of ROP do not occur after 3 months of age.

      e. **Treatment** for severe manifestations of ROP has included photocoagulation, diathermy, cryotherapy, and vitrectomy, although none has proved to be effective.

F. Infectious diseases

  1. Environment

      a. **Neonates are particularly vulnerable to infection.** They have decreased cellular and humoral defense immune systems and are at increased risk for colonization and nosocomial infection.

      b. **Prevention.** Infectious transmission can be reduced by using separate equipment and isolettes for each infant, by hand washing before and after each contact, and by wearing cover gowns.

  2. Risk factors for infection. Prolonged rupture of membranes is associated with a high incidence of amnionitis and subsequent ascending bacterial and viral infection in the neonate. Maternal fever, maternal leukocytosis, and fetal tachycardia are also associated with neonatal infection.

  3. Laboratory studies include Gram's stain of gastric aspirate, complete blood count with differential, and blood cultures. A lumbar puncture for culture and analysis of CSF may be indicated. If appropriate, viral cultures should be obtained.

  4. Neonatal sepsis

      a. Organisms responsible for infections soon after birth are usually acquired in utero or during passage through the birth canal. These can include group B β-hemolytic streptococci, *Escherichia coli, Listeria,* and herpes. Later-onset infections can be caused by *Staphylococcus aureus* and *Staphylococcus epidermidis.*

      b. **The clinical features of sepsis** include respiratory failure, seizures, and shock. Often subtle signs, including respiratory distress, apnea, irritability, or poor feeding, are seen first and warrant evaluation.

      c. **Laboratory studies** should include cultures of blood, urine, and CSF; complete blood count; platelet count; urinalysis; and chest radiograph.

      d. **Antibiotic coverage** with ampicillin or oxacillin and an aminoglycoside is begun and continued for 48 to 72 hours. If culture results are positive, treatment should continue as indicated by the severity and location of infection. Aminoglycoside serum levels should be monitored and dosages adjusted to prevent toxicity.

SELECTED REFERENCES

Avery GB. Neonatology. *Pathophysiology and management of the newborn,* 3rd ed. Philadelphia: JB Lippincott, 1987.

Barry JE, Auldist AW. The Vater association; one end of a spectrum of anomalies. *Am J Dis Child* 1974;128:769–771.

Drummond WH, Gregory GA, Heymann MA, et al. The independent effects of hyperventilation, tolazoline, and dopamine on infants with persistent pulmonary hypertension. *J Pediatr* 1981;98:603–611.

Gersony W, Peckham G, Ellison R, et al. Effects of indomethacin in premature infants with patent ductus arteriosus: results of a national collaborative study. *J Pediatr* 1983;102:895–906.

Hammerman C, Aramburo MJ. Prolonged indomethacin therapy for the prevention of recurrences of patent ductus arteriosus. *J Pediatr* 1990;117:771–776.

Insoft RM, Sanderson IR, Walker WA. Development of immune function in the intestine and its role in neonatal diseases. *Pediatr Clin North Am* 1996;43:551–571.

Kurth CD, Spitzer AR, Broennle AM, et al. Postoperative apnea in premature infants. *Anesthesiology* 1987;66:483–488.

Liu LM, Cote CJ, Goudsouzian NG, et al. Life-threatening apnea in infants recovering from anesthesia. *Anesthesiology* 1983;59:506–510.

Peckham GJ, Fox WW. Physiologic factors affecting pulmonary artery pressure in infants with persistent pulmonary hypertension. *J Pediatr* 1978;93:1005–1010.

Roberts Jr JD, Cote C, Todres ID. Neonatal emergencies. In: Cote C, Ryan J, eds. *Practice of anesthesia for infants and children,* 2nd ed. Philadelphia: WB Saunders, 1992.

Roberts Jr JD, Shaul PW. Advances in the treatment of persistent pulmonary hypertension of the newborn. *Pediatr Clin North Am* 1993;40:983–1004.

Roberts Jr JD, Fineman JR, Morin FC, 3rd. Inhaled nitric oxide and persistent pulmonary hypertension. The Inhaled Nitric Oxide Study Group. *N Engl J Med* 1997;336:605–610.

Rudolph AM, Yuan S. Response of the pulmonary vasculature to hypoxia and H^+ ion concentration changes. *J Clin Invest* 1966;45:399–411.

Shannon DC, Gotay F, Stein IM. Prevention of apnea and bradycardia in low-birthweight infants. *Pediatrics* 1975;55:589–594.

Soll RF, Hoekstra RE, Fangman JJ, et al. Multicenter trial of single-dose modified bovine surfactant extract (Survanta) for prevention of respiratory distress syndrome. Ross Collaborative Surfactant Prevention Study Group. *Pediatrics* 1990;85:1092–1102.

Volpe JJ *Neurology of the newborn,* 3rd ed. Philadelphia: WB Saunders, 1995.

Obstetrics and Gynecology

Kevin C. Dennehy

I. **Introduction.** The obstetric patient population is mostly a healthy one, but several conditions contracted during pregnancy are associated with significant morbidity and mortality. The gynecologic patient population represents extremes of age and often has significant comorbid disease. This chapter primarily discusses obstetric illnesses and, when appropriate, critical care of the gynecologic patient.

II. **Hyperemesis gravidarum** is characterized by excessive nausea and vomiting, not related to other pathology, that occurs for the first time before the 20th week of gestation and is severe enough to cause weight loss, dehydration, and electrolyte and acid-base disturbances. It can result in oliguria, ketonuria, hypochloremic metabolic alkalosis, and hemoconcentration. Rarely, confusion, coma and death from hepatorenal failure will occur if appropriate treatment is not instituted.

    A. **The incidence** of hyperemesis gravidarum varies from 0.3% to 1.5% of pregnancies. The disorder is self-limiting; it does not extend beyond the duration of the pregnancy, but can recur in subsequent pregnancies; its cause is unknown.

    B. **Liver function tests** may be abnormal with the alkaline phosphatase being increased above the normal elevation expected during pregnancy. Bilirubin and aminotransferases may also be mildly elevated. Serum levels of 5′ nucleotidase and γ-glutamyl transpeptidase should remain normal in the absence of liver disease.

    C. **Other conditions that can mimic hyperemesis gravidarum** (e.g., peptic ulcer disease, intestinal obstruction, cholecystitis, intracranial pathology, genitourinary pathology, drug toxicity, and hydatidiform mole) should be excluded.

    D. **Treatment** is aimed initially at correcting fluid and electrolyte abnormalities, followed by insulin administration for patients suffering from diabetic ketoacidosis (DKA).

    E. **Many antiemetics** have been used with variable success at controlling nausea and vomiting. Cyclizine, meclizine, chlorpromazine, doxylamine plus pyridoxine, diphenhydramine, dimenhydrinate, and metoclopramide in the third trimester have all been used safely during pregnancy. The risk of teratogenic effects of drugs administered during the first trimester must be balanced by the adverse effects of maternal dehydration, ketosis, and malnutrition on the fetus.

F. **Nutritional support** includes adequate calories, vitamins, especially thiamine to prevent the development of Wernicke-Korsakoff's disease, and trace elements. Enteral feeding may work by preventing the mother from seeing or smelling food, but parenteral nutrition may be necessary.

III. **Preeclampsia and eclampsia**

A. **Preeclampsia** is characterized by hypertension (systolic blood pressure > 140 mm Hg or > 30 mm Hg above prepregnant values; diastolic blood pressure > 90 mm Hg or > 15 mm Hg above prepregnant values), proteinuria (≥300 mg/24 hours or ≥1+ on urine dipstick), and peripheral edema occurring usually after the 20th week of pregnancy. Hyperuricemia (serum urate > 5.5 mg/dl) is present in almost all cases. **Severe preeclampsia** is characterized by a blood pressure of more than 160/110 mm Hg, proteinuria (≥5 g/24 hours or ≥3+ on urine dipstick), oliguria (urine output < 400 ml/24 hours), epigastric or right upper quadrant pain, visual or cerebral disturbances, and occasionally pulmonary edema. **Eclampsia** is defined by the presence of seizures in a patient with preeclampsia. The cause of eclampsia is unknown. Immunologic incompatibility between the placenta and the maternal organs or a defect in trophoblastic invasion into the uterus have been postulated to produce an imbalance of placental prostaglandin release or nitric oxide synthesis. This results in endothelial dysfunction manifested as vasospasm, altered vascular permeability, and activation of the coagulation system.

B. **Effects on specific organ systems**

1. **Cardiovascular.** Total body water is increased, but intravascular volume may be reduced by 30% to 40%. Central venous pressure is usually low. Myocardial function varies from hyperdynamic to depressed. A pulmonary artery catheter may be useful to monitor filling pressures and myocardial function in patients developing left ventricular failure or pulmonary edema.

2. **Neurologic.** Seizure threshold is decreased and central nervous system (CNS) irritability is increased, presumably because of increased brain water, cerebral vasospasm, or thrombotic occlusion of the cerebral microcirculation. Hyperreflexic deep tendon reflexes are expected.

3. **Renal.** Injury to renal vascular endothelium results in proteinuria. Swelling of glomerular cells termed "endotheliosis" results in a reduction in glomerular filtration and creatinine clearance.

4. **Hepatic** involvement can range from mild edema to periportal hemorrhages, subcapsular hematoma, and, rarely, spontaneous hepatic rupture. Initial signs include epigastric tenderness with elevations in hepatic transaminase level and a reduction in synthetic function.

5. **Hematologic. Thrombocytopenia** (platelet count <150,000/L/mm³), which occurs in 15% of patients with preeclampsia, reflects increased platelet consumption. A qualitative defect in platelet function also may be present. A low grade consumptive coagulopathy and primary fibrinolysis are common.

C. **Therapy**

1. **Goals**

   a. Control of hypertension and replacement of intravascular volume will reduce CNS irritability and improve organ perfusion.

   b. Eliminate the cause of the preeclampsia through delivery of the fetus. The timing of delivery depends on the clinical condition of the mother and the viability of the fetus. Provided hypotension is avoided, the antihypertensive agents mentioned below provide good control of blood pressure with minimal effects on uterine blood flow.

2. **Pharmacologic therapy**

   a. **Magnesium sulfate** (loading dose of 2–4 g IV over 15 minutes followed by an infusion of 1–3 g/h) produces vasodilation and acts as an anticonvulsant. It is effective in preventing the recurrence of seizures in eclampsia and in seizure prophylaxis in preeclampsia. The infusion rate is reduced with renal insufficiency. The therapeutic range is a serum magnesium level of 4 to 8 mEq/L. Levels of 7 to 10 mEq/L result in loss of deep tendon reflexes. Levels in excess of 10 mEq/L can produce respiratory depression and heart block. In case of an overdose, calcium gluconate administration will reverse the harmful skeletal muscle effects. Magnesium therapy is usually continued for 24 hours after delivery because eclampsia can develop in up to 20% of cases in the postpartum period.

   b. **Labetalol,** administered in bolus doses of 5 to 10 mg IV every 5 to 10 minutes (or by infusion), is usually well tolerated. The combined α and β blockade rapidly reduces blood pressure and produces minimal reflex tachycardia.

   c. **Hydralazine** (5–10 mg IV every 15 minutes as needed) dilates arteriolar smooth muscle. The peak antihypertensive effect occurs in 10 to 20 minutes following IV administration. Reflex tachycardia and postural hypotension are common.

   d. **Sodium nitroprusside** is a fast-acting, direct vasodilator with a very short duration of action used to treat hypertensive crises. Because of concern regarding fetal cyanide toxicity (the fetal liver has less thiosulfate substrate for rhodanase detoxification of cyanide than the maternal liver), infusion duration should be limited to that time of immediate danger to the mother.

IV. **HELLP syndrome**
A. **HELLP syndrome** is characterized by **h**emolysis, **e**levated **l**iver enzymes and **l**ow **p**latelets. It usually occurs in association with preeclampsia, but can occur without hypertension and proteinuria. The cause is unknown. Intravascular platelet activation and microvascular endothelial damage are pathologic hallmarks.
  1. **Symptoms** include malaise, nausea, vomiting, and epigastric or right upper quadrant pain.
  2. **Diagnosis** relies on the demonstration of:
    a. An abnormal peripheral blood smear and an elevated bilirubin level (> 1.2 mg/dl).
    b. Aspartate aminotransferase more than 70 U/L and lactate dehydrogenase more than 600 U/L.
    c. Platelet count less than 100,000/mm^3.
  3. **Differential diagnosis** includes hepatitis, gall bladder disease, acute fatty liver of pregnancy, and thrombotic thrombocytopenic purpura. All patients have evidence of diffuse intravascular coagulation (DIC). Severe DIC is extremely rare.
  4. **Treatment** is supportive along with immediate delivery. The abnormal laboratory values return to normal in 2 to 7 days. Maternal and fetal morbidity increase with increasing disease severity.

V. **Acute fatty liver of pregnancy**
A. This idiopathic condition is characterized by a short history of malaise, anorexia, persistent nausea or vomiting, heartburn, upper abdominal pain, mild jaundice, fevers, and hematemesis. Some patients will have concomitant diabetes insipidus. This condition may be caused by a defect in mitochondrial β-oxidation of fatty acids causing microvesicular steatosis of the liver. The incidence has been reported to vary from 1 of 6,600 to 1 of 15,900 deliveries. Half of these patients are nulliparous and the average maternal age is 27 years. The average gestation is 37.5 weeks with a predominance of male fetuses (3–5:1) and an increased incidence with twins. The maternal and fetal mortality rates are 10% and 20%, respectively. Morbidity and mortality are caused by DIC with fibrin-induced organ dysfunction, gastrointestinal hemorrhage, renal failure, acute pancreatitis, and fulminant hepatic failure.
B. **Laboratory findings** include elevated transaminases, bilirubin, prothrombin time, partial thromboplastin time (aPTT), blood urea nitrogen (BUN), creatinine, and white blood cell count; and decreased fibrinogen and glucose levels. Tests of acute or chronic viral hepatitis should be performed to exclude an infectious cause. The gall bladder should be imaged to

exclude choledocholithiasis. A liver biopsy can be helpful in the diagnosis of questionable cases, but should be considered carefully if coagulation studies are abnormal.

C. **Delivery of the fetus** is necessary to halt progression of the condition. Although most patients do not develop problems with excess bleeding, occasionally hemorrhage can be severe. Laboratory values return toward normal values 5 to 7 days following delivery.

VI. **Acute respiratory distress syndrome in pregnancy**

A. **Acute respiratory distress syndrome (ARDS)** is characterized by acute bilateral pulmonary infiltrates on chest radiograph and marked intrapulmonary shunting of blood with an arterial oxygen tension to inspired oxygen concentration ratio (PaO_2/FIO_2) less than 200 in the absence of evidence of fluid overload (i.e., a pulmonary artery occlusion pressure less than 18 mm Hg), in the presence of defined risk factors (Chapter 20).

B. **Common causes of ARDS during pregnancy** include infections (e.g., urinary tract infections, viral causes, endometritis, amnionitis), preeclampsia or eclampsia, acute fatty liver of pregnancy, tocolytic therapy with β-agonists, aspiration during anesthesia, and massive hemorrhage.

C. **The clinical course** is variable. Increased intraabdominal pressures during pregnancy will be transmitted to the diaphragm and reduce thoracic compliance and functional residual capacity. The physiologic anemia of pregnancy and reduced venous return (caused by inferior vena caval compression) can reduce oxygen delivery to peripheral tissues.

D. **Pulmonary and hemodynamic management** goals and techniques are generally as outlined in Chapters 4 and 20. Of note, little information is available regarding the use of prone positioning during pregnancy as a ventilatory strategy to improve matching of ventilation to perfusion. The use of vasoactive drugs also has not been extensively studied in pregnancy. Alpha-adrenergic-agonists can decrease uteroplacental blood flow, but may be necessary to treat maternal hypotension. Extracorporeal lung support (Chapter 14) and inhaled nitric oxide (Chapter 20) may be useful adjunctive therapies in selected patients.

E. **Obstetric management.** The timing and the route of neonatal delivery are determined on an individual basis. The mother should be monitored for signs of active labor and the fetus for signs of fetal distress. If delivery is indicated, some authors recommend vaginal delivery and reserve cesarean section for obstetric indications. Successful vaginal deliveries during mechanical ventilation for ARDS have been reported.

F. **Morbidity in the parturient with acute respiratory failure** is significant. A prolonged course of mechanical ventilation, however, does not imply increased maternal mortality. In one series, six of nine mothers intubated for more than 40 days survived.

VII. **Asthma**

A. **Asthma** continues to be a cause of maternal mortality. Because of its prevalence in the general population (~4%), it is the most common respiratory complaint in pregnancy. It is characterized by reversible airway obstruction, airway inflammation, and increased bronchial smooth muscle reactivity to a variety of stimuli (Chapter 21).

B. **Treatment of the asthmatic parturient** is the same as for the nonpregnant patient. β-Adrenergic agonists, inhaled corticosteroids, sodium cromoglycate, theophylline, oral corticosteroids, and inhaled ipratropium have all been used during pregnancy. The effect of these drugs on the fetus is considered to be less than the resultant effects of inadequately treated asthma. Theophylline levels should be followed closely during the third trimester, as clearance is reduced 25% to 30%.

C. **Approximately 10% of asthmatic patients** will have an exacerbation of their asthma during labor. Supplemental doses of corticosteroids (hydrocortisone 50–100 mg every 8 hours during labor) should be administered to those who have been receiving steroids. Prostaglandin $F_{2\alpha}$ causes broncho-constriction and should be avoided as a treatment for uterine atony.

D. **The overall perinatal prognosis** is comparable to that of the nonasthmatic population if asthma is well managed.

VIII. **Diabetic ketoacidosis in the pregnant patient**

A. **DKA** is characterized by insulin deficiency, hyperglycemia, acidosis, and dehydration (Chapter 26). Early and frequent antenatal screening for diabetes mellitus has reduced the morbidity associated with the development of DKA during pregnancy. The fetal mortality was as high as 90% prior to 1975, but more recently is reported to be 35%.

B. **The cause** of the adverse effects of DKA on the fetus is unknown. Maternal dehydration and acidosis can cause fetal hypoxia through impaired uterine blood flow. Maternal hypokalemia can cause fetal cardiac dysrhythmias. The relative catabolic state that exists during pregnancy results in relative hypoglycemia, hypoinsulinemia, hyperketonemia, and protein catabolism. Therefore, DKA can develop at lower serum glucose levels than it does in the nonpregnant diabetic patient.

C. **Clinical features** of DKA are the same in the pregnant patient as in the nonpregnant patient; they range from vomiting, polyuria, and polydipsia to disorientation and coma.

D. **Laboratory abnormalities** include hyperglycemia, acidosis (arterial pH < 7.3, serum HCO_3 < 15 mEq/L with an anion gap > 12 mEq/L) and ketonemia. Serum osmolality and plasma glucose values, although variable, usually are more than 280 mOsm/kg and more than 300 mg/dl, respectively.

E. **Management.** Baseline laboratory data including complete blood count, electrolytes, serum creatinine, BUN, serum phosphorus, and serum magnesium should be obtained. A **source of infection** should be sought and appropriate cultures should be done. Antibiotic therapy is directed toward a specific source or begun empirically if infection is suspected. General management following admission to an intensive care unit (ICU) is detailed in Table 40-1 and Chapter 26. Specific measures concerning fluid, electrolyte, and insulin administration are detailed in Table 40-2.

F. **Obstetric management.** Preterm contractions and abnormal fetal biophysical profiles can revert to normal following treatment of the underlying maternal condition. Magnesium should be used for tocolysis, if necessary. β-Adrenergic agonists promote glycogenolysis and lipolysis and can aggravate the DKA. Corticosteroids administered to promote fetal lung maturity can have similar adverse effects. Maternal stabilization with the fetus in utero is probably the best course. An emergency cesarean section offers minimal benefit to the fetus and exposes the parturient to the increased risks of an operative delivery.

IX. **Cardiovascular disease**
   A. **Valvular heart disease (Chapter 18)**
      1. **Severe or critical aortic stenosis (AS)** is characterized by an aortic valve area less than 0.4 cm^2 (normal is 2.6–3.5 cm^2) and a systolic pressure gradient greater than 50 mm Hg with normal cardiac output. Severe AS has been reported to result in a maternal mortality rate of 17%. (See Chapter 18 for details concerning diagnosis and management.)
         a. It is recommended that these patients undergo corrective surgery prior to becoming pregnant.

Table 40-1. General considerations for the management of diabetic ketoacidosis in pregnancy

1. Admit to intensive care unit.
2. Position patient with left lateral tilt and monitor fetal heart rate.
3. Ensure airway protection if comatose.
4. Ensure adequate oxygenation.
5. Obtain baseline laboratory data.
6. Place central venous and arterial catheters as indicated.
7. Monitor urine output.
8. Search for source of infection (blood, urine cultures).

Table 40-2.   Correction of abnormalities associated with diabetic ketoacidosis (DKA) in pregnancy

Fluids
1. 0.9% saline at 1 L/h for first 1–2 h.
2. 0.45% saline at 1 L/h for first 1–2 h if Na^+ >155 mEq/L, serum Osm >320 mosm/kg or pH <7.0.
3. 0.45% saline at 250–400 ml/h after first 1–2 h of fluid replacement.
4. Add 5% dextrose to fluids and reduce infusion to 150 ml/h as serum glucose reaches 200 mg/dl.

Insulin
1. Administer IV loading dose of 0.4 IU/kg regular insulin.
2. Administer continuous infusion at 6–10 IU/h.
3. Double infusion rate if no response within 1 h.
4. Decrease infusion to 1–2 IU/h as serum glucose decreases to 250 mg/dl.
5. Continue infusion at reduced rate for 12–24 h after DKA has resolved.

Potassium
1. KCl at 40 mEq/h if serum potassium <3.0 mEq/L.
2. KCl at 20 mEq/h if serum potassium is normal.
3. Withhold KCl if serum potassium ≥6 mEq/L.
4. Monitor electrocardiogram if oliguric.

Bicarbonate
1. Add 2 ampoules of 8.4% $NaHCO_3$ to each liter of 0.45% saline if pH <7.0. Solution approaches isotonicity.

   b. Percutaneous balloon valvuloplasty may be necessary during pregnancy or postpartum.
   c. Antibiotic prophylaxis should be administered during labor and delivery.
2. **Aortic regurgitation (AR)** is more common in women of childbearing age than AS; 75% of cases are caused by previous rheumatic fever (Chapter 18).
   a. Acute AR can follow rupture of the valvular apparatus caused by endocarditis, trauma, or aortic dissection from cystic medial necrosis of the aorta. The result is an increase in left ventricular end-diastolic volume (LVEDV) and left ventricular end-diastolic pressure with left ventricular failure and eventual development of pulmonary edema. If this occurs acutely, emergency surgery may be necessary to save the life of the mother.
   b. Antibiotic prophylaxis should be administered during labor and delivery.
   c. Treatment with digoxin, salt restriction, and diuretics may be necessary during pregnancy and continued into the postpartum period.

3. **Severe mitral stenosis (MS)** is characterized by a mitral valve area less than 1 cm^2 (normal is 4–6 cm^2) and is common following rheumatic fever. Approximately 90% of pregnant women who have rheumatic heart disease have MS (Chapter 18).

    a. **β-Blocker administration** has been shown to reduce the incidence of maternal pulmonary edema without adverse effect on the fetus or neonate.

    b. **The autotransfusion** that occurs at delivery can result in severe volume overload and pulmonary edema. Intravenous nitroglycerin and diuresis may attenuate these rapid changes. Because of the fixed nature of blood flow from the left atrium to the left ventricle, hypovolemia and reduced venous return, including aortocaval compression, must be prevented.

    c. Those patients with MS who are asymptomatic prior to becoming pregnant usually tolerate pregnancy well. Those with preexisting pulmonary edema have a higher incidence of mortality during or after pregnancy.

    d. **Closed mitral valvotomy or balloon valvuloplasty** may be necessary during pregnancy and is performed if maternal symptoms warrant. Mortality rate is approximately 2% to 3% following valvotomy. It is a palliative procedure that may allow completion of the pregnancy.

    e. **Antibiotic prophylaxis** should be administered during labor and delivery.

4. **Mitral regurgitation (MR)** can occur secondary to rheumatic heart disease, myxomatous degeneration, congenital causes, endocarditis, hypertrophic cardiomyopathy, trauma, or, occasionally, following spontaneous chordal rupture. Mortality related to MR is low in pregnancy, unless MS coexists. Chronic, severe MR results in increased left atrial pressure (Chapter 18). Antibiotic prophylaxis should be administered during labor and delivery.

5. **Mitral valve prolapse** appears to be well tolerated during pregnancy with no increased risk of obstetric or fetal complications. Mitral regurgitation can occur, however, and require treatment. Antibiotic prophylaxis should also be administered.

6. **Prosthetic cardiac valves** are associated with special risks during pregnancy.

    a. Despite the replacement of a malfunctioning heart valve with a mechanical or bioprosthetic valve, some degree of myocardial, valvular, or pulmonary dysfunction usually persists.

      b. **Thromboembolic phenomena** are a concern. All obstetric patients with mechanical valves and those with bioprosthetic valves, who are also in atrial fibrillation or have demonstrated thromboembolism, should receive anticoagulation.

      c. Women with **porcine heterograft valves** and no risk factors do not require anticoagulation. For this reason, porcine heterografts are considered the best choice for valve replacement in women of childbearing age, although these valves can fail earlier than mechanical valves.

      d. **Warfarin** is teratogenic and should not be administered during pregnancy.

      e. **Endocarditis** is a potentially serious problem for the obstetric patient with a prosthetic valve. She should receive antibiotic prophylaxis for any genitourinary procedure performed during pregnancy.

   7. **Cardiopulmonary bypass (CPB)** occasionally is necessary for progressive heart failure secondary to valve dysfunction, prosthetic valve failure, trauma, massive pulmonary embolism, or coronary revascularization. These cases are rare. Maternal mortality is reportedly less than 5%. Fetal mortality, however, is 30% to 50%, which is thought to be related to the preexisting condition of the mother and the abnormal blood flow and hypothermia associated with CPB. Should CPB be necessary shortly after vaginal delivery or cesarean section, the anticoagulation can cause profuse bleeding from the surgical site or the site of placental implantation. Inhibition of fibrinolysis using aprotinin has been reported to reduce bleeding complications associated with CPB in the early puerperium.

B. **Congenital heart disease**

   1. Women born with congenital heart disease are surviving to childbearing age.

      a. **Common congenital lesions** include left-to-right shunts, tetralogy of Fallot (TOF), and coarctation of the aorta.

      b. **Left-to-right intracardiac shunting** can occur via an atrial septal defect (ASD), a ventricular septal defect (VSD), or a patent ductus arteriosus (PDA).

      c. **De-airing of all intravenous (IV) lines** and injections must be ensured.

      d. **Shunt reversal and paradoxical embolism** can occur in association with straining at delivery or with the reduction in systemic vascular resistance (SVR) following regional blockade. Mild degrees of shunting are generally well tolerated and mortality in this group is less than 1%.

2. **Tetralogy of Fallot (TOF)** involves a VSD, right ventricular hypertrophy, right ventricular outflow tract (RVOT) obstruction, and an aorta that overrides the right and left ventricles. Very few of these women survive to childbearing age without surgical correction. Correction usually involves closure of the VSD and widening of the RVOT. Reduction in SVR will increase the right-to-left shunting. The mortality rate in corrected TOF is less than 1% but is 5% to 15% if the TOF has not been corrected.

3. **Uncorrected coarctation of the aorta** places patients at risk for left ventricular failure, aortic rupture or dissection, and endocarditis during pregnancy. The mortality rate in this group is 5% to 15%. The coarctation is usually located just distal to the left subclavian artery and patients have a gradient between blood pressure measured in the upper and lower limbs. Fetal mortality approaches 20%.

   a. The condition is associated with intracranial aneurysms and bicuspid aortic valves.

   b. **Invasive monitoring** proximal and distal to the coarctation will allow measurement of uterine perfusion pressure and maintenance of the preexisting gradient if interventions are planned.

   c. **Antibiotic prophylaxis** should be administered.

C. **Coronary artery disease (Chapter 17)**

1. **The risk of myocardial infarction** (MI) during pregnancy has been estimated to be between 1 per 10,000 and 1.5 per 100,000 deliveries. Most occur in the third trimester. The incidence of MI in this patient population appears to be increasing along with mean maternal age. More than half of women suffering an MI during pregnancy are aged at least 35 years.

2. Approximate occurrences of **MI** are 40% secondary to coronary atherosclerosis; 10% from coronary aneurysms or obstruction; 30% to 40% from coronary thrombosis; and 10% in those with normal coronary arteries. Smoking and cocaine use are significant cofactors. The mortality rate is approximately 30% with the greatest risk of death occurring immediately following infarction and if the MI occurs around the time of delivery. An MI occurring in association with severe preeclampsia is associated with a particularly poor prognosis.

3. **Investigations** should include serial electrocardiograms (ECG), cardiac enzymes, tests of coagulation, full blood count, BUN, creatinine level, and electrolytes. An echocardiogram can be useful to establish ventricular and valvular function. Cardiac catheterization may demonstrate a coro-

nary lesion and be followed by correction by percutaneous transluminal coronary angioplasty or
coronary bypass grafting.

   4. **Systemic thrombolytic therapy** has been asso-
      ciated with significant maternal bleeding, prema-
      ture labor, and dysfunctional uterine contractions.
      Little or no information is available on the use of
      intracoronary lytic therapy, dipyridamole, or as-
      pirin administration following MI in the pregnant
      patient. The use of inotropes and an intraaortic
      balloon pump may be necessary.

   5. **Adjunctive therapy** includes administration of
      β-blockers, heparin, nitroglycerin, oxygen, and lat-
      eral uterine displacement. The timing and method
      of delivery should be determined on a case-by-case
      basis.

D. **Pulmonary hypertension** is present when the mean
   pulmonary artery pressure is more than 25 mm Hg.

   1. **Primary pulmonary hypertension (PPH)** is a
      progressively fatal disease of unknown cause.
      Estimates of the incidence of PPH range from 1 to
      2 per million of the general population. The patho-
      physiology involves pulmonary vasoconstriction,
      vascular wall remodeling, and thrombosis, which
      can produce right ventricular failure (RVF) and
      death. RVF can rapidly ensue when pregnancy-
      induced increases of blood volume and cardiac out-
      put are superimposed on preexisting PPH.

      a. **Diagnosis** is based on the demonstration of el-
         evated pulmonary artery pressures by cardiac
         catheterization or echocardiography.

      b. **Management** should be individualized in
         each case and a multidisciplinary team ap-
         proach adopted. It has been suggested that
         these patients be admitted to the hospital 4
         to 8 weeks before delivery. **Oxygen,** either
         continuous or for a few hours each day and at
         night, has been recommended. **Anticoagu-
         lation** with either subcutaneous or IV he-
         parin may prevent pulmonary emboli (PE).
         Minute PE can be fatal in established pul-
         monary hypertension. **Specific pulmonary
         vasodilator therapy** has been attempted.
         High-dose calcium channel blockade (20 mg
         nifedipine orally every hour until an effect is
         seen); inhaled nitric oxide at 20 to 80 ppm;
         and inhaled or IV prostacyclin can be useful
         if the patient has some reversibility of pul-
         monary vasoconstriction. Monitoring with a
         pulmonary artery (PA) catheter is useful to
         determine the effects of drug administration.
         Systemic arterial pressure should be main-
         tained greater than PA pressure to ensure
         adequate coronary perfusion of the right ven-
         tricle. **Heart–lung or lung transplanta-
         tion** should be considered early in those pa-

tients who do not respond to pulmonary vasodilator therapy and urgently in those with critically low cardiac output. End-stage right ventricular failure usually does not respond well to inotrope administration.

2. **Secondary pulmonary hypertension** can develop from long-standing mitral valve disease, Eisenmenger's syndrome, or untreated ASD, VSD, PDA, or TOF. The mortality rate in these patients is 25% to 50%. Causes of death include embolism, dysrhythmia, right ventricular failure, myocardial infarction, and hypotension.

E. **Peripartum cardiomyopathy** is characterized by heart failure of unknown etiology, but may be due to myocarditis arising from an infectious, autoimmune, or idiopathic process. Its incidence is 1 in 1,300 to 1 of 15,000 pregnancies, most commonly in obese, black, multiparous women aged more than 30 years. It is estimated that 250 to 1,350 women will develop peripartum cardiomyopathy each year.

1. **Diagnosis** is based on evidence of left ventricular dysfunction (i.e., left ventricular ejection fraction < 45%), symptoms of heart failure that manifest in the last month of pregnancy or within 5 months of delivery, and no other apparent cause of heart failure. These patients have an increased incidence of premature births and low-birthweight babies.

2. **Treatment** involves fluid restriction, modest daily exercise, amlodipine, hydralazine, nitrates, digoxin, diuretics, α-blockers, angiotensin-converting enzyme inhibitors or angiotensin II receptor blockers, and anticoagulation. Low dose β-blockers can be added postpartum. Inotropes can be added for those unresponsive to other therapies. Cardiac transplantation can be considered for those with progressive disease. Those patients who received transplants demonstrated an increased left ventricular end-diastolic diameter and a trend toward decreased left ventricular ejection fraction. Immunosuppressive therapy has not been shown to be of benefit.

   a. Interpretation of data from follow-up studies is difficult because of the small numbers of patients who develop peripartum cardiomyopathy. Some studies suggest that 50% of patients will have spontaneous resolution of their symptoms; others suggest that 93% have progressive or persistent cardiomyopathy with eventual death or transplant as an endpoint. Subsequent pregnancies in those who recover have been uneventful in 75% and resulted in temporary deterioration in 25%. Subsequent pregnancies in those with persistent cardiomyopathy have resulted in death in up to 50% of these patients.

X.   Neurologic problems

A. **Stroke.** The risk of stroke during pregnancy has been estimated at 5.6 per 100,000 deliveries. Ischemic and hemorrhagic strokes are responsible for approximately one third and two thirds of events, respectively. Transient ischemic attacks and cerebral infarction are five times more common during pregnancy and the early puerperium than in the nonpregnant patient.

1. **Common signs and symptoms** include severe headaches, weakness, aphasia, and visual disturbances. Evaluation should proceed urgently with computed tomography, angiography, or magnetic resonance imaging (Chapter 29).

2. **Reversible causes** include carotid artery or cerebral venous thrombosis or a leaking aneurysm or arteriovenous (AV) malformation. These can be successfully treated surgically or recanalization may be possible by using thrombolytics and interventional radiologic procedures. Surgical management of aneurysms, but not AV malformations, has been associated with significantly lower maternal and fetal mortality. Care is supportive, but there are case reports of delivery by cesarean section at the time of aneurysm clipping.

3. The risk of **aneurysms** bleeding increases as pregnancy progresses. Some authors recommend urgent delivery should subarachnoid hemorrhage (SAH) occur during labor. Treatment of arterial spasm with nimodipine to prevent ischemic stroke following SAH has also been recommended. The prognosis following SAH is very serious with maternal mortality rate being as high as 80%.

B. **Status epilepticus** is characterized by a seizure lasting longer than 30 minutes or recurrent seizures without intervening recovery.

1. **Generalized tonic–clonic seizures** are those seen most commonly during pregnancy; however, petit mal and focal seizures of the temporal lobe and motor cortex status epilepticus also occur. Other causes, including eclampsia, encephalitis, meningitis, tumor, drug withdrawal, local anesthetic toxicity, and intracranial hemorrhage, should be excluded.

2. When related to a preexisting epileptic focus, status epilepticus usually occurs in the second half of pregnancy and is associated with subtherapeutic levels of anticonvulsant drugs. Absorption of anticonvulsants falls, metabolism usually increases, and plasma protein binding falls. This results in a greater decrease in total blood anticonvulsant levels and a lesser decrease in free, or unbound, drug. Free drug levels should be monitored, if possible, during pregnancy.

3. **Treatment goals** include maintaining an adequate airway and ensuring adequate oxygenation

while attempting to determine the cause and stop the seizure. The patient should be placed in the **lateral position** and supplemental oxygen administered. Blood should be sent for a toxicology screen and determinations of concentrations of glucose, electrolytes, and calcium. Administer 50 ml of 50% dextrose and 100 mg of thiamine IV, followed by an anticonvulsant of choice (benzodiazepines and barbiturates are used most commonly) until a seizure-free interval is achieved. A long-acting anticonvulsant can then be administered.

4. **The pharmacokinetics of phenytoin** loading in preeclamptic patients have been determined. Therapeutic free phenytoin levels can be achieved with a loading dose of 10 mg/kg initially, followed by 5 mg/kg 2 hours later.

5. **For intractable seizure activity,** electroencephalographic monitoring, suppression of seizure activity with high-dose barbiturates (20 mg/kg phenobarbital), tracheal intubation, and mechanical ventilation may be necessary.

XI. **Hematologic problems**

A. **Thromboembolic disease** is the leading cause of maternal mortality. Changes in the coagulation system during pregnancy result in a hypercoagulable state, but pregnant patients without risk factors have a low incidence of spontaneous venous thrombosis (0.5–3/1,000). The risk of recurrence has been reported to be between 7.5% to 12%.

1. **Risk factors** include increased age and parity, obesity, prolonged bed rest, surgery, acquired or congenital hypercoagulable states, and postphlebitic syndrome. The American College of Chest Physicians recommendations for antithrombotic therapy during pregnancy are listed in Table 40-3.

2. Controlled trials of thrombolytic therapy during pregnancy have not been performed. Use is generally restricted to hemodynamically unstable patients with acute pulmonary embolus (PE) or patients with extensive iliofemoral thrombosis and a low risk of bleeding (Chapter 22). The risk of maternal hemorrhage is increased, and greatest if these agents are given at the time of delivery. The pregnancy loss rate has been reported to be 5.8% following lytic therapy.

B. **Antepartum hemorrhage**

1. The causes of antepartum hemorrhage include:
   a. Placenta previa and vasa previa.
   b. Placental abruption.
   c. Uterine rupture.

2. The incidence of **placenta previa** is approximately 1 in 200 pregnancies. It is associated with multiparity, increased maternal age, previous cesarean section or uterine surgery, and previous

Table 40-3.   The American College of Chest Physicians guidelines for antithrombotic therapy during pregnancy

Condition	Recommendation
Previous venous thrombosis or PE prior to current pregnancy	Heparin (5,000 IU every 12 h or adjusted to produce a heparin level of 0.1–0.2 IU/ml) throughout pregnancy followed by warfarin postpartum for 4–6 wk.
Venous thrombosis or PE during current therapy	Heparin in full IV doses for 5–10 d, followed by SC injections every 12 h to prolong 6-h postinjection aPTT into the therapeutic range until delivery; warfarin can then be used postpartum.
Planning pregnancy in patients who are being treated with long-term oral anticoagulants	Either heparin SC every 12 h to prolong 6-h postinjection aPTT into the therapeutic range Or Frequent pregnancy tests and substitute heparin (as above) for warfarin when pregnancy is achieved.
Mechanical heart valves	Either heparin SC every 12 h to prolong 6-h postinjection aPTT into the therapeutic range Or Adjusted dose SC heparin until the 13th week, warfarin (target INR 2.5–3.0) until the middle of the third trimester, then adjusted dose SC heparin until delivery. The addition of aspirin (80–100 mg PO) daily to either regimen should be considered.
APLA and >1 previous pregnancy loss	Either aspirin plus prednisone Or Aspirin plus heparin Or Aspirin alone
APLA and 0 or 1 previous pregnancy loss	Low dose aspirin during the second and third trimester.
APLA and previous venous thrombosis	Heparin SC every 12 h to prolong 6-h postinjection aPTT into the therapeutic range.
APLA without previous venous thrombosis	Either clinical surveillance combined with intermittent pneumatic compression or elastic stockings Or Heparin (5,000 IU) every 12 h throughout pregnancy.

APLA, antiphospholipid antibodies; IU, international units; IV, intravenous; PE, pulmonary embolism; PO, orally; aPTT, activated partial thromboplastin time; SC, subcutaneous.
Adapted from Ginsburg JS, Hirsh J. Use of antithrombotic agents during pregnancy. *Chest* 1998;115:524S–530S, with permission.

placenta previa. Bleeding is painless and usually stops spontaneously on the first occasion. Subsequent hemorrhage can be more profuse and lead to shock. Up to 10% of patients have a co-existing placental abruption. Diagnosis is confirmed by ultrasound or, occasionally, a double set-up examination, in which preparations are made for possible immediate delivery. Investigations include complete blood count, coagulation tests, and assessment of fetal lung maturity. Cross-matched blood should be available. Preparation should be made for a large volume resuscitation because these patients can bleed spontaneously or secondary to placental incision during cesarean section, and an increased risk of placenta accreta, increta, or percreta exists.

3. The cause of **placental abruption** (separation of the placenta before delivery) is unknown. Risk factors include hypertension, increased maternal age, tobacco and cocaine use, trauma, prolonged rupture of membranes, and history of previous abruption. The incidence is approximately 1% of pregnancies. The amount of vaginal bleeding can underestimate the true blood loss as a large hematoma may have formed at the placental site. Complications include fetal distress or death, shock, DIC, and acute renal failure.

4. **Uterine rupture** occurs following previous uterine surgery, trauma, inappropriate use of oxytocin; in grand multiparous patients; and secondary to tumors, uterine anomaly, and fetal macrosomia or malposition. Anterior rupture and extension into the uterine vessels laterally results in massive hemorrhage. Uterine repair can be possible, but hysterectomy may be necessary.

C. **Postpartum hemorrhage.** Blood loss following vaginal delivery is 300 to 600 ml and 500 to 1000 ml following cesarean section. Any bleeding in excess of this is considered excessive.

1. **Primary postpartum hemorrhage** occurs in the first 24 hours following delivery. **Secondary postpartum hemorrhage** occurs after 24 hours to 6 weeks postpartum.

2. **Causes** include uterine atony, trauma, retained placenta; placenta accreta, increta, or percreta; and uterine inversion.

3. **Management** includes the ability to administer large volume resuscitation, continual assessment of the effectiveness of transfusion by following the hematocrit and coagulation tests, and correction of the obstetric cause of the problem.

4. **Pharmacologic treatment of uterine atony** includes IV infusion of oxytocin, ergometrine [100–250 µg, usually administered intramuscularly (IM)] with preexisting hypertension being a

relative contraindication, or 15-methyl $PGF_{2\alpha}$ (250 μg administered intramyometrial or IM), which can cause or aggravate bronchospasm. Correction of obstetric cause usually requires surgery, but can be amenable to radiologic embolization.

XII. **Amniotic fluid embolism (AFE)** has an incidence of approximately 3/100,000 live births. The mortality rate is as high as 80% with most deaths occurring in the first few hours.

   A. **Clinical features** consist of rapid onset of hypotension and dyspnea, followed by development of coagulopathy (probably from the presence of factor X activator, circulating trophoblast, or hemorrhage caused by uterine atony), seizures, and cardiopulmonary arrest.

   B. **The cause** is unclear. Intravenous injection of autologous amniotic fluid does not produce the syndrome, and the amount of particulate matter found in the pulmonary vasculature does not correlate with the severity of the presentation. Unidentified vasoactive substances that cause intense PA vasoconstriction and right ventricular failure may be present in amniotic fluid. Pulmonary hypertension is of short duration in those patients resuscitated from AFE, because their PA pressures are near normal once monitoring has begun.

   C. **Treatment** involves aggressive resuscitation methods. Tracheal intubation, mechanical ventilation, and establishment of the ability to administer large volumes of IV fluids and blood products should be performed. Early consultation with a hematologist and the blood bank may facilitate treatment of the coagulopathy. Monitoring should include peripheral arterial and PA catheters. Inotropic support of the heart, with or without an intraaortic balloon pump, may be necessary.

   D. **Other sequelae** include neurologic injury, ARDS, acute renal failure, and hepatic failure. Successful pregnancies have been reported in two patients who survived AFE.

XIII. **Infectious complications**

   A. **Toxic shock syndrome (TSS)** is caused by infection with *Staphylococcus aureus* and release of toxin from the bacteria. TSS can develop following postpartum infections; with the use of contraceptive sponges or diaphragms; or with the use of tampons during menstruation. The mortality rate approximates 2% to 3%.

      1. **Clinical features of TSS** include a fever of ≥38.9°C; diffuse, macular erythroderma; desquamation, particularly of the palms and soles 1 to 2 weeks after onset of the illness; and systemic hypotension. Evidence of other organ system involvement can include vomiting, diarrhea, mucous membrane hyperemia, myalgia with elevated creatine phosphokinase levels, and disorientation or alterations in level of consciousness. Progression to multiple organ failure can occur with hepa-

tic and renal dysfunction, thrombocytopenia, and ARDS.

2. **Diagnosis of TSS** is based on the constellation of signs and symptoms. No specific diagnostic test is available. Differentiation between TSS **and toxic epidermal necrolysis (TEN)** can be difficult. Examination of the roof of a bulla reveals only epidermal cell layers above the stratum granulosum, whereas in TEN the roof is composed of the entire epidermis. This distinction is important because glucocorticoid administration may offer benefits in TEN but can aggravate TSS.

3. **General principles of therapy** include removing all foreign bodies, draining accessible collections of pus, administering IV antimicrobials, and looking for metastatic foci of infection. The peak serum antibiotic level should be documented to be eight or more times the minimal inhibitory concentration of the organism in all severe infections. Until susceptibility data are available, the choice of antibiotic for severe infections should ensure activity against all strains of *S. aureus*. A reasonable choice would be to administer vancomycin (30 mg/kg/d) in three divided doses. If the organism is found to be β-lactamase negative, therapy can be changed to penicillin G or nafcillin or continued with vancomycin if the patient is allergic to penicillin.

B. **Chorioamnionitis** occurs in approximately 1% of all pregnancies. Clinical signs include temperature more than 38°C, maternal or fetal tachycardia, and uterine tenderness with or without foul smelling amniotic fluid. Ascending infection from the maternal genital tract is the most common cause, but blood-borne spread via the placenta has also been implicated. The infection is usually polymicrobial with bacteroides, group B streptococcus and *Escherichia coli* organisms predominating. Maternal bacteremia occurs in 10% of patients.

1. **Maternal complications** include postpartum infection, sepsis, postpartum hemorrhage, and death. **Neonatal complications** include pneumonia, meningitis, sepsis, and death.

2. **Treatment** is based on antepartum antibiotic administration and results in reduced maternal and neonatal morbidity when compared with postpartum antibiotic therapy. A combination of ampicillin and gentamicin is generally effective.

C. **Pyelonephritis** is common during pregnancy. Clinical features of acute pyelonephritis include fever, rigors, flank pain, dysuria, frequency, pyuria, and leukocytosis. Bacteremia is documented in 10% to 15% of cases. Common causative organisms include *E. coli*, *Klebsiella* spp, and *Proteus* spp. Pyelonephritis is associated with an increased risk of preterm labor and delivery and pulmonary injury leading to ARDS. Excessive fluid administration and the concomitant use of tocolytics are associated with pulmonary injury. Hospitalization and IV antibiotic therapy are usually required.

XIV. Miscellaneous

   A. Local anesthetic (LA) toxicity following regional anesthesia in nonpregnant, adult patients is greatest, depending on the type of regional block performed (e.g., caudal > supraclavicular brachial plexus > interscalene brachial plexus > axillary brachial plexus > epidural).

   1. Total serum bupivacaine levels greater than 4 μg/ml and total serum lidocaine levels greater than 10 μg/ml have been associated with cardiac toxicity. The serum concentration of ropivacaine that produces toxic manifestations is similar to that of bupivacaine, but the dose required to produce these levels is 40% to 50% greater for ropivacaine, probably because of its shorter elimination half-life and faster clearance. Local anesthetic toxicity is exacerbated by hypoxia, acidosis, hyponatremia, and hyperkalemia.

   2. The pregnant patient is more susceptible to LA toxicity because of reduced levels of α_1-acid glycoprotein, which results in increased levels of free LA in the blood.

   3. Clinical features are manifested sequentially by convulsions, hypotension, apnea, and, finally, circulatory collapse. Provisions for airway management and ventilation should be available should seizures occur.

   4. Therapy. Should cardiovascular collapse occur, norepinephrine and epinephrine are the drugs indicated for resuscitation. Norepinephrine use can be associated with fewer ventricular dysrhythmias following resuscitation. Various degrees of atrioventricular conduction blockade can persist following resuscitation. If ventricular dysrhythmias or asystole persists, then give **bretylium** (350 mg IV, followed by 700 mg IV after 5 to 15 minutes). Resuscitation should be continued for at least 45 minutes following the administration of bretylium. **Phenytoin** (7 mg/kg) has been shown to be useful for the treatment of resistant ventricular dysrhythmias associated with bupivacaine toxicity in neonates. No single drug is optimal for treating the various manifestations of bupivacaine-induced cardiac toxicity. Most recommendations have been extrapolated from animal research. The optimal treatment of toxic manifestations is prevention. This can be achieved by administration of small fractionated doses and attention to the total dose administered. Toxicity appears to be additive if a combination of local anesthetics is administered.

B. **Cardiopulmonary resuscitation of the pregnant patient (Chapter 15)**

1. **Cardiac arrest** in the pregnant patient is a rare event, estimated to occur in 1 of 30,000 deliveries. The cause includes amniotic fluid embolism, pulmonary embolism, eclampsia, drug toxicity, aortic dissection, trauma, and hemorrhage. Cardiopulmonary resuscitation (CPR) should include early airway protection by endotracheal intubation.

2. **Major mechanical changes** secondary to the enlarging uterus and its contents produce alterations in cardiopulmonary physiology, with peak effects noted in the second and third trimesters. With the patient supine, the gravid uterus obstructs the inferior vena caval (IVC) return in the later stages of pregnancy, which will reduce cardiac output. The uterus may be displaced to the left, reducing the obstructive effect of the gravid uterus on the IVC, by providing 30° of left lateral tilt to the abdomen. The compressive force that can be generated on the sternum during CPR at this angle is reduced to 80% of the force generated in the supine position.

3. **Cesarean delivery of the fetus** has been recommended if CPR has not been successful within the first 4 to 5 minutes. This recommendation is based on anecdotal case reports describing successful CPR following delivery of the near term fetus. Neonatal survival following perimortem cesarean section has been quoted to be between 50% to 70%, with good neurologic outcome provided the delivery occurs within 5 minutes of maternal arrest. The lower limit of gestational age for the beneficial effect of emergent delivery of the fetus during CPR is unknown. A case of resuscitative delivery at 32 weeks' gestation has been reported.

4. **Venous access** during CPR should be placed above the diaphragm.

5. **Emergent thoracotomy and open cardiac massage** has been advocated if no response occurs during closed-chest CPR.

C. **Supine hypotensive syndrome** is caused by aortocaval compression by the gravid uterus and must be considered when caring for the pregnant patient in the intensive care setting. In the supine position, both the IVC and the aorta are compressed by the uterus. Compression of the IVC by the gravid uterus is evident as early as 13 to 16 weeks gestation. This results in reduced femoral artery pressures, increased femoral vein and IVC pressures, reduced venous return to the heart, reduced stroke volume and cardiac output, compensatory tachycardia, and hypotension (~5% of women at term experiencing bradycardia). Uterine and lower extremity blood flow decreases. Proper positioning of the pregnant patient to maintain left lateral displacement of the uterus is mandatory.

D. **Anticoagulant therapy** during pregnancy is used for the treatment of acute thromboembolic events and for prophylaxis of patients with a history of thromboembolism or thrombosis, valvular heart disease, or antiphospholipid antibody syndrome. Prospective data regarding anticoagulant therapy in pregnancy is difficult to obtain, because pregnant women are usually excluded from many prospective studies. Table 40-3 lists the recommendations of the American College of Chest Physicians (Chapters 12 and 22).

1. **Warfarin, or coumadin,** crosses the placenta and has the potential to cause both bleeding and teratogenicity in the fetus. The rate of fetal loss from coumadin use ranges from 8% to 50%. Treatment with coumadin during pregnancy is usually restricted to patients with mechanical heart valves whose fetus is between 12 and 34 weeks of gestation. The significant failure rate of heparin anticoagulation must be balanced against the risk of increased bleeding during a traumatic delivery if the mother has been anticoagulated with coumadin. The incidence of adverse outcomes is reported as 16.9% with coumadin compared with 3% with heparin. Warfarin can be given to lactating mothers, because little or none diffuses into breast milk.

2. **Heparin** is the anticoagulant of choice during pregnancy because it is a large, charged molecule and does not cross the placenta. **Heparin requirements increase** during pregnancy because of increases in heparin binding proteins, plasma volume, renal clearance, and degradation by the placenta. It is difficult, therefore, to maintain an anticoagulant effect with subcutaneous heparin administration throughout the pregnancy. Doses as high as 20,000 U every 8 hours may be necessary to maintain a therapeutic aPTT 1.5–2.5 times control. Subcutaneous administration of heparin via a programmable pump may prove beneficial, but further studies are needed.

3. **Low molecular weight heparin (LMWH)** is derived from standard heparin by either chemical or enzymatic depolymerization to yield fragments that are approximately one third the size of heparin. The dose–response relationship of LMWH has been shown to be more predictable, obviating the need to monitor anticoagulant activity. LMWH does not cross the placenta. Unfortunately, experience with the use of LMWH during pregnancy is limited.

4. **Thrombolytic therapy** during pregnancy has been relatively contraindicated because of the concerns of maternal and fetal hemorrhage, particularly at delivery or within the first 1 to 2 weeks postpartum. Streptokinase and tissue plasmino-

gen activator do not cross the placenta in animals. Although little is known about human placental transfer, they are not thought to be teratogenic. Preterm delivery and fetal loss are other concerns.

5. **The choice of anticoagulant therapy** is based on the indication.

    a. **Acute thromboembolism** requires IV heparin anticoagulation for 5 to 10 days, followed by subcutaneous heparin to prolong the aPTT at least 1.5 times control throughout the dosing interval. An alternative strategy is to aim for an aPTT peak of 2 to 2.5 times control 2 to 3 hours following heparin administration and a trough at least 10 to 15 seconds above control. Prophylaxis, should be continued for 6 weeks into the postpartum period, during which warfarin can be administered. No guidelines exist for the use of LMWH for this indication.

    b. **Prophylaxis** for patients who have had a previous thromboembolic event is generally recommended, but treatment strategies proposed by the various working groups are contradictory. Patients with risk factors (e.g., a previous deep venous thrombosis, a positive family history of thrombosis, or chronic venous insufficiency) should probably receive prophylaxis. Others can be monitored with periodic ultrasound surveillance of the deep veins. Heparin (7,500–10,000 U subcutaneously twice daily during pregnancy and continued postpartum) can be used for prophylaxis. The aPTT should be checked early in pregnancy to ensure that it is not excessively prolonged and later in pregnancy to ensure that it is sufficiently prolonged. The aPTT can become significantly prolonged at term because of reduced heparinase activity from placental aging; no guidelines exist for the use of LMWH for this indication.

    c. **Prophylaxis for patients with mechanical heart valves** can involve heparin administration throughout the pregnancy. Warfarin can be substituted during the second and third trimesters and then replaced with heparin at the time of delivery.

SELECTED REFERENCES

Anonymous. Special resuscitation situations. *Resuscitation* 1997;34: 129–149.

Barbour LA. Current concepts of anticoagulant therapy in pregnancy. *Obstet Gynecol Clin North Am* 1997;24:499–521.

Chien PFW, Khan KS, Arnott N. Magnesium sulphate in the treatment of eclampsia and pre-eclampsia: an overview of the evidence from randomised trials. *Br J Obstet Gynaecol* 1996;103:1085–1091.

Datta S. *Anesthetic and obstetric management of high-risk pregnancy,* 2nd ed. St. Louis: Mosby, 1996.

Donaldson JO. Neurologic emergencies in pregnancy. *Obstet Gynecol Clin North Am* 1991;18:199–212.

Ginsburg JS, Hirsh J. Use of antithrombotic agents during pregnancy. *Chest* 1998;115:524S–530S.

Sibai BM. Treatment of hypertension in pregnant women. *N Engl J Med* 1996;335:257–265.

Thornhill ML, Camann WR. Cardiovascular disease. In: Chestnut DH, ed. *Obstetric anesthesia: principles and practice.* St. Louis: Mosby, 1994:746–779.

Wood AJJ. Drugs in pregnancy. *N Engl J Med* 1998;338:1128–1137.

IV

Appendices

Supplemental Drug Information

Abciximab (ReoPro)

Indications: Prevents thrombus formation after percutaneous transluminal coronary angioplasty (PTCA) and after stent placement.

Dosage: Bolus (0.25 mg/kg) administered 10–60 minutes prior to PTCA.

Effect: Glycoprotein IIB/IIIA inhibitor; prevents platelet adhesion and aggregation.

Onset: Less than 10 minutes.

Duration: Platelet function usually recovers within 48 hours of discontinuation.

Clearance: Remains in circulation for 15 days or more in a platelet-bound state.

Comments: Anaphylaxis can occur; hypotension with bolus dose. Bleeding complications and thrombocytopenia are common side effects.

Acetazolamide (Diamox)

Indications: Respiratory acidosis with metabolic alkalosis; alternative antiepileptic agent; increased intraocular and intracranial pressures.

Dosage: 125–500 mg IV over 1 to 2 minutes or PO not to exceed 2 g in 24 hours.

Effect: Carbonic anhydrase inhibitor that increases the excretion of bicarbonate ions.

Onset: 2 hours (extended release tablet) or 2 minutes IV.

Duration: Extended release capsule: 18–24 hours; tablet: 8–12 hours; IV: 4–5 hours.

Clearance: 70% to 100% excreted unchanged in the urine within 24 hours.

Comments: May increase insulin requirements in diabetic patients, cause renal calculi in patients with past history of calcium stones. May cause hypokalemia, thrombocytopenia, aplastic anemia, increased urinary excretion of uric acid, and hyperglycemia. Initial dose can produce marked diuresis. Tolerance to desired effects of acetazolamide occurs in 2–3 days. Rare hypersensitivity reaction in patients with sulfa allergies.

Acyclovir (Zovirax)

Indications: Treatment of initial and prophylaxis of recurrent
                  mucosal and cutaneous **1:** herpes simplex (HSV-1
                  and HSV-2) infections, **2:** HSV encephalitis, **3:**
                  varicella zoster infections, herpes zoster, genital
                  herpes, and **4:** varicella-zoster infections in im-
                  munocompromised patients.

Dosage: Can vary with specific indication.
                  Adult **1:** IV: 750 mg/m²/d divided q8h or 15
                  mg/kg/d divided q8h for 5–10 days.
                  2: IV: 1,500 mg/m²/d divided q8h or 30 mg/kg/d di-
                  vided q8h for 10 days.
                  3: IV: 1,500 mg/m²/d divided q8h or 30 mg/kg/d di-
                  vided q8h for 5–10 days.
                  PO: 600–800 mg/dose 5 times/d for 7–10 days or
                  1,000 mg q6h for 5 days.
                  4: IV: 7.5 mg/kg/dose q8h.
                  PO: 800 mg q4h (5 times/d) for 7–10 days.
                  Pediatric **1:** IV: 750 mg/m²/d divided q8h or 15
                  mg/kg/d divided q8h for 5–10 days.
                  2: IV: 1,500 mg/m²/d divided q8h or 30 mg/kg/d di-
                  vided q8h for 10 days.
                  3: IV: 1,500 mg/m²/d divided q8h or 30 mg/kg/d di-
                  vided q8h for 5–10 days.
                  PO: 10–20 mg/kg/dose (≤ 800 mg) 4 times/d.
                  4: IV: 7.5 mg/kg/dose q8h.
                  PO: 250–600 mg/m²/dose 4–5 times/d.
                  Neonate: HSV infection: IV: 1,500 mg/m²/d divided
                  q8h or 30 mg/kg/d divided q8h for 10–14 days.

Effect: Antiviral; inhibits herpes DNA synthesis
Onset: PO: within 1.5–2 hours; IV: within 1 hour.
Duration: Half-life: neonates: 4 hours; children 1–12 years:
                  2–3 hours; adults: 3 hours.
Clearance: Primary route is the kidney (30% to 90% of a dose
                  excreted unchanged); hemodialysis removes ~ 60%
                  of the dose; removal by peritoneal dialysis is to a
                  much lesser extent.
Comments: Dosage should be reduced in patients with renal
                  impairment; use with caution in patients with pre-
                  existing renal disease or in those receiving other
                  nephrotoxic drugs concurrently; use with caution
                  in patients with underlying neurologic abnormali-
                  ties and in patients with serious renal, hepatic, or
                  electrolyte abnormalities or substantial hypoxia.

Adenosine (Adenocard)

Indications: Paroxysmal supraventricular tachycardia, Wolff-
                  Parkinson-White syndrome.

Dosage:	Adult: 6–12 mg IV bolus.
	Pediatric: 50 µg/kg IV.
Effect:	Slow or temporary cessation of AV node conduction and conduction through reentrant pathways.
Onset:	Immediate.
Duration:	< 10 seconds.
Clearance:	RBC and endothelial cell metabolism.
Comments:	The effects of adenosine are antagonized by methylxanthines such as theophylline. Adenosine is contraindicated in patients with second- or third-degree heart block or sick sinus syndrome. When large doses are given by infusion, hypotension can occur. Not effective in atrial flutter or fibrillation. Asystole for 3–6 seconds is common.

Albuterol (Proventil, Ventolin)

Indications:	Bronchospasm.
Dosage:	Aerosolized: 2.5 mg in 3 ml saline via nebulizer.
	180 or 200 µg (2 puffs) via inhaler.
	PO: 2.5 mg.
	Pediatric: 0.1 mg/kg (syrup 2 mg/5 ml).
Effect:	β_2-receptor agonist.
Onset:	Immediate.
Duration:	3–6 hours.
Clearance:	Hepatic metabolism; renal elimination.
Comments:	Possible β-adrenergic overload, tachydysrhythmias.

Aminocaproic acid (Amicar)

Indications:	Hemorrhage due to fibrinolysis.
Dosage:	5 g/100–250 ml of NSS IV to load followed by 1 g/h infusion.
Effect:	Stabilizes clot formation by inhibiting plasminogen activators and plasmin.
Clearance:	Primarily renal elimination.
Comments:	Contraindicated in disseminated intravascular coagulation.

Aminophylline (theophylline ethylenediamine)

| Indications: | Bronchospasm, infantile apneic spells. |

Dosage: Adult: LOAD: 5.0 mg/kg IV at < 25 mg/min.
MAINT: 0.5–0.7 mg/kg/h IV.
Lower dose in elderly, CHF, hepatic disease.
Pediatric: 1 month to 1 year: 0.16–0.7 mg/kg/h.
1–9 years: 0.8 mg/kg/h.

Effect: Inhibits phosphodiesterase and adenosine antagonism, resulting in bronchodilation with positive inotropic and chronotropic effects.

Onset: Rapid.

Duration: 6–12 hours.

Clearance: Hepatic metabolism, renal elimination (10% unchanged).

Comments: May cause tachydysrhythmias. Therapeutic concentration, 10–20 µg/ml. Each mg/kg raises concentration approximately 2 µg/ml. Aminophylline 100 mg = theophylline 80 mg.

Amiodarone (Cordarone)

Indications: Refractory or recurrent ventricular tachycardia or ventricular fibrillation. Supraventricular tachycardias and atrial fibrillation.

Dosage: LOAD: 800–1,600 mg/d PO × 1–3 weeks; then 600–800 mg/d PO × 4 weeks.
MAINT: 100–400 mg/d PO.
IV: 150 mg over 10 minutes (15 mg/min); 360 mg over the next 6 hours (1 mg/min); then 540 mg over the next 18 hours (0.5 mg/min).

Effect: Depresses the sinoatrial node and prolongs the PR, QRS, and QT intervals and produces α-and β-adrenergic blockade.

Onset: PO: 2 days.

Duration: Weeks to months.

Clearance: Biliary elimination.

Comments: May cause severe sinus bradycardia, ventricular dysrhythmias, AV block, liver and thyroid function test abnormalities, hepatitis, and cirrhosis. Pulmonary fibrosis can result from long-term use. Increases serum levels of digoxin, oral anticoagulants, diltiazem, quinidine, procainamide, and phenytoin.

Amrinone (Inocor)

Indication: Acute ventricular failure.

Dosage: 0.75 mg/kg IV bolus over several minutes, then infuse at 5–10 µg/kg/min; infusion mixtures (usually 100 mg in 250 ml) must not contain dextrose.

Effect:	Inhibition of phosphodiesterase increases cardiac output, contractility, and direct vasodilation.
Onset:	10 minutes.
Duration:	30 minutes to 12 hours (dose-dependent).
Clearance:	Variable hepatic metabolism; renal or fecal excretion.
Comments:	May cause hypotension, thrombocytopenia, anaphylaxis (contains sulfites).

Aprotinin (Trasylol)

Indications:	Prophylactic reduction in perioperative blood loss in patients undergoing cardiopulmonary bypass.
Dosage:	Supplied as 10,000 KIU (kallikrein inhibitor units)/ml or 1.4 mg/ml.
	Test dose (1 ml) followed by:
	LOAD: 1–2 million KIU (100–200 ml) IV over 20–30 minutes.
	"Pump Prime": 1–2 million KIU.
	MAINT: 250,000–500,000 KIU/h (25–50 ml/h).
Effect:	Protease inhibitor of trypsin, plasmin, and kallikrein; antifibrinolytic; protects glycoprotein Ib receptor on platelets during cardiopulmonary bypass.
Clearance:	Renal elimination.
Comments:	Rapid administration may cause transient hypotension and ananphylactic reaction in < 0.5% of patients.

Atenolol (Tenormin)

Indications:	Hypertension, angina, after myocardial infarction (MI).
Dosage:	PO: 50–100 mg/d.
	IV: 5 mg prn.
Effect:	β_1-selective adrenergic receptor blockade
Onset:	PO: 30–60 minutes; IV: 5 minutes.
Duration:	PO: > 24 hours; IV: 12–24 hours.
Clearance:	Renal, intestinal elimination unchanged.
Comments:	High doses block β_2-adrenergic receptors. Relatively contraindicated in CHF, asthma, and heart block. Caution in patients on calcium channel blockers. Rebound angina can occur with abrupt cessation.

Atropine

Indications:	**1:** Antisialagogue. **2:** Bradycardia.
Dosage:	Adult **1:** 0.2–0.4 mg IV. **2:** 0.4–1.0 mg IV. Pediatric **1:** 0.01 mg/kg/dose IV/IM (< 0.4 mg). **2:** 0.02 mg/kg/dose IV (< 0.4 mg).
Effect:	Competitive blockade of acetylcholine at muscarinic receptors.
Onset:	Rapid.
Duration:	Variable.
Clearance:	50%–70% hepatic metabolism, renal elimination.
Comments:	May cause tachydysrhythmias, AV dissociation, premature ventricular contractions, dry mouth, or urinary retention. CNS effects occur at high doses.

Azathioprine (Imuran)

Indications:	**1:** Adjunct to prevent rejection in allotransplantation. **2:** Rheumatoid arthritis.
Dosage:	May vary with specific indication. Adult **1:** Renal transplantation: PO, IV: 200–300 mg/d to start; maintenance dose: 50–200 mg/d. **2:** Rheumatoid arthritis: PO: 50–100 mg/d for 6–8 weeks; increase by 0.5 mg/kg q4 weeks until response or up to 200 mg/d; maintenance therapy should be the lowest effective dose. Pediatric **1:** Renal transplantation: PO, IV: 3–5 mg/kg/d to start; maintenance dose: 1–3 mg/kg/d.
Effect:	Antimetabolite, immunosupressant.
Clearance:	Extensively metabolized by hepatic xanthine oxidase to 6-mercaptopurine (active).
Comments:	Dosage should be reduced for WBC < 4,000 cells/mm^3 and/or held for WBC < 3,000 cells/mm^3. Azathioprine metabolism is competitively inhibited by allopurinol and dosage reduction is required. Use with caution in patients with liver disease, renal impairment; chronic immunosuppression increases the risk of neoplasia; a mutagenic potential exists for both men and women and with possible hematologic toxicities.

Bicarbonate, sodium (NaHCO$_3$)

Indications:	Metabolic acidosis.

Dosage: IV dose in mEq $NaHCO_3$ = [base deficit × wt (kg) × 0.3] (subsequent doses titrated against patient's pH).
Effect: H^+ neutralization.
Onset: Rapid.
Duration: Variable.
Clearance: Plasma metabolism; pulmonary, renal elimination.
Comments: May cause metabolic alkalosis, hypercarbia, hyperosmolality. Can decrease cardiac output, systemic vascular resistance, and myocardial contractility. In neonates, can cause intraventricular hemorrhage. Crosses placenta. An 8.4% solution is ~ 1.0 mEq/ml; a 4.2% solution is ~ 0.5 mEq/ml.

Bretylium (Bretylol)

Indications: Ventricular fibrillation, ventricular tachycardia.
Dosage: LOAD: 5–10 mg/kg IV in 50–100 ml of 5% D/W over 10–20 minutes; repeated once after 1–2 hours prn.
              MAINT: 5–10 mg/kg IV in 50–100 ml of 5% D/W over 10–20 minutes q6h or, preferably, as constant infusion, 1–2 mg/min.
              In life-threatening dysrhythmias may give LOAD dose q15–30 minutes prn to 30 mg/kg (undiluted).
Onset: Ventricular fibrillation: minutes.
              Ventricular tachycardia: 30–60 minutes.
Duration: 6–24 hours.
Effect: Initially, release of norepinephrine into circulation, followed by prevention of synaptic release of norepinephrine; suppression of ventricular fibrillation and ventricular dysrhythmias; increase in myocardial contractility (direct effect).
Clearance: 90% renal excretion unchanged.
Comments: May cause initial hypertension and ectopy, followed by a decrease in systemic vascular resistance with hypotension (potentiated by quinidine or procainamide), increased sensitivity to catecholamines, aggravation of digoxin-induced dysrhythmias, or drowsiness.

Bumetanide (Bumex)

Indications: Edema, hypertension, intracranial hypertension.
Dosage: 0.5–1.0 mg IV, repeated to a maximum of 10 mg/d.
Effect: Loop diuretic with principal effect on the ascending limb of the loop of Henle. Causes increased excretion of Na^+, K^+, Cl^-, and H_2O.

Onset:	Immediate, peak 15–30 minutes.
Duration:	2–4 hours.
Clearance:	Hepatic metabolism; 81% renal excretion (45% unchanged).
Comments:	May cause electrolyte imbalance, dehydration, and deafness. Patients who are allergic to sulfonamides may show hypersensitivity to bumetanide. Effective in renal insufficiency.

Calcium chloride ($CaCl_2$), Calcium gluconate (Kalcinate)

Indications:	Hypocalcemia, hyperkalemia, hypermagnesemia.
Dosage:	Calcium chloride: 5–10 mg/kg IV prn (10% $CaCl_2$ = 1.36 mEq Ca^{2+}/ml).
	Calcium gluconate: 15–30 mg/kg IV prn (10% calcium gluconate = 0.45 mEq Ca^{2+}/ml).
Effect:	Maintenance of cell membrane integrity, muscular excitation-contraction coupling, glandular stimulation-secretion coupling, and enzyme function; increases blood pressure.
Onset:	Rapid.
Duration:	Variable.
Clearance:	Incorporated into muscle, bone, and other tissues; rapid onset; variable duration.
Comments:	May cause bradycardia or dysrhythmia (especially with digitalis). Irritating to veins. Ca^{2+} less available with calcium gluconate than with calcium chloride because of the binding of gluconate.

Captopril (Capoten)

Indications:	Hypertension, CHF.
Dosage:	LOAD: 12.5–25.0 mg PO bid.
	MAINT: 25–150 mg PO bid.
Effect:	Angiotensin I-converting enzyme inhibition decreases angiotensin II and aldosterone levels; reduces both preload and afterload in patients with CHF.
Onset:	15–60 minutes, peak 60–90 minutes.
Duration:	4–6 hours.
Clearance:	Hepatic metabolism; 95% renal elimination (40% to 50% unchanged).
Comments:	Can be used in hypertensive emergency. May cause neutropenia, agranulocytosis, hypotension, or bronchospasm. Avoid in pregnant patients.

Exaggerated response in renal artery stenosis and when used with diuretics.

Cimetidine (Tagamet)

Indications:	Pulmonary aspiration prophylaxis (reduction of gastric volume and acidity), gastroesophageal reflux, gastric acid hypersecretion; anaphylaxis prophylaxis.
Dosage:	300 mg q6h IV/IM/PO (q12h in renal failure).
Effect:	Antagonism of histamine action on H_2 receptors, with inhibition of gastric acid secretion.
Onset:	45–90 minutes.
Duration:	4–5 hours.
Clearance:	Hepatic metabolism; 75% renal elimination unchanged (IV dose).
Comments:	May cause small increase in creatinine; increase in concentration of many drugs caused by inhibition of oxidative drug metabolism. Confusion or somnolence with repeated dosing. Venous irritation.

Chlorothiazide (Diuril)

Indications:	Edema, heart failure, acute or chronic renal failure, hypertension.
Dosage:	Adult: 250 to 500 mg IV bolus at 50–100 mg/min, 2,000 mg maximum over 24 hours.
Pediatric:	PO, 20 mg/kg/d in two divided doses q12h.
Effect:	Thiazide diuretic.
Onset:	2 hours.
Duration:	PO: 6–12 hours; IV: ~ 2 hours.
Clearance:	Renal elimination.
Comments:	Enhances activity of antihypertensives, digoxin. May enhance activity of loop diuretics in renal failure. May increase insulin requirements in diabetic patients.

Citrate, sodium dihydrate/citric acid monohydrate (Bicitra)

Indications:	Gastric acid neutralization.

Dosage:	15 ml in 15 ml water PO (500 mg sodium citrate; citric acid 334 mg/5 ml).
Effect:	Absorbed and metabolized to sodium bicarbonate.
Clearance:	Oxidation; 5% excreted in urine unchanged.
Comments:	Contraindicated in patients with sodium restriction or severe renal impairment. Do not use with aluminum-based antacids.

Clonidine (Catapres)

Indications:	Hypertension.
Dosage:	0.1–1.2 mg/d PO in divided doses (2.4 mg/d maximum dose); also available as a transdermal patch delivering 0.1, 0.2, or 0.3 mg/d for 7 days.
Effect:	Central α_2-adrenergic agonist, resulting in decrease in systemic vascular resistance and heart rate.
Onset:	30–60 minutes; peak 2–4 hours.
Duration:	8 hours.
Clearance:	50% hepatic metabolism; elimination 20% biliary, 80% renal.
Comments:	Abrupt withdrawal may cause rebound hypertension or dysrhythmias. Can cause drowsiness, nightmares, restlessness, anxiety, or depression. Intravenous injection may cause transient peripheral α-adrenergic stimulation.

Dantrolene (Dantrium)

Indications:	Malignant hyperthermia (MH), skeletal muscle spasticity.
Dosage:	Prophylactic IV treatment is generally not recommended. If signs of MH syndrome develop: 3 mg/kg IV bolus; if syndrome persists after 30 minutes, repeat dose, up to 10 mg/kg.
Effect:	Reduction of Ca^{2+} release from sarcoplasmic reticulum.
Onset:	30 minutes.
Duration:	8 hours.
Clearance:	Hepatic metabolism; renal elimination.
Comments:	Mix 20 mg in 60 ml of sterile water. Dissolves slowly into solution. Can cause muscle weakness, gastrointestinal (GI) upset, drowsiness, sedation, or abnormal liver function (chronically). Additive effect with neuromuscular blocking agents. Tissue irritant.

Desmopressin acetate (DDAVP)

Indications:	**1:** Coagulation improvement in von Willebrand's disease, hemophilia A, renal failure. **2:** Antidiuretic.
Dosage:	Adult **1:** 0.3 μg/kg IV (diluted 50 ml NSS), infused over 15–30 minutes. **2:** 2–4 μg/d usually in two divided doses. Pediatric **1:** < 10 kg: dilute adult dose in 10 ml NSS. > 10 kg: see adult dose.
Onset:	Minutes; peak 15–30 minutes.
Duration:	3 hours for von Willebrand's disease; 4–24 hours for hemophilia A.
Effect:	Increases plasma levels of factor VIII activity by causing release of von Willebrand's factor from endothelial cells; increases renal water reabsorption.
Clearance:	Renal elimination.
Comments:	Chlorpropamide, carbamazepine, and clofibrate potentiate the antidiuretic effect. Repeat doses every 12–24 hours will have diminished effect compared with initial dose.

Dexamethasone (Decadron)

Indications:	Cerebral edema from CNS tumors; airway edema.
Dosage:	LOAD: 10 mg IV. MAINT: 4 mg IV q6h (tapered over 6 days).
Onset:	Minutes IV.
Duration:	4–6 hours IV.
Effect:	See hydrocortisone. Has 25 times the glucocorticoid potency of hydrocortisone; minimal mineralocorticoid effect.
Clearance:	Primarily hepatic metabolism; renal elimination.
Comments:	See hydrocortisone.

Dextran 40 (Rheomacrodex)

Indications:	Inhibition of platelet aggregation; improvement of blood flow in low-flow states (e.g., vascular surgery); intravascular volume expander.
Dosage:	Adult: LOAD: 30–50 ml IV over 30 minutes. MAINT: 15–30 ml/h IV (10% solution). Pediatric: < 20 ml/kg/24 h of 10% dextran.
Effect:	Immediate, short-lived plasma volume expansion; adsorption to RBC surface preventing RBC aggre-

gation and decreasing blood viscosity and platelet adhesiveness.

Onset:	Rapid.
Duration:	4–8 hours.
Clearance:	100% renal elimination.
Comments:	Administer Promit (dextran monomer), 20 ml IV, prior to giving dextran 40 to minimize the risk of anaphylaxis. May cause volume overload, anaphylaxis, bleeding tendency, interference with blood cross-matching, or false elevation of blood sugar. Can cause renal failure.

Digoxin (Lanoxin)

Indications:	Heart failure, tachydysrhythmias, atrial fibrillation, atrial flutter.
Dosage:	Adult: LOAD: 0.5–1.0 mg/d IV or PO in divided doses. MAINT: 0.125–0.5 mg IV or PO every day. Pediatric (IV/IM in divided doses): LOAD: Total daily doses usually divided into two or more doses. Neonates: 15–30 µg/kg/d. 1 month to 2 years: 30–50 µg/kg/d. 2–5 years: 25–35 µg/kg/d. 5–10 years: 15–30 µg/kg/d. > 10 years: 8–12 µg/kg/d. MAINT: 20%–35% of LOAD every day (reduce in renal failure).
Effect:	Increase in myocardial contractility; decrease in conduction in AV node and Purkinje fibers.
Onset:	15–30 minutes.
Duration:	2–6 days.
Clearance:	Renal elimination (50%–70% unchanged).
Comments:	May cause GI intolerance, blurred vision, ECG changes, or dysrhythmias. Toxicity potentiated by hypokalemia, hypomagnesemia, hypercalcemia. Cautious use in Wolff-Parkinson-White syndrome and with defibrillation. Heart block potentiated by β-blockade and calcium channel blockade.

Diltiazem (Cardizem)

Indications:	Angina pectoris, variant angina from coronary artery spasm, atrial fibrillation or flutter, paroxysmal supraventricular tachycardia, hypertension.
Dosage:	PO: 30–60 mg q6h. IV: 20 mg bolus then 10 mg/h infusion.

Effect:	Calcium channel antagonist that slows conduction through sinoatrial and AV nodes, dilates coronary and peripheral arterioles, and reduces myocardial contractility.
Onset:	PO: 1–3 hours, IV: 1–3 minutes.
Duration:	PO: 4–24 hours, IV: 1–3 hours.
Clearance:	Primarily hepatic metabolism; renal elimination.
Comments:	May cause bradycardia and heart block. May interact with β-blockers and digoxin to impair contractility. Causes transiently elevated liver function tests. Avoid use in patients with accessory tracts, AV block, IV β-blockers, or ventricular tachycardia. Active metabolite one fourth to one half coronary dilation effect.

Diphenhydramine (Benadryl)

Indications:	Allergic reactions, drug-induced extrapyramidal reactions, sedation.
Dosage:	Adult: 10–50 mg IV q6–8h. Pediatric: 5.0 mg/kg/d IV in four divided doses (maximum 300 mg)
Effect:	Antagonism of histamine action on H_1 receptors; anticholinergic; CNS depression.
Onset:	Rapid.
Duration:	4–6 hours.
Clearance:	Hepatic metabolism; renal excretion.
Comments:	May cause hypotension, tachycardia, dizziness, urinary retention.

Dobutamine (Dobutrex)

Indications:	Heart failure, hypotension.
Dosage:	Infusion mix: 250 mg in 250 ml of 5% D/W or NSS. Start infusion at 2 µg/kg/min. 5–20 µg/kg/min titrated to effect.
Effect:	1–2 minutes.
Onset:	Rapid.
Duration:	< 5 minutes.
Clearance:	Hepatic metabolism; renal elimination.
Comments:	May cause hypertension, dysrhythmias, or myocardial ischemia. Can increase ventricular rate in atrial fibrillation.

Dopamine (Intropin)

Indications:	**1:** Hypotension, heart failure.
	2: Oliguria.
Dosage:	Infusion mix: 200–800 mg in 250 ml of 5% D/W or NSS.
	1: Infusion at 5–20 µg/kg/min IV titrated to effect.
	2: Infusion at 1–3 µg/kg/min IV.
Effect:	Dopaminergic, α- and β-adrenergic agonist.
Onset:	5 minutes.
Duration:	< 10 minutes.
Clearance:	MAO/COMT metabolism.
Comments:	May cause hypertension, dysrhythmias, or myocardial ischemia. Primarily dopaminergic effects (increased renal blood flow) at 1–5 µg/kg/min. Primarily α- and β-adrenergic effects at ≥ 10 µg/kg/min.

Doxazosin (Cardura)

Indications:	Hypertension.
Dosage:	Starting 1 mg PO every day, may be slowly increased (over weeks) to 4 to 16 mg PO every day, depending on the individual patient's response.
Effect:	α_1 (postjunctional) adrenergic antagonist.
Onset:	Within 1–2 hours.
Duration:	1 day.
Clearance:	Hepatic metabolism predominates.
Comments:	Significant "first-dose" effect with marked postural hypotension and dizziness. Maximal reductions of blood pressure with 2 to 6 hours of dosing.

Droperidol (Inapsine)

Indications:	**1:** Nausea, vomiting.
	2: Agitation, sedation, adjunct to anesthesia.
Dosage:	Adult **1:** 0.625–2.5 mg IV prn.
	2: 2.5–10 mg IV prn.
	Pediatric **1:** 0.05–0.06 mg/kg q4–6h.
Effect:	Dopamine (D_2) receptor antagonist. Apparent psychic indifference to environment, catatonia, antipsychotic, antiemetic.
Onset:	3–10 minutes.
Duration:	3–6 hours.

Clearance: Hepatic metabolism; renal excretion.
Comments: May cause anxiety, extrapyramidal reactions, or hypotension (from moderate α-adrenergic and dopaminergic antagonism). Residual effects can persist ≥ 24 hours. Potentiates other CNS depressants.

Enalapril/Enalaprilat (Vasotec)

Indications: Hypertension, CHF.
Dosage: PO: LOAD: 2.5–5.0 mg every day.
              MAINT: 10–40 mg every day.
              IV: 0.125–5.0 mg q6h (as enalaprilat).
Effect: Angiotensin-converting enzyme inhibitor; synergistic with diuretics.
Onset: 1 hour.
Duration: 6–24 hours.
Clearance: Hepatic metabolism of enalapril to active metabolite (enalaprilat); renal or fecal elimination.
Comments: Causes increased serum potassium, increased renal blood flow, volume-responsive hypotension. Subsequent doses are additive in effect. Can cause angioedema, blood dyscrasia, cough, lithium toxicity, or worsening of renal impairment.

Ephedrine

Indication: Hypotension.
Dosage: 5–50 mg IV prn.
Effect: α- and β-adrenergic stimulation; norepinephrine release at sympathetic nerve endings.
Onset: Rapid.
Duration: 1 hour.
Clearance: Mostly renal elimination, unchanged.
Comments: May cause hypertension, dysrhythmias, myocardial ischemia, CNS stimulation, decrease in uterine activity or mild bronchodilation. Avoid giving to patients taking MAO inhibitors. Minimal effect on uterine blood flow. Tachyphylaxis with repeated dosing.

Epinephrine (Adrenalin)

Indications: **1:** Heart failure, hypotension, cardiac arrest.
2: Bronchospasm, anaphylaxis.
Dosage: Infusion mix: 1 mg in 250 ml of 5% D/W or NSS.
Adult **1:** 0.1–1 mg IV or intracardiac q5min prn or
1 mg intratracheal.
2: 0.1–0.5 mg SC; 0.l–0.25 mg IV; or 0.25–1.5
µg/min IV infusion.
Pediatric **1:** Neonates: 0.01–0.03 mg/kg q 3–5 min-
utes.
Children: 0.01 mg/kg IV or intratracheal q3–5 min.
(Up to 5 ml 1:10,000 solution.)
2: 0.01 mg/kg IV up to 0.5 mg.
0.01 mg/kg SC q 15 min × 2 doses; up to 1 mg/dose.
Onset: Rapid.
Duration: 1–2 minutes.
Effect: α- and β-adrenergic agonist.
Clearance: MAO/COMT metabolism.
Comments: May cause hypertension, dysrhythmias, or
myocardial ischemia. Topical or local injection
(1:80,000–1:500,000) causes vasoconstriction.
Crosses the placenta.

Epinephrine, racemic (Vaponefrin)

Indications: Airway edema, bronchospasm.
Dosage: Adult: Inhaled via nebulizer: 0.5 ml of 2.25% solu-
tion in 2.5–3.5 ml of NSS q1–4h prn.
Pediatric: Inhaled via nebulizer: 0.5 ml of 2.25% so-
lution in 2.5–3.5 ml of NSS q4h prn.
Effect: Mucosal vasoconstriction (see also epinephrine).
Comments: See epinephrine.
Clearance: See epinephrine.

Ergonovine (Ergotrate)

Indication: Postpartum hemorrhage due to uterine atony.
Dosage: IV: (emergency only): 0.2 mg in 5 ml of NSS over ≥
1 minute.
IM: 0.2 mg q2–4h prn for < 5 doses.
Then PO: 0.2–0.4 mg q6–12h × 2 days or prn.

Effect:	Constriction of uterine and vascular smooth muscle.
Onset:	PO 6–15 minutes; IM 2–3 minutes; IV 1 minute.
Duration:	PO/IM 3 hours; IV 45 minutes.
Clearance:	Hepatic metabolism; renal elimination.
Comments:	May cause hypertension from systemic vasoconstriction (especially in eclampsia and hypertension), dysrhythmias, coronary spasm, uterine tetany, or GI upset. Intravenous route is only used in emergencies. Overdosage may cause convulsions or stroke.

Esmolol (Brevibloc)

Indications:	Supraventricular tachydysrhythmias, myocardial ischemia.
Dosage:	Start with 5 to 10 mg IV bolus and increase every 3 minutes prn to total 100–300 mg; infusion 1–15 mg/min.
Effect:	Selective β_1-adrenergic blockade.
Onset:	Rapid.
Duration:	10–20 minutes following discontinuation.
Clearance:	Degraded by RBC esterases; renal elimination.
Comments:	May cause bradycardia, AV conduction delay, hypotension, CHF; β_2 activity at high doses.

Ethacrynic acid (Edecrin)

Indications:	Edema, CHF, acute or chronic renal failure.
Dosage:	Adult: PO: 50–200 mg/d in 1–2 divided doses. IV: 25–100 mg IV over 5–10 minutes; 24-hour cumulative dose: 400 mg. Pediatric: PO: 25 mg/d to start, increase by 25 mg/d until response is obtained; maximum: 3 mg/kg/d. IV: 1 mg/kg/dose; repeat doses with caution because of potential for ototoxicity.
Effect:	Diuretic.
Onset:	PO: within 30 minutes; IV: 5 minutes.
Duration:	PO: 12 hours; IV: 2 hours.
Clearance:	Hepatically metabolized to active cysteine conjugate (35% to 40%); 30% to 60% excreted unchanged in bile and urine.
Comments:	May potentiate the activity of antihypertensives, neuromuscular blocking agents, and digoxin, and increase insulin requirements in diabetic patients.

Famotidine (Pepcid)

Indications:	Pulmonary aspiration prophylaxis, peptic ulcer disease.
Dosage:	20 mg IV/PO q12h (dilute in 1–10 ml of 5% D/W or NSS).
Effect:	Antagonism of histamine action on H_2 receptors.
Onset:	1 hour.
Duration:	8–12 hours.
Clearance:	30%–35% hepatic metabolism; 65%–70% renal elimination.
Comments:	May cause confusion. Rapid IV administration may increase risk of cardiac dysrythmias and hypotension.

Flumazenil (Romazicon)

Indication:	**1:** Reversal of benzodiazepine sedation. **2:** Benzodiazepine overdose.
Dosage:	**1:** 0.2–1.0 mg IV every 20 minutes at 0.2 mg/min. **2:** 3–5 mg IV at 0.5 mg/min.
Effect:	Competitive antagonism of CNS benzodiazepine receptor.
Onset:	1–2 minutes.
Duration:	1–2 hours (dose-dependent).
Clearance:	100% hepatic metabolism; 90% to 95% renal elimination of metabolite.
Comments:	Duration of action dependent on dose and duration of action of administered benzodiazepine and on dose of flumazenil. May induce CNS excitation including seizures, acute withdrawal, nausea, dizziness, agitation. Does not reverse non–benzodiazepine-induced CNS depression.

Folic acid (Folacin; Folate)

Indications:	Megaloblastic and macrocytic anemias.
Dosage:	Adult: PO, IM, IV, SC: initial dose: 1 mg/d. MAINT: 0.5 mg/d; pregnant and lactating women: 0.8 mg/d. Pediatric: PO, IM, IV, SC: initial dose: 1 mg/d. MAINT: 1–10 years: 0.1–0.3 mg/d. Infants: 15 µg/kg/d or 50 µg/d.
Effect:	Vitamin B complex substrate.

Onset: Within 0.5–1 hour.
Clearance: Enterohepatic recirculation.
Comments: Folic acid may alleviate the hematologic compli-
              cations of pernicious anemia while allowing neu-
              rologic sequelae to occur. Therefore, it should be
              administered with extreme caution to patients
              with undiagnosed anemia. May produce allergic
              reactions.

Furosemide (Lasix)

Indications: Edema, hypertension, intracranial hypertension,
              renal failure, hypercalcemia.
Dosage: Adult: 2–40 mg IV (initial dose, dosage individual-
              ized).
              Pediatric: 1–2 mg/kg/d.
Effect: Increase in excretion of Na^+, Cl^-, K^+, PO_4^{3-}, Ca^{2+},
              and H_2O by inhibiting reabsorption in loop of
              Henle.
Onset: 5 minutes.
Duration: 2 hours.
Clearance: Hepatic metabolism; 88% renal elimination.
Comments: May cause electrolyte imbalance, dehydration,
              transient hypotension, deafness, hyperglycemia, or
              hyperuricemia. Sulfa-allergic patients may exhibit
              hypersensitivity to furosemide.

Ganciclovir (Cytovene)

Indications: Treatment of cytomegalovirus (CMV) retinitis in
              immunocompromised individuals; treatment of
              CMV colitis and pneumonitis.
Dosage: Adult and pediatric: Initial: 5 mg/kg q12h for 14–
              21 days followed by 5 mg/kg/d as a single dose for
              the duration of patient's immunosuppression; ad-
              just dose for renal impairment.
Effect: Antiviral.
Onset: Oral absorption increased with food.
Duration: Half-life: 1.7–5.8 hours; increases with impaired
              renal function.
Clearance: Most (94% to 99%) excreted as unchanged drug in
              the urine.
Comments: Dosage adjustment or interruption of ganciclovir
              therapy may be necessary in patients with neu-
              tropenia or thrombocytopenia and patients with
              impaired renal function.

Filgrastim (G-CSF, granulocyte-colony stimulating factor, neupogen)

Indications: Neutropenia secondary to immunosuppressive drug therapy.

Dosage: Adult and pediatric: Initial dosing recommendations: 5 µg/kg/d administered SC or IV; doses can be increased in increments of 5 µg/kg as titrated to patient response, according to the duration and severity of the absolute neutrophil count (ANC) nadir.

Effect: Promotes neutrophil production.

Onset: Rapid elevation in neutrophil counts within the first 24 hours, reaching a plateau in 3–5 days.

Duration: ANC decreases by 50% within 2 days after discontinuing G-CSF; white counts return to the normal range in 4–7 days.

Clearance: Systemically metabolized.

Comments: Filgrastim dosage should be adjusted to coincide with available single use containers (300 µg, 480 µg) wherever possible.

Glucagon

Indications: **1:** Duodenal or choledochal relaxation. **2:** Refractory beta blocker toxicity

Dosage: **1:** 0.25–0.5 mg IV q20min prn. **2:** 5 mg IV bolus, then 1–5 mg/hr titrated to patient response.

Effect: Catecholamine release. Positive inotrope and chronotrope.

Onset: 45 seconds.

Duration: 9–25 minutes (dose-dependent).

Clearance: Hepatic and renal proteolysis.

Comments: May cause anaphylaxis, nausea, vomiting, hyperglycemia, or positive inotropic and chronotropic effects. High doses potentiate oral anticoagulants. Use with caution in presence of insulinoma or pheochromocytoma.

Glycopyrrolate (Robinul)

Indications: **1:** Decrease GI motility, antisialagogue.
2: Bradycardia.

Dosage: Adult: **1:** IV/IM/SC: 0.1–0.2 mg; PO: 1–2 mg.
2: 0.1–0.2 mg/dose IV.
Pediatric: 0.004–0.008 mg/kg IV/IM up to 0.1 mg.

Effect: See atropine.
Onset: IV: 1–4 minutes; IM: 30–45 minutes.
Duration: IV: 2–4 hours; IM: 2–7 hours.
Clearance: Renal elimination.
Comments: See atropine. Does not cross blood–brain barrier or placenta. Better antisialagogue with less chronotropy than atropine. Erratic oral absorption.

Haloperidol (Haldol)

Indications: Psychosis, agitation.
Dosage: 0.5–2 mg IV prn (dosage highly individualized).
Effect: Antipsychotic effects due to dopamine (D_2) receptor antagonism; CNS depression.
Onset: IV peak effect < 20 minutes.
Duration: IV half-life 14 hours.
Clearance: Hepatic metabolism; renal or biliary elimination.
Comments: May cause extrapyramidal reactions or very mild α-adrenergic antagonism. Can precipitate neuroleptic malignant syndrome. Contraindicated in Parkinson's disease, toxic CNS depression, and coma.

Heparin (Lipo-Hepin, Liquaemin Sodium, Panheprin)

Indications: **1:** Anticoagulation for thrombosis, thromboembolism.
               2: Cardiopulmonary bypass.
               3: Disseminated intravascular coagulation.
               4: Thromboembolism prophylaxis.
Dosage: Adult: **1:** LOAD: 75 U/kg IV.
               MAINT: 18 U/kg/h IV; titrate dosage with partial thromboplastin time or activated clotting time.
               2: LOAD: 300 U/kg IV.
               MAINT: 100 U/kg/h IV; titrate with coagulation tests.
               3: LOAD: 50–100 U/kg IV.
               Pediatric: LOAD: 50 U/kg IV.
               MAINT: 15–25 U/kg/h IV; titrate with coagulation tests.
               4: 5000 units q 8–12 h SC.
Effect: Potentiates action of antithrombin III; blockade of conversion of prothrombin and activation of other coagulation factors.

Onset:	IV immediate; SC 1–2 hours.
Duration:	Half-life 1–6 hours; increases with dose.
Clearance:	Primarily by reticuloendothelial uptake, hepatic biotransformation.
Comments:	May cause bleeding, thrombocytopenia, allergic reactions, or diuresis (36–48 hours after a large dose). Half-life increased in renal failure and decreased in thromboembolism and liver disease. Does not cross the placenta. Reversed by protamine.

Hydralazine (Apresoline)

Indication:	Hypertension.
Dosage:	2.5–20.0 mg IV q4h or prn (dosage individualized).
Effect:	Relaxation of vascular smooth muscle (arteriole > venule).
Onset:	5–20 min, peak effect 10–80 minutes.
Duration:	2–6 hours.
Clearance:	Extensive hepatic metabolism; renal elimination.
Comments:	May cause hypotension (diastolic > systolic), reflex tachycardia, systemic lupus erythematosus syndrome. Increases coronary, splanchnic, cerebral, and renal blood flows.

Hydrocortisone (Solu-Cortef)

Indications:	Adrenal insufficiency, inflammation cerebral edema from CNS tumors, asthma.
Dosage:	10–100 mg IV q8h Physiologic replacement: IV: 0.25–0.35 mg/kg/day PO: 0.5–0.75 mg/kg/day
Effect:	Antiinflammatory and antiallergic effect; mineralocorticoid effect; stimulation of gluconeogenesis; inhibition of peripheral protein synthesis; membrane stabilizing effect.
Onset:	1 hour.
Duration:	6–8 hours (dose- or route-dependent).
Clearance:	Hepatic metabolism; renal elimination.
Comments:	May cause adrenocortical insufficiency (Addison's crisis) with abrupt withdrawal, delayed wound healing, CNS disturbances, osteoporosis, or electrolyte disturbances.

Hydroxyzine (Vistaril, Atarax)

Indications: Anxiety, nausea and vomiting, allergies, sedation.
Dosage: PO: 25–200 mg q6–8h.
               IM: 25–100 mg q4–6h.
               Not an IV drug.
Effect: Antagonism of histamine action on H_1 receptors, CNS depression, antiemetic.
Onset: 15–60 minutes.
Duration: 4–6 hours.
Clearance: Hepatic (P-450) metabolism; renal elimination.
Comments: May cause dry mouth. Minimal cardiorespiratory depression. Intravenous injection may cause thrombosis. Crosses the placenta.

Indocyanine green (Cardio-Green)

Indications: Cardiac output measurement by indicator dye dilution.
Dosage: 5 mg IV (diluted in 1 ml of normal saline) rapidly injected into central circulation.
Effect: Almost complete binding to plasma protein with distribution within plasma volume.
Onset: Immediate.
Duration: Minutes.
Clearance: Hepatic elimination.
Comments: May cause allergic reactions or transient increase in bilirubin. Absorption spectra changed by heparin. Cautious use in patients with iodine allergy (contains 5% sodium iodide).

Insulin

Indications: **1:** Hyperglycemia.
               2: Diabetic ketoacidosis.
Dosage: **1:** Individualized: usually 5–10 U IV/SC prn (regular insulin).
               2: LOAD: 10–20 U IV (regular insulin).
               MAINT: 0.05–0.1 U/kg/h IV (regular insulin), titrated against plasma glucose level.
Effect: Facilitation of glucose transport intracellularly; shift of K^+ and Mg^{2+} intracellular.
Onset: SC: regular: 30 minutes; Semilente: 30 minutes; NPH: 1–2 hours; Lente: 1–4 hours; PZI: 4–6 hours; Ultralente: 4–6 hours.

Duration: SC: Regular 5–7 hours; Semilente: 12–16 hours; NPH: 18–24 hours; Lente: 18–28 hours; PZI: 24–36 hours; Ultralente: 30–36 hours.

Clearance: Hepatic and renal metabolism; 30% to 80% renal elimination; unchanged insulin is reabsorbed.

Comments: May cause hypoglycemia, allergic reactions, or synthesis of insulin antibodies. May be absorbed by plastic in IV tubing. When initiating insulin therapy, use Humulin rather than beef or pork insulin to minimize the development of antibodies.

Isoproterenol (Isuprel)

Indications: Heart failure, bradycardia.
Dosage: Adult: 2 μg/min titrated up to 10 μg/min IV.
Pediatric: Start at 0.1 μg/kg/min; titrate to effect.
Effect: β-adrenergic agonist; chronotropy, inotropy.
Onset: Immediate.
Duration: 1 hour.
Clearance: Hepatic and pulmonary metabolism; 40% to 50% renal excretion unchanged.
Comments: May cause dysrhythmias, myocardial ischemia, hypertension, or CNS excitation.

Isordil (Isosorbide dinitrate)

Indications: Angina, hypertension, MI, CHF.
Dosage: 5–20 mg PO q6h.
Effect: See nitroglycerin.
Onset: 15–40 minutes.
Duration: 4–6 hours.
Clearance: Nearly 100% hepatic metabolism; renal elimination.
Comments: See nitroglycerin. Tolerance may develop.

Ketorolac (Toradol)

Indications: Nonsteroidal, antiinflammatory analgesic (NSAID) for moderate pain; useful adjunct for severe pain when used with parenteral or epidural opioids.
Dosage: PO: 10 mg q4–6h.
               IM/IV: 30–60 mg, then 15–30 mg q6h.

Effect: Limits prostaglandin synthesis by cyclooxygenase inhibition.
Onset: 30–60 minutes.
Duration: 4–6 hours.
Clearance: < 50% hepatic metabolism; renal metabolism; 91% renal elimination.
Comments: Adverse effects are similar to those with other NSAIDs: peptic ulceration, bleeding, decreased renal blood flow. Duration of treatment not to exceed 5 days.

Labetalol (Normodyne, Trandate)

Indications: Hypertension, angina, (controlled hypotension).
Dosage: IV: increments of 5–10 mg at 5-minute intervals, to 40–80 mg/dose.
                Infusion: 5 mg/ml mix; start at 0.05 µg/kg/min.
Effect: Selective α_1-adrenergic blockade with nonselective β-adrenergic blockade; ratio of α/β blockade = 1 : 7.
Onset: Minutes.
Duration: 2–12 hours.
Clearance: Hepatic metabolism; renal elimination.
Comments: May cause bradycardia, AV conduction delays, bronchospasm in asthmatics, and postural hypotension. Crosses the placenta.

Levothyroxine (Synthroid)

Indications: Hypothyroidism.
Dosage: Adjust according to individual requirements and response.
                Pediatric, PO:
                0–6 months: 25–50 µg/d or 8–10 µg/kg/d.
                6–12 months: 50–75 µg/d or 6–8 µg/kg/d.
                1–5 years: 75–100 µg/d or 5–6 µg/kg/d.
                6–12 years: 100–150 µg/d or 4–5 µg/kg/d.
                > 12 years: > 150 µg/d or 2–3 µg/kg/d.
                IV: 75% of oral dose.
                Adults, PO:
                0.1–0.2 mg/d.
                IV: 75% of adult oral dose.
Effect: Exogenous thyroxine.
Onset: PO: 3–5 days; IV within 6–8 hours.
Duration: Peak effect at ~ 24 hours.
Clearance: Metabolized in the liver to triiodothyronine (active); eliminated in feces and urine.

Comments: Contraindicated with recent MI or thyrotoxicosis, or uncorrected adrenal insufficiency. Phenytoin may decrease levothyroxine levels. Increases effects of oral anticoagulants. Tricyclic antidepressants may increase toxic potential of both drugs. Intravenous therapy can be given at 75% of the oral dose.

Lidocaine (Xylocaine)

Indications: **1:** Ventricular dysrhythmias.
2: Cough suppression.
3: Local anesthesia.

Dosage: Adult **1:** LOAD: 1 mg/kg IV × 2 (2nd dose 20–30 minutes after 1st dose).
MAINT: 15–50 µg/kg/min IV (1–4 mg/min).
2: 1 mg/kg IV.
3: 5 mg/kg maximal dose for infiltration or conduction block.
Pediatric **1:** LOAD: 0.5–1 mg/kg IV (2nd dose 20–30 minutes after 1st dose).
MAINT: 15–50 µg/kg/min IV.

Effect: Antidysrhythmic effect; sedation; neural blockade; decrease conductance of sodium channels.

Onset: Rapid.

Duration: 5–20 minutes.

Clearance: Hepatic metabolism to active or toxic metabolites; renal elimination (10% unchanged).

Comments: May cause dizziness, seizures, disorientation, heart block (with myocardial conduction defect), or hypotension. Crosses the placenta. Therapeutic concentration = 1–5 mg/L. Avoid in patients with Wolff-Parkinson-White syndrome.

Magnesium sulfate

Indications: **1:** Preeclampsia or eclampsia.
2: Hypomagnesemia.
3: Polymorphic ventricular tachycardia (torsades de pointes).

Dosage: Adult **1:** LOAD: 1–4 g (32 mEq) IV (10 or 20% solution).
MAINT: 1–3 ml/min (4 g/250 ml of 5% D/W or NSS).
2: 1 g (8 mEq) q6h × 4 doses.

3: 1–2 g in 10 ml 5% dextrose in water (5% D/W) over 1–2 minutes; 5–10 g may be administered for refractory dysrhythmias.

Effect:	To replete serum magnesium; for the prevention and treatment of seizures or hyperreflexia associated with preeclampsia or eclampsia.
Onset:	Rapid.
Duration:	4–6 hours.
Clearance:	100% renal elimination for IV route.
Comments:	Potentiates neuromuscular blockade (both depolarizing and nondepolarizing agents). Potentiates CNS effects of anesthetics, hypnotics, and opioids. Toxicity occurs with serum concentration ≥ 10 mEq/L. Avoid in patients with heart block. May alter cardiac conduction in digitalized patients. Caution in patients with renal failure.

Mannitol (Osmitrol)

Indications:	**1:** Increased intracranial pressure. **2:** Oliguria, or anuria associated with acute renal injury.
Dosage:	Adult **1:** 0.25–1.0 g/kg IV as 20% solution over 30–60 minutes (in acute situation; can give bolus of 12.5–25.0 g over 5–10 minutes). **2:** 0.2 g/kg test dose over 3–5 minutes, then 50–100 g IV over 30 minutes if adequate response. Pediatric **1:** 0.2 g/kg test dose, with maintenance of 2 g/kg over 30–60 minutes.
Effect:	Increase in serum osmolality, which reduces cerebral edema and lowers intracranial and intraocular pressure; also causes osmotic diuresis and transient expansion of intravascular volume.
Onset:	15 minutes.
Duration:	2–3 hours.
Clearance:	Renal elimination; onset 15 minutes; duration 2–3 hours.
Comments:	Rapid administration can cause vasodilation and hypotension. May worsen or cause pulmonary edema, intracranial hemorrhage, systemic hypertension, or rebound intracranial hypertension.

Metaproterenol (Alupent)

Indication:	Bronchospasm.
Dosage:	Inhaled (metered aerosol): 2–3 puffs (0.65 mg/puff) q3–4h prn (maximum 12 puffs/d).

Inhaled intermittent positive-pressure breathing: 0.2–0.3 ml of 5% solution in 2.5 ml of NSS q4h.

Effect: β-adrenergic stimulation (mostly β_2), resulting in bronchodilation.

Onset: 1–10 minutes.

Duration: 1–5 hours.

Clearance: Hepatic or intestinal metabolism; renal elimination.

Comments: May cause dysrhythmias, hypertension, CNS stimulation, nausea, vomiting, or inhibition of uterine contractions. Tachyphylaxis can occur.

Methylene blue (methylthionine chloride, Urolene Blue)

Indications: **1:** Surgical marker for genitourinary surgery.
2: Methemoglobinemia.

Dosage: **1:** 100 mg (10 ml of 1% solution) IV.
2: 1–2 mg/kg IV of 1% solution over 10 minutes; repeat q1h prn.

Effect: Low dose promotes conversion of methemoglobin to hemoglobin; high dose promotes conversion of hemoglobin to methemoglobin; less useful than sodium nitrate and amyl nitrite.

Onset: Immediate.

Clearance: Tissue reduction; urinary and biliary elimination.

Comments: May cause RBC destruction (prolonged use), hypertension, bladder irritation, nausea, diaphoresis. May inhibit nitrate-induced coronary artery relaxation. Interferes with pulse oximetry for 1–2 minutes. Can cause hemolysis in patients with glucose 6 phosphate dehydrogenase deficiency.

Methylergonovine (Methergine)

Indication: Postpartum hemorrhage.

Dosage: IV (EMERGENCY ONLY, after delivery of placenta): 0.2 mg in 5 ml of NSS/dose over ≥ 1 minute.
IM: 0.2 mg q2–4h prn (< 5 doses).
PO (after IM or IV doses): 0.2–0.4 mg q6–12h × 2–7 days.

Onset: IV, immediate.
IM, 2–5 minutes (maximal response after 30 minutes).
PO, 5–10 minutes.

Duration: 1–3 hours.

Clearance: Hepatic metabolism; renal elimination.
Comments: See ergonovine. Hypertensive response less marked than with ergonovine.

Methylprednisolone (Solu-Medrol)

Indications: See hydrocortisone. Spinal cord injury.
Dosage: Adult: 40–60 mg IV q6h. Higher doses in transplant patients.
              Pediatric: 0.16–0.8 mg/kg/day.
              Status asthmaticus: LOAD: 2 mg/kg.
              MAINT: 0.5–1 mg/kg q6h.
              Spinal cord injury: LOAD: 30 mg/kg IV over 15 min; after 45 min begin MAINT: 5.4 mg/kg/hr × 23 or 47h.
Effect: See hydrocortisone; has five times the glucocorticoid potency of hydrocortisone; almost no mineralocorticoid activity.
Onset: Minutes.
Duration: 6 hours.
Clearance: Hepatic metabolism; renal elimination (dose- or route-dependent).
Comments: See hydrocortisone.

Metoclopramide (Reglan)

Indications: Gastroesophageal reflux, diabetic gastroparesis, premedication for patients needing pulmonary aspiration prophylaxis, antiemetic.
Dosage: Adult IV: 10 mg; PO: 10 mg.
              Pediatric: 0.1 mg/kg.
Effect: Facilitates gastric emptying by increasing GI motility and lowering esophageal sphincter tone; antiemetic effects are secondary to antagonism of central and peripheral dopamine receptors.
Onset: IV: 1–3 minutes; PO: 30–60 minutes to peak effect.
Duration: 1–2 hours.
Kinetics: Hepatic metabolism; renal elimination.
Comments: Avoid in patients with GI obstruction, pheochromocytoma, and Parkinson's disease. Extrapyramidal reactions in 0.2% to 1% of patients. May exacerbate depression.

Metoprolol (Lopressor)

Indications: Hypertension, angina pectoris, dysrhythmia, hypertrophic cardiomyopathy, MI, pheochromocytoma.
Dosage: 25–100 mg PO q6–12h. 5 mg IV bolus q2 minutes, up to 15 mg.
Effect: β_1-adrenergic blockade (β_2-adrenergic antagonism at high doses).
Onset: 15 minutes.
Duration: 6 hours.
Clearance: See labetolol.
Comments: May cause bradycardia, clinically significant bronchoconstriction (with doses > 100 mg/d), dizziness, fatigue, insomnia. May increase risk of heart block. Crosses the placenta and blood-brain barrier.

Milrinone (Primacor)

Indications: CHF.
Dosage: LOAD: 50 µg/kg IV over 10 minutes.
               MAINT: Titrate 0.375–0.750 µg/kg/min to effect.
Effect: Phosphodiesterase inhibition causing positive inotropy, vasodilation.
Onset: Immediate.
Duration: 2–3 hours.
Clearance: Renal elimination.
Comments: Short-term therapy. May increase ventricular ectopy and aggravate outflow tract obstruction in IHSS. Not recommended for acute MI.

Nadolol (Corgard)

Indications: Angina pectoris, hypertension.
Dosage: 40–240 mg/d PO.
Effect: Nonselective β-adrenergic blockade.
Onset: 1–2 hours.
Duration: > 24 hours.
Clearance: No hepatic metabolism; renal elimination.
Comments: May cause severe bronchospasm in susceptible patients (see propranolol).

Naloxone (Narcan)

Indications:	Reversal of systemic opioid effects.
Dosage:	Adult: 0.04– to 0.4–mg doses IV, titrated q2–3 minutes.
	Pediatric: 1–10 µg/kg (in increments) IV q2–3 minutes (up to 0.4 mg).
Effect:	Antagonism of opioid effects by competitive inhibition.
Onset:	Rapid.
Duration:	Dose-dependent, lasting 20–60 minutes.
Clearance:	95% hepatic metabolism; primarily renal elimination.
Comments:	May cause reversal of analgesia, hypertension, dysrhythmias, rare pulmonary edema, delirium, or withdrawal syndrome (in opioid-dependent patients). Renarcotization may occur because antagonist has short duration. Caution in hepatic failure.

Nifedipine (Procardia)

Indications:	Coronary artery spasm, hypertension, myocardial ischemia.
Dosage:	PO: 10–40 mg tid; SL: 10–20 mg (extracted from capsule).
Effect:	Blockade of slow calcium channels in heart; systemic and coronary vasodilation and increase in myocardial perfusion.
Onset:	PO: 20 minutes; SL: 1–5 minutes.
Duration:	4–24 hours.
Clearance:	Hepatic metabolism.
Comments:	May cause reflex tachycardia, GI upset, or mild negative inotropic effects. Little effect on automaticity and atrial conduction. May be useful in asymmetric septal hypertrophy. Drug solution is light sensitive. May rapidly produce severe hypotension in susceptible patients, especially with sublingual administration.

Nitric oxide (INOmax)

Indications:	Hypoxemic respiratory failure of the newborn; pulmonary hypertension.
Dosage:	1–40 ppm by continuous inhalation.

Effect: Cyclic guanosine monophosphate-mediated pulmonary vasodilation of ventilated lung regions.
Onset: 1–3 minutes.
Duration: For duration of inhalation.
Clearance: Bound to hemoglobin; metabolized to nitrates or nitrites.
Comments: Efficacy in adults uncertain.

Nitroglycerin (glycerol trinitrate, Nitrostat, Nitrol, Nitro-Bid, Nitrolingual)

Indications: Angina, myocardial ischemia or infarction, hypertension, CHF, controlled hypotension, esophageal spasm.
Dosage: Intravenous infusion initially at 10 µg/min; titrate to effect. Customary mix: 30–50 mg in 250 ml of 5% D/W or NSS;
               SL: 0.15–0.6 mg/dose;
               Topical: 2% ointment, 0.5– 2.5 inches q6–8h.
Effect: Smooth muscle relaxation by enzymatic release of NO, causing systemic, coronary, and pulmonary vasodilation (veins > arteries); bronchodilation; biliary, GI, and genitourinary tract relaxation.
Onset: IV: 1–2 minutes; SL: 1–3 minutes; PO: 1 hour; topical: 30 minutes
Duration: IV: 10 minutes; SL: 30–60 minutes; PO: 8–12 hours; topical: 8–24 hours.
Clearance: Nearly complete hepatic metabolism; renal elimination.
Comments: May cause reflex tachycardia, hypotension, headache. Tolerance with chronic use may be avoided with a 10- to 12-hour nitrate-free period. May be absorbed by plastic in IV tubing. May cause methemoglobinemia at very high doses.

Nitroprusside (Nipride, Nitropress)

Indications: Hypertension, controlled hypotension, CHF.
Dosage: IV infusion initially at 0.1 µg/kg/min, then titrated against patient response to maximum 10 µg/kg/min.
               Customary mix: 50 mg in 250 ml of 5% D/W or NSS.
Effect: Direct NO donor causing smooth muscle relaxation (arterial > venous).
Onset: 1–2 minutes.

Duration: 1–10 minutes after stopping infusion.
Clearance: RBC and tissue metabolism; renal elimination.
Comments: May cause excessive hypotension, reflex tachycar-
                dia. Accumulation of cyanide with liver dysfunc-
                tion; thiocyanate with kidney disfunction. Cyanide
                or thiocyanate buildup with prolonged infusion.
                Avoid with Leber's hereditary optic atrophy, to-
                bacco amblyopia, hypothyroidism, or vitamin B_{12}
                deficiency. Solution and powder are light sensitive
                and must be wrapped in opaque material.

Norepinephrine (Levarterenol, Levophed)

Indication: Hypotension.
Dosage: 1–8 µg/min IV; start at 1–8 µg/min, then titrate to
                desired effect.
                Customary mix: 4 mg in 250 ml of 5% D/W or NSS.
Effect: Both α- and β-adrenergic activity, with α-adrener-
                gic-agonism predominating.
Onset: Rapid.
Duration: 1–2 minutes following discontinuation.
Clearance: MAO/COMT metabolism.
Comments: May cause hypertension, dysrhythmias, myocar-
                dial ischemia, increased uterine contractility, con-
                stricted microcirculation, or CNS stimulation.

Octreotide (Sandostatin)

Indication: **1:** Upper GI tract bleeding, acute variceal hemor-
                rhage.
                2: Control of symptoms in patients with metastatic
                carcinoid and vasoactive intestinal peptide-secreting
                tumors (VIPomas); pancreatic tumors, gastrinoma,
                secretory diarrhea.
                3: Unlabeled uses include AIDS-associated secretory
                diarrhea, cryptosporidiosis, Cushing's syndrome,
                insulinomas, small bowel fistulas, postgastrectomy
                dumping syndrome, chemotherapy-induced diar-
                rhea, graft-versus-host disease (GVHD)-induced
                diarrhea, Zollinger-Ellison syndrome.
Dosage: **1:** Adults: IV bolus: 25–50 µg followed by continu-
                ous IV infusion of 25–50 µg/h.
                2, 3: Adults: SC: Initial: 50 µg 1–2 times/d; titrate
                dose based on patient tolerance and response.
                Carcinoid: 100–600 µg/d in 2–4 divided doses;
                VIPomas: 200–300 µg/d in 2–4 divided doses.
                Diarrhea: Initial: IV: 50–100 µg q8h; increase by

100 µg/dose at 48-hour intervals; maximal dose: 500 µg q8h.
Pediatric: 1–10 µg/kg q12h beginning at the low end of the range and increasing by 0.3 µg/kg/dose at 3-day intervals.

Effect: Somatostatin analogue that suppresses release of serotonin, gastrin, vasoactive intestinal peptide, insulin, glucagon, and secretin.
Onset: IV: minutes.
Duration: 6–12 hours.
Clearance: Hepatic and renal (32% eliminated unchanged); decreased in renal failure.
Comments: May cause nausea, decreased GI motility, transient hyperglycemia. Duration of therapy should be no longer than 72 hours because of lack of efficacy beyond this time.

Omeprazole (Losec, Prilosec)

Indications: Gastric acid hypersecretion or gastritis; gastroesophageal reflux.
Dosage: 20–40 mg PO every day.
Effect: Inhibition of H^+ secretion by irreversibly binding H^+/K^+ adenosine triphosphatase (ATPase).
Onset: 1 hour.
Duration: > 24 hours.
Clearance: Extensive hepatic metabolism: 72% to 80% renal elimination; 18% to 23% fecal elimination.
Comments: Increases secretion of gastrin. More rapid healing of gastric ulcers than with H_2 blockers. Effective in ulcers resistant to H_2 blocker therapy. Inhibits some cytochrome P450 enzymes.

Ondansetron hydrochloride (Zofran)

Indications: Perioperative nausea, vomiting (prevention, treatment).
Dosage: Adult IV: Perioperative 4 mg undiluted over > 30 seconds; PO: 8 mg.
               Pediatric: 4 mg PO.
Effect: Selective 5-HT$_3$ receptor antagonist.
Onset: 30 minutes.
Duration: 4–8 hours.
Clearance: 95% hepatic; 5% renal excretion.
Comments: Used in much higher doses for chemotherapy-induced nausea. Mild side effects include headache and reversible transaminase elevation.

Oxytocin (Pitocin, Syntocinon)

Indications:	**1:** Postpartum hemorrhage, uterine atony.
	2: Augmentation of labor.
Dosage:	**1:** IV infusion at rate necessary to control atony (e.g., 0.02–0.04 U/min).
	2: Labor induction: 0.0005–0.002 U/min.
	Customary mix: 10–40 U in 1,000 ml of crystalloid.
Effect:	Reduces postpartum blood loss by contraction of uterine smooth muscle; renal, coronary, and cerebral vasodilation.
Onset:	Immediate.
Duration:	1 hour.
Clearance:	Tissue metabolism; renal elimination.
Comments:	May cause uterine tetany and rupture, fetal distress, or anaphylaxis. Intravenous bolus can cause hypotension, tachycardia, and dysrhythmia.

Pentamadine (Pentam)

Indications:	**1:** Treatment and **2:** prevention of pneumonia caused by *Pneumocystis carinii*.
Dosage:	**1:** Adult and pediatric: 4 mg/kg/d IM or IV for 14 days. Adults: Inhalation of 300 mg every 4 weeks via nebulizer.
	2: Pediatric: Inhalation of 300 mg q3–4 weeks via nebulizer.
Effect:	Antiprotozoal.
Duration:	Terminal half-life 6.4–9.4 hours; may be prolonged in patients with severe renal impairment.
Clearance:	33% to 66% excreted unchanged in urine.
Comments:	Concomitant use of nephrotoxic drugs may increase risk of nephrotoxicity.

Phenobarbital

Indications:	**1:** Sedative or hypnotic.
	2: Anticonvulsant.
Dosage:	**1:** Adults and pediatric 1–3 mg/kg PO IM, IV.
	2: Adults, infants, and pediatric.
	LOAD: 10–20 mg/kg IV, additional 5 mg/kg doses

q15–30 min for contol of status epilepticus; maximal 30 mg/kg.

MAINT: 3–5 mg/kg/d PO; IV in divided doses.

Onset: 5 minutes; allow 60–90 minutes for full sedative effect.

Duration: 10–12 hours; half-life may be > 100 hours.

Clearance: Hepatic metabolism; 25% to 50% renal elimination unchanged.

Comments: May cause hypotension and multiple drug interactions by induction of hepatic enzyme systems. Therapeutic anticonvulsant concentration of 15–40 µg/ml at trough (just before next dose).

Phenoxybenzamine (Dibenzyline)

Indication: Preoperative preparation for pheochromocytoma resection.

Dosage: 10–40 mg/d PO titrated (start at 10 mg/d and increase dosage by 10 mg/d q4d prn).

Effect: Nonselective noncompetitive α-adrenergic antagonist.

Onset: Hours.

Duration: 3–4 days.

Clearance: Hepatic metabolism; renal or biliary excretion.

Comments: May cause orthostatic hypotension (which may be refractory to norepinephrine), and reflex tachycardia. Nasal congestion expected.

Phentolamine (Regitine)

Indications: **1:** Hypertension from catecholamine excess as in pheochromocytoma.
2: Extravasation of α-agonist.

Dosage: **1:** 1–5 mg IV prn for hypertension.
2: 5–10 mg in 10 ml of NSS SC into affected area within 12 hours.

Effect: Nonselective, competitive α-adrenergic antagonist.

Onset: Minutes.

Duration: Half-life 19 minutes.

Clearance: Unknown metabolism; 10% renal elimination unmetabolized.

Comments: May cause hypotension, reflex tachycardia, cerebrovascular spasm, dysrhythmias, stimulation of GI tract, or hypoglycemia.

Phenylephrine (Neo-Synephrine)

Indication: Hypotension.
Dosage: IV infusion initially at 10 µg/min, then titrated for response; IV bolus: 40–100 µg/dose.
              Customary mix: 10–30 mg in 250 ml of 5% D/W or NSS.
Effect: α-adrenergic agonist.
Onset: Rapid.
Duration: 5–20 minutes.
Clearance: Hepatic metabolism; renal elimination.
Comments: May cause hypertension, reflex bradycardia, constricted microcirculation, uterine contraction, or uterine vasoconstriction.

Phenytoin (diphenylhydantoin, Dilantin)

Indications: 1: Seizures.
              2: Digoxin-induced dysrhythmias.
              3: Refractory ventricular tachycardia.
Dosage: Adult: 1: LOAD: 10–15 mg/kg IV at < 50 mg/min (up to 1,000 mg cautiously, with ECG monitoring); for neurosurgical prophylaxis: 100–200 mg IV q4h (IV < 50 mg/min). MAINT: 100–300 mg IV q8–12h.
              2, 3: For dysrhythmias: 50–100 mg IV at < 50 mg/min q10–15 min until dysrhythmia is abolished, side effects occur, or maximal dose 10–15 mg/kg is given.
              Pediatric: 1: LOAD: 15–18 mg/kg IV at a rate of 0.5–1.5 mg/kg/minute. MAINT: 4–8 mg/kg/day IV or PO in divided doses q8–12h.
              Fosphenytoin can be subsituted for phenytoin for IV or IM injection. Fosphenytoin injections appear to be better tolerated and have fewer side effects compared with phenytoin, which uses propylene glycol as a vehicle. Fosphenytoin is a prodrug of phenytoin with 1.5 g of fosphenytoin yielding 1 g of phenytoin. Fosphenytoin is prescribed as phenytoin equivalent units (PE).
Effect: Anticonvulsant effect via membrane stabilization; antidysrhythmic effects similar to those of quinidine or procainamide.
Onset: 3–5 minutes.
Duration: Dose-dependent; half-life is dose-dependent in therapeutic range.
Clearance: Hepatic metabolism; renal elimination (enhanced by alkaline urine).
Comments: May cause nystagmus, diplopia, ataxia, drowsiness, gingival hyperplasia, GI upset, hyperglycemia, or hepatic microsomal enzyme induc-

tion. Intravenous bolus can cause bradycardia, hypotension, respiratory arrest, cardiac arrest, CNS depression. Is a tissue irritant. Crosses the placenta. Significant interpatient variation in dose needed to achieve therapeutic concentration = 7.5–20.0 µg/ml. Determination of unbound phenytoin levels may be helpful in patients with renal failure or hypoalbuminemia.

Phosphorus (Phospho-Soda; Neutra-Phos; potassium phosphate; sodium phosphate)

Indications:	**1:** Treatment and prevention of hypophosphatemia; **2:** short-term treatment of constipation; **3:** evacuation of the colon for rectal and bowel examinations.
Dosage:	**1:** Mild to moderate hypophosphatemia. Children < 4 years: PO: 250 mg (phosphorus) 3–4 times/d. > 4 years and adults: PO: 250–500 mg (phosphorus) 3 times/d for 3 days; IV: 0.08–0.15 mmol/kg over 6 hours. Moderate to severe hypophosphatemia: IV: Children < 4 years: 0.15–0.3 mmol/kg over 6 hours. > 4 years and adults: 0.15–0.25 mmol/kg over 6–12 hours. Usual adult dose: 10 mmol IV over 6h or 6mmol PO 3–4 times/day. **2:** Laxative (Fleet Phospho-Soda): PO: Children 5–9 years: 5 ml as a single dose. 10–12 years: 10 ml as a single dose. Children > 12 years and adults: 20–30 ml as a single dose. **3:** Colonoscopy preparation regimen: (Fleet-Phospho-Soda): PO: adults: 45 ml diluted to 90 ml with water the evening prior to the examination. Repeat the dose again the following morning.
Effect:	Electrolyte replacement.
Onset:	Cathartic: 3–6 hours.
Clearance:	80% of dose reabsorbed by the kidneys.
Comments:	Infuse doses of IV phosphate over a 4- to 6-hour period; risks of rapid IV infusion include hypocalcemia, hypotension, muscular irritability, calcium deposits, renal function deterioration, and hyperkalemia. Orders for IV phosphate preparations should be written in millimole (1 mmol = 31 mg). Use with caution in patients with cardiac disease and renal insufficiency. Do not give with magnesium- and aluminum-containing antacids or sucralfate, which can bind with phosphate.

Physostigmine (Antilirium)

Indications:	Postoperative delirium, tricyclic antidepressant overdose, reversal of CNS effects of anticholinergic drugs.
Dosage:	0.5–2.0 mg IV q15min prn.
Effect:	Inhibition of cholinesterase, central and peripheral cholinergic effects.
Onset:	Rapid.
Duration:	30–60 minutes.
Clearance:	Cholinesterase metabolism.
Comments:	May cause bradycardia, tremor, convulsions, hallucinations, psychiatric or CNS depression, mild ganglionic blockade, or cholinergic crisis. Crosses blood–brain barrier. Antagonized by atropine. Contains sulfite.

Potassium (KCl)

Indication:	Hypokalemia, digoxin toxicity.
Dosage:	Adult: 20 mEq of KCl administered IV over 30–60 min; usual infusion 10 mEq/h. Pediatric: 0.02 mEq/kg/min.
Effect:	To correct severe hypokalemia.
Onset:	Immediate.
Duration:	Variable.
Clearance:	Renal.
Comments:	Bolus administration may cause cardiac arrest; not to exceed 1 mEq/min in adults. A central venous line is preferable for administration.

Procainamide (Pronestyl)

Indications:	Atrial and ventricular dysrhythmias.
Dosage:	LOAD: 500–1000 mg IV over 30 min or until toxicity or desired effect occurs; stop if $\geq$ 50% QRS widening or PR lengthening occurs. MAINT: 1–4 mg/h.
Effect:	Class IA antidysrhythmic; blocks sodium channels.
Onset:	Immediate.
Duration:	Half-life 2.5–4.5 hours, depending on acetylator phenotype.
Clearance:	25% hepatic conversion to active metabolite N-acetyl-procainamide (NAPA), a class III antidys-

rhythmic; renal elimination (50% to 60% unchanged).

Comments: May cause increased ventricular response in atrial tachydysrhythmias unless predigitalized, asystole (with AV block), myocardial depression, CNS excitement, blood dyscrasia, lupus syndrome with positive ANA, liver damage. Intravenous administration can cause hypotension from vasodilation, accentuated by general anesthesia. Decrease LOAD by one third in CHF or shock. Therapeutic concentration = 4–8 mg/L. Contains sulfite.

Prochlorperazine (Compazine)

Indications:	Nausea and vomiting.
Dosage:	5–10 mg/dose IV (≤ 40 mg/d); 5–10 mg IM q2–4h prn; 25 mg PR q12h prn.
Effect:	Central dopamine (D_2) antagonist with neuroleptic and antiemetic effects; also antimuscarinic and antihistaminic (H_1) effects.
Onset:	Rapid.
Duration:	3–4 hours.
Clearance:	Hepatic metabolism; renal or biliary elimination.
Comments:	May cause hypotension (especially when given IV), extrapyramidal reactions, neuroleptic malignant syndrome, leukopenia, or cholestatic jaundice. Contains sulfites. Caution in liver disease. Less sedating than chlorpromazine.

Promethazine (Phenergan)

Indications:	Allergies, anaphylaxis, nausea and vomiting, sedation.
Dosage:	Adult: 12.5–50.0 mg IV, IM, PO, PR q4–6h prn. Pediatric: 0.1–1 mg/kg IV, IM, PO, PR q4–6h PM.
Effect:	Antagonist of H_1, D_2, and muscarinic receptors; antiemetic, and sedative.
Onset:	3–5 minutes.
Duration:	2–4 hours.
Clearance:	Hepatic metabolism; renal elimination.
Comments:	May cause mild hypotension or mild anticholinergic effects. Crosses the placenta. Extrapyramidal effects rare. Contains sulfite. Intraarterial injection can cause gangrene.

Propranolol (Inderal)

Indications:	Hypertension, atrial and ventricular dysrhythmias, myocardial ischemia or infarction, hypertension, thyrotoxicosis, hypertrophic cardiomyopathy, migraine headache.
Dosage:	Adult: Test dose of 0.25–0.5 mg IV, then titrate ≤ 1 mg/ min to effect.
	PO: 10–40 mg q6–8h, increased prn.
	Pediatric: 0.05–0.1 mg/kg IV over 10 minutes.
Effect:	Nonspecific β-adrenergic blockade.
Onset:	IV: 2 minutes, PO: 30 minutes.
Duration:	IV: 1–6 hours, PO: 6 hours.
Clearance:	Hepatic metabolism; renal elimination.
Comments:	May cause bradycardia, AV dissociation, and hypoglycemia. Bronchospasm, CHF, and drowsiness can occur with low doses. Crosses the placenta and blood–brain barrier. Abrupt withdrawal can precipitate rebound angina.

Prostaglandin E_1 (Alprostadil, Prostin VR)

Indications:	Pulmonary vasodilator, maintenance of patent ductus arteriosus.
Dosage:	Starting dose 0.05–0.1 µg/kg/min. Titrate to effect or maximum of 0.6 µg/kg/min.
	Customary mix: 500 µg/250 ml of NSS or 5% D/W.
Effect:	Prostaglandin E_1 will cause vasodilation, inhibition of platelet aggregation, vascular smooth muscle relaxation, uterine and intestinal smooth muscle stimulation.
Onset:	Immediate.
Duration:	60 minutes.
Clearance:	Pulmonary metabolism; renal elimination.
Comments:	May cause hypotension, apnea, flushing, and bradycardia.

Protamine

Indication:	Reversal of the effects of heparin.
Dosage:	1 mg/100 U of heparin activity IV at ≤ 5 mg/min.
Effect:	Polybasic compound forms complex with polyacidic heparin.
Onset:	30 seconds to 1 minute.
Duration:	2 hours, dependent on body temperature.

Clearance: Fate of heparin–protamine complex is unknown.
Comments: May cause myocardial depression and peripheral
                vasodilation with sudden hypotension or bradycar-
                dia. May cause severe pulmonary hypertension,
                particularly in the setting of cardiopulmonary by-
                pass. Protamine–heparin complex antigenically
                active. Transient reversal of heparin may be fol-
                lowed by rebound heparinization. Can cause anti-
                coagulation if given in excess relative to amount of
                circulating heparin (controversial). Monitor re-
                sponse with partial thromboplastin time or acti-
                vated clotting time.

Quinidine gluconate (Quinaglute)

Indications: Atrial and ventricular dysrhythmias.
Dosage: For acute dysrhythmias: LOAD: 500–1000 mg IV
                in 100 ml of 5% D/W (over 30 to 60 min): stop IV in-
                fusion if dysrhythmia is gone or toxicity occurs
                (25–50% QRS widening, HR > 120, or loss of P
                waves). MAINT: Quinidine gluconate sustained re-
                lease tablets 324 mg PO tid.
                Therapeutic concentration = 3–6 mg/L.
Effect: Class IA antidysrythmic; blocks Na channels.
Onset: IV: 4–6 minutes.
Duration: PO: 6–12 hours.
Clearance: Hepatic metabolism; renal elimination (10% to
                50% unchanged).
Comments: May cause hypotension (from vasodilation and neg-
                ative inotropic effects), increased ventricular re-
                sponse in atrial tachydysrhythmias, AV block, QT
                prolongation, CHF, mild anticholinergic effects, in-
                crease in serum digoxin level, cinchonism, or GI
                upset. Hemolysis in G-6-P-D deficient patients. Can
                potentiate action of oral anticoagulants.

Ranitidine (Zantac)

Indications: Duodenal and gastric ulcers, reduction of gastric
                volume, raising gastric pH; esophageal reflux.
Dosage: IV: 50–100 mg q8h; PO: 150–300 mg q12h.
Effect: Histamine H_2-receptor antagonist; inhibits basal,
                nocturnal, and stimulated gastric acid secretion.
Onset: IV: rapid; PO: 1–3 hours.
Duration: IV: 6–8 hours; PO: 12 hours.
Clearance: 70% renal elimination unchanged.
Comments: Doses should be reduced by 50% with renal failure.

Ritodrine (Yutopar)

Indication: Tocolysis (inhibition of preterm labor).
Dosage: IV (infusion): 0.1–0.35 mg/min.
                Customary mix: 150 mg in 5% D/W.
Effect: β_2-selective adrenergic agonist that decreases uterine contractility.
Onset: 5 minutes.
Duration: 2 hours.
Clearance: Renal elimination (70% to 90% unchanged); some hepatic metabolism.
Comments: Dose-related increases in maternal and fetal heart rate and blood pressure because of β_1 stimulation. Crosses the placenta. Pulmonary edema can occur, particularly in patients given corticosteroids. May cause increased insulin resistance. Potentiation of dysrhythmias and hypotension by magnesium sulfate, volatile general anesthetics, and meperidine. Hypertension can be potentiated by atropine. Contains sulfite. Contraindicated in eclampsia, pulmonary hypertension, and hyperthyroidism.

Scopolamine (Hyoscine)

Indications: Antisialagogue; amnesia, sedation, antiemetic, antimotion sickness.
Dosage: 0.3–0.6 mg IV/IM.
Effect: Peripheral and central cholinergic (muscarinic) antagonism.
Onset: Rapid.
Duration: Variable.
Clearance: Hepatic metabolism; renal elimination.
Comments: Excessive CNS depression can be reversed by physostigmine. Can cause excitement or delirium, transient tachycardia, hyperthermia, urinary retention. Crosses the blood-brain barrier and placenta.

Streptokinase (Kabikinase, Streptase)

Indications: **1:** Thrombolytic agent used in treatment of recent severe or massive deep vein thrombosis, pulmonary emboli. **2:** myocardial infarction. **3:** Occluded arteriovenous cannulas.
Dosage: Adult **1:** Thromboses: 250,000 U IV over 30 minutes, then 100,000 U/h for 24–72 hours.

2: Myocardial infarction: 1.5 million U IV over 1 hour; if hypotension develops, decrease infusion rate by 50%; standard concentration is 1.5 million U/250 ml.

3: Cannula occlusion: 250,000 U into cannula, clamp for 2 hours, then aspirate contents and flush with normal saline.

Pediatric: Safety and efficacy not established; limited studies have used 3,500–4,000 U/kg over 30 minutes followed by 1,000–1,500 units/kg/h.

Effect:	Thrombolytic agent.
Onset:	Activation of plasminogen occurs almost immediately.
Duration:	Fibrinolytic effects last only a few hours, whereas anticoagulant effects can persist for 12–24 hours.
Clearance:	Eliminated by circulating antibodies and via the reticuloendothelial system.
Comments:	Best results are realized if used within 5–6 hours of MI; has been demonstrated to be effective up to 12 hours after coronary artery occlusion and onset of symptoms; give aspirin (325 mg) at the start of streptokinase infusion; begin heparin therapy (800–1000 U/h) at the end of streptokinase infusion. Avoid IM injections and vascular punctures at noncompressible sites before, during, and after therapy. Contraindicated with recent administration of streptokinase (antibodies to streptokinase remain for 3–6 months after initial dose), recent streptococcus infection; active internal bleeding, recent cerebrovascular accident (within 2 months), or intracranial or intraspinal surgery. Relatively contraindicated following major surgery within the last 10 days, GI bleeding, recent trauma, or severe hypertension.

Terbutaline (Brethine, Bricanyl)

Indications:	**1:** Bronchospasm.
	2: Tocolysis (inhibition of premature labor).
Dosage:	**1:** Adult: 0.25 mg SC; repeat in 15 minutes prn (use < 0.5 mg/4 h); 2.5–5.0 mg PO q6h prn (< 15.0 mg/d). Pediatric: 3.5–5.0 μg/kg SC.
	2: 10 μg/min IV infusion; titrate to a maximal dose of 80 μg/min.
Effect:	β_2-selective adrenergic agonist.
Onset:	SC < 15 minutes; PO < 30 minutes.
Duration:	SC 1.5–4 hours; PO 4–8 hours.
Clearance:	Hepatic metabolism; renal elimination.
Comments:	May cause dysrhythmias, pulmonary edema, hypertension, hypokalemia, or CNS excitement.

Thiamine (Vitamin B$_1$; Betalin)

Indications:	Treatment of thiamine deficiency including beriberi, Wernicke's encephalopathy syndrome, peripheral neuritis associated with pellagra, and pregnancy.
Dosage:	Adult: Noncritically ill thiamine deficiency: 5–50 mg/d PO for 1 month. Beriberi: 5–50 mg IM 3 times/d for 2 weeks, then switch to 5–50 mg PO every day for 1 month. Severe deficiency: 50–100 mg IM or slow IV over 5 minutes, repeated daily until oral therapy can be substituted; 300 mg maximal 24-hour dose. Recommended daily allowance: 1.4 mg (male); 1 mg (female). Pediatric: Noncritically ill thiamine deficiency: 10–50 mg/d PO in divided doses for 2 weeks followed by 5–10 mg/d for 1 month. Beriberi: 10–25 mg/d IM for 2 weeks, then 5–10 mg PO every day for 1 month. Recommended daily allowance for infants and children: 0.3–1.4 mg.
Effect:	Vitamin supplement.
Clearance:	Eliminated unchanged in urine and as pyrimidine, after body storage sites become saturated.
Comments:	Single vitamin B$_1$ deficiency is rare, suspect multiple vitamin deficiencies. The IV route of administration is not preferred because of the increased incidence of side effects.

Thiosulfate, sodium

Indication:	Cyanide toxicity, cisplatin-induced nephrotoxicity.
Dosage:	Adult: 50 ml of a 25% solution IV over 10 minutes; may repeat with 50% of initial dose if signs of cyanide toxicity recur. Pediatric: 7–10 g/m^2 ($\sim$ 250 mg/kg) (maximum $\leq$ 12.5 g).
Effect:	Facilitates conversion of cyanide to less-toxic thiocyanate by rhodanese.
Clearance:	Renal elimination.
Comments:	Give after amyl nitrite and sodium nitrite.

Tissue plasminogen activator (tissue plasminogen activator, recombinant; tPA, Alteplase, Activase)

Indications:	**1:** Lysis of thrombi in coronary arteries in hemodynamically unstable patients with acute MI. **2:** Management of acute massive pulmonary embolism (PE) in adults. **3:** Acute embolic stroke.
Dosage:	**1:** LOAD: 15 mg (30 ml of the infusion) IV over 1 minute followed by 0.75 mg/kg (not to exceed 50 mg) given over 30 minutes; start maintenance infusion immediately after loading dose: 0.5 mg/kg up to 35 mg/h for 1 hour; total dose not to exceed 100 mg
	2: 100 mg continuous infusion over 2 hours.
	3: Total dose of 0.9 mg/kg (maximum 90 mg) administer 10% as a bolus and the remainder over 60 minutes.
Effect:	Tissue-type plasminogen activator (tPA).
Onset:	Rapid.
Duration:	80% cleared within 10 minutes of discontinuing infusion.
Clearance:	Rapid hepatic clearance.
Comments:	Alteplase has not been demonstrated to be superior to streptokinase for thrombolysis in acute MI. Aspirin (325 mg) should be given at the initiation of therapy; heparin should be started (1,000 U/h) by continuous infusion 1 hour from the initiation of alteplase. Doses > 150 mg have been associated with an increased incidence of intracranial hemorrhage. Use within 6 hours of coronary occlusion for best results. Contraindicated with active internal bleeding, history of hemorrhagic stroke, intracranial neoplasm, aneurysm, or recent (within 2 months) intracranial or intraspinal surgery or trauma. Should be used with caution in patients who have received chest compressions, and in patients who are currently receiving heparin, coumadin, or antiplatelet drugs.

Trimethaphan (Arfonad)

Indications:	Hypertension, controlled hypotension.
Dosage:	1–4 mg/min IV × 5–10 minutes, then titrated (usually about 1 mg/min).
	Customary mix: 500 mg in 500 ml of 5% D/W.
Effect:	Blocks nicotinic receptors at autonomic ganglia; vasodilation.

Onset: Immediate.
Duration: 10–15 minutes.
Clearance: Possible pseudocholinesterase metabolism; renal
              elimination (mostly unchanged).
Comments: Mild decrease in cardiac contractility thought to be
              useful in patients with dissecting aortic aneurysms.
              May cause prolonged hypotension (especially with
              high doses), bradycardia in elderly, tachycardia in
              the young. Histamine release, urinary retention,
              mydriasis, tachyphylaxis. Potentiation of the ef-
              fects of succinylcholine.

Tromethamine (Tris buffer; THAM)

Indications: Metabolic acidosis.
Dosage: Adult and pediatric: Dose depends on buffer base
              deficit; tromethamine ml of 0.3 M solution = body
              weight (kg) × base deficit (mEq/L) × 1.1.
              Pediatric: Maximal recommended pediatric dose:
              33–40 ml/kg/d or 500 mg/kg/dose.
              1 meq of THAM (0.3 M tromethamine) = 3.3 ml =
              120 mg tromethamine.
Effect: Organic proton acceptor (buffer).
Onset: Rapid.
Duration: Hours.
Clearance: Rapidly eliminated by kidneys (> 75% in 3 hours).
Comments: Use with caution in patients with renal impair-
              ment or chronic respiratory acidosis.

Urokinase (Abbokinase)

Indications: Treatment of: (1) recent MI, (2) deep vein throm-
              bosis, (3) severe or massive pulmonary emboli, (4)
              occluded IV cannulas, (5) liquify loculated pleural
              effusions and empyemas.
Dosage: Adults:
              1: Myocardial infarction: 6,000 U/min intracoro-
              nary for up to 2 hours.
              2: Deep vein thrombosis: 4,400 U/kg/h IV for 12
              hours.
              3: Clot lysis: (large vessel thrombi).
              LOAD: 4,000 U/kg/dose IV over 10 minutes.
              MAINT: 4,000–6,000 U/kg/h adjusted to achieve
              clot lysis or patency of affected vessel; doses up to
              50,000 U/ kg/h have been used.
              Therapy should be initiated as soon as possible
              after diagnosis of thrombi and continued until clot
              is dissolved (usually 24–72 hours).

4: Occluded IV catheters: 5,000 U into the catheter, then aspirate; may repeat every 5 minutes for 30 minutes, if still occluded; cap and leave in catheter for 30 minutes to 1 hour, then aspirate contents and flush with normal saline.

5: 80,000 U/50 ml instilled into a chest tube.

Effect: Thrombolytic agent.

Onset: Fibrinolysis occurs rapidly.

Duration: 4 or more hours.

Clearance: Cleared by the liver with a small amount excreted in urine and bile.

Comments: Contraindicated with recent streptococcal infection, any internal bleeding, cerebrovascular accident (within 2 months), or brain carcinoma. Use with caution in patients with severe hypertension, recent lumbar puncture, or in those receiving IM injections. Increased bleeding with anticoagulants, antiplatelet drugs, aspirin, indomethacin, dextran. Avoid IM injections and vascular punctures at noncompressible sites before, during, and after therapy.

Vasopressin (antidiuretic hormone, Pitressin)

Indications: **1:** Diabetes insipidus.

2: Upper GI hemorrhage.

Dosage: **1:** 5–10 U IM/SC q 8–12 h. 2.4–10 U/hr by IV infusion.

2: 0.1–0.4 U/min by IV infusion.

Effect: Increases in urine osmolality and decreases in urine volume; smooth muscle contraction; constriction in splanchnic, coronary, muscle, and skin vasculature.

Onset: Immediate.

Duration: 2–8 hours.

Clearance: Hepatic and renal metabolism; renal elimination.

Comments: May cause oliguria, water intoxication, pulmonary edema; hypertension, dysrhythmias, myocardial ischemia; abdominal cramps (from increased peristalsis); anaphylaxis; contraction of gallbladder, urinary bladder, or uterus; vertigo, or nausea. Patients with coronary artery disease are often treated with concurrent nitroglycerin.

Verapamil (Isoptin, Calan)

Indications:	Supraventricular tachycardia, atrial fibrillation or flutter, Wolff-Parkinson-White syndrome, Lown-Ganong-Levine syndrome.
Dosage:	Adult: 2.5–10.0 mg (75–150 µg/kg) IV over ≥ 2 minutes; if no response in 30 minutes, repeat 10 mg (150 µg/kg). PO: 80–120 mg q6–8h
	Pediatric: 0–1 year: 0.1–0.2 mg/kg IV.
	1–15 years: 0.1–0.3 mg/kg IV; repeat once if no response in 30 minutes.
Effect:	Blockade of slow calcium channels in heart; prolongation of PR and AH intervals with negative inotropy and chronotropy; systemic and coronary vasodilatation.
Onset:	PO: 1–2 hours; IV: 1–5 minutes.
Duration:	PO: 8–24 hours; IV: 10 minutes to 2 hours.
Clearance:	Hepatic metabolism; renal elimination.
Comments:	May cause severe bradycardia, AV block (especially with concomitant β-blockade), excessive hypotension, or CHF. May increase ventricular response to atrial fibrillation or flutter in patients with accessory tracts. Active metabolite has 20% antihypertensive effect.

Vitamin K/Phytonadione (AquaMEPHYTON)

Indications:	Deficiency of vitamin K-dependent clotting factors, reversal of warfarin effect.
Dosage:	IV: 1–10 mg at ≤ 1 mg/min.
	IM/SQ/PO: 2.5–10 mg; if 8 hours after IV/IM/SQ dose, prothrombin time is not improved, repeat dose prn.
Effect:	Promotion of synthesis of clotting factors II, VII, IX, X.
Onset:	PO: 6–12 hours; IV: 1–2 hours.
Clearance:	Hepatic metabolism.
Comments:	Excessive dose can make patient refractory to further oral anticoagulation. May fail with hepatocellular disease. Rapid IV bolus can cause profound hypotension, fever, diaphoresis, bronchospasm, anaphylaxis, and pain at injection site. Crosses the placenta.

Warfarin (Coumadin, Panwarfin, Athrombin-k)

Indications:	Anticoagulation.
Dosage:	LOAD: 10–15 mg PO.
	MAINT: 2–10 mg PO; titrated to prothrombin time.
Effect:	Interferes with utilization of vitamin K by the liver and inhibits synthesis of factors II, VII, IX, X.
Onset:	12–72 hours.
Duration:	2–5 days.
Clearance:	Hepatic metabolism; renal elimination.
Comments:	May be potentiated by ethanol, antibiotics, chloral hydrate, cimetidine, dextran, diazoxide, ethacrynic acid, glucagon, methyldopa, monoamine oxidase inhibitors, phenytoin, prolonged use of narcotics, quinidine, sulfonamides, thyroid hormone, CHF, hyperthermia, liver disease, malabsorption, and so on. May be antagonized by barbiturates, chlordiazepoxide, haloperidol, oral contraceptives, hypothyroidism, hyperlipidemia. Crosses the placenta.

ANC, absolute neutrophil count; AV, atrioventricular; CHF, congestive heart failure; CMV, cytomegalovirus; CNS, central nervous system; COMT, catechol-O-methyltransferase; D/W, dextrose in water; ECG, electrocardiogram; GI, gastrointestinal; IM, intramuscularly; IV, intravenously; MAO, monoamine oxidase; MD, maintenance dose; NPH, neutral protamine Hagedorn; NSS, normal saline solution; PO, orally; prn, as needed or indicated; PZI, protamine zinc insulin; RBCs, red blood cells; SL, sublingually; SC, subcutaneously; $t_{1/2}$, redistribution half-life; WBC, white blood cells.

See chapters 5 and 6 for specific information concerning sedative and analgesic drugs. See chapter 7 for neuromuscular blocking drugs. Adapted from Wald S, Lerdahl D, Rosow C. Appendix of commonly used drugs. In: Hurford WE, Bailin MT, Davison JL, et al. *Clinical anesthesia procedures of the Massachusetts General Hospital,* 5th ed. Philadelphia: Lippincott-Raven, 1998:689–731; and the *Massachusetts General Hospital Formulary,* 1999.

Common intravenous antibiotics

Drug	Usual adult IV dose[a]	Usual dose interval	Comments
Amikacin	300 mg	q 8 h	Preferred for infections resistant to other aminoglycosides.
Amphotericin B (Fungizone)	Initial dose: 0.25 mg/kg administered over 6 h; dose should be gradually increased, ranging up to 1 mg/kg/d or 1.5 mg/kg on alternate days	q 1–2 d	Broad-spectrum antifungal. Initial test dose: 1 mg infused over 30 min to 1 h. Do not exceed 1.5 mg/kg/d. Because of the nephrotoxic potential of amphotericin, other nephrotoxic drugs should be avoided.
Ampicillin	1 g	q 4 h	May induce interstitial nephritis. Combined with sulbactam in Unasyn.
Ampicillin–sulbactam (Unasyn)	3 g	q 6 h	Not effective against *Pseudomonas* spp.
Aztreonam	1 g	q 8 h	Can be used for patients allergic to penicillins or cephalosporins.
Cefazolin (Ancef, Kefzol)	1 g	q 4–8 h	First generation cephalosporin. Adjust dosage in renal disease.
Cefotetan (Cefotan)	1–2 g	q 12 h	Second generation cephalosporin. Possible disulfiram-like reaction.
Ceftazidime	1 g	q 8 h	Preferred for *Pseudomonas aeruginosa* infections and neutropenic patients with fever.
Ceftriaxone	1 g	q 24 h	Preferred for empiric coverage for bacterial meningitis.
Cefuroxime	750 mg	q 8 h	Preferred for community-acquired pneumonia.
Chloramphenicol	0.25–1 g	q 6 h	Adjust dose according to serum concentration.

Common intravenous antibiotics *continued*

Drug	Usual adult IV dose	Usual dose interval	Comments
Ciprofloxacin	400 mg	q 12 h	Good absorption via oral route (500 mg q 12 h).
Clindamycin (Cleocin)	600 mg	q 8 h	Associated with *Clostridium difficile* colitis. May prolong neuromuscular blockade.
Doxycycline	100 mg	q 12 h	Possible hepatoxicity. Can cause benign intracranial hypertension with vitamin A. See tetracycline.
Erythromycin	0.5–1 g	q 6 h	Bacteriostatic. Gastritis with oral route. Venous irritation.
Fluconazole	200–400 mg	q 24 h	Well absorbed orally.
Gentamicin	60–120 mg (3–5 mg/kg/d)	q 8–12 h	Decrease dosage in renal failure. Renal ototoxicity. Precipitates with heparin. Can cause or prolong neuromuscular blockade.
Imipenem–cilastatin	500 mg	q 6 h	Preferred for multiple drug-resistant, gram-negative bacterial infections. Can cause seizures, especially in renal failure.
Levofloxacin	500 mg	q d	Pure *L*-isomer of ofloxacin. Well absorbed orally.
Meropenem	0.5–1 g	q 8 h	Less likely to cause seizures than imipenem.
Metronidazole (Flagyl)	500 mg	q 6 h	Possible disulfram-like reaction; leukopenia, convulsions, acute toxic psychosis with disulfram.
Nafcillin	1–2 g	q 4 h	Preferred for anti-staphylococcal coverage.
Penicillin G[b]	500,000–2,000,000 U	q 4 h	Hypersensitivity is common. Can induce seizures at high doses and induce interstitial nephritis.
Piperacillin	4 g	q 6 h	Usually combined with aminoglycoside for treatment of *Pseudomonas*.

continued

Drug	Dose	Interval	Notes
Piperacillin–tazobactam (Zosyn)	3.375 g	q 6 h	Tazobactam expands activity of piperacillin to include β-lactamase producing strains of *S. aureus*, *Haemophilus influenzae, Enterobacteriaceae, Pseudomonas, Klebsiella, Citrobacter, Serratia, Bacteroides*, and other gram-negative anaerobes.
Tetracycline	250–500 mg	q 12 h	Contraindicated in pediatrics (tooth discoloration). Antagonism with penicillins. Crosses placenta.
Ticarcillin	3 g	q 4 h	Antipseudomonal penicillin of choice. Can cause bleeding abnormalities.
Ticarcillin–clavulanate (Timentin)	3.1 g	q 4 h	
Trimethoprim/ sulfamethoxazole (Bactrim, Septra)	8–10 mg/kg/d (based on trimethoprim component)	q 6–12 h	Allergic reactions common. Interferes with secretion of creatinine and potassium; values may increase.
Tobramycin	60–120 mg (3–5 mg/kg/d)	q 8 h	See gentamicin.
Vancomycin (Vancocin)	500 mg–1 g	q 6–12 h	Preferred for oxacillin-resistant staphylococcal infections and patients with penicillin allergy. Decrease dose in renal disease. Histamine release ("red man"), renal damage, deafness. May precipitate with other medications.

[a] Adult doses are those usually given to healthy 70-kg patients and can vary with the patient's condition or concomitant drug intake. Older or debilitated patients may require smaller doses.

[b] 5% to 10% of penicillin-allergic patients will react to cephalosporins.

Laboratory values for blood

Chemistry

Albumin	3.1–4.3 g/dl
Alkaline phosphatase	
Male	45–115 U/L
Female	30–100 U/L
Ammonia, plasma	12–48 μmol/L
Amylase, serum	53–123 U/L
Anion gap (calculated)	5–15 mmol/L
Arterial blood gas tensions and pH	
P_{O_2}	80–100 mm Hg
P_{CO_2}	35–45 mm Hg
pH	7.35–7.45
Bicarbonate (CO_2)	22–26 mmol/L
Bilirubin, direct	≤0.4 mg/dl
Bilirubin, total	≤1.0 mg/dl
Blood urea nitrogen (BUN)	8–25 mg/dl
Calcium	8.5–10.5 mg/dl
Calcium, ionized	1.14–1.30 mmol/L
Chloride	100–108 mmol/L
Cholesterol	
Desirable	<200 mg/dl
Borderline	200–239 mg/dl
High	>239 mg/dl
Creatine phosphokinase (CPK)	
Male	60–400 U/L
Female	40–150 U/L
Creatinine	0.6–1.5 mg/dl
Globulin	2.6–4.1 g/dl
Glucose (fasting)	70–110 mg/dl
Iron, serum	30–160 μg/dl
Lactate dehydrogenase (LDH)	110–210 U/L
Lactic acid, plasma	0.5–2.2 mmol/L
Lipase, serum	3–19 U/dl
Magnesium	1.4–2.0 mEq/L
Osmolality	280–296 mOsm/kg
Phosphorus	2.6–4.5 mg/dl
Potassium	3.5–5.0 mmol/L
Protein, total	6.0–8.0 g/dl
SGOT [aspartate aminotransferase (AST)]	
Male	10–40 U/L
Female	9–25 U/L
SGPT [alanine aminotransferase ALT)]	
Male	10–55 U/L
Female	7–30 U/L
Sodium	135–145 mmol/L
Thyroid function tests	
Thyroid hormone binding index	0.77–1.23
T_3	60–181 ng/dl
T_4	4.5–10.9 μg/dl
TSH	0.5–5.0 μU/ml

continued

Laboratory values *Continued*

Total iron binding capacity (TIBC)	228–428 µg/dl
Triglycerides (fasting)	40–150 mg/dl
Uric acid	
Male	3.6–8.5 mg/dl
Female	2.3–6.6 mg/dl
Venous blood gas tensions, mixed	
Po_2	50 mm Hg
Pco_2	40–50 mm Hg
pH	7.32–7.42

Hematology and coagulation values

D-dimer	0.0–0.5 µg/ml
Erythrocyte count (RBC)	
Male	$4.5–5.3 \times 10^6/mm^3$
Female	$4.1–5.1 \times 10^6/mm^3$
Erythrocyte sedimentation rate (ESR)	
Male	1–17 mm/h
Female	1–25 mm/h
Ferritin, serum	20–300 ng/ml
Fibrin split products (FSP)	0–2.5 µg/ml
Fibrinogen	175–400 mg/dl
Hematocrit	
Male	37%–49%
Female	36%–46%
Hemoglobin	
Male	13–18 g/dl
Female	12–16 g/dl
Leukocyte count (WBC)	$4.5–11.0 \times 10^3/mm^3$
Neutrophils	45%–75%
Bands	0%–5%
Lymphocytes	16%–46%
Monocytes	4%–11%
Eosinophils	0%–8%
Basophils	0%–3%
Mean corpuscular hemoglobin (MCH)	25–35 pg/cell
Mean corpuscular volume (MCV)	78–100 µm³
Partial thromboplastin time, activated (aPTT)	22.1–34.1 sec
Platelet count	$150–350 \times 10^3/mm^3$
Prothrombin time (PT)	11.2–13.2 sec
Reticulocyte count	0.5%–2.5%

Reference: Kratz A, Lewandrowski B. Case records of the Massachussets General Hospital. Weekly clinicopathological exercises. Normal reference laboratory values. *N Engl J Med* 1998;339:1063–1072

Subject Index

Numbers followed by the letter f *indicate figures; numbers followed by the letter* t *indicate tables.*